# Atlas
# of
# Human
# Anatomy

*F. Netter, M.D.*

# ATLAS

# HUMAN

# OF
# ANATOMY
## Second Edition

## by FRANK H. NETTER, M.D.

Arthur F. Dalley II, Ph.D., *Consulting Editor*

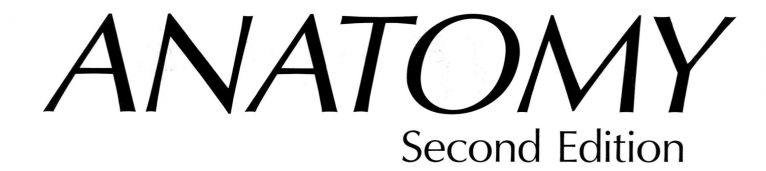 NOVARTIS

*EAST HANOVER, NEW JERSEY*

Copies of *Atlas of Human Anatomy, The Netter (formerly CIBA) Collection of Medical Illustrations,
Clinical Symposia* reprints and color slides of all illustrations are available from Novartis Medical Education,
call 800-631-1181




Library of Congress Cataloging–in–Publication Data

Netter, Frank H. (Frank Henry), 1906–1991
     Atlas of human anatomy / by Frank H. Netter: Arthur F. Dalley II,
   consulting editor.
        p.   cm,
     Includes bibliographies and index.
     ISBN 0-914168-80-0—ISBN 0-914168-81-9 (pbk.)
     1. Anatomy, Human–Atlases. I. Dalley II, Arthur F. II. Title.
     [DNLM: 1. Anatomy–atlases. QS 17 N474a]
   QM25. N46 1989
   611: 0022–dc20
   DNLM/DLC
   for Library of Congress                                97–075710
                                                              CIP

First Printing, 1989
Second Printing, 1990
Third Printing, 1991
Fourth Printing, 1992
Fifth Printing, 1996
Sixth Printing, 1997
Seventh Printing, 1997


ISBN 0-914168-80-0
Library of Congress Catalog No: 97-075710


Printed in U.S.A.


Book printed offset by Hoechstetter Printing Company Inc.
Binding by The Riverside Group
Color separations by PAGE Imaging, Inc.
Composition by Granite Graphics

*To my dear wife, Vera*

Other books by FRANK H. NETTER, M.D.

*THE NETTER COLLECTION OF MEDICAL ILLUSTRATIONS*

Nervous System, Part I: Anatomy and Physiology

Nervous System, Part II: Neurologic and Neuromuscular Disorders

Reproductive System

Digestive System, Part I: Upper Digestive Tract

Digestive System, Part II: Lower Digestive Tract

Digestive System, Part III: Liver, Biliary Tract, and Pancreas

Endocrine System and Selected Metabolic Diseases

Heart

Kidneys, Ureters, and Urinary Bladder

Respiratory System

Musculoskeletal System, Part I: Anatomy, Physiology, and Metabolic Disorders

Musculoskeletal System, Part II: Developmental Disorders, Tumors,
    Rheumatic Diseases, and Joint Replacement

Musculoskeletal System, Part III: Trauma, Evaluation, and Management

# INTRODUCTION

I have often said that my career as a medical artist for almost 50 years has been a sort of "command performance" in the sense that it has grown in response to the desires and requests of the medical profession. Over these many years, I have produced almost 4,000 illustrations, mostly for *The CIBA (now Netter) Collection of Medical Illustrations* but also for *Clinical Symposia*. These pictures have been concerned with the varied subdivisions of medical knowledge such as gross anatomy, histology, embryology, physiology, pathology, diagnostic modalities, surgical and therapeutic techniques and clinical manifestations of a multitude of diseases. As the years went by, however, there were more and more requests from physicians and students for me to produce an atlas purely of gross anatomy. Thus, this atlas has come about, not through any inspiration on my part but rather, like most of my previous works, as a fulfillment of the desires of the medical profession.

It involved going back over all the illustrations I had made over so many years, selecting those pertinent to gross anatomy, classifying them and organizing them by system and region, adapting them to page size and space and arranging them in logical sequence. Anatomy of course does not change, but our understanding of anatomy and its clinical significance does change, as do anatomical terminology and nomenclature. This therefore required much updating of many of the older pictures and even revision of a number of them in order to make them more pertinent to today's ever-expanding scope of medical and surgical practice. In addition, I found that there were gaps in the portrayal of medical knowledge as pictorialized in the illustrations I had previously done, and this necessitated my making a number of new pictures that are included in this volume.

In creating an atlas such as this, it is important to achieve a happy medium between complexity and simplification. If the pictures are too complex, they may be difficult and confusing to read; if oversimplified, they may not be adequately definitive or may even be misleading. I have therefore striven for a middle course of realism without the clutter of confusing minutiae. I hope that the students and members of the medical and allied professions will find the illustrations readily understandable, yet instructive and useful.

At one point, the publisher and I thought it might be nice to include a foreword by a truly outstanding and renowned anatomist, but there are so many in that category that we could not make a choice. We did think of men like Vesalius, Leonardo da Vinci, William Hunter and Henry Gray, who of course are unfortunately unavailable, but I do wonder what their comments might have been about this atlas.

Frank H. Netter, M.D.
(1906–1991)

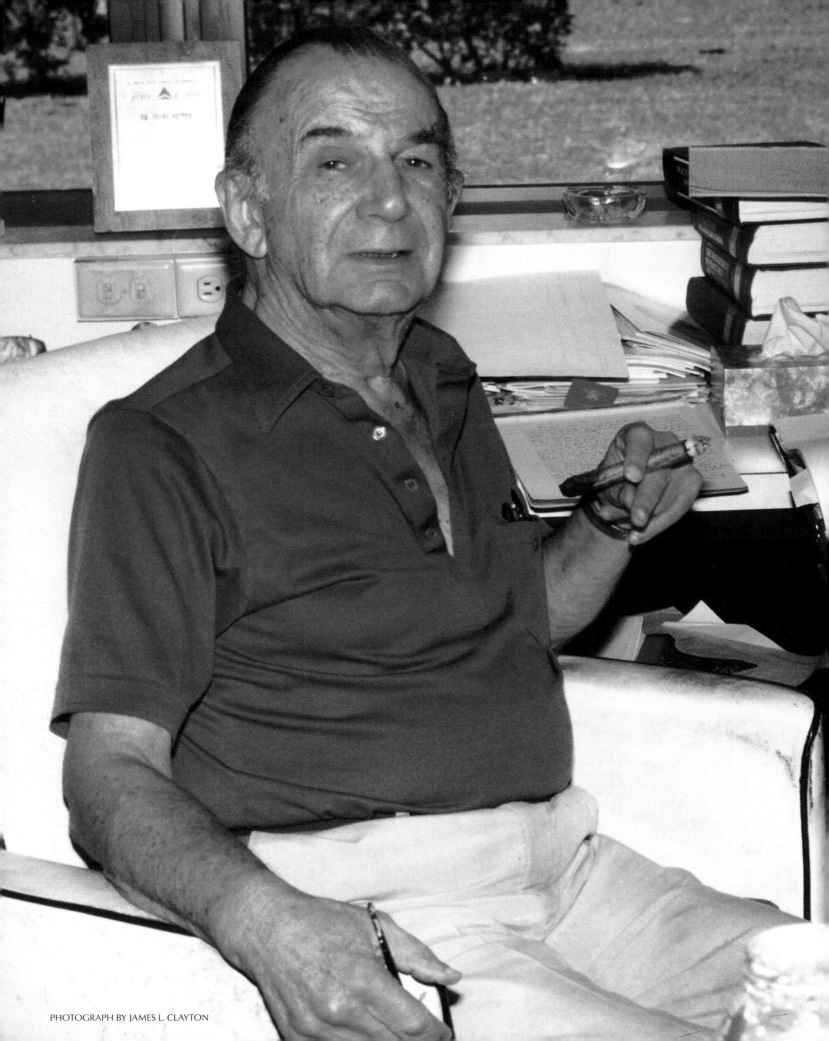

PHOTOGRAPH BY JAMES L. CLAYTON

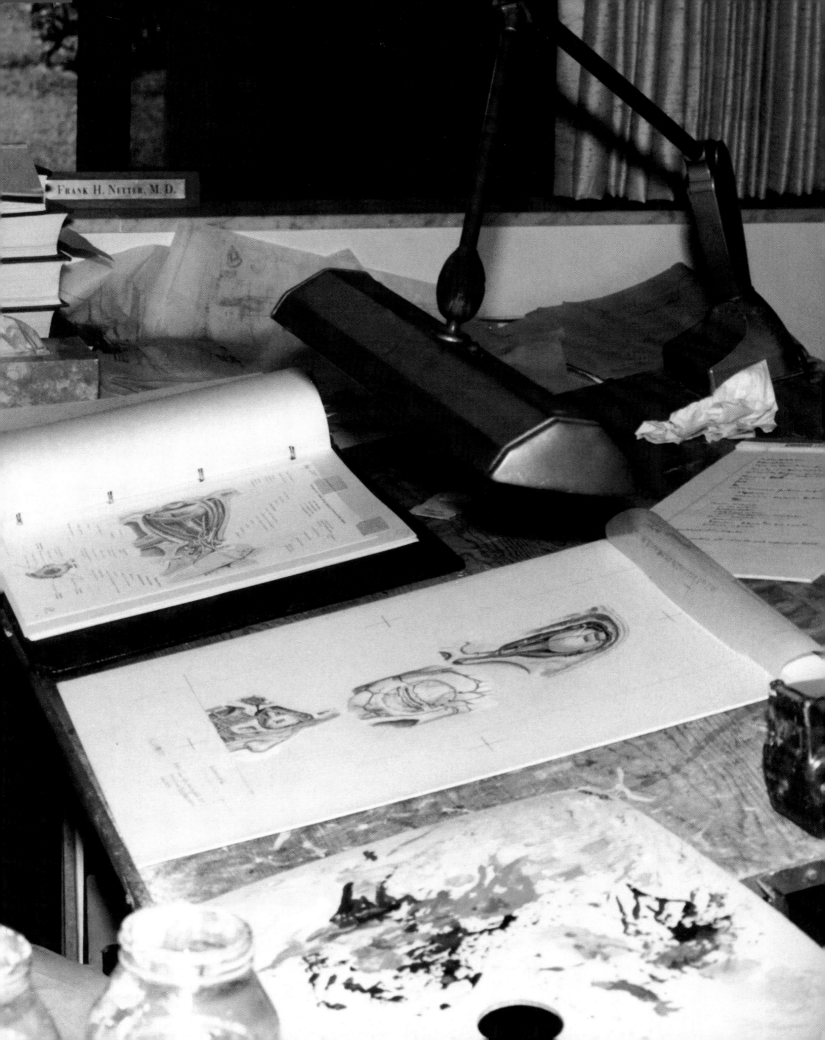

# ACKNOWLEDGMENTS

Throughout the many years that he was creating *The Netter (formerly CIBA) Collection of Medical Illustrations,* Dr. Frank Netter dreamed of producing a one-volume collection of normal anatomy illustrations that would encompass all regions of the human body. In 1989, two years before his death, he realized his dream with the publication of the first edition of the *Atlas of Human Anatomy.* The phenomenal, worldwide success of his *Atlas* far exceeded the hopes of Dr. Netter and his consulting editor, Dr. Sharon Oberg-Colacino, and the wildest expectations of the publisher. Soon after its publication, the book became the best-selling anatomy atlas in U.S. medical schools and has clearly remained the "students' choice" since then because of the clarity, focus, and beauty of the illustrations. In addition, the *Atlas* sells in over 60 countries and has been translated into at least seven languages.

But time moves on and all things change; hence our decision to publish a second edition of the *Atlas.* For this task, we were fortunate to work with Dr. Arthur F. Dalley II, professor of anatomy at Creighton University School of Medicine and President of the American Association of Clinical Anatomists. Dr. Dalley led the forces in scrutinizing, updating, and editing the artwork, terminology, and voluminous index, with almost relentless care and precision. It was a privilege for the publishing staff of the *Atlas* to work with Dr. Dalley, a dedicated anatomist, tireless worker, and exceptional writer.

Completion of a project like this requires the work of many people with diverse skills and a wealth of talent and single-minded dedication to see their tasks through to the end. We have had just such people working together on this book, and they have done so with enthusiasm, tenacity, and great care. Dr. Carlos Machado has skillfully and artistically modified some of Dr. Netter's illustrations and painted new cross sections for this edition: his accuracy and superb artistic style provide an exciting preview of the future in medical illustration. Special thanks are due Sandra Purrenhage, Gina Dingle, Thomas Moore, and Nicole Friedman of the Editorial Development staff and Michelle Jahn and Kathleen Buckley of Production, all of whom moved mountains to ensure the accuracy, quality, and timeliness of this edition.

Of course, we at Novartis remain especially indebted to Frank H. Netter, M.D., whose extraordinary illustrations continue to inspire us. It is our hope that countless generations of students will learn the complexities of the human body from these illustrations, and that this book will continue to be a prized reference wherever the intricacies of human anatomy are discussed.

Peter Carlin
Novartis Medical Education

# PREFACE TO THE SECOND EDITION

The release in 1989 of the first edition of Dr. Frank Netter's "personal Sistine Chapel"—the *Atlas of Human Anatomy*—was a major event in the history of the teaching and learning of anatomy. Almost instantly, the *Atlas of Human Anatomy* became the top-selling anatomical atlas in the world and clearly became the students' choice universally. It has retained that position ever since. At the core of that success, of course, is the remarkable artwork and style of Dr. Netter, rendered in consultation with many of the century's outstanding anatomists, skillfully edited and published through the teamwork of Novartis Medical Education, in consultation with Dr. Sharon Colacino (now Oberg) for the first edition. Joining the Novartis team for the development of the "sister" Netter products (*Interactive Atlas of Human Anatomy* and *Interactive Atlas of Clinical Anatomy* CD-ROMs) and now the second edition of the *Atlas of Human Anatomy* book is the fulfillment of a nearly lifelong dream for me. I am delighted to have the opportunity to continue this tradition of quality as we strive to improve the education, learning, and applied knowledge of healthcare providers for the new century.

It is a testimony to the high quality of the first edition that a decade later record sales and course adoptions continue to increase annually. In view of this success, why a new edition? We intend to make the best-seller even better! In doing so, however, we have made a conscious effort not to significantly increase the overall size of the book or the level of detail, or alter the style of presentation, which students have clearly told us are some key reasons for the first edition's success.

The most noticeable changes are the importing of additional Netter illustrations (e.g., see Plates 288, 430, 432, and 512) and the addition of new artwork rendered masterfully in the Netter style by Novartis artist Carlos Machado, M.D. (see the new section on cross-sectional anatomy, Plates 511 through 525). These new plates and illustrations significantly enhance the usefulness of the *Atlas* in the contemporary anatomy curriculum and in practice, adding meaningful detail and helping the student to learn and understand cross-sectional anatomy, essential to the interpretation of the new medical imaging techniques. To accommodate the additional plates at least in part, several plates on variations of abdominal vasculature have been condensed. The common variations are still addressed; reference to *The Netter* (formerly *CIBA*) *Collection of Medical Illustrations* is recommended for treatment of the more rare anomalies.

Dr. Machado has made changes on a number of plates to correct anatomical errors and especially to update anatomical detail consistent with current knowledge, gained largely through the use of medical imaging techniques in studying the anatomy in the living. In particular, the section on the pelvis and perineum has been extensively revised, replacing the outdated concepts of the trilaminar "U.G. diaphragm" or "deep perineal pouch" and the planar external urethral sphincter with current concepts.

Labeling has also been improved by making the terminology consistent throughout the book and updating it to the most current standard for anatomical terminology. I am grateful to have had the assistance of Dr. Duane Haines (central nervous system), and especially Dr. Robert Leonard (everything else!) in this formidable task. Internationally, the Latin form of terminology has been replaced with more user-friendly anglicized forms (English equivalents), in both common usage and scholarly endeavors. Where the new terminology is a marked change from that previously employed, we have retained the previous term in parenthesis to ease the transition (e.g., fibular (peroneal) nerve). While most anatomists favor use of descriptive anatomical terminology, many clinicians are reluctant to forego the tradition of the eponym. Thus the more common eponyms have also been retained parenthetically. The index—which, as Dr. Netter remarked in reference to the first edition, "is a book in itself"—has been thoroughly revised and updated to reflect the consistently applied, revised terminology. Accuracy of leader line placement has been increased even further, and leaders have been modified where necessary to delineate more clearly the labeled structures. The efforts of proofreader Nicole Friedman, who worked with me as we sacrificed our eyesight verifying the accuracy of the 32,000 leader lines running from as many labels, are also greatly appreciated.

Thanks to project editors Gina Dingle and Thomas Moore for their oversight (and insights), and to "the boss," team leader Sandy Purrenhage, for cracking that whip and getting the job done mostly on schedule (reason be damned!). Special thanks to my wife, Muriel Dalley (still Dalley), for keeping the home fires burning, and for the patience she and our boys have had with me, my projects, and my office hours.

Arthur F. Dalley II, Ph.D.
Professor of Anatomy

# CONTENTS

## Section I   HEAD AND NECK

| | |
|---|---|
| BONES AND LIGAMENTS | Plates 1 – 16 |
| SUPERFICIAL FACE | Plates 17 – 21 |
| NECK | Plates 22 – 30 |
| NASAL REGION | Plates 31 – 44 |
| ORAL REGION | Plates 45 – 56 |
| PHARYNX | Plates 57 – 67 |
| THYROID GLAND AND LARYNX | Plates 68 – 75 |
| ORBIT AND CONTENTS | Plates 76 – 86 |
| EAR | Plates 87 – 93 |
| MENINGES AND BRAIN | Plates 94 – 109 |
| CRANIAL AND CERVICAL NERVES | Plates 110 – 129 |
| CEREBRAL VASCULATURE | Plates 130 – 141 |

## Section II   BACK AND SPINAL CORD

| | |
|---|---|
| BONES AND LIGAMENTS | Plates 142 – 147 |
| SPINAL CORD | Plates 148 – 159 |
| MUSCLES AND NERVES | Plates 160 – 166 |

## Section III   THORAX

| | |
|---|---|
| MAMMARY GLAND | Plates 167 – 169 |
| BODY WALL | Plates 170 – 183 |
| LUNGS | Plates 184 – 199 |
| HEART | Plates 200 – 217 |
| MEDIASTINUM | Plates 218 – 230 |

## Section IV   ABDOMEN

| | |
|---|---|
| BODY WALL | Plates 231 – 250 |
| PERITONEAL CAVITY | Plates 251 – 257 |
| VISCERA (GUT) | Plates 258 – 268 |
| VISCERA (ACCESSORY ORGANS) | Plates 269 – 281 |
| VISCERAL VASCULATURE | Plates 282 – 299 |
| INNERVATION | Plates 300 – 310 |
| KIDNEYS AND SUPRARENAL GLANDS | Plates 311 – 329 |

## Section V    PELVIS AND PERINEUM

| | |
|---|---|
| BONES AND LIGAMENTS | Plates 330 – 332 |
| PELVIC FLOOR AND CONTENTS | Plates 333 – 343 |
| FEMALE STRUCTURES | Plates 344 – 353 |
| MALE STRUCTURES | Plates 354 – 362 |
| RECTUM | Plates 363 – 368 |
| VASCULATURE | Plates 369 – 379 |
| INNERVATION | Plates 380 – 390 |

## Section VI    UPPER LIMB

| | |
|---|---|
| SHOULDER AND AXILLA | Plates 391 – 401 |
| ARM | Plates 402 – 406 |
| ELBOW AND FOREARM | Plates 407 – 421 |
| WRIST AND HAND | Plates 422 – 440 |
| NEUROVASCULATURE | Plates 441 – 452 |

## Section VII    LOWER LIMB

| | |
|---|---|
| HIP AND THIGH | Plates 453 – 471 |
| KNEE | Plates 472 – 477 |
| LEG | Plates 478 – 487 |
| ANKLE AND FOOT | Plates 488 – 501 |
| NEUROVASCULATURE | Plates 502 – 510 |

## Section VIII    CROSS-SECTIONAL ANATOMY

| | |
|---|---|
| SKIN | Plate 511 |
| CROSS-SECTION OVERVIEW | Plate 512 |
| THORAX | Plates 513 – 516 |
| ABDOMEN | Plates 517 – 522 |
| MALE PELVIS | Plate 523 |
| THORAX | Plates 524 – 525 |

REFERENCES

INDEX

# Section I
# HEAD AND NECK

**BONES AND LIGAMENTS**
*Plates 1 – 16*

1. Skull: Anterior View
2. Skull: Lateral View
3. Skull: Midsagittal Section
4. Calvaria
5. Cranial Base: Inferior View
6. Bones of Cranial Base: Superior View
7. Foramina of Cranial Base: Superior View
8. Skull of Newborn
9. Bony Framework of Head and Neck
10. Mandible
11. Temporomandibular Joint
12. Cervical Vertebrae: Atlas and Axis
13. Cervical Vertebrae (*continued*)
14. External Craniocervical Ligaments
15. Internal Craniocervical Ligaments
16. Atlantooccipital Junction

**SUPERFICIAL FACE**
*Plates 17 – 21*

17. Superficial Arteries and Veins of Face and Scalp
18. Cutaneous Nerves of Head and Neck
19. Facial Nerve Branches and Parotid Gland
20. Muscles of Facial Expression: Anterior View
21. Muscles of Facial Expression: Lateral View

**NECK**
*Plates 22 – 30*

22. Muscles of Neck: Lateral View
23. Muscles of Neck: Anterior View
24. Infrahyoid and Suprahyoid Muscles
25. Scalene and Prevertebral Muscles

26. Superficial Veins and Cutaneous
    Nerves of Neck
27. Cervical Plexus In Situ
28. Subclavian Artery
29. Carotid Arteries
30. Fascial Layers of Neck

**NASAL REGION**
*Plates 31 – 44*
31. Nose
32. Lateral Wall of Nasal Cavity
33. Lateral Wall of Nasal Cavity
    (*continued*)
34. Medial Wall of Nasal Cavity
    (Nasal Septum)
35. Maxillary Artery
36. Arteries of Nasal Cavity
37. Nerves of Nasal Cavity
38. Nerves of Nasal Cavity (*continued*)
39. Autonomic Innervation of Nasal Cavity
40. Ophthalmic ($V_1$) and
    Maxillary ($V_2$) Nerves
41. Mandibular Nerve ($V_3$)
42. Paranasal Sinuses
43. Paranasal Sinuses (*continued*)
44. Paranasal Sinuses:
    Changes With Age

**ORAL REGION**
*Plates 45 – 56*
45. Inspection of Oral Cavity
46. Roof of Mouth
47. Floor of Mouth
48. Muscles Involved in Mastication
49. Muscles Involved in Mastication
    (*continued*)

50. Teeth
51. Teeth (*continued*)
52. Tongue
53. Tongue (*continued*)
54. Tongue and Salivary Glands: Sections
55. Salivary Glands
56. Afferent Innervation of Mouth
    and Pharynx

**PHARYNX**
*Plates 57 – 67*
57. Pharynx: Median Section
58. Fauces
59. Muscles of Pharynx: Median (Sagittal)
    Section
60. Pharynx: Opened Posterior View
61. Muscles of Pharynx: Partially Opened
    Posterior View
62. Muscles of Pharynx: Lateral View
63. Arteries of Oral and
    Pharyngeal Regions
64. Veins of Oral and Pharyngeal Regions
65. Nerves of Oral and
    Pharyngeal Regions
66. Lymph Vessels and Nodes of
    Head and Neck
67. Lymph Vessels and Nodes of
    Pharynx and Tongue

**THYROID GLAND AND LARYNX**
*Plates 68 – 75*
68. Thyroid Gland: Anterior View
69. Thyroid Gland and Pharynx:
    Posterior View
70. Parathyroid Glands
71. Cartilages of Larynx

72. Intrinsic Muscles of Larynx
73. Action of Intrinsic Muscles of Larynx
74. Nerves of Larynx
75. Inspection of Larynx

**ORBIT AND CONTENTS**
*Plates 76 – 86*
76. Eyelids
77. Lacrimal Apparatus
78. Fascia of Orbit and Eyeball
79. Extrinsic Eye Muscles
80. Arteries and Veins of Orbit
    and Eyelids
81. Nerves of Orbit
82. Eyeball
83. Anterior and Posterior
    Chambers of Eye
84. Iridocorneal Angle of Anterior
    Chamber of Eye
85. Lens and Supporting Structures
86. Intrinsic Arteries and Veins of Eye

**EAR**
*Plates 87 – 93*
87. Pathway of Sound Reception
88. External Ear and Tympanic Cavity
89. Tympanic Cavity
90. Bony and Membranous Labyrinths
91. Bony and Membranous Labyrinths
    (*continued*)
92. Orientation of Labyrinth in Skull
93. Pharyngotympanic (Auditory) Tube

**MENINGES AND BRAIN**
*Plates 94 – 109*
94. Meninges and Diploic Veins

96. Meningeal Arteries
96. Meninges and Superficial
    Cerebral Veins
97. Dural Venous Sinuses
98. Dural Venous Sinuses
    (*continued*)
99. Cerebrum: Lateral Views
100. Cerebrum: Medial Views
101. Cerebrum: Inferior View
102. Ventricles of Brain
103. Circulation of Cerebrospinal Fluid
104. Basal Nuclei (Ganglia)
105. Thalamus
106. Hippocampus and Fornix
107. Cerebellum
108. Brainstem
109. Fourth Ventricle and Cerebellum

**CRANIAL AND CERVICAL NERVES**
*Plates 110 – 129*
110. Cranial Nerve Nuclei in Brainstem:
    Schema
111. Cranial Nerve Nuclei in Brainstem:
    Schema (*continued*)
112. Cranial Nerves (Motor and Sensory
    Distribution): Schema
113. Olfactory Nerve (I): Schema
114. Optic Nerve (II) (Visual Pathway):
    Schema
115. Oculomotor, Trochlear and Abducent
    Nerves (III, IV and VI): Schema
116. Trigeminal Nerve (V): Schema
117. Facial Nerve (VII): Schema
118. Vestibulocochlear Nerve (VIII):
    Schema
119. Glossopharyngeal Nerve (IX): Schema

120. Vagus Nerve (X): Schema
121. Accessory Nerve (XI): Schema
122. Hypoglossal Nerve (XII): Schema
123. Cervical Plexus: Schema
124. Autonomic Nerves in Neck
125. Autonomic Nerves in Head
126. Ciliary Ganglion: Schema
127. Pterygopalatine and Submandibular Ganglia: Schema
128. Otic Ganglion: Schema
129. Taste Pathways: Schema

**CEREBRAL VASCULATURE**
*Plates 130 – 141*
130. Arteries to Brain and Meninges
131. Arteries to Brain: Schema
132. Arteries of Brain: Inferior Views
133. Cerebral Arterial Circle (Willis)
134. Arteries of Brain: Frontal View and Section
135. Arteries of Brain: Lateral and Medial Views
136. Arteries of Posterior Cranial Fossa
137. Veins of Posterior Cranial Fossa
138. Deep Veins of Brain
139. Subependymal Veins of Brain
140. Hypothalamus and Hypophysis
141. Arteries and Veins of Hypothalamus and Hypophysis

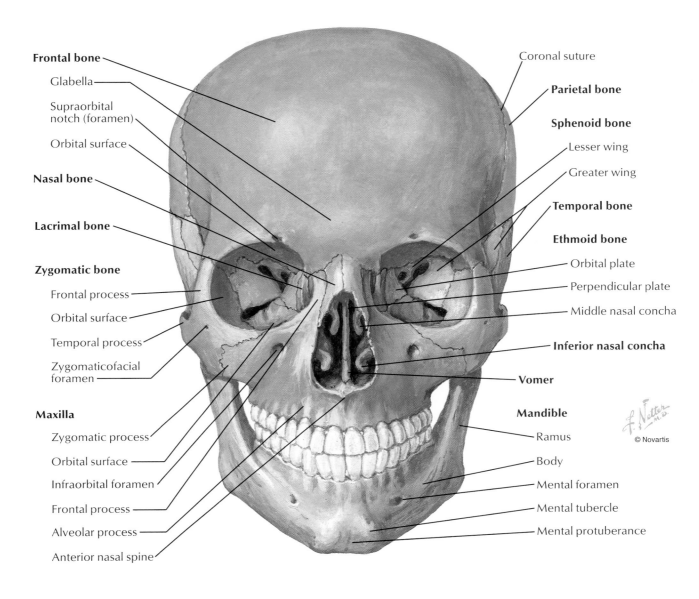

Frontal bone
Glabella
Supraorbital notch (foramen)
Orbital surface
Nasal bone
Lacrimal bone

Zygomatic bone
Frontal process
Orbital surface
Temporal process
Zygomaticofacial foramen

Maxilla
Zygomatic process
Orbital surface
Infraorbital foramen
Frontal process
Alveolar process
Anterior nasal spine

Coronal suture
Parietal bone
Sphenoid bone
Lesser wing
Greater wing
Temporal bone
Ethmoid bone
Orbital plate
Perpendicular plate
Middle nasal concha
Inferior nasal concha
Vomer
Mandible
Ramus
Body
Mental foramen
Mental tubercle
Mental protuberance

© Novartis

### Right orbit: frontal and slightly lateral view

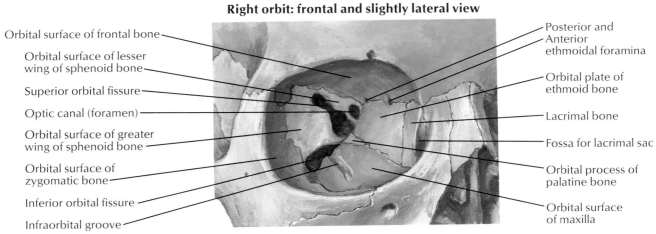

Orbital surface of frontal bone
Orbital surface of lesser wing of sphenoid bone
Superior orbital fissure
Optic canal (foramen)
Orbital surface of greater wing of sphenoid bone
Orbital surface of zygomatic bone
Inferior orbital fissure
Infraorbital groove

Posterior and Anterior ethmoidal foramina
Orbital plate of ethmoid bone
Lacrimal bone
Fossa for lacrimal sac
Orbital process of palatine bone
Orbital surface of maxilla

**BONES AND LIGAMENTS**

*PLATE 1*

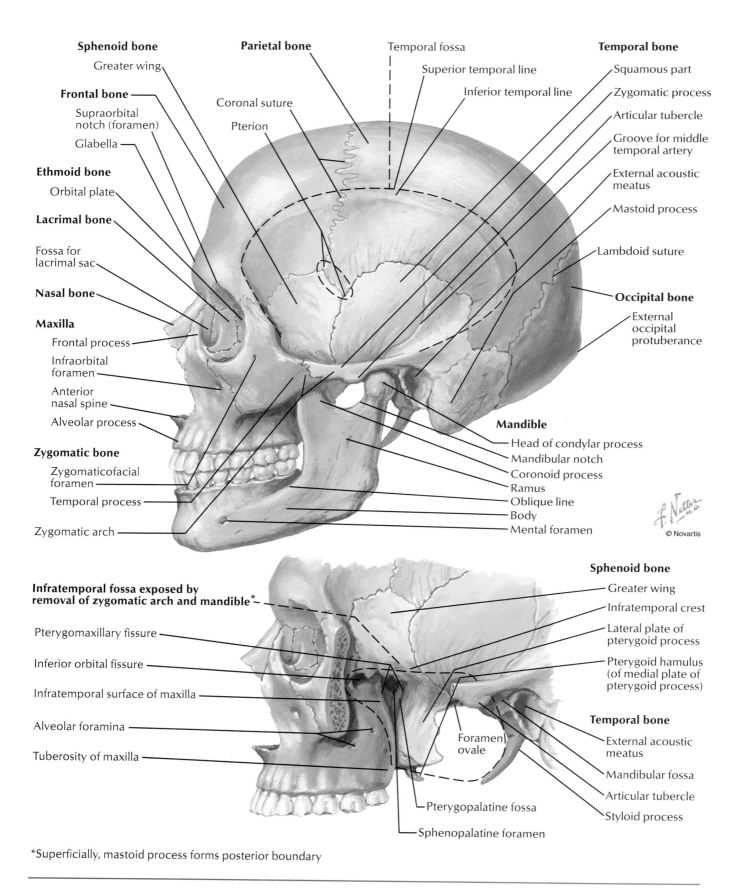

**Sphenoid bone**
Greater wing

**Frontal bone**
Supraorbital notch (foramen)
Glabella

**Ethmoid bone**
Orbital plate

**Lacrimal bone**
Fossa for lacrimal sac

**Nasal bone**

**Maxilla**
Frontal process
Infraorbital foramen
Anterior nasal spine
Alveolar process

**Zygomatic bone**
Zygomaticofacial foramen
Temporal process
Zygomatic arch

**Parietal bone**
Coronal suture
Pterion

Temporal fossa
Superior temporal line
Inferior temporal line

**Temporal bone**
Squamous part
Zygomatic process
Articular tubercle
Groove for middle temporal artery
External acoustic meatus
Mastoid process
Lambdoid suture

**Occipital bone**
External occipital protuberance

**Mandible**
Head of condylar process
Mandibular notch
Coronoid process
Ramus
Oblique line
Body
Mental foramen

© Novartis

**Infratemporal fossa exposed by removal of zygomatic arch and mandible** *

Pterygomaxillary fissure

Inferior orbital fissure

Infratemporal surface of maxilla

Alveolar foramina

Tuberosity of maxilla

**Sphenoid bone**
Greater wing
Infratemporal crest
Lateral plate of pterygoid process
Pterygoid hamulus (of medial plate of pterygoid process)

**Temporal bone**
External acoustic meatus
Mandibular fossa
Articular tubercle
Styloid process

Foramen ovale

Pterygopalatine fossa

Sphenopalatine foramen

*Superficially, mastoid process forms posterior boundary

**PLATE 2**                    **HEAD AND NECK**

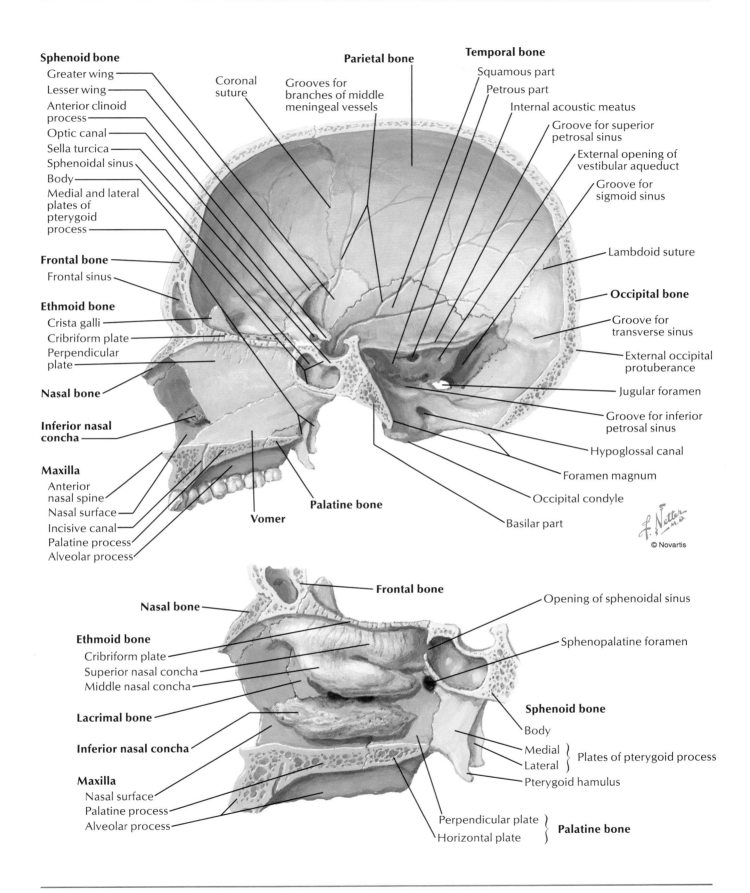

**Sphenoid bone**
Greater wing
Lesser wing
Anterior clinoid process
Optic canal
Sella turcica
Sphenoidal sinus
Body
Medial and lateral plates of pterygoid process

**Frontal bone**
Frontal sinus

**Ethmoid bone**
Crista galli
Cribriform plate
Perpendicular plate

**Nasal bone**

**Inferior nasal concha**

**Maxilla**
Anterior nasal spine
Nasal surface
Incisive canal
Palatine process
Alveolar process

Coronal suture

Grooves for branches of middle meningeal vessels

**Parietal bone**

**Temporal bone**
Squamous part
Petrous part
Internal acoustic meatus
Groove for superior petrosal sinus
External opening of vestibular aqueduct
Groove for sigmoid sinus

Lambdoid suture

**Occipital bone**
Groove for transverse sinus
External occipital protuberance
Jugular foramen
Groove for inferior petrosal sinus
Hypoglossal canal
Foramen magnum
Occipital condyle
Basilar part

**Palatine bone**

**Vomer**

**Frontal bone**

**Nasal bone**

**Ethmoid bone**
Cribriform plate
Superior nasal concha
Middle nasal concha

**Lacrimal bone**

**Inferior nasal concha**

**Maxilla**
Nasal surface
Palatine process
Alveolar process

Opening of sphenoidal sinus

Sphenopalatine foramen

**Sphenoid bone**
Body
Medial } Plates of pterygoid process
Lateral }
Pterygoid hamulus

Perpendicular plate }
**Palatine bone**
Horizontal plate }

© Novartis

# *Calvaria*

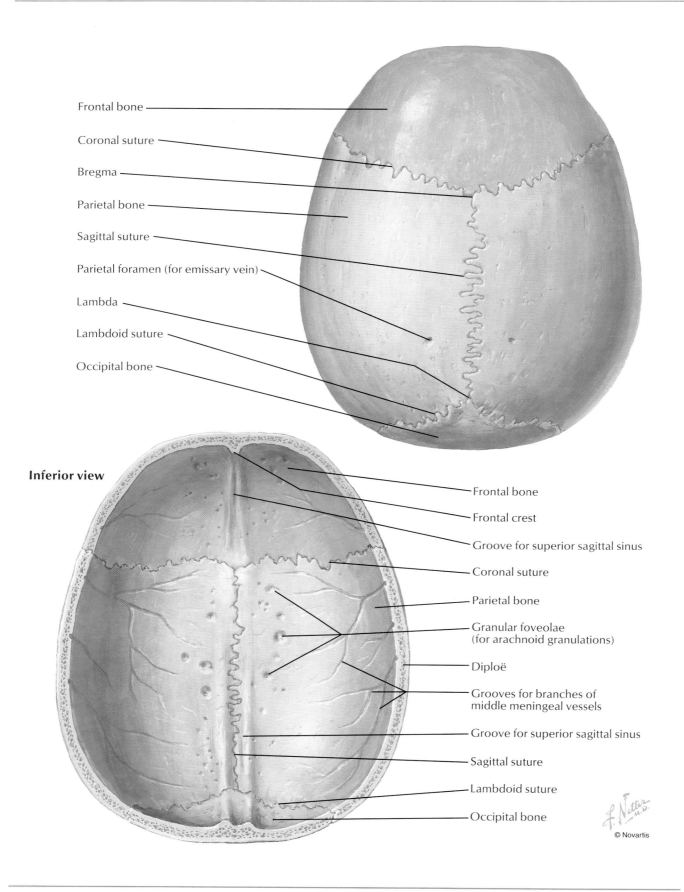

Frontal bone

Coronal suture

Bregma

Parietal bone

Sagittal suture

Parietal foramen (for emissary vein)

Lambda

Lambdoid suture

Occipital bone

**Inferior view**

Frontal bone

Frontal crest

Groove for superior sagittal sinus

Coronal suture

Parietal bone

Granular foveolae
(for arachnoid granulations)

Diploë

Grooves for branches of
middle meningeal vessels

Groove for superior sagittal sinus

Sagittal suture

Lambdoid suture

Occipital bone

© Novartis

*PLATE 4*

**HEAD AND NECK**

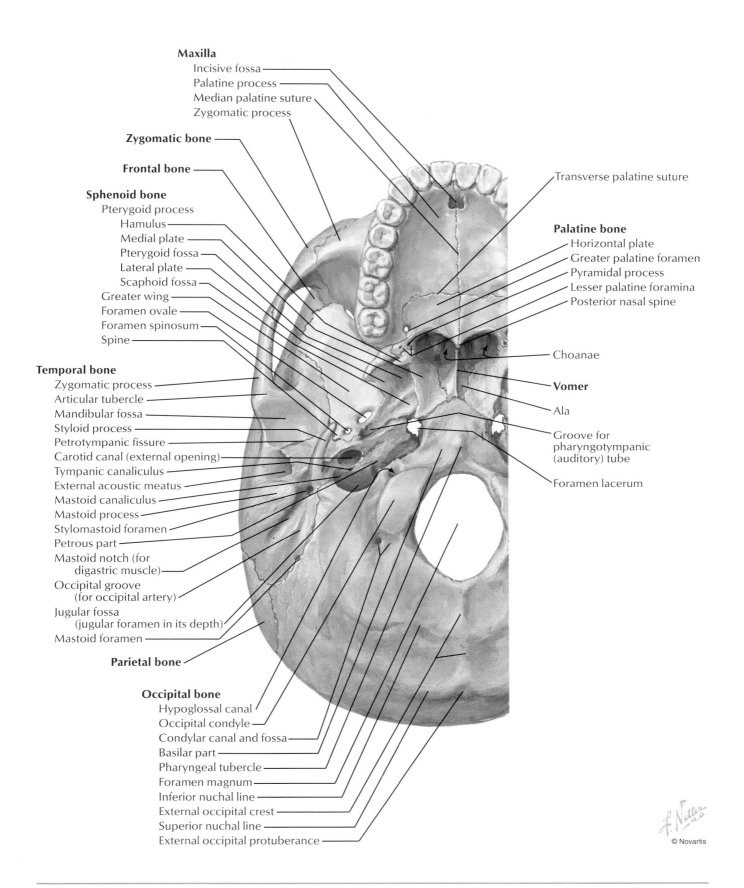

**Maxilla**
Incisive fossa
Palatine process
Median palatine suture
Zygomatic process

**Zygomatic bone**

**Frontal bone**

**Sphenoid bone**
Pterygoid process
Hamulus
Medial plate
Pterygoid fossa
Lateral plate
Scaphoid fossa
Greater wing
Foramen ovale
Foramen spinosum
Spine

**Temporal bone**
Zygomatic process
Articular tubercle
Mandibular fossa
Styloid process
Petrotympanic fissure
Carotid canal (external opening)
Tympanic canaliculus
External acoustic meatus
Mastoid canaliculus
Mastoid process
Stylomastoid foramen
Petrous part
Mastoid notch (for digastric muscle)
Occipital groove (for occipital artery)
Jugular fossa (jugular foramen in its depth)
Mastoid foramen

**Parietal bone**

**Occipital bone**
Hypoglossal canal
Occipital condyle
Condylar canal and fossa
Basilar part
Pharyngeal tubercle
Foramen magnum
Inferior nuchal line
External occipital crest
Superior nuchal line
External occipital protuberance

Transverse palatine suture

**Palatine bone**
Horizontal plate
Greater palatine foramen
Pyramidal process
Lesser palatine foramina
Posterior nasal spine

Choanae

**Vomer**

Ala

Groove for pharyngotympanic (auditory) tube

Foramen lacerum

# Bones of Cranial Base: Superior View

**Frontal bone**
Groove for superior sagittal sinus
Frontal crest
Groove for anterior meningeal vessels
Foramen cecum
Superior surface of orbital part

**Ethmoid bone**
Crista galli
Cribriform plate

**Sphenoid bone**
Lesser wing
Anterior clinoid process
Greater wing
Groove for middle meningeal
vessels (frontal branches)
Body
Jugum
Prechiasmatic groove
Sella turcica { Tuberculum sellae
Hypophyseal fossa
Dorsum sellae
Posterior clinoid process
Carotid groove (for int. carotid a.)
Clivus

**Temporal bone**
Squamous part
Petrous part
Groove for lesser petrosal nerve
Groove for greater petrosal nerve
Arcuate eminence
Trigeminal impression
Groove for superior petrosal sinus
Groove for sigmoid sinus

**Parietal bone**
Groove for middle meningeal
vessels (parietal branches)
Mastoid angle

**Occipital bone**
Clivus
Groove for inferior petrosal sinus
Basilar part
Groove for posterior meningeal vessels
Condyle
Groove for transverse sinus
Groove for occipital sinus
Internal occipital crest
Internal occipital protuberance
Groove for superior sagittal sinus

Anterior
cranial
fossa

Middle
cranial
fossa

Posterior
cranial
fossa

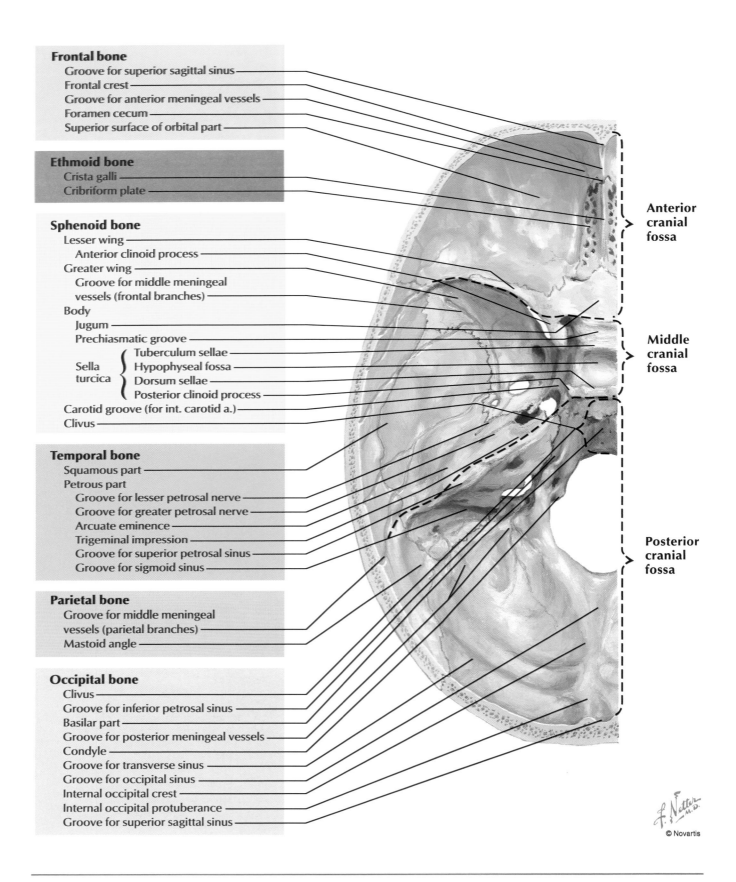

© Novartis

**PLATE 6**

**HEAD AND NECK**

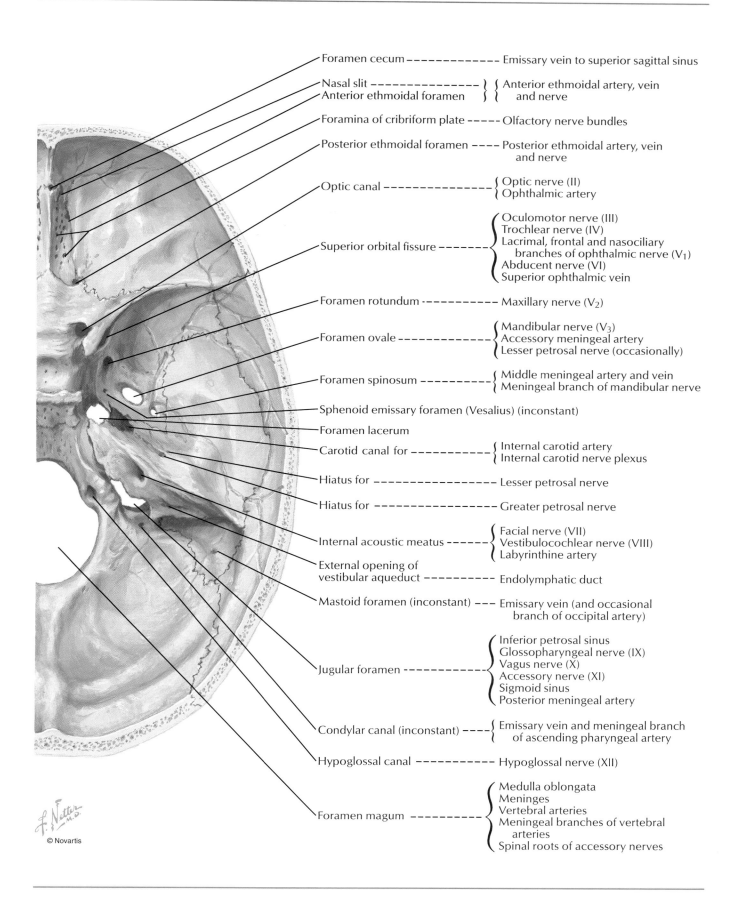

Foramen cecum -------------- Emissary vein to superior sagittal sinus

Nasal slit --------------- } { Anterior ethmoidal artery, vein
Anterior ethmoidal foramen } {   and nerve

Foramina of cribriform plate ----- Olfactory nerve bundles

Posterior ethmoidal foramen ---- Posterior ethmoidal artery, vein
  and nerve

Optic canal --------------- { Optic nerve (II)
{ Ophthalmic artery

Superior orbital fissure ------- { Oculomotor nerve (III)
{ Trochlear nerve (IV)
{ Lacrimal, frontal and nasociliary
{   branches of ophthalmic nerve (V₁)
{ Abducent nerve (VI)
{ Superior ophthalmic vein

Foramen rotundum ---------- Maxillary nerve (V₂)

Foramen ovale ------------- { Mandibular nerve (V₃)
{ Accessory meningeal artery
{ Lesser petrosal nerve (occasionally)

Foramen spinosum ---------- { Middle meningeal artery and vein
{ Meningeal branch of mandibular nerve

Sphenoid emissary foramen (Vesalius) (inconstant)

Foramen lacerum

Carotid canal for ---------- { Internal carotid artery
{ Internal carotid nerve plexus

Hiatus for ---------------- Lesser petrosal nerve

Hiatus for ---------------- Greater petrosal nerve

Internal acoustic meatus ------ { Facial nerve (VII)
{ Vestibulocochlear nerve (VIII)
{ Labyrinthine artery

External opening of
vestibular aqueduct --------- Endolymphatic duct

Mastoid foramen (inconstant) --- Emissary vein (and occasional
  branch of occipital artery)

Jugular foramen ----------- { Inferior petrosal sinus
{ Glossopharyngeal nerve (IX)
{ Vagus nerve (X)
{ Accessory nerve (XI)
{ Sigmoid sinus
{ Posterior meningeal artery

Condylar canal (inconstant) ---- { Emissary vein and meningeal branch
{   of ascending pharyngeal artery

Hypoglossal canal ---------- Hypoglossal nerve (XII)

Foramen magum --------- { Medulla oblongata
{ Meninges
{ Vertebral arteries
{ Meningeal branches of vertebral
{   arteries
{ Spinal roots of accessory nerves

*f. Netter*
M.D.
© Novartis

# Skull of Newborn

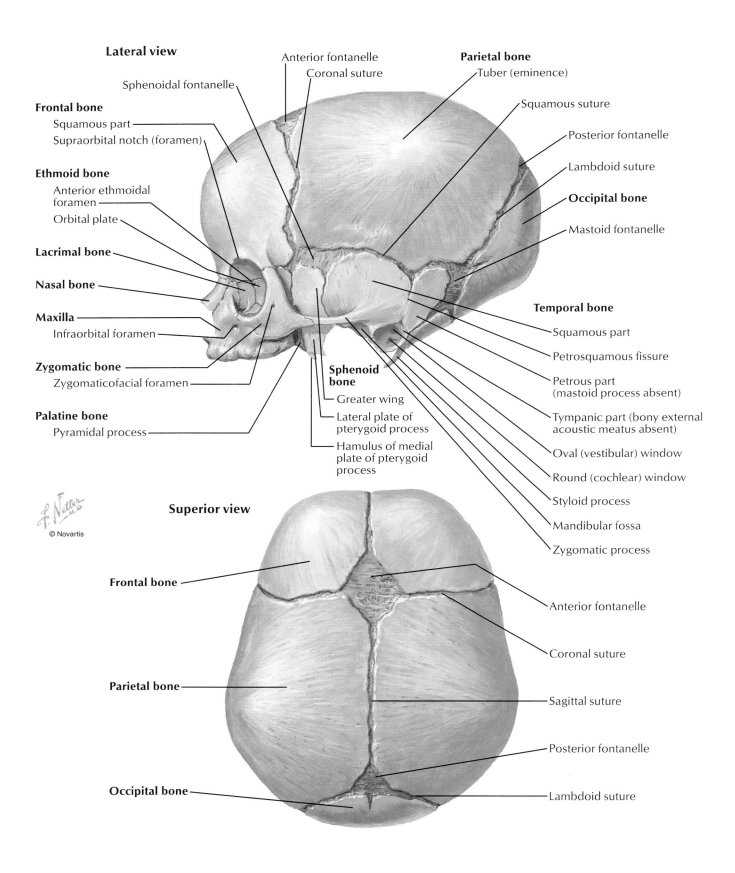

**Lateral view**

Anterior fontanelle

Coronal suture

Sphenoidal fontanelle

**Parietal bone**

Tuber (eminence)

**Frontal bone**

Squamous part

Supraorbital notch (foramen)

Squamous suture

Posterior fontanelle

Lambdoid suture

**Ethmoid bone**

Anterior ethmoidal foramen

Orbital plate

**Occipital bone**

Mastoid fontanelle

**Lacrimal bone**

**Nasal bone**

**Maxilla**

Infraorbital foramen

**Temporal bone**

Squamous part

Petrosquamous fissure

**Zygomatic bone**

Zygomaticofacial foramen

**Sphenoid bone**

Greater wing

Lateral plate of pterygoid process

Hamulus of medial plate of pterygoid process

Petrous part (mastoid process absent)

Tympanic part (bony external acoustic meatus absent)

Oval (vestibular) window

Round (cochlear) window

**Palatine bone**

Pyramidal process

Styloid process

Mandibular fossa

Zygomatic process

**Superior view**

**Frontal bone**

Anterior fontanelle

Coronal suture

**Parietal bone**

Sagittal suture

Posterior fontanelle

**Occipital bone**

Lambdoid suture

f. Netter M.D.
© Novartis

*PLATE 8*

**HEAD AND NECK**

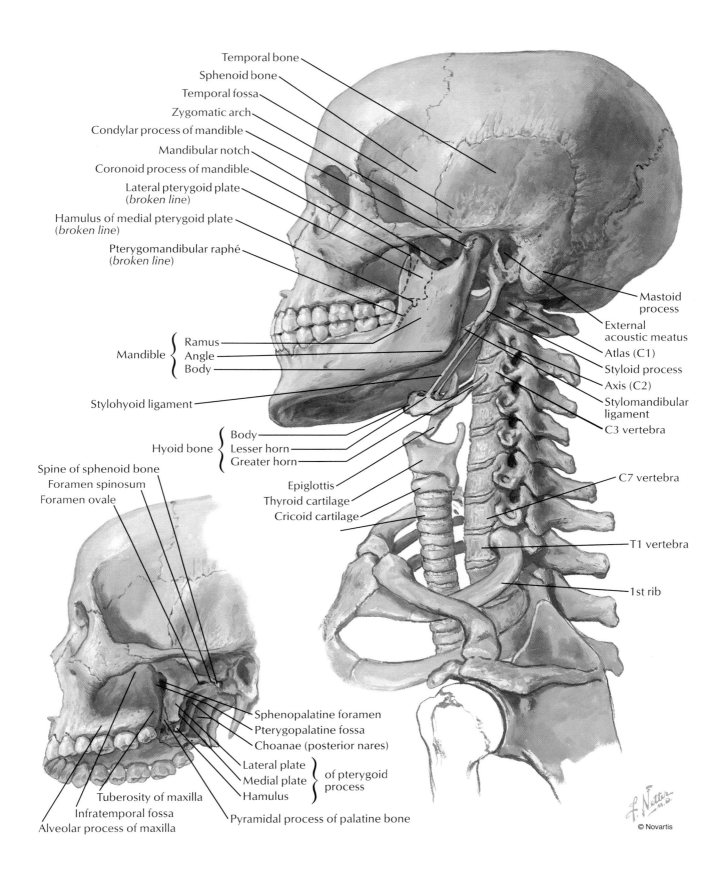

Temporal bone
Sphenoid bone
Temporal fossa
Zygomatic arch
Condylar process of mandible
Mandibular notch
Coronoid process of mandible
Lateral pterygoid plate (*broken line*)
Hamulus of medial pterygoid plate (*broken line*)
Pterygomandibular raphé (*broken line*)

Mastoid process
External acoustic meatus
Atlas (C1)
Styloid process
Axis (C2)
Stylomandibular ligament
C3 vertebra

Mandible { Ramus
Angle
Body

Stylohyoid ligament

Hyoid bone { Body
Lesser horn
Greater horn

Epiglottis
Thyroid cartilage
Cricoid cartilage

C7 vertebra

T1 vertebra

1st rib

Spine of sphenoid bone
Foramen spinosum
Foramen ovale

Sphenopalatine foramen
Pterygopalatine fossa
Choanae (posterior nares)
Lateral plate }
Medial plate } of pterygoid process
Hamulus }
Pyramidal process of palatine bone

Tuberosity of maxilla
Infratemporal fossa
Alveolar process of maxilla

*f. Netter*

© Novartis

# Mandible

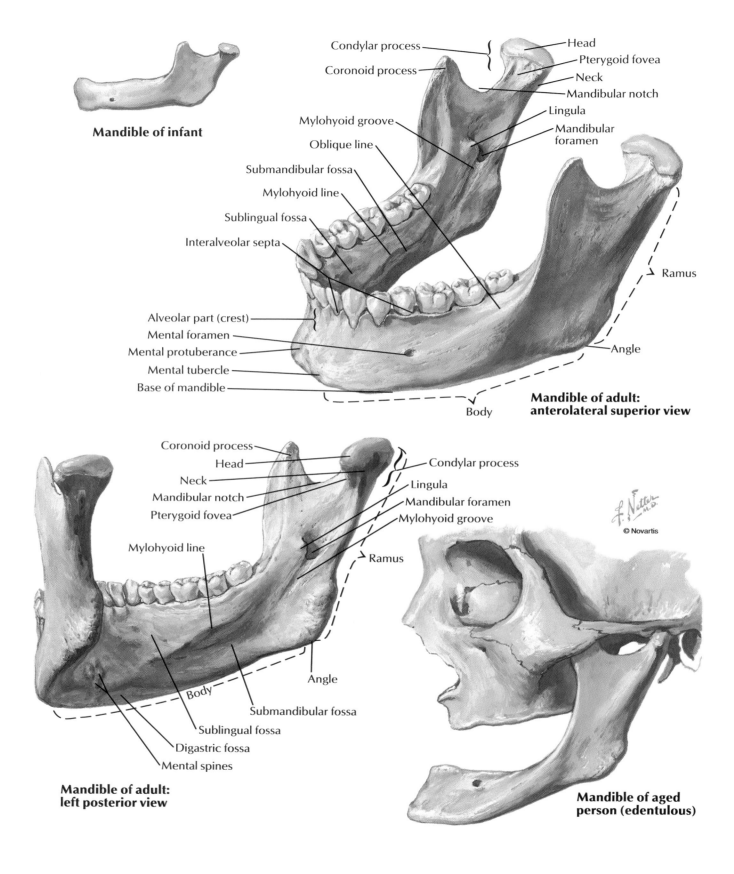

**Mandible of infant**

Condylar process
Coronoid process

Head
Pterygoid fovea
Neck
Mandibular notch
Lingula
Mandibular foramen

Mylohyoid groove
Oblique line
Submandibular fossa
Mylohyoid line
Sublingual fossa
Interalveolar septa

Ramus

Alveolar part (crest)
Mental foramen
Mental protuberance
Mental tubercle
Base of mandible

Angle

**Mandible of adult: anterolateral superior view**

Body

Coronoid process
Head
Neck
Mandibular notch
Pterygoid fovea

Condylar process
Lingula
Mandibular foramen
Mylohyoid groove

Mylohyoid line

Ramus

Angle
Body
Submandibular fossa
Sublingual fossa
Digastric fossa
Mental spines

**Mandible of adult: left posterior view**

**Mandible of aged person (edentulous)**

**PLATE 10**

**HEAD AND NECK**

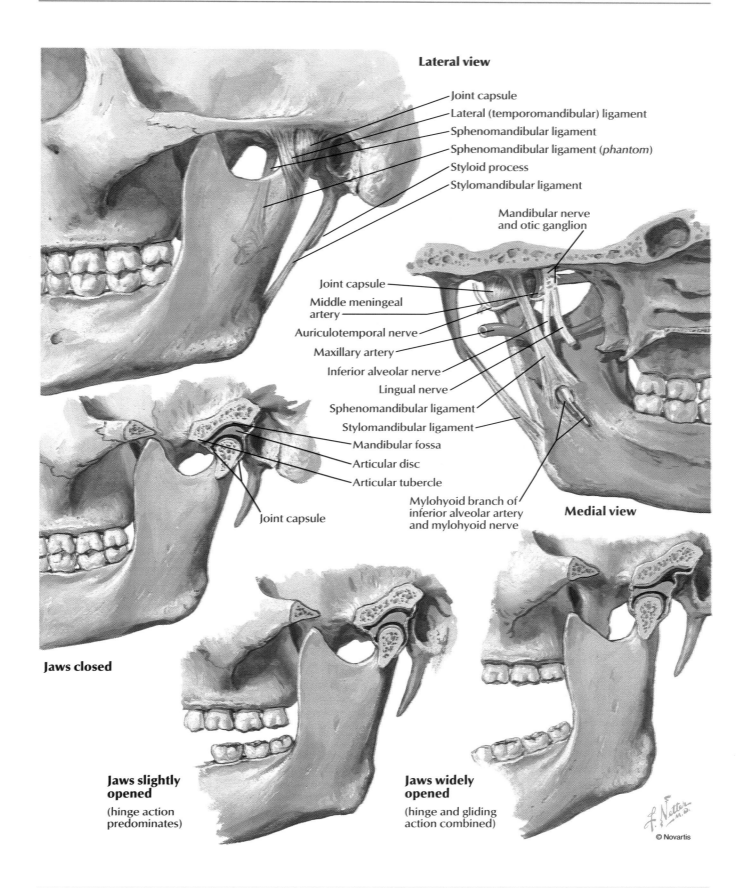

**Lateral view**

Joint capsule
Lateral (temporomandibular) ligament
Sphenomandibular ligament
Sphenomandibular ligament (*phantom*)
Styloid process
Stylomandibular ligament

Mandibular nerve and otic ganglion

Joint capsule
Middle meningeal artery
Auriculotemporal nerve
Maxillary artery
Inferior alveolar nerve
Lingual nerve
Sphenomandibular ligament
Stylomandibular ligament
Mandibular fossa
Articular disc
Articular tubercle

Joint capsule

Mylohyoid branch of inferior alveolar artery and mylohyoid nerve

**Medial view**

**Jaws closed**

**Jaws slightly opened**

(hinge action predominates)

**Jaws widely opened**

(hinge and gliding action combined)

© Novartis

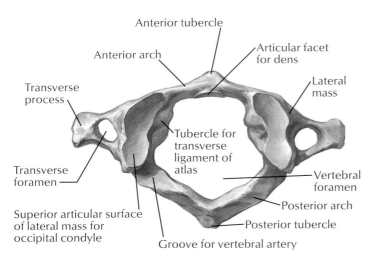

Anterior tubercle

Anterior arch

Articular facet for dens

Transverse process

Lateral mass

Tubercle for transverse ligament of atlas

Transverse foramen

Vertebral foramen

Superior articular surface of lateral mass for occipital condyle

Posterior arch

Posterior tubercle

Groove for vertebral artery

**Atlas (C1): superior view**

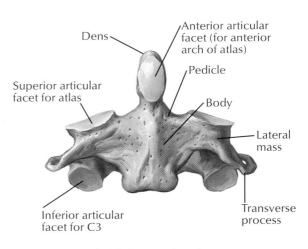

Dens

Anterior articular facet (for anterior arch of atlas)

Superior articular facet for atlas

Pedicle

Body

Lateral mass

Inferior articular facet for C3

Transverse process

**Axis (C2): anterior view**

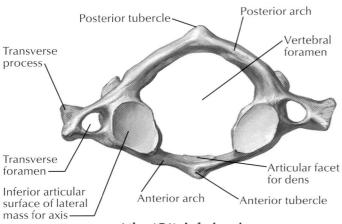

Posterior tubercle

Posterior arch

Transverse process

Vertebral foramen

Transverse foramen

Articular facet for dens

Inferior articular surface of lateral mass for axis

Anterior arch

Anterior tubercle

**Atlas (C1): inferior view**

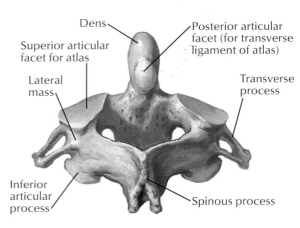

Dens

Posterior articular facet (for transverse ligament of atlas)

Superior articular facet for atlas

Lateral mass

Transverse process

Inferior articular process

Spinous process

**Axis (C2): posterosuperior view**

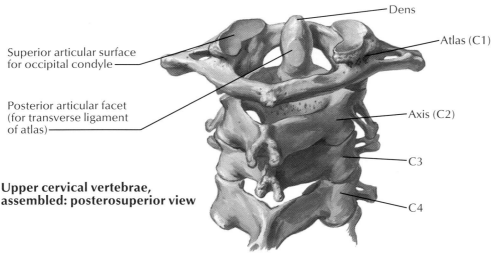

Dens

Atlas (C1)

Superior articular surface for occipital condyle

Posterior articular facet (for transverse ligament of atlas)

Axis (C2)

C3

C4

**Upper cervical vertebrae, assembled: posterosuperior view**

© Novartis

**PLATE 12**

**HEAD AND NECK**

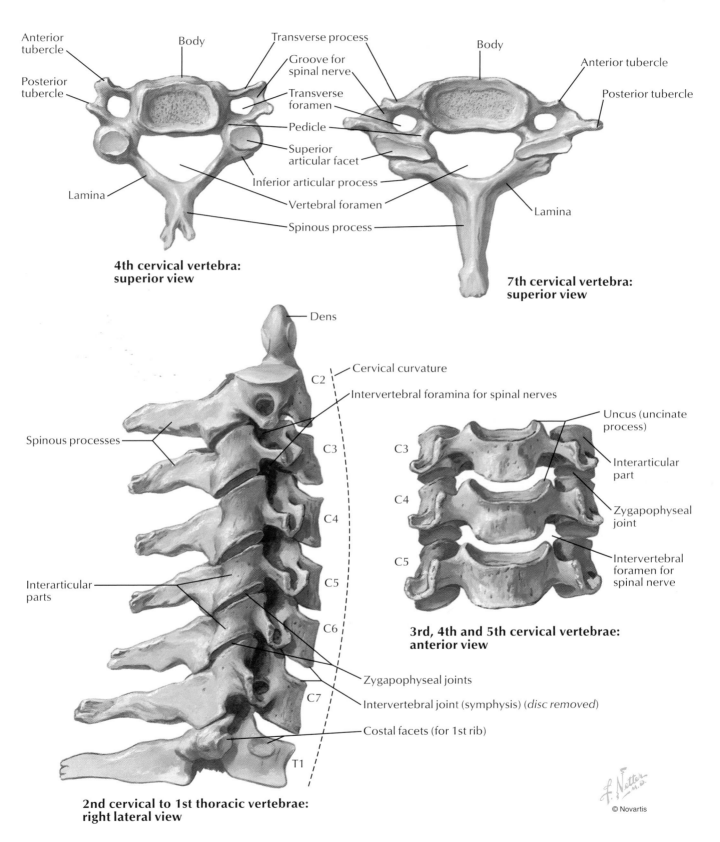

Anterior tubercle · Body · Transverse process · Groove for spinal nerve · Transverse foramen · Pedicle · Superior articular facet · Inferior articular process · Vertebral foramen · Spinous process

Posterior tubercle · Lamina

**4th cervical vertebra: superior view**

Body · Anterior tubercle · Posterior tubercle · Lamina

**7th cervical vertebra: superior view**

Dens

Cervical curvature · C2 · Intervertebral foramina for spinal nerves · C3 · C4 · C5 · C6 · C7 · T1

Spinous processes

Interarticular parts

Zygapophyseal joints · Intervertebral joint (symphysis) (*disc removed*) · Costal facets (for 1st rib)

**2nd cervical to 1st thoracic vertebrae: right lateral view**

Uncus (uncinate process) · Interarticular part · Zygapophyseal joint · Intervertebral foramen for spinal nerve

C3 · C4 · C5

**3rd, 4th and 5th cervical vertebrae: anterior view**

© Novartis

# *External Craniocervical Ligaments*

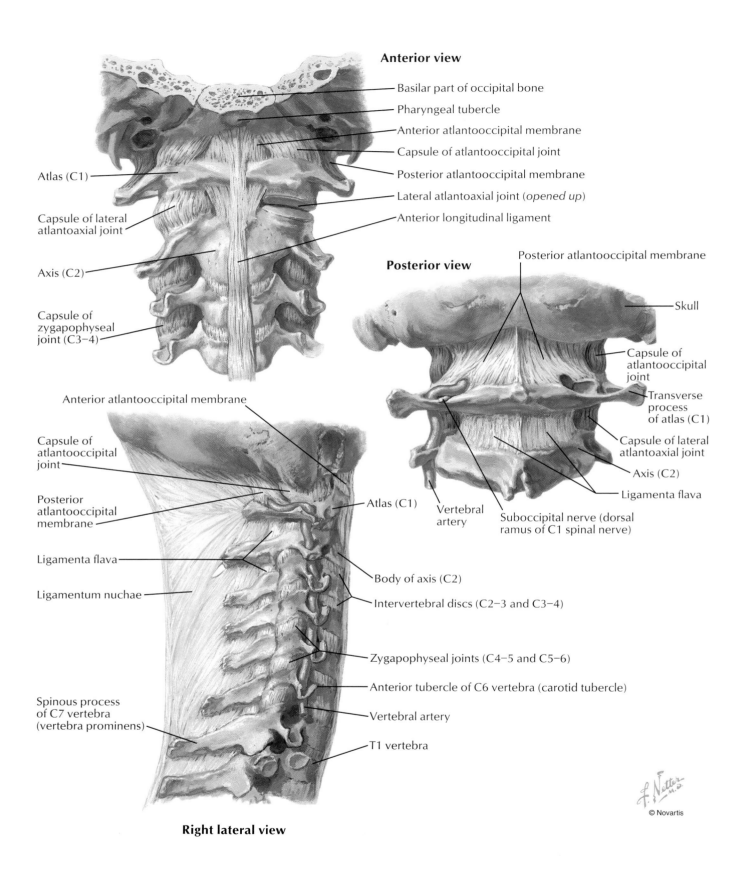

**Anterior view**

Basilar part of occipital bone

Pharyngeal tubercle

Anterior atlantooccipital membrane

Capsule of atlantooccipital joint

Posterior atlantooccipital membrane

Lateral atlantoaxial joint (*opened up*)

Anterior longitudinal ligament

Atlas (C1)

Capsule of lateral atlantoaxial joint

Axis (C2)

Capsule of zygapophyseal joint (C3–4)

**Posterior view**

Posterior atlantooccipital membrane

Skull

Capsule of atlantooccipital joint

Transverse process of atlas (C1)

Capsule of lateral atlantoaxial joint

Axis (C2)

Ligamenta flava

Vertebral artery

Suboccipital nerve (dorsal ramus of C1 spinal nerve)

Anterior atlantooccipital membrane

Capsule of atlantooccipital joint

Posterior atlantooccipital membrane

Ligamenta flava

Ligamentum nuchae

Atlas (C1)

Body of axis (C2)

Intervertebral discs (C2–3 and C3–4)

Zygapophyseal joints (C4–5 and C5–6)

Anterior tubercle of C6 vertebra (carotid tubercle)

Vertebral artery

Spinous process of C7 vertebra (vertebra prominens)

T1 vertebra

© Novartis

**Right lateral view**

**PLATE 14**

**HEAD AND NECK**

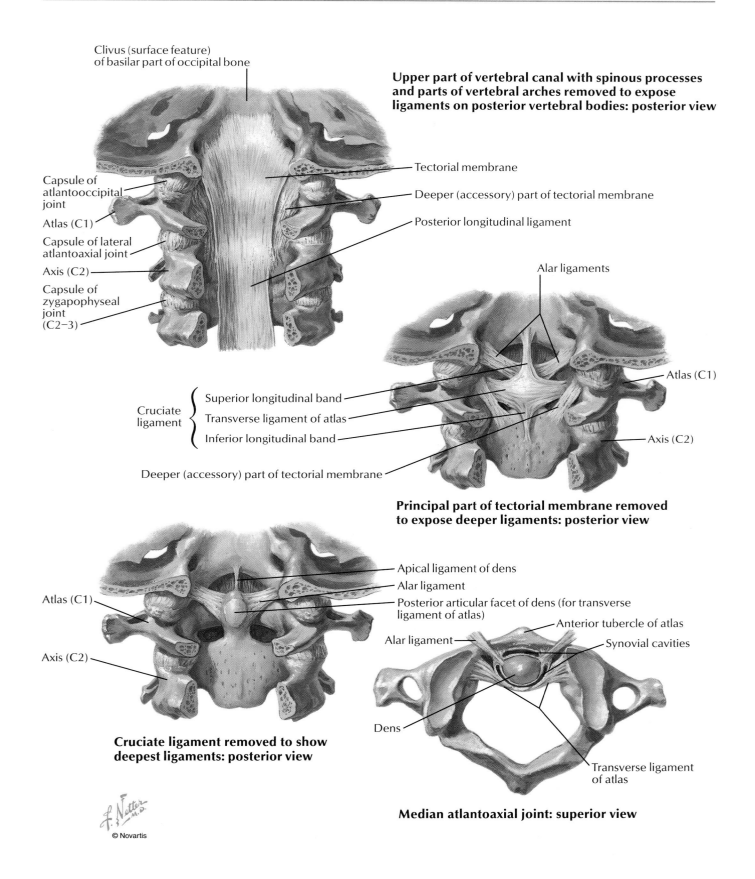

Clivus (surface feature) of basilar part of occipital bone

**Upper part of vertebral canal with spinous processes and parts of vertebral arches removed to expose ligaments on posterior vertebral bodies: posterior view**

Capsule of atlantooccipital joint

Atlas (C1)

Capsule of lateral atlantoaxial joint

Axis (C2)

Capsule of zygapophyseal joint (C2–3)

Tectorial membrane

Deeper (accessory) part of tectorial membrane

Posterior longitudinal ligament

Alar ligaments

Atlas (C1)

Cruciate ligament
- Superior longitudinal band
- Transverse ligament of atlas
- Inferior longitudinal band

Axis (C2)

Deeper (accessory) part of tectorial membrane

**Principal part of tectorial membrane removed to expose deeper ligaments: posterior view**

Atlas (C1)

Axis (C2)

Apical ligament of dens

Alar ligament

Posterior articular facet of dens (for transverse ligament of atlas)

Anterior tubercle of atlas

Alar ligament

Synovial cavities

Dens

Transverse ligament of atlas

**Cruciate ligament removed to show deepest ligaments: posterior view**

**Median atlantoaxial joint: superior view**

© Novartis

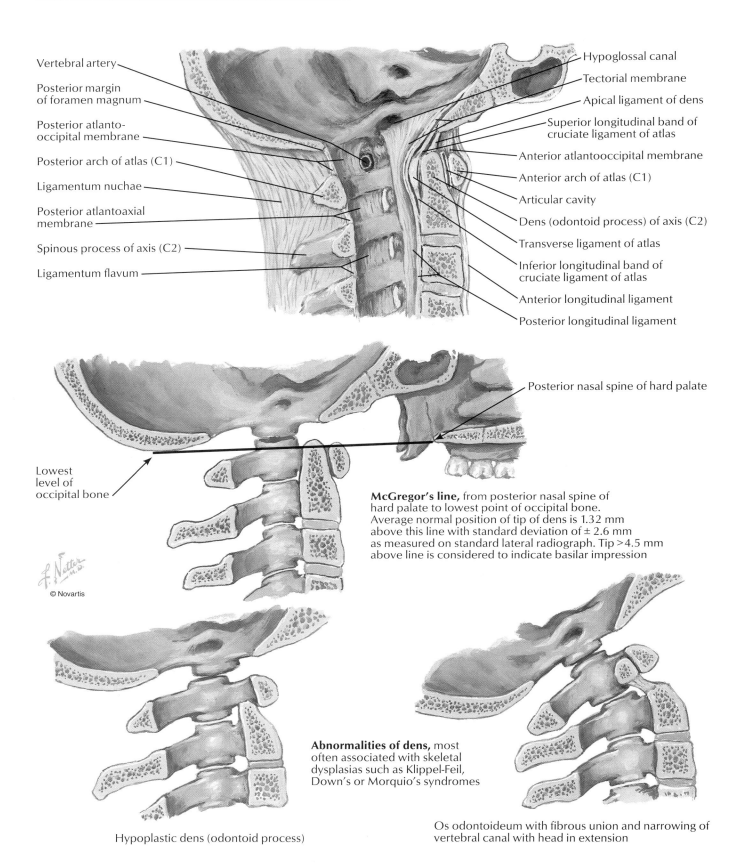

Vertebral artery

Posterior margin
of foramen magnum

Posterior atlanto-
occipital membrane

Posterior arch of atlas (C1)

Ligamentum nuchae

Posterior atlantoaxial
membrane

Spinous process of axis (C2)

Ligamentum flavum

Hypoglossal canal

Tectorial membrane

Apical ligament of dens

Superior longitudinal band of
cruciate ligament of atlas

Anterior atlantooccipital membrane

Anterior arch of atlas (C1)

Articular cavity

Dens (odontoid process) of axis (C2)

Transverse ligament of atlas

Inferior longitudinal band of
cruciate ligament of atlas

Anterior longitudinal ligament

Posterior longitudinal ligament

Posterior nasal spine of hard palate

Lowest
level of
occipital bone

**McGregor's line,** from posterior nasal spine of
hard palate to lowest point of occipital bone.
Average normal position of tip of dens is 1.32 mm
above this line with standard deviation of ± 2.6 mm
as measured on standard lateral radiograph. Tip >4.5 mm
above line is considered to indicate basilar impression

F. Netter
© Novartis

**Abnormalities of dens,** most
often associated with skeletal
dysplasias such as Klippel-Feil,
Down's or Morquio's syndromes

Hypoplastic dens (odontoid process)

Os odontoideum with fibrous union and narrowing of
vertebral canal with head in extension

**PLATE 16**

**HEAD AND NECK**

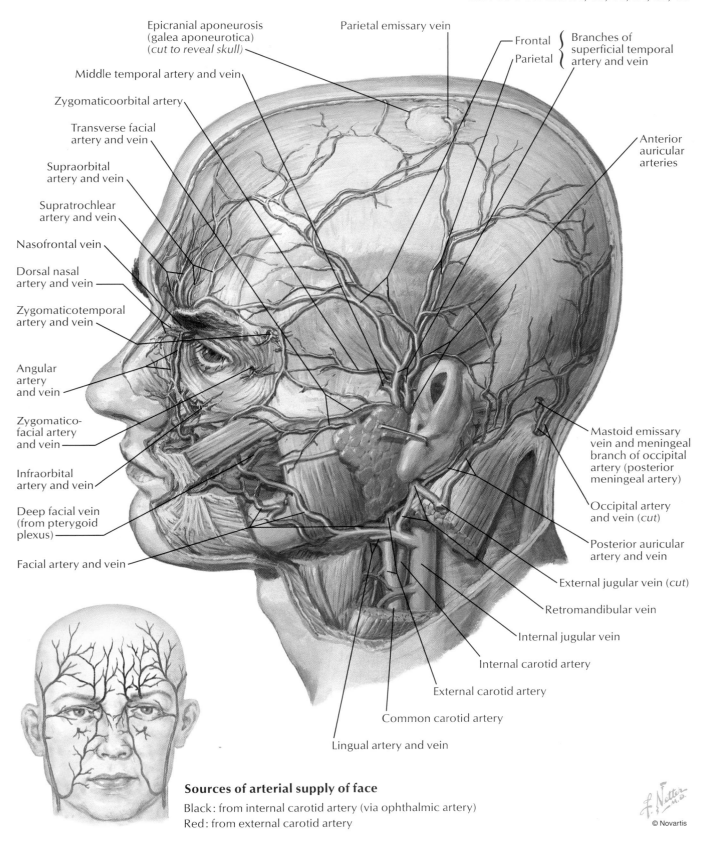

Epicranial aponeurosis
(galea aponeurotica)
(*cut to reveal skull*)

Middle temporal artery and vein

Zygomaticoorbital artery

Transverse facial artery and vein

Supraorbital artery and vein

Supratrochlear artery and vein

Nasofrontal vein

Dorsal nasal artery and vein

Zygomaticotemporal artery and vein

Angular artery and vein

Zygomatico-facial artery and vein

Infraorbital artery and vein

Deep facial vein (from pterygoid plexus)

Facial artery and vein

Parietal emissary vein

Frontal
Parietal } Branches of superficial temporal artery and vein

Anterior auricular arteries

Mastoid emissary vein and meningeal branch of occipital artery (posterior meningeal artery)

Occipital artery and vein (*cut*)

Posterior auricular artery and vein

External jugular vein (*cut*)

Retromandibular vein

Internal jugular vein

Internal carotid artery

External carotid artery

Common carotid artery

Lingual artery and vein

**Sources of arterial supply of face**

Black: from internal carotid artery (via ophthalmic artery)
Red: from external carotid artery

© Novartis

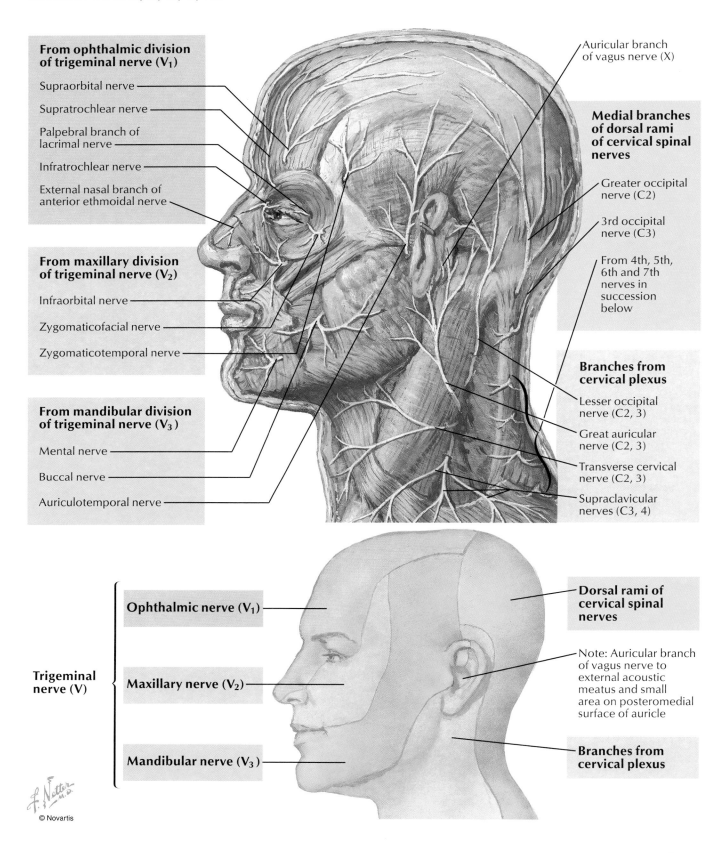

**From ophthalmic division of trigeminal nerve (V₁)**

Supraorbital nerve

Supratrochlear nerve

Palpebral branch of lacrimal nerve

Infratrochlear nerve

External nasal branch of anterior ethmoidal nerve

**From maxillary division of trigeminal nerve (V₂)**

Infraorbital nerve

Zygomaticofacial nerve

Zygomaticotemporal nerve

**From mandibular division of trigeminal nerve (V₃)**

Mental nerve

Buccal nerve

Auriculotemporal nerve

Auricular branch of vagus nerve (X)

**Medial branches of dorsal rami of cervical spinal nerves**

Greater occipital nerve (C2)

3rd occipital nerve (C3)

From 4th, 5th, 6th and 7th nerves in succession below

**Branches from cervical plexus**

Lesser occipital nerve (C2, 3)

Great auricular nerve (C2, 3)

Transverse cervical nerve (C2, 3)

Supraclavicular nerves (C3, 4)

Ophthalmic nerve (V₁)

Maxillary nerve (V₂)

Mandibular nerve (V₃)

Trigeminal nerve (V)

Dorsal rami of cervical spinal nerves

Note: Auricular branch of vagus nerve to external acoustic meatus and small area on posteromedial surface of auricle

Branches from cervical plexus

© Novartis

**PLATE 18**

**HEAD AND NECK**

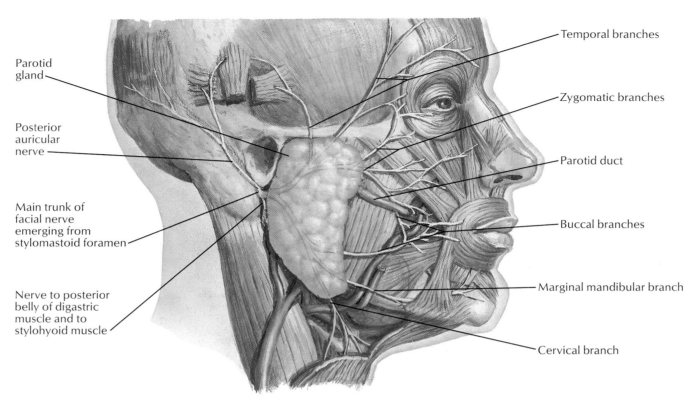

Parotid gland

Posterior auricular nerve

Main trunk of facial nerve emerging from stylomastoid foramen

Nerve to posterior belly of digastric muscle and to stylohyoid muscle

Temporal branches

Zygomatic branches

Parotid duct

Buccal branches

Marginal mandibular branch

Cervical branch

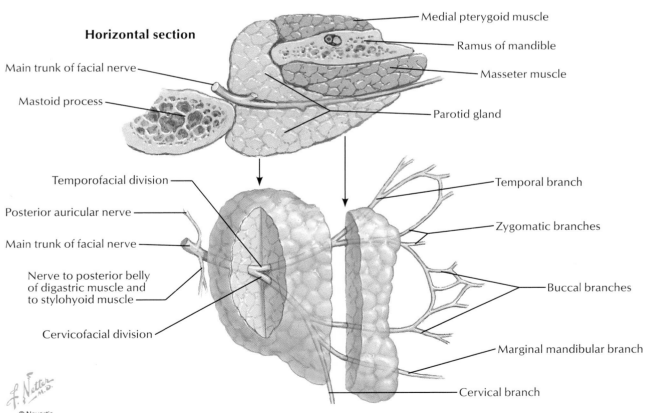

**Horizontal section**

Main trunk of facial nerve

Mastoid process

Medial pterygoid muscle

Ramus of mandible

Masseter muscle

Parotid gland

Temporofacial division

Posterior auricular nerve

Main trunk of facial nerve

Nerve to posterior belly of digastric muscle and to stylohyoid muscle

Cervicofacial division

Temporal branch

Zygomatic branches

Buccal branches

Marginal mandibular branch

Cervical branch

© Novartis

# Muscles of Facial Expression: Anterior View

SEE ALSO PLATE 48

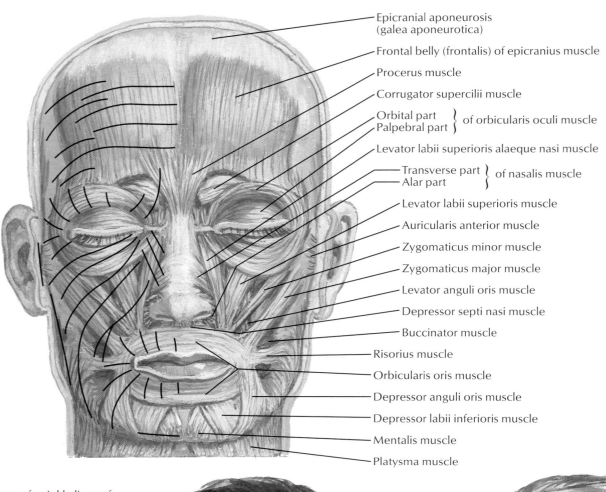

Epicranial aponeurosis
(galea aponeurotica)

Frontal belly (frontalis) of epicranius muscle

Procerus muscle

Corrugator supercilii muscle

Orbital part  } of orbicularis oculi muscle
Palpebral part

Levator labii superioris alaeque nasi muscle

Transverse part } of nasalis muscle
Alar part

Levator labii superioris muscle

Auricularis anterior muscle

Zygomaticus minor muscle

Zygomaticus major muscle

Levator anguli oris muscle

Depressor septi nasi muscle

Buccinator muscle

Risorius muscle

Orbicularis oris muscle

Depressor anguli oris muscle

Depressor labii inferioris muscle

Mentalis muscle

Platysma muscle

Course of wrinkle lines of skin is transverse to fiber direction of facial muscles. Elliptical incisions for removal of skin tumors conform to direction of wrinkle lines

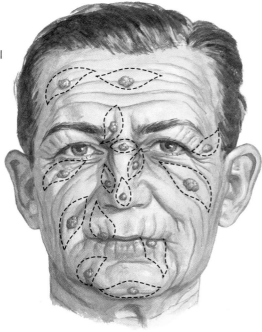

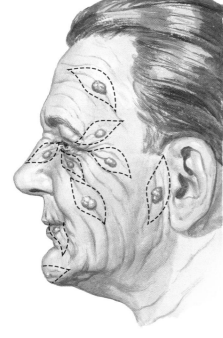

© Novartis

**PLATE 20**

**HEAD AND NECK**

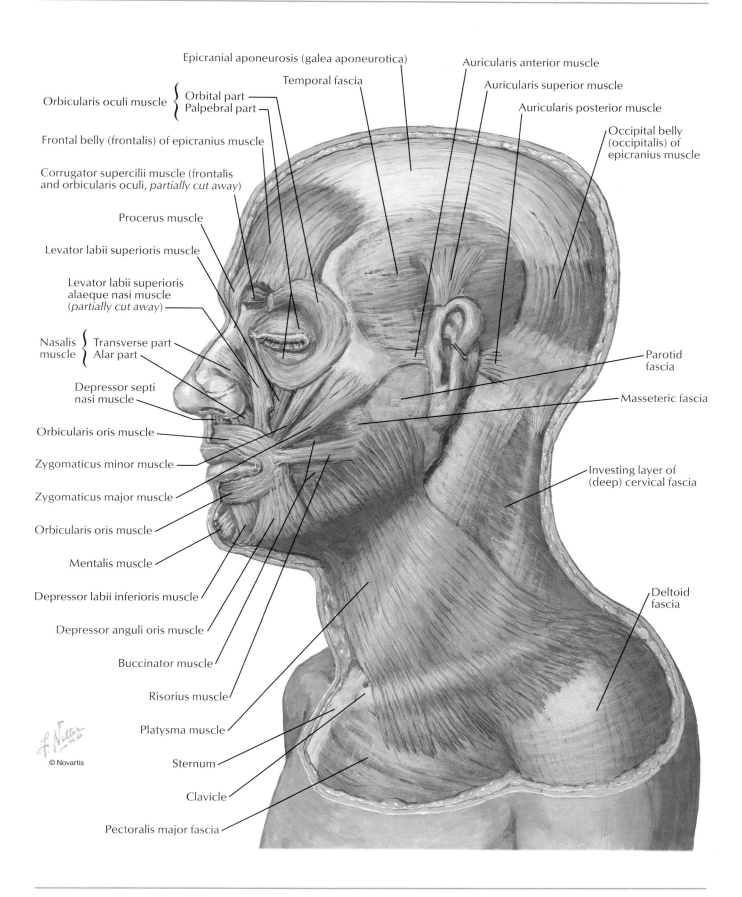

Epicranial aponeurosis (galea aponeurotica)

Temporal fascia

Auricularis anterior muscle

Auricularis superior muscle

Auricularis posterior muscle

Occipital belly (occipitalis) of epicranius muscle

Orbicularis oculi muscle { Orbital part Palpebral part

Frontal belly (frontalis) of epicranius muscle

Corrugator supercilii muscle (frontalis and orbicularis oculi, *partially cut away*)

Procerus muscle

Levator labii superioris muscle

Levator labii superioris alaeque nasi muscle (*partially cut away*)

Nasalis muscle { Transverse part Alar part

Depressor septi nasi muscle

Orbicularis oris muscle

Zygomaticus minor muscle

Zygomaticus major muscle

Orbicularis oris muscle

Mentalis muscle

Depressor labii inferioris muscle

Depressor anguli oris muscle

Buccinator muscle

Risorius muscle

Platysma muscle

Sternum

Clavicle

Pectoralis major fascia

Parotid fascia

Masseteric fascia

Investing layer of (deep) cervical fascia

Deltoid fascia

© Novartis

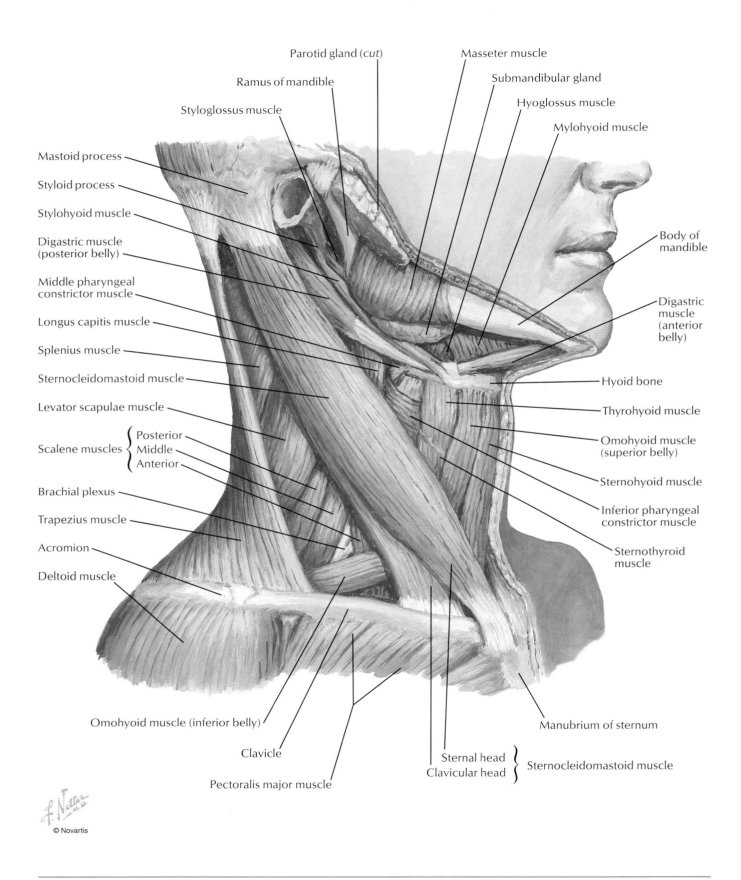

Parotid gland (*cut*)

Masseter muscle

Ramus of mandible

Submandibular gland

Styloglossus muscle

Hyoglossus muscle

Mylohyoid muscle

Mastoid process

Styloid process

Stylohyoid muscle

Body of mandible

Digastric muscle (posterior belly)

Digastric muscle (anterior belly)

Middle pharyngeal constrictor muscle

Longus capitis muscle

Splenius muscle

Sternocleidomastoid muscle

Hyoid bone

Levator scapulae muscle

Thyrohyoid muscle

Scalene muscles { Posterior Middle Anterior

Omohyoid muscle (superior belly)

Brachial plexus

Sternohyoid muscle

Trapezius muscle

Inferior pharyngeal constrictor muscle

Acromion

Deltoid muscle

Sternothyroid muscle

Omohyoid muscle (inferior belly)

Manubrium of sternum

Clavicle

Sternal head } Sternocleidomastoid muscle
Clavicular head }

Pectoralis major muscle

© Novartis

**PLATE 22**

**HEAD AND NECK**

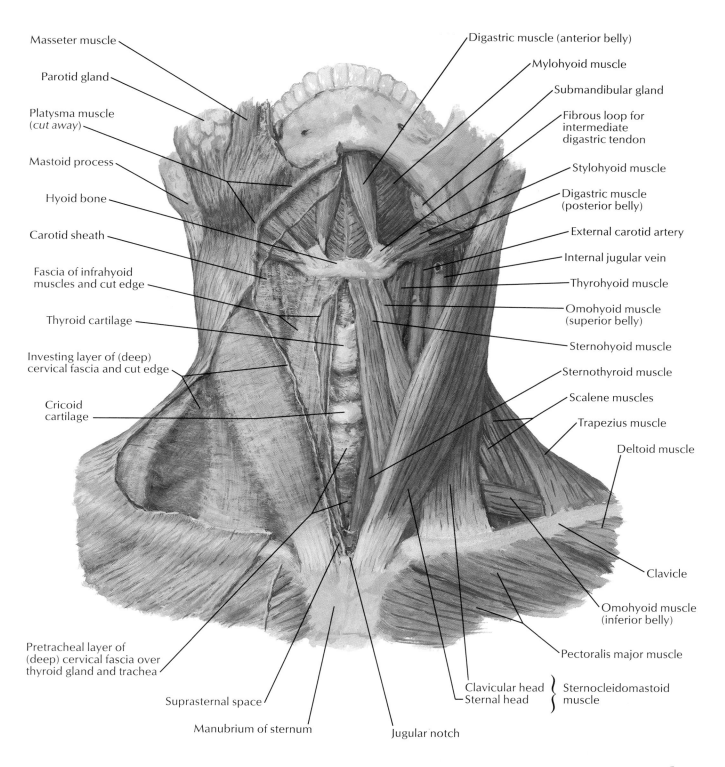

Masseter muscle

Parotid gland

Platysma muscle (*cut away*)

Mastoid process

Hyoid bone

Carotid sheath

Fascia of infrahyoid muscles and cut edge

Thyroid cartilage

Investing layer of (deep) cervical fascia and cut edge

Cricoid cartilage

Pretracheal layer of (deep) cervical fascia over thyroid gland and trachea

Suprasternal space

Manubrium of sternum

Digastric muscle (anterior belly)

Mylohyoid muscle

Submandibular gland

Fibrous loop for intermediate digastric tendon

Stylohyoid muscle

Digastric muscle (posterior belly)

External carotid artery

Internal jugular vein

Thyrohyoid muscle

Omohyoid muscle (superior belly)

Sternohyoid muscle

Sternothyroid muscle

Scalene muscles

Trapezius muscle

Deltoid muscle

Clavicle

Omohyoid muscle (inferior belly)

Pectoralis major muscle

Clavicular head
Sternal head } Sternocleidomastoid muscle

Jugular notch

*SEE ALSO PLATE 47*

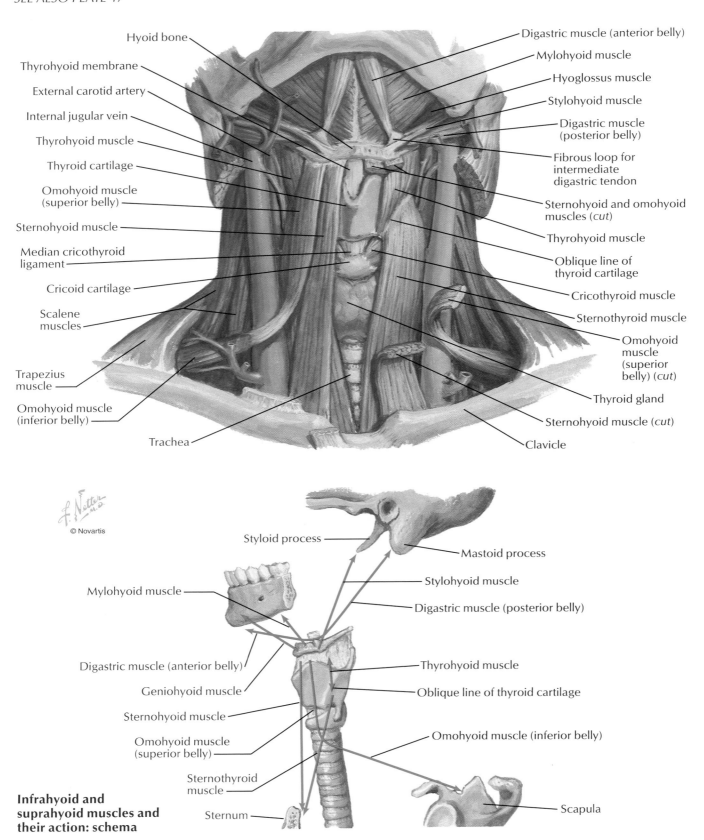

Hyoid bone

Thyrohyoid membrane

External carotid artery

Internal jugular vein

Thyrohyoid muscle

Thyroid cartilage

Omohyoid muscle (superior belly)

Sternohyoid muscle

Median cricothyroid ligament

Cricoid cartilage

Scalene muscles

Trapezius muscle

Omohyoid muscle (inferior belly)

Trachea

Digastric muscle (anterior belly)

Mylohyoid muscle

Hyoglossus muscle

Stylohyoid muscle

Digastric muscle (posterior belly)

Fibrous loop for intermediate digastric tendon

Sternohyoid and omohyoid muscles (*cut*)

Thyrohyoid muscle

Oblique line of thyroid cartilage

Cricothyroid muscle

Sternothyroid muscle

Omohyoid muscle (superior belly) (*cut*)

Thyroid gland

Sternohyoid muscle (*cut*)

Clavicle

© Novartis

Styloid process

Mastoid process

Mylohyoid muscle

Stylohyoid muscle

Digastric muscle (posterior belly)

Digastric muscle (anterior belly)

Geniohyoid muscle

Sternohyoid muscle

Omohyoid muscle (superior belly)

Sternothyroid muscle

Sternum

Thyrohyoid muscle

Oblique line of thyroid cartilage

Omohyoid muscle (inferior belly)

Scapula

**Infrahyoid and suprahyoid muscles and their action: schema**

**PLATE 24**

**HEAD AND NECK**

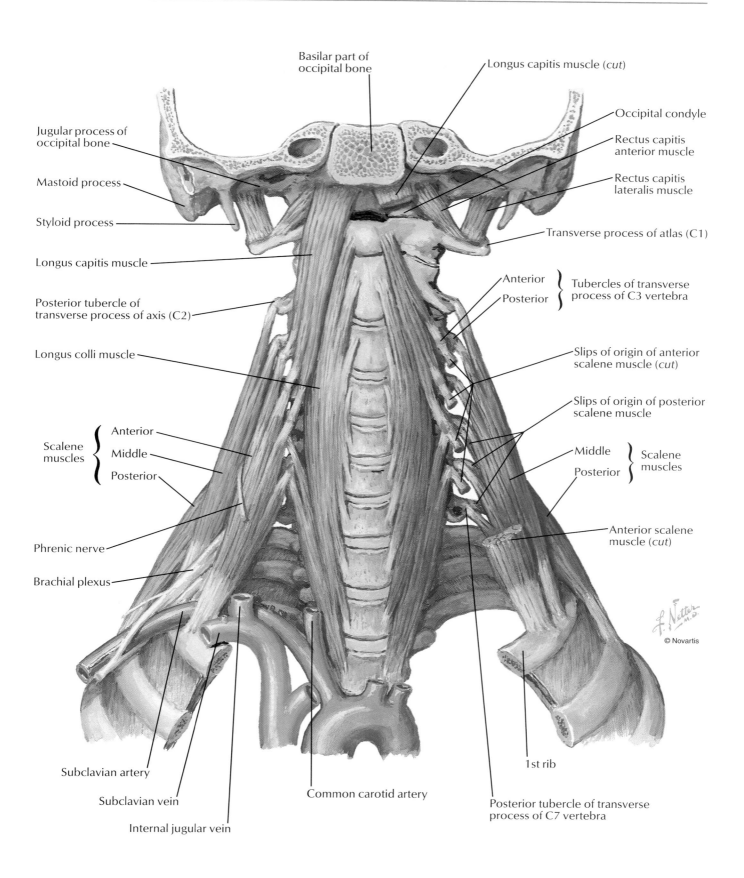

Basilar part of occipital bone

Longus capitis muscle (*cut*)

Occipital condyle

Jugular process of occipital bone

Rectus capitis anterior muscle

Mastoid process

Rectus capitis lateralis muscle

Styloid process

Transverse process of atlas (C1)

Longus capitis muscle

Anterior
Posterior
Tubercles of transverse process of C3 vertebra

Posterior tubercle of transverse process of axis (C2)

Slips of origin of anterior scalene muscle (*cut*)

Longus colli muscle

Slips of origin of posterior scalene muscle

Anterior
Middle
Posterior
Scalene muscles

Middle
Posterior
Scalene muscles

Anterior scalene muscle (*cut*)

Phrenic nerve

Brachial plexus

1st rib

Subclavian artery

Subclavian vein

Common carotid artery

Internal jugular vein

Posterior tubercle of transverse process of C7 vertebra

# Superficial Veins and Cutaneous Nerves of Neck

*FOR DEEP VEINS OF NECK SEE PLATE 64*

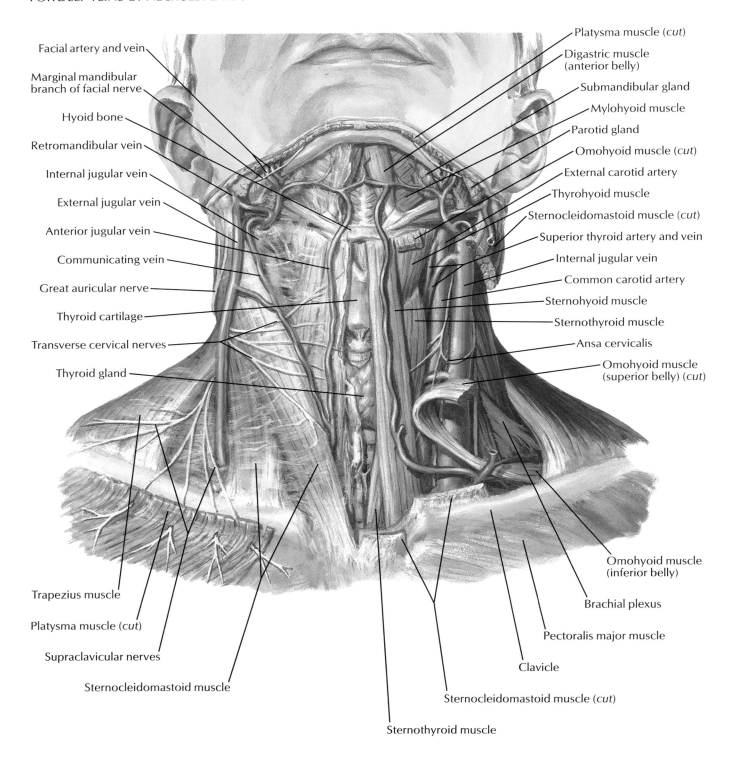

Facial artery and vein

Marginal mandibular branch of facial nerve

Hyoid bone

Retromandibular vein

Internal jugular vein

External jugular vein

Anterior jugular vein

Communicating vein

Great auricular nerve

Thyroid cartilage

Transverse cervical nerves

Thyroid gland

Trapezius muscle

Platysma muscle (*cut*)

Supraclavicular nerves

Sternocleidomastoid muscle

Sternothyroid muscle

Platysma muscle (*cut*)

Digastric muscle (anterior belly)

Submandibular gland

Mylohyoid muscle

Parotid gland

Omohyoid muscle (*cut*)

External carotid artery

Thyrohyoid muscle

Sternocleidomastoid muscle (*cut*)

Superior thyroid artery and vein

Internal jugular vein

Common carotid artery

Sternohyoid muscle

Sternothyroid muscle

Ansa cervicalis

Omohyoid muscle (superior belly) (*cut*)

Omohyoid muscle (inferior belly)

Brachial plexus

Pectoralis major muscle

Clavicle

Sternocleidomastoid muscle (*cut*)

© Novartis

**PLATE 26**

**HEAD AND NECK**

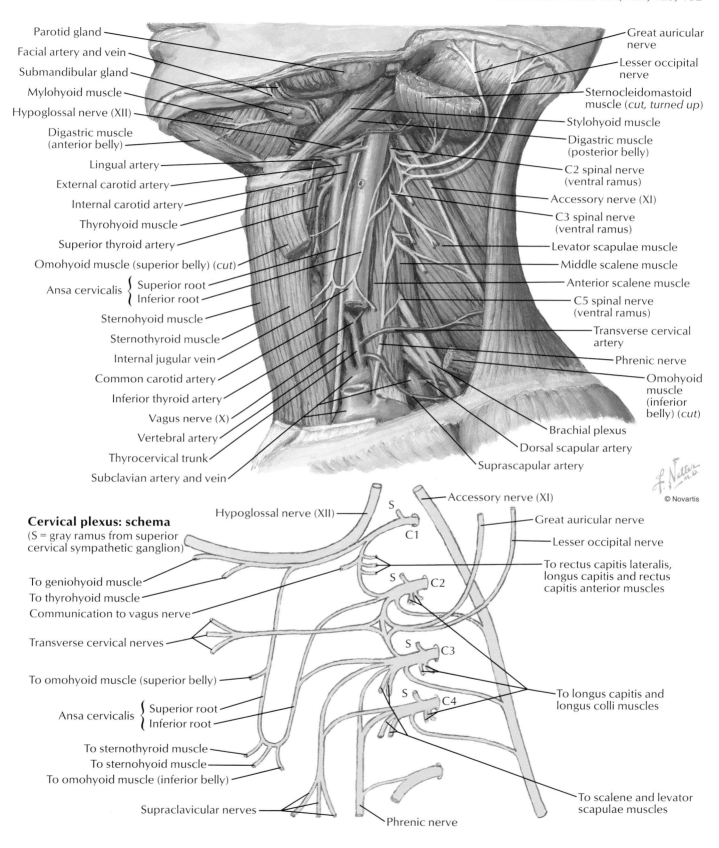

Parotid gland

Facial artery and vein

Submandibular gland

Mylohyoid muscle

Hypoglossal nerve (XII)

Digastric muscle (anterior belly)

Lingual artery

External carotid artery

Internal carotid artery

Thyrohyoid muscle

Superior thyroid artery

Omohyoid muscle (superior belly) (cut)

Ansa cervicalis { Superior root / Inferior root

Sternohyoid muscle

Sternothyroid muscle

Internal jugular vein

Common carotid artery

Inferior thyroid artery

Vagus nerve (X)

Vertebral artery

Thyrocervical trunk

Subclavian artery and vein

Great auricular nerve

Lesser occipital nerve

Sternocleidomastoid muscle (cut, turned up)

Stylohyoid muscle

Digastric muscle (posterior belly)

C2 spinal nerve (ventral ramus)

Accessory nerve (XI)

C3 spinal nerve (ventral ramus)

Levator scapulae muscle

Middle scalene muscle

Anterior scalene muscle

C5 spinal nerve (ventral ramus)

Transverse cervical artery

Phrenic nerve

Omohyoid muscle (inferior belly) (cut)

Brachial plexus

Dorsal scapular artery

Suprascapular artery

© Novartis

**Cervical plexus: schema**
(S = gray ramus from superior cervical sympathetic ganglion)

To geniohyoid muscle

To thyrohyoid muscle

Communication to vagus nerve

Transverse cervical nerves

To omohyoid muscle (superior belly)

Ansa cervicalis { Superior root / Inferior root

To sternothyroid muscle

To sternohyoid muscle

To omohyoid muscle (inferior belly)

Supraclavicular nerves

Hypoglossal nerve (XII)

Accessory nerve (XI)

Great auricular nerve

Lesser occipital nerve

To rectus capitis lateralis, longus capitis and rectus capitis anterior muscles

To longus capitis and longus colli muscles

To scalene and levator scapulae muscles

Phrenic nerve

S   C1

S   C2

S   C3

S   C4

# Subclavian Artery

*SEE ALSO PLATE 398*

**Right anterior dissection**

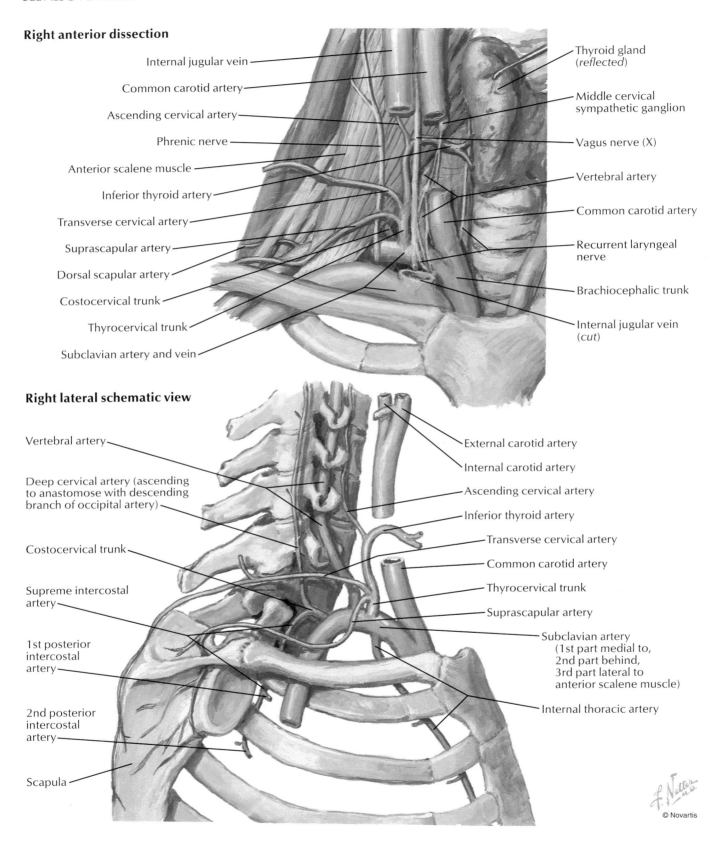

Internal jugular vein

Common carotid artery

Ascending cervical artery

Phrenic nerve

Anterior scalene muscle

Inferior thyroid artery

Transverse cervical artery

Suprascapular artery

Dorsal scapular artery

Costocervical trunk

Thyrocervical trunk

Subclavian artery and vein

Thyroid gland (*reflected*)

Middle cervical sympathetic ganglion

Vagus nerve (X)

Vertebral artery

Common carotid artery

Recurrent laryngeal nerve

Brachiocephalic trunk

Internal jugular vein (*cut*)

**Right lateral schematic view**

Vertebral artery

Deep cervical artery (ascending to anastomose with descending branch of occipital artery)

Costocervical trunk

Supreme intercostal artery

1st posterior intercostal artery

2nd posterior intercostal artery

Scapula

External carotid artery

Internal carotid artery

Ascending cervical artery

Inferior thyroid artery

Transverse cervical artery

Common carotid artery

Thyrocervical trunk

Suprascapular artery

Subclavian artery (1st part medial to, 2nd part behind, 3rd part lateral to anterior scalene muscle)

Internal thoracic artery

**PLATE 28**                                              **HEAD AND NECK**

© Novartis

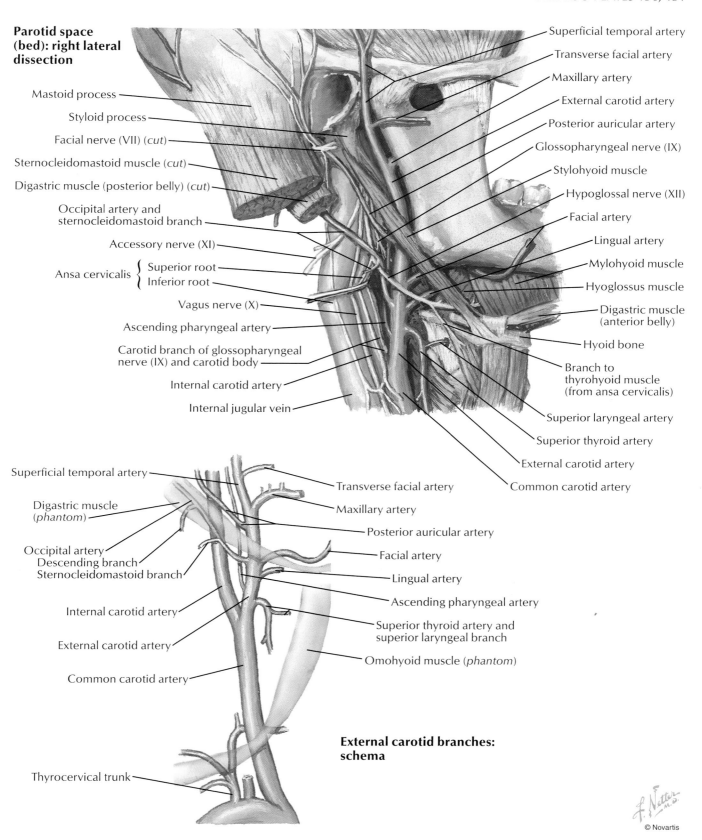

**Parotid space (bed): right lateral dissection**

Mastoid process

Styloid process

Facial nerve (VII) (*cut*)

Sternocleidomastoid muscle (*cut*)

Digastric muscle (posterior belly) (*cut*)

Occipital artery and sternocleidomastoid branch

Accessory nerve (XI)

Ansa cervicalis { Superior root / Inferior root

Vagus nerve (X)

Ascending pharyngeal artery

Carotid branch of glossopharyngeal nerve (IX) and carotid body

Internal carotid artery

Internal jugular vein

Superficial temporal artery

Transverse facial artery

Maxillary artery

External carotid artery

Posterior auricular artery

Glossopharyngeal nerve (IX)

Stylohyoid muscle

Hypoglossal nerve (XII)

Facial artery

Lingual artery

Mylohyoid muscle

Hyoglossus muscle

Digastric muscle (anterior belly)

Hyoid bone

Branch to thyrohyoid muscle (from ansa cervicalis)

Superior laryngeal artery

Superior thyroid artery

External carotid artery

Common carotid artery

Superficial temporal artery

Digastric muscle (*phantom*)

Occipital artery

Descending branch

Sternocleidomastoid branch

Internal carotid artery

External carotid artery

Common carotid artery

Thyrocervical trunk

Transverse facial artery

Maxillary artery

Posterior auricular artery

Facial artery

Lingual artery

Ascending pharyngeal artery

Superior thyroid artery and superior laryngeal branch

Omohyoid muscle (*phantom*)

**External carotid branches: schema**

© Novartis

# Fascial Layers of Neck

FOR CONTENTS OF CAROTID SHEATH SEE PLATES 63, 64, 65

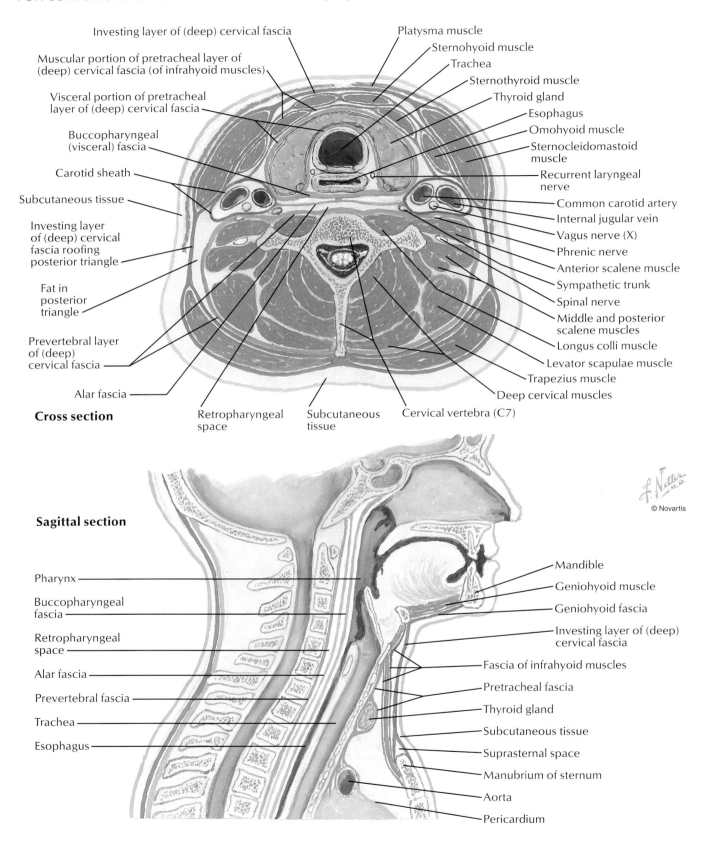

**Cross section**

Investing layer of (deep) cervical fascia

Muscular portion of pretracheal layer of (deep) cervical fascia (of infrahyoid muscles)

Visceral portion of pretracheal layer of (deep) cervical fascia

Buccopharyngeal (visceral) fascia

Carotid sheath

Subcutaneous tissue

Investing layer of (deep) cervical fascia roofing posterior triangle

Fat in posterior triangle

Prevertebral layer of (deep) cervical fascia

Alar fascia

Retropharyngeal space

Subcutaneous tissue

Cervical vertebra (C7)

Platysma muscle

Sternohyoid muscle

Trachea

Sternothyroid muscle

Thyroid gland

Esophagus

Omohyoid muscle

Sternocleidomastoid muscle

Recurrent laryngeal nerve

Common carotid artery

Internal jugular vein

Vagus nerve (X)

Phrenic nerve

Anterior scalene muscle

Sympathetic trunk

Spinal nerve

Middle and posterior scalene muscles

Longus colli muscle

Levator scapulae muscle

Trapezius muscle

Deep cervical muscles

**Sagittal section**

Pharynx

Buccopharyngeal fascia

Retropharyngeal space

Alar fascia

Prevertebral fascia

Trachea

Esophagus

Mandible

Geniohyoid muscle

Geniohyoid fascia

Investing layer of (deep) cervical fascia

Fascia of infrahyoid muscles

Pretracheal fascia

Thyroid gland

Subcutaneous tissue

Suprasternal space

Manubrium of sternum

Aorta

Pericardium

PLATE 30

**Anterolateral view**

Frontal bone

Nasal bones

Frontal process of maxilla

Lateral process of
septal nasal cartilages

Septal cartilage

Minor alar cartilage

Accessory nasal cartilage

Major alar cartilage

Lateral crus

Medial crus

Septal nasal cartilage

Anterior nasal spine of maxilla

Alar fibrofatty tissue

Infraorbital foramen

**Inferior view**

Major alar cartilage

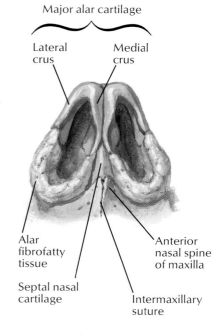

Lateral
crus

Medial
crus

Alar
fibrofatty
tissue

Septal nasal
cartilage

Anterior
nasal spine
of maxilla

Intermaxillary
suture

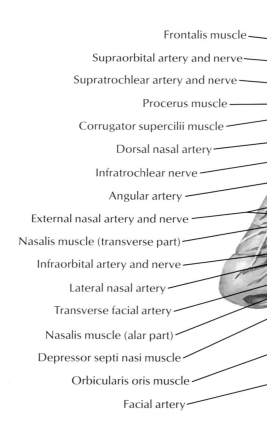

Frontalis muscle

Supraorbital artery and nerve

Supratrochlear artery and nerve

Procerus muscle

Corrugator supercilii muscle

Dorsal nasal artery

Infratrochlear nerve

Angular artery

External nasal artery and nerve

Nasalis muscle (transverse part)

Infraorbital artery and nerve

Lateral nasal artery

Transverse facial artery

Nasalis muscle (alar part)

Depressor septi nasi muscle

Orbicularis oris muscle

Facial artery

© Novartis

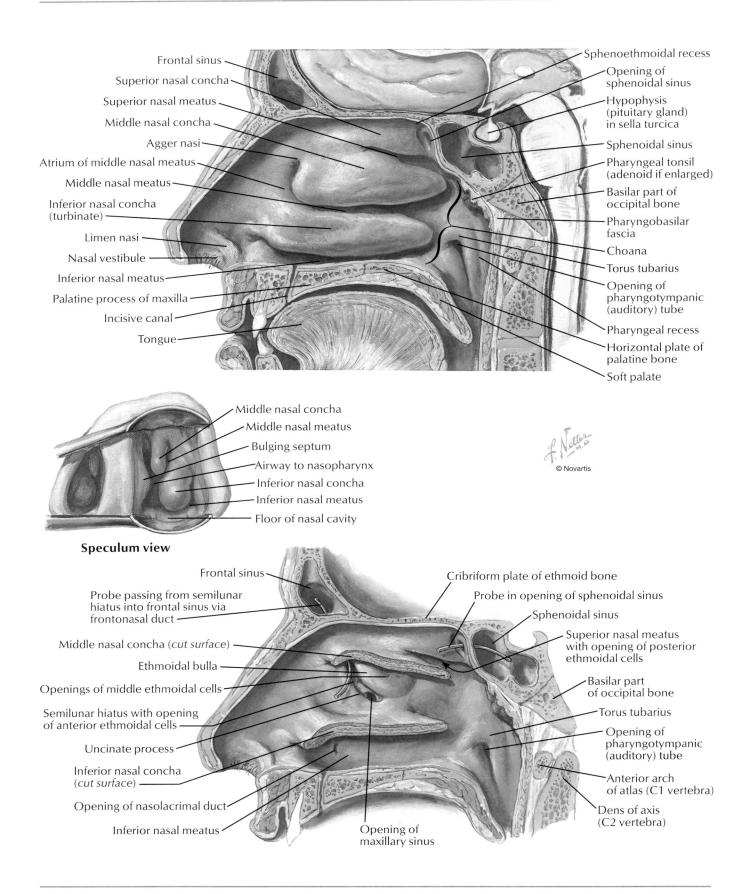

Frontal sinus

Superior nasal concha

Superior nasal meatus

Middle nasal concha

Agger nasi

Atrium of middle nasal meatus

Middle nasal meatus

Inferior nasal concha (turbinate)

Limen nasi

Nasal vestibule

Inferior nasal meatus

Palatine process of maxilla

Incisive canal

Tongue

Sphenoethmoidal recess

Opening of sphenoidal sinus

Hypophysis (pituitary gland) in sella turcica

Sphenoidal sinus

Pharyngeal tonsil (adenoid if enlarged)

Basilar part of occipital bone

Pharyngobasilar fascia

Choana

Torus tubarius

Opening of pharyngotympanic (auditory) tube

Pharyngeal recess

Horizontal plate of palatine bone

Soft palate

Middle nasal concha

Middle nasal meatus

Bulging septum

Airway to nasopharynx

Inferior nasal concha

Inferior nasal meatus

Floor of nasal cavity

**Speculum view**

Frontal sinus

Probe passing from semilunar hiatus into frontal sinus via frontonasal duct

Middle nasal concha (*cut surface*)

Ethmoidal bulla

Openings of middle ethmoidal cells

Semilunar hiatus with opening of anterior ethmoidal cells

Uncinate process

Inferior nasal concha (*cut surface*)

Opening of nasolacrimal duct

Inferior nasal meatus

Opening of maxillary sinus

Cribriform plate of ethmoid bone

Probe in opening of sphenoidal sinus

Sphenoidal sinus

Superior nasal meatus with opening of posterior ethmoidal cells

Basilar part of occipital bone

Torus tubarius

Opening of pharyngotympanic (auditory) tube

Anterior arch of atlas (C1 vertebra)

Dens of axis (C2 vertebra)

**PLATE 32**

**HEAD AND NECK**

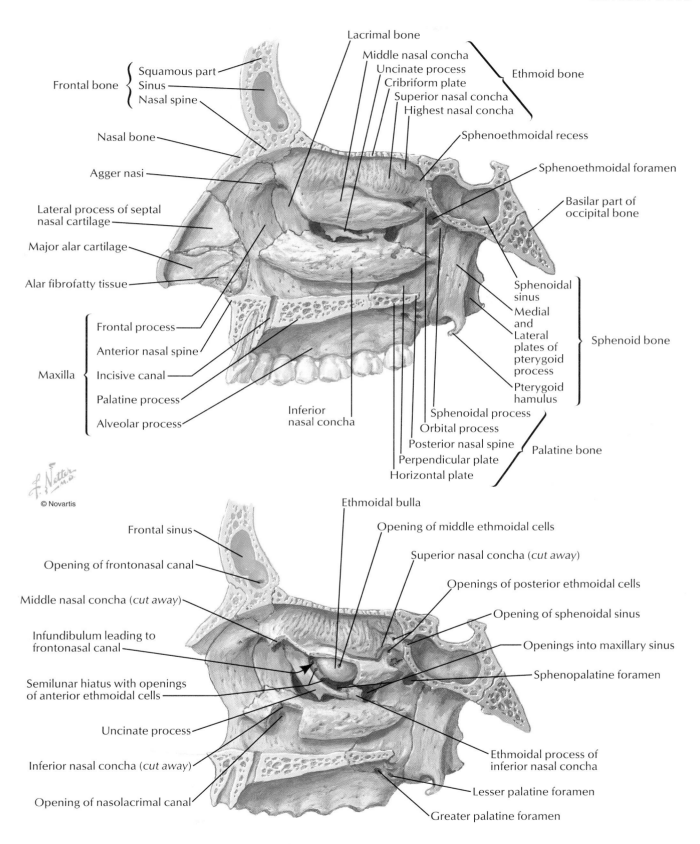

Lacrimal bone

Frontal bone
- Squamous part
- Sinus
- Nasal spine

Middle nasal concha
Uncinate process
Cribriform plate
Superior nasal concha
Highest nasal concha

Ethmoid bone

Nasal bone

Sphenoethmoidal recess

Agger nasi

Sphenoethmoidal foramen

Lateral process of septal nasal cartilage

Basilar part of occipital bone

Major alar cartilage

Alar fibrofatty tissue

Sphenoidal sinus

Medial and Lateral plates of pterygoid process

Sphenoid bone

Maxilla
- Frontal process
- Anterior nasal spine
- Incisive canal
- Palatine process
- Alveolar process

Pterygoid hamulus

Inferior nasal concha

Sphenoidal process
Orbital process
Posterior nasal spine
Perpendicular plate
Horizontal plate

Palatine bone

© Novartis

Ethmoidal bulla

Frontal sinus

Opening of middle ethmoidal cells

Opening of frontonasal canal

Superior nasal concha (*cut away*)

Middle nasal concha (*cut away*)

Openings of posterior ethmoidal cells

Infundibulum leading to frontonasal canal

Opening of sphenoidal sinus

Semilunar hiatus with openings of anterior ethmoidal cells

Openings into maxillary sinus

Sphenopalatine foramen

Uncinate process

Inferior nasal concha (*cut away*)

Ethmoidal process of inferior nasal concha

Lesser palatine foramen

Opening of nasolacrimal canal

Greater palatine foramen

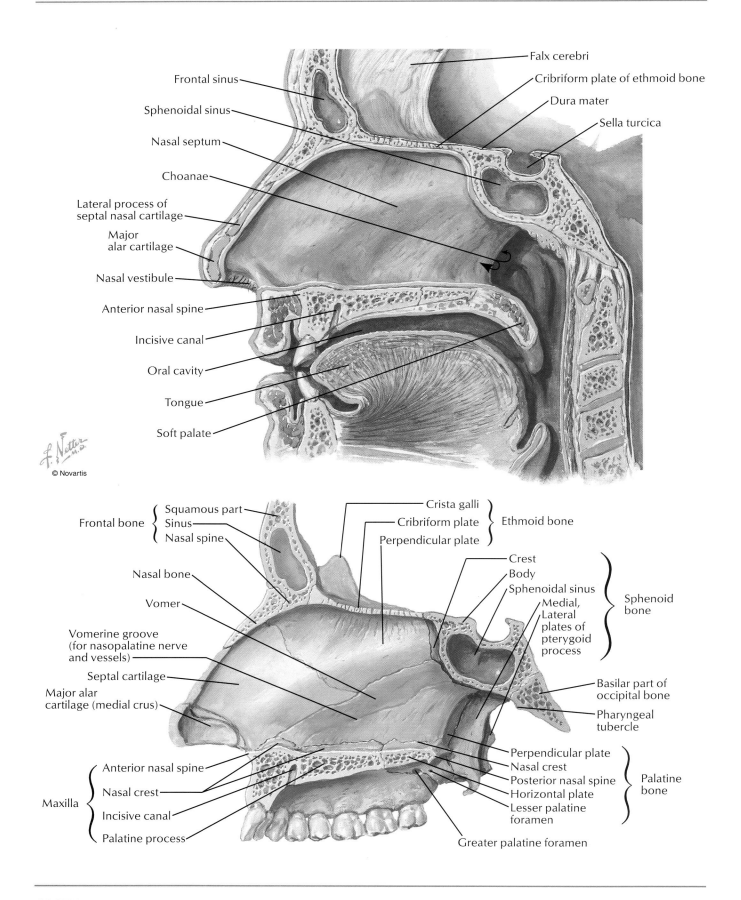

Falx cerebri

Frontal sinus

Cribriform plate of ethmoid bone

Sphenoidal sinus

Dura mater

Nasal septum

Sella turcica

Choanae

Lateral process of
septal nasal cartilage

Major
alar cartilage

Nasal vestibule

Anterior nasal spine

Incisive canal

Oral cavity

Tongue

Soft palate

© Novartis

Frontal bone { Squamous part
Sinus
Nasal spine

Crista galli
Cribriform plate        Ethmoid bone
Perpendicular plate

Nasal bone

Crest
Body
Sphenoidal sinus
Medial,
Lateral
plates of
pterygoid
process        Sphenoid
bone

Vomer

Vomerine groove
(for nasopalatine nerve
and vessels)

Septal cartilage

Major alar
cartilage (medial crus)

Basilar part of
occipital bone

Pharyngeal
tubercle

Perpendicular plate
Nasal crest
Posterior nasal spine        Palatine
Horizontal plate        bone
Lesser palatine
foramen

Anterior nasal spine

Nasal crest

Maxilla {

Incisive canal

Palatine process

Greater palatine foramen

**PLATE 34**                                                    **HEAD AND NECK**

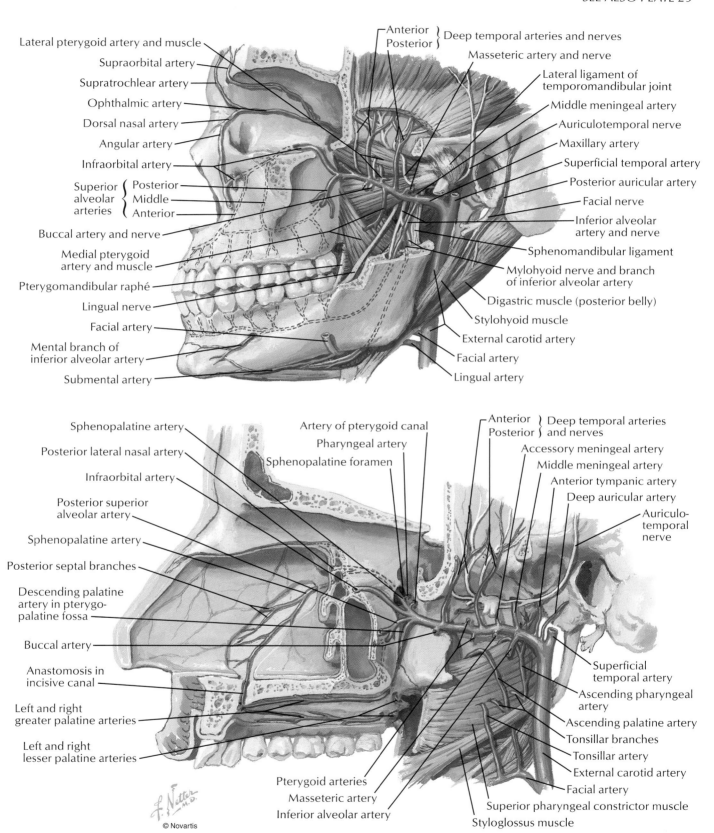

Lateral pterygoid artery and muscle

Supraorbital artery

Supratrochlear artery

Ophthalmic artery

Dorsal nasal artery

Angular artery

Infraorbital artery

Superior alveolar arteries { Posterior / Middle / Anterior

Buccal artery and nerve

Medial pterygoid artery and muscle

Pterygomandibular raphé

Lingual nerve

Facial artery

Mental branch of inferior alveolar artery

Submental artery

Anterior } Deep temporal arteries and nerves
Posterior }

Masseteric artery and nerve

Lateral ligament of temporomandibular joint

Middle meningeal artery

Auriculotemporal nerve

Maxillary artery

Superficial temporal artery

Posterior auricular artery

Facial nerve

Inferior alveolar artery and nerve

Sphenomandibular ligament

Mylohyoid nerve and branch of inferior alveolar artery

Digastric muscle (posterior belly)

Stylohyoid muscle

External carotid artery

Facial artery

Lingual artery

Sphenopalatine artery

Posterior lateral nasal artery

Infraorbital artery

Posterior superior alveolar artery

Sphenopalatine artery

Posterior septal branches

Descending palatine artery in pterygo-palatine fossa

Buccal artery

Anastomosis in incisive canal

Left and right greater palatine arteries

Left and right lesser palatine arteries

Artery of pterygoid canal

Pharyngeal artery

Sphenopalatine foramen

Anterior } Deep temporal arteries
Posterior } and nerves

Accessory meningeal artery

Middle meningeal artery

Anterior tympanic artery

Deep auricular artery

Auriculo-temporal nerve

Superficial temporal artery

Ascending pharyngeal artery

Ascending palatine artery

Tonsillar branches

Tonsillar artery

External carotid artery

Facial artery

Superior pharyngeal constrictor muscle

Pterygoid arteries

Masseteric artery

Inferior alveolar artery

Styloglossus muscle

© Novartis

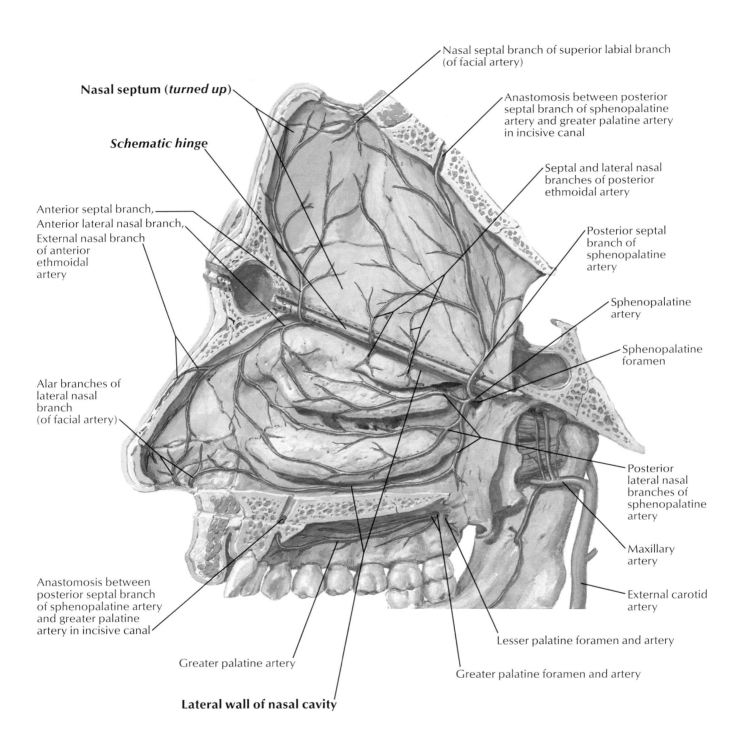

Nasal septal branch of superior labial branch (of facial artery)

Nasal septum (*turned up*)

Anastomosis between posterior septal branch of sphenopalatine artery and greater palatine artery in incisive canal

*Schematic hinge*

Septal and lateral nasal branches of posterior ethmoidal artery

Anterior septal branch, Anterior lateral nasal branch, External nasal branch of anterior ethmoidal artery

Posterior septal branch of sphenopalatine artery

Sphenopalatine artery

Sphenopalatine foramen

Alar branches of lateral nasal branch (of facial artery)

Posterior lateral nasal branches of sphenopalatine artery

Maxillary artery

External carotid artery

Anastomosis between posterior septal branch of sphenopalatine artery and greater palatine artery in incisive canal

Greater palatine artery

Lateral wall of nasal cavity

Lesser palatine foramen and artery

Greater palatine foramen and artery

*PLATE 36*

**HEAD AND NECK**

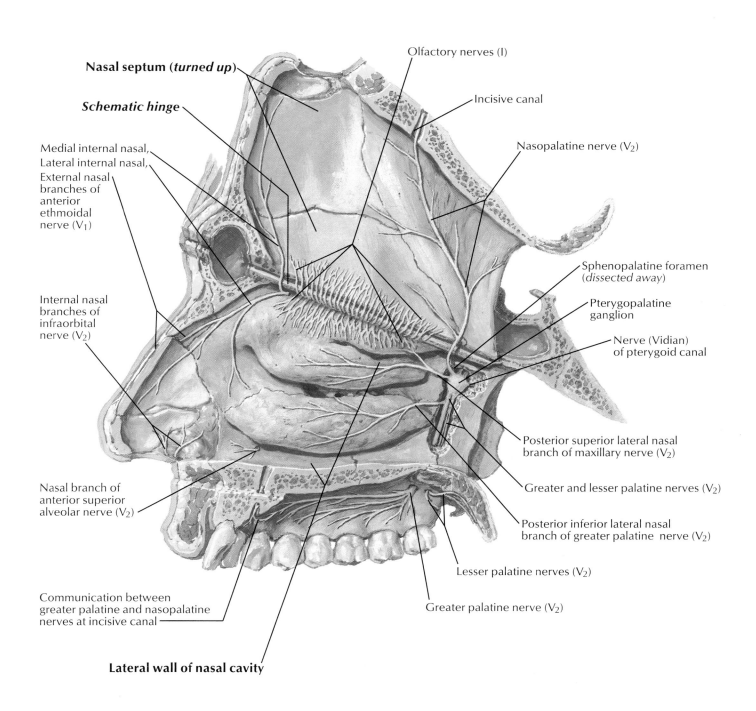

Nasal septum (*turned up*)

*Schematic hinge*

Medial internal nasal,
Lateral internal nasal,
External nasal
branches of
anterior
ethmoidal
nerve (V₁)

Internal nasal
branches of
infraorbital
nerve (V₂)

Nasal branch of
anterior superior
alveolar nerve (V₂)

Communication between
greater palatine and nasopalatine
nerves at incisive canal

**Lateral wall of nasal cavity**

Olfactory nerves (I)

Incisive canal

Nasopalatine nerve (V₂)

Sphenopalatine foramen
(*dissected away*)

Pterygopalatine
ganglion

Nerve (Vidian)
of pterygoid canal

Posterior superior lateral nasal
branch of maxillary nerve (V₂)

Greater and lesser palatine nerves (V₂)

Posterior inferior lateral nasal
branch of greater palatine nerve (V₂)

Lesser palatine nerves (V₂)

Greater palatine nerve (V₂)

© Novartis

# Nerves of Nasal Cavity (continued)

SEE ALSO PLATE 113

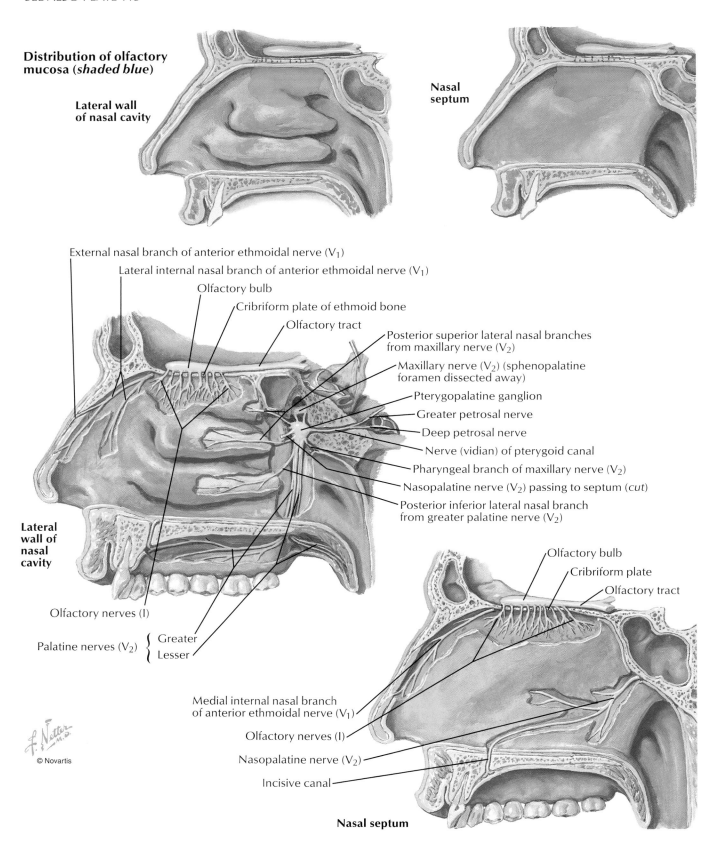

**Distribution of olfactory mucosa (*shaded blue*)**

Lateral wall of nasal cavity

Nasal septum

External nasal branch of anterior ethmoidal nerve (V₁)

Lateral internal nasal branch of anterior ethmoidal nerve (V₁)

Olfactory bulb

Cribriform plate of ethmoid bone

Olfactory tract

Posterior superior lateral nasal branches from maxillary nerve (V₂)

Maxillary nerve (V₂) (sphenopalatine foramen dissected away)

Pterygopalatine ganglion

Greater petrosal nerve

Deep petrosal nerve

Nerve (vidian) of pterygoid canal

Pharyngeal branch of maxillary nerve (V₂)

Nasopalatine nerve (V₂) passing to septum (*cut*)

Posterior inferior lateral nasal branch from greater palatine nerve (V₂)

Lateral wall of nasal cavity

Olfactory nerves (I)

Palatine nerves (V₂) { Greater Lesser

Olfactory bulb

Cribriform plate

Olfactory tract

Medial internal nasal branch of anterior ethmoidal nerve (V₁)

Olfactory nerves (I)

Nasopalatine nerve (V₂)

Incisive canal

**Nasal septum**

**PLATE 38**

© Novartis

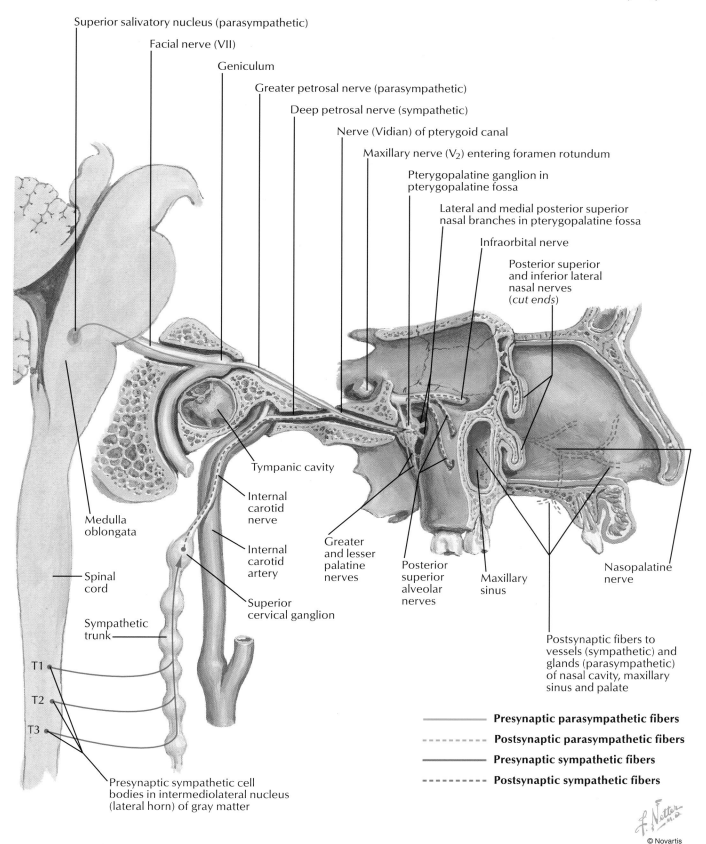

Superior salivatory nucleus (parasympathetic)

Facial nerve (VII)

Geniculum

Greater petrosal nerve (parasympathetic)

Deep petrosal nerve (sympathetic)

Nerve (Vidian) of pterygoid canal

Maxillary nerve (V₂) entering foramen rotundum

Pterygopalatine ganglion in pterygopalatine fossa

Lateral and medial posterior superior nasal branches in pterygopalatine fossa

Infraorbital nerve

Posterior superior and inferior lateral nasal nerves (*cut ends*)

Tympanic cavity

Internal carotid nerve

Internal carotid artery

Greater and lesser palatine nerves

Posterior superior alveolar nerves

Maxillary sinus

Nasopalatine nerve

Medulla oblongata

Spinal cord

Sympathetic trunk

Superior cervical ganglion

Postsynaptic fibers to vessels (sympathetic) and glands (parasympathetic) of nasal cavity, maxillary sinus and palate

T1

T2

T3

Presynaptic sympathetic cell bodies in intermediolateral nucleus (lateral horn) of gray matter

**Presynaptic parasympathetic fibers**

**Postsynaptic parasympathetic fibers**

**Presynaptic sympathetic fibers**

**Postsynaptic sympathetic fibers**

© Novartis

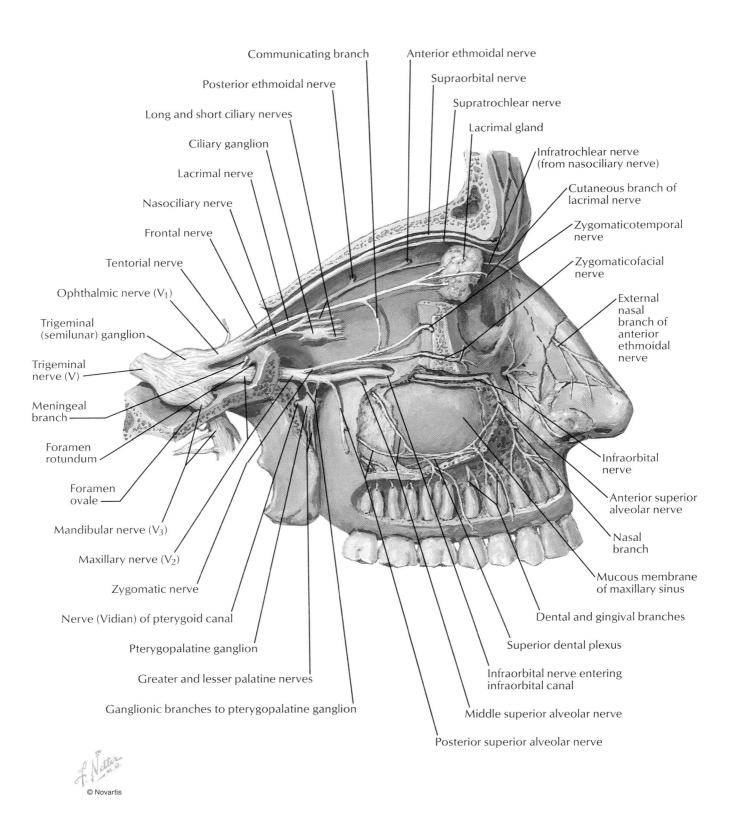

Communicating branch

Posterior ethmoidal nerve

Long and short ciliary nerves

Ciliary ganglion

Lacrimal nerve

Nasociliary nerve

Frontal nerve

Tentorial nerve

Ophthalmic nerve (V₁)

Trigeminal (semilunar) ganglion

Trigeminal nerve (V)

Meningeal branch

Foramen rotundum

Foramen ovale

Mandibular nerve (V₃)

Maxillary nerve (V₂)

Zygomatic nerve

Nerve (Vidian) of pterygoid canal

Pterygopalatine ganglion

Greater and lesser palatine nerves

Ganglionic branches to pterygopalatine ganglion

Anterior ethmoidal nerve

Supraorbital nerve

Supratrochlear nerve

Lacrimal gland

Infratrochlear nerve (from nasociliary nerve)

Cutaneous branch of lacrimal nerve

Zygomaticotemporal nerve

Zygomaticofacial nerve

External nasal branch of anterior ethmoidal nerve

Infraorbital nerve

Anterior superior alveolar nerve

Nasal branch

Mucous membrane of maxillary sinus

Dental and gingival branches

Superior dental plexus

Infraorbital nerve entering infraorbital canal

Middle superior alveolar nerve

Posterior superior alveolar nerve

© Novartis

**PLATE 40**

**HEAD AND NECK**

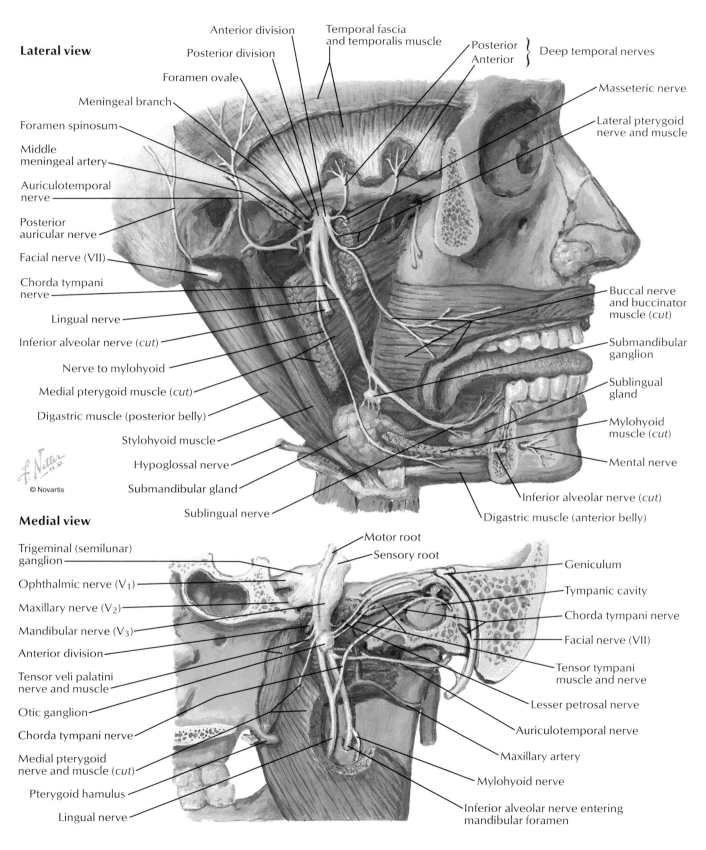

**Lateral view**

Anterior division
Posterior division
Foramen ovale
Meningeal branch
Foramen spinosum
Middle meningeal artery
Auriculotemporal nerve
Posterior auricular nerve
Facial nerve (VII)
Chorda tympani nerve
Lingual nerve
Inferior alveolar nerve (*cut*)
Nerve to mylohyoid
Medial pterygoid muscle (*cut*)
Digastric muscle (posterior belly)
Stylohyoid muscle
Hypoglossal nerve
Submandibular gland
Sublingual nerve

Temporal fascia and temporalis muscle
Posterior
Anterior } Deep temporal nerves
Masseteric nerve
Lateral pterygoid nerve and muscle
Buccal nerve and buccinator muscle (*cut*)
Submandibular ganglion
Sublingual gland
Mylohyoid muscle (*cut*)
Mental nerve
Inferior alveolar nerve (*cut*)
Digastric muscle (anterior belly)

**Medial view**

Trigeminal (semilunar) ganglion
Ophthalmic nerve (V₁)
Maxillary nerve (V₂)
Mandibular nerve (V₃)
Anterior division
Tensor veli palatini nerve and muscle
Otic ganglion
Chorda tympani nerve
Medial pterygoid nerve and muscle (*cut*)
Pterygoid hamulus
Lingual nerve

Motor root
Sensory root
Geniculum
Tympanic cavity
Chorda tympani nerve
Facial nerve (VII)
Tensor tympani muscle and nerve
Lesser petrosal nerve
Auriculotemporal nerve
Maxillary artery
Mylohyoid nerve
Inferior alveolar nerve entering mandibular foramen

*f. Netter M.D.*
© Novartis

**NASAL REGION**

*PLATE 41*

# *Paranasal Sinuses*

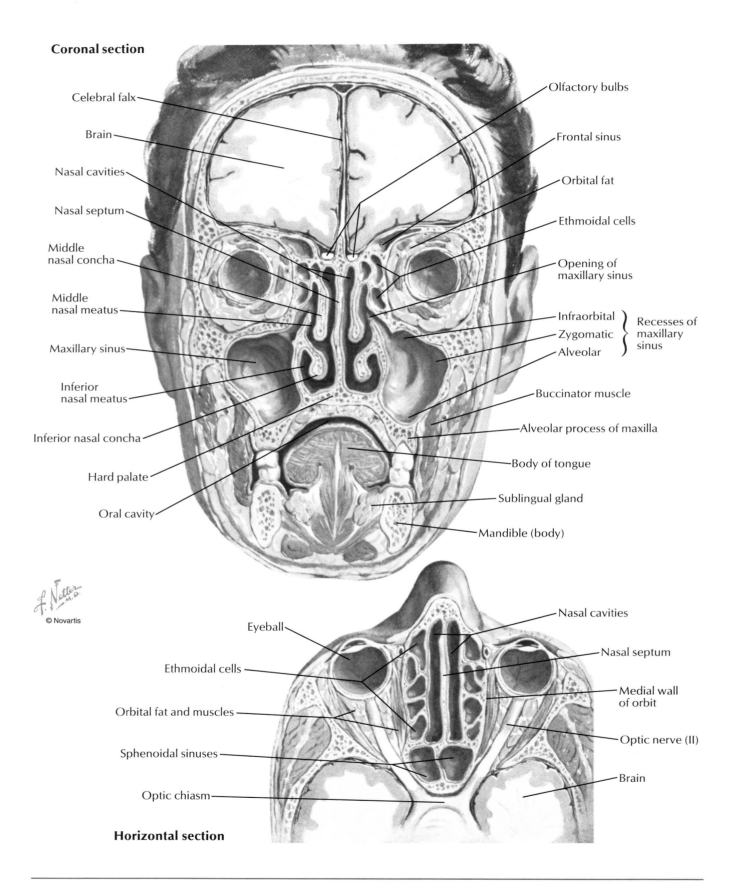

**Coronal section**

Celebral falx

Brain

Nasal cavities

Nasal septum

Middle nasal concha

Middle nasal meatus

Maxillary sinus

Inferior nasal meatus

Inferior nasal concha

Hard palate

Oral cavity

Olfactory bulbs

Frontal sinus

Orbital fat

Ethmoidal cells

Opening of maxillary sinus

Infraorbital  ⎫
Zygomatic    ⎬ Recesses of maxillary sinus
Alveolar     ⎭

Buccinator muscle

Alveolar process of maxilla

Body of tongue

Sublingual gland

Mandible (body)

*f. Netter* M.D.
© Novartis

Eyeball

Ethmoidal cells

Orbital fat and muscles

Sphenoidal sinuses

Optic chiasm

**Horizontal section**

Nasal cavities

Nasal septum

Medial wall of orbit

Optic nerve (II)

Brain

*PLATE 42*                                                    **HEAD AND NECK**

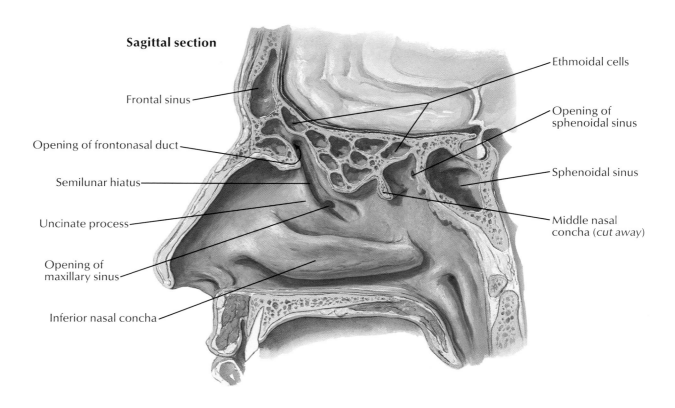

**Sagittal section**

Frontal sinus

Opening of frontonasal duct

Semilunar hiatus

Uncinate process

Opening of
maxillary sinus

Inferior nasal concha

Ethmoidal cells

Opening of
sphenoidal sinus

Sphenoidal sinus

Middle nasal
concha (*cut away*)

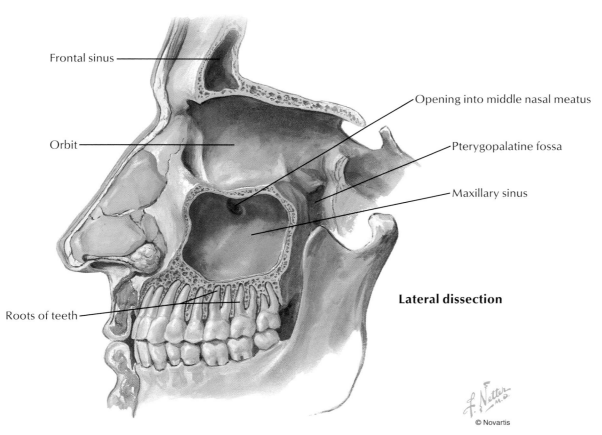

Frontal sinus

Orbit

Roots of teeth

Opening into middle nasal meatus

Pterygopalatine fossa

Maxillary sinus

**Lateral dissection**

© Novartis

# Paranasal Sinuses: Changes With Age

## Bones of nasal cavity and paranasal sinuses at birth

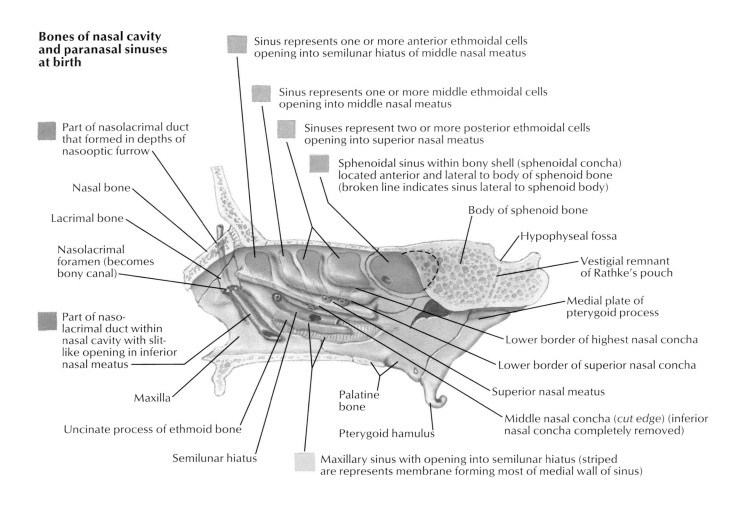

Sinus represents one or more anterior ethmoidal cells opening into semilunar hiatus of middle nasal meatus

Sinus represents one or more middle ethmoidal cells opening into middle nasal meatus

Sinuses represent two or more posterior ethmoidal cells opening into superior nasal meatus

Sphenoidal sinus within bony shell (sphenoidal concha) located anterior and lateral to body of sphenoid bone (broken line indicates sinus lateral to sphenoid body)

Part of nasolacrimal duct that formed in depths of nasooptic furrow

Nasal bone

Lacrimal bone

Nasolacrimal foramen (becomes bony canal)

Body of sphenoid bone

Hypophyseal fossa

Vestigial remnant of Rathke's pouch

Medial plate of pterygoid process

Lower border of highest nasal concha

Lower border of superior nasal concha

Superior nasal meatus

Middle nasal concha (*cut edge*) (inferior nasal concha completely removed)

Part of naso-lacrimal duct within nasal cavity with slit-like opening in inferior nasal meatus

Maxilla

Uncinate process of ethmoid bone

Semilunar hiatus

Palatine bone

Pterygoid hamulus

Maxillary sinus with opening into semilunar hiatus (striped are represents membrane forming most of medial wall of sinus)

## Growth of frontal and maxillary sinuses throughout life

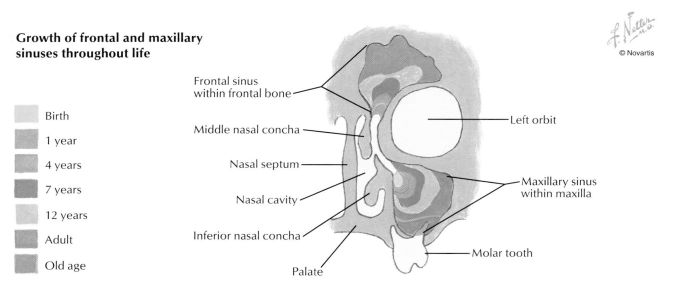

Birth

1 year

4 years

7 years

12 years

Adult

Old age

Frontal sinus within frontal bone

Middle nasal concha

Nasal septum

Nasal cavity

Inferior nasal concha

Palate

Left orbit

Maxillary sinus within maxilla

Molar tooth

PLATE 44

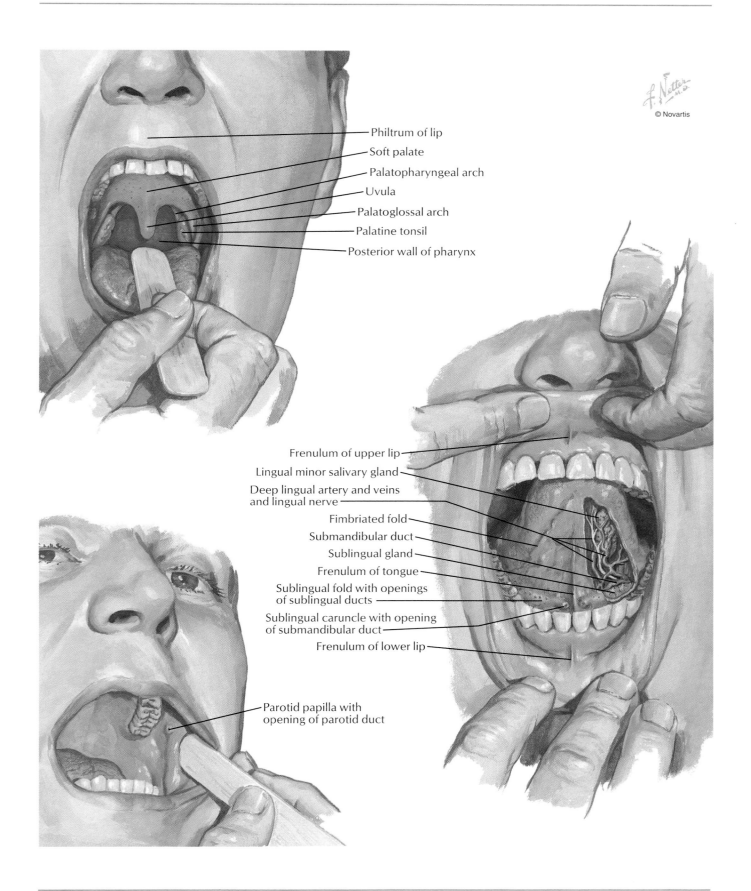

Philtrum of lip

Soft palate

Palatopharyngeal arch

Uvula

Palatoglossal arch

Palatine tonsil

Posterior wall of pharynx

© Novartis

Frenulum of upper lip

Lingual minor salivary gland

Deep lingual artery and veins and lingual nerve

Fimbriated fold

Submandibular duct

Sublingual gland

Frenulum of tongue

Sublingual fold with openings of sublingual ducts

Sublingual caruncle with opening of submandibular duct

Frenulum of lower lip

Parotid papilla with opening of parotid duct

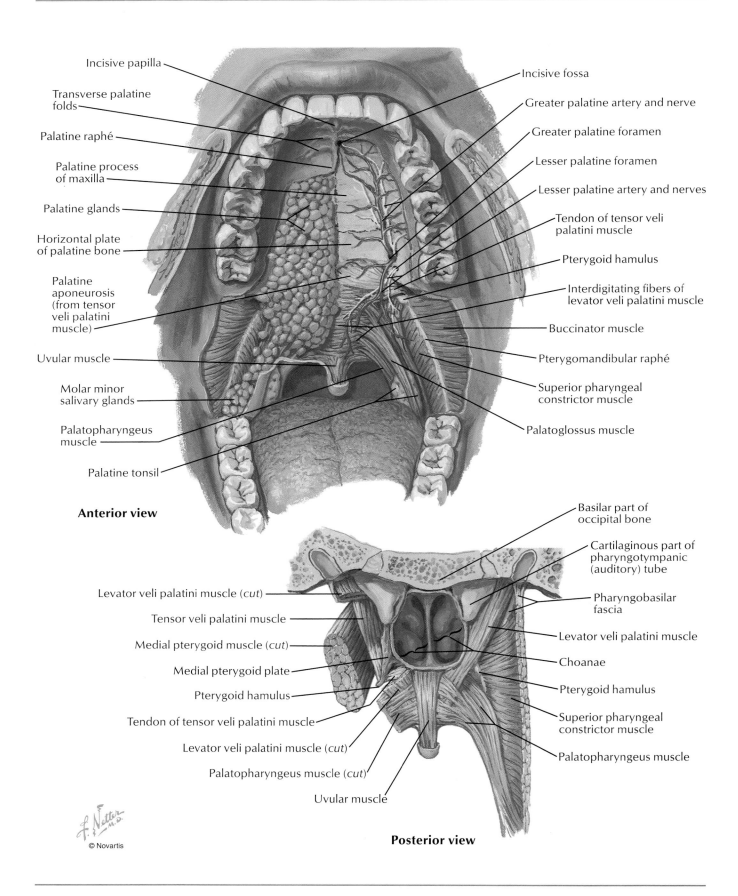

Incisive papilla

Transverse palatine folds

Palatine raphé

Palatine process of maxilla

Palatine glands

Horizontal plate of palatine bone

Palatine aponeurosis (from tensor veli palatini muscle)

Uvular muscle

Molar minor salivary glands

Palatopharyngeus muscle

Palatine tonsil

**Anterior view**

Incisive fossa

Greater palatine artery and nerve

Greater palatine foramen

Lesser palatine foramen

Lesser palatine artery and nerves

Tendon of tensor veli palatini muscle

Pterygoid hamulus

Interdigitating fibers of levator veli palatini muscle

Buccinator muscle

Pterygomandibular raphé

Superior pharyngeal constrictor muscle

Palatoglossus muscle

Levator veli palatini muscle (*cut*)

Tensor veli palatini muscle

Medial pterygoid muscle (*cut*)

Medial pterygoid plate

Pterygoid hamulus

Tendon of tensor veli palatini muscle

Levator veli palatini muscle (*cut*)

Palatopharyngeus muscle (*cut*)

Uvular muscle

Basilar part of occipital bone

Cartilaginous part of pharyngotympanic (auditory) tube

Pharyngobasilar fascia

Levator veli palatini muscle

Choanae

Pterygoid hamulus

Superior pharyngeal constrictor muscle

Palatopharyngeus muscle

**Posterior view**

© Novartis

**PLATE 46**      **HEAD AND NECK**

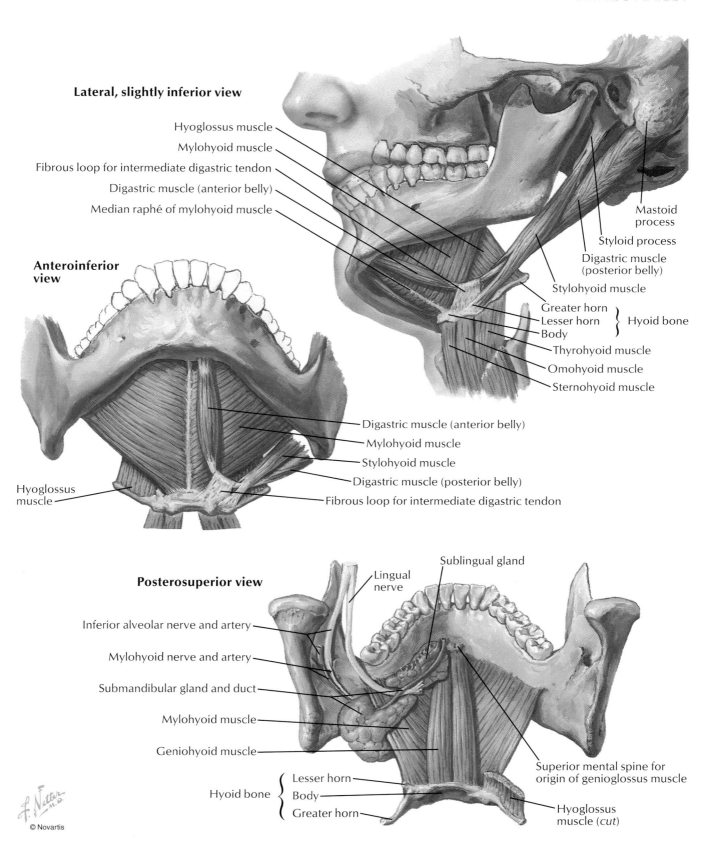

**Lateral, slightly inferior view**

Hyoglossus muscle
Mylohyoid muscle
Fibrous loop for intermediate digastric tendon
Digastric muscle (anterior belly)
Median raphé of mylohyoid muscle

Mastoid process
Styloid process
Digastric muscle (posterior belly)
Stylohyoid muscle
Greater horn
Lesser horn } Hyoid bone
Body
Thyrohyoid muscle
Omohyoid muscle
Sternohyoid muscle

**Anteroinferior view**

Digastric muscle (anterior belly)
Mylohyoid muscle
Stylohyoid muscle
Digastric muscle (posterior belly)
Fibrous loop for intermediate digastric tendon
Hyoglossus muscle

**Posterosuperior view**

Lingual nerve
Sublingual gland

Inferior alveolar nerve and artery
Mylohyoid nerve and artery
Submandibular gland and duct
Mylohyoid muscle
Geniohyoid muscle

Superior mental spine for origin of genioglossus muscle

Hyoid bone {
Lesser horn
Body
Greater horn

Hyoglossus muscle (*cut*)

© Novartis

# Muscles Involved in Mastication

*FOR FACIAL MUSCLES SEE PLATES 20, 21*

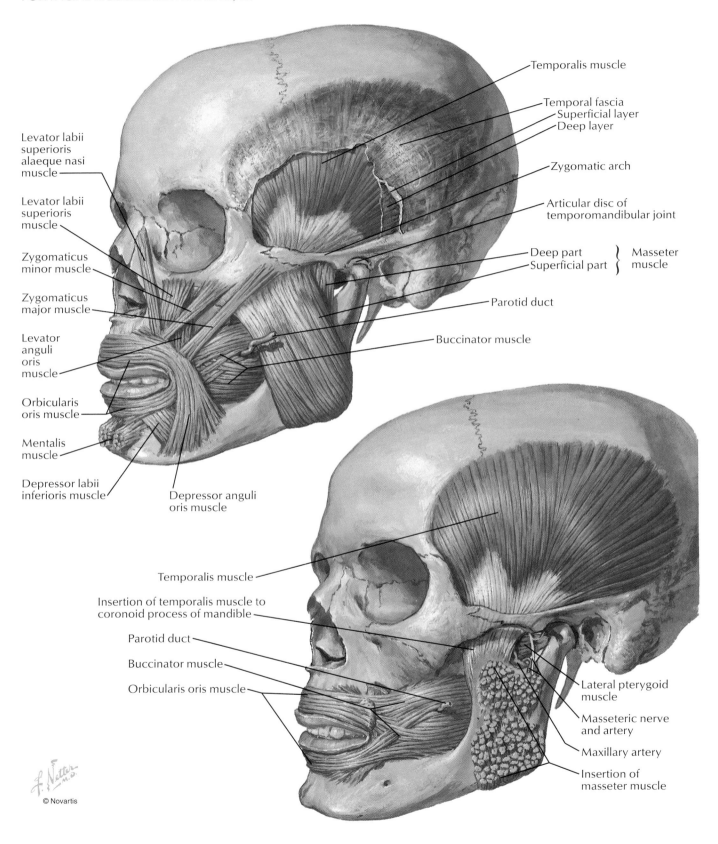

Temporalis muscle

Temporal fascia
Superficial layer
Deep layer

Zygomatic arch

Articular disc of temporomandibular joint

Deep part ⎫ Masseter
Superficial part ⎭ muscle

Parotid duct

Buccinator muscle

Levator labii superioris alaeque nasi muscle

Levator labii superioris muscle

Zygomaticus minor muscle

Zygomaticus major muscle

Levator anguli oris muscle

Orbicularis oris muscle

Mentalis muscle

Depressor labii inferioris muscle

Depressor anguli oris muscle

Temporalis muscle

Insertion of temporalis muscle to coronoid process of mandible

Parotid duct

Buccinator muscle

Orbicularis oris muscle

Lateral pterygoid muscle

Masseteric nerve and artery

Maxillary artery

Insertion of masseter muscle

© Novartis

**PLATE 48**

**HEAD AND NECK**

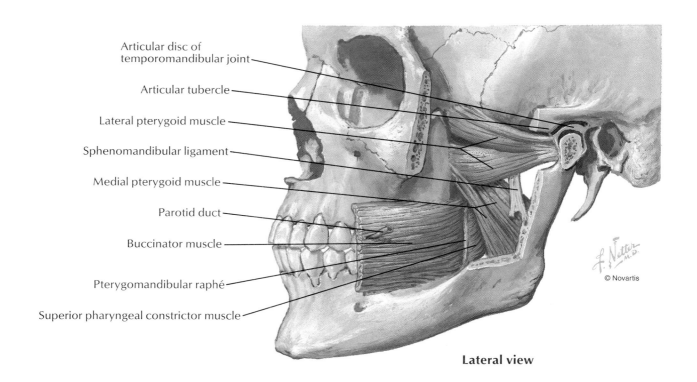

Articular disc of
temporomandibular joint

Articular tubercle

Lateral pterygoid muscle

Sphenomandibular ligament

Medial pterygoid muscle

Parotid duct

Buccinator muscle

Pterygomandibular raphé

Superior pharyngeal constrictor muscle

**Lateral view**

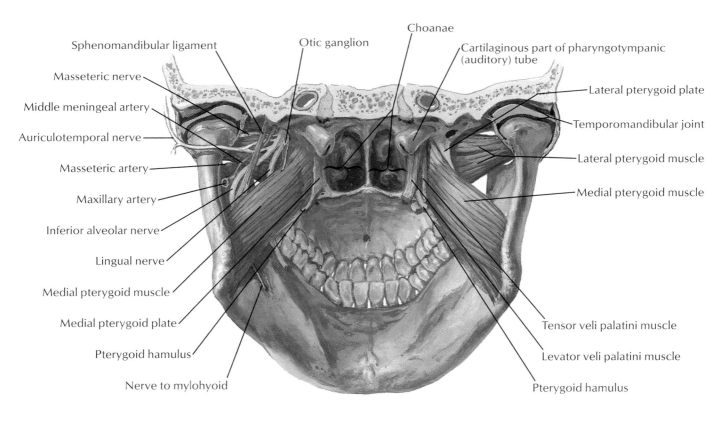

Sphenomandibular ligament

Otic ganglion

Choanae

Cartilaginous part of pharyngotympanic
(auditory) tube

Masseteric nerve

Middle meningeal artery

Auriculotemporal nerve

Masseteric artery

Maxillary artery

Inferior alveolar nerve

Lingual nerve

Medial pterygoid muscle

Medial pterygoid plate

Pterygoid hamulus

Nerve to mylohyoid

Lateral pterygoid plate

Temporomandibular joint

Lateral pterygoid muscle

Medial pterygoid muscle

Tensor veli palatini muscle

Levator veli palatini muscle

Pterygoid hamulus

**Posterior view**

# Teeth

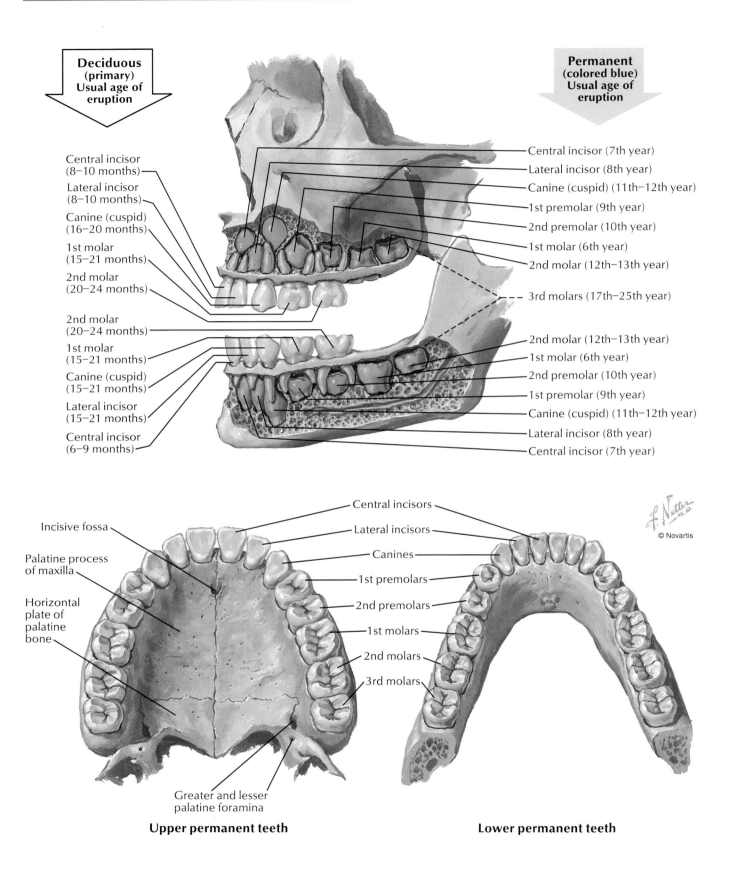

Central incisor (8–10 months)
Lateral incisor (8–10 months)
Canine (cuspid) (16–20 months)
1st molar (15–21 months)
2nd molar (20–24 months)

2nd molar (20–24 months)
1st molar (15–21 months)
Canine (cuspid) (15–21 months)
Lateral incisor (15–21 months)
Central incisor (6–9 months)

Central incisor (7th year)
Lateral incisor (8th year)
Canine (cuspid) (11th–12th year)
1st premolar (9th year)
2nd premolar (10th year)
1st molar (6th year)
2nd molar (12th–13th year)

3rd molars (17th–25th year)

2nd molar (12th–13th year)
1st molar (6th year)
2nd premolar (10th year)
1st premolar (9th year)
Canine (cuspid) (11th–12th year)
Lateral incisor (8th year)
Central incisor (7th year)

Incisive fossa
Palatine process of maxilla
Horizontal plate of palatine bone
Greater and lesser palatine foramina

Central incisors
Lateral incisors
Canines
1st premolars
2nd premolars
1st molars
2nd molars
3rd molars

**Upper permanent teeth**

**Lower permanent teeth**

**PLATE 50**

**HEAD AND NECK**

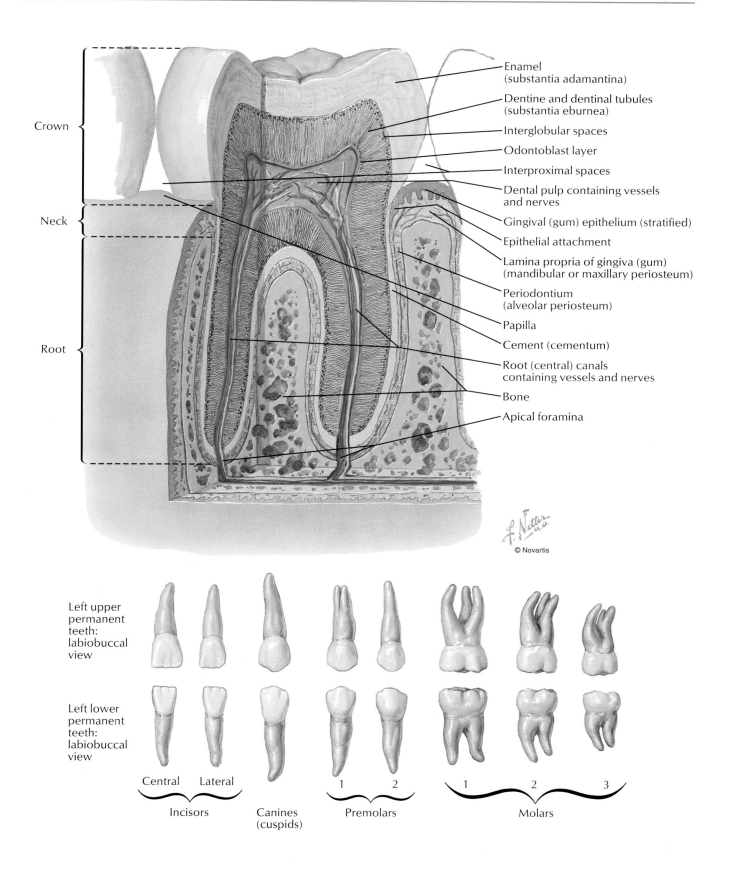

Crown

Neck

Root

Enamel
(substantia adamantina)

Dentine and dentinal tubules
(substantia eburnea)

Interglobular spaces

Odontoblast layer

Interproximal spaces

Dental pulp containing vessels
and nerves

Gingival (gum) epithelium (stratified)

Epithelial attachment

Lamina propria of gingiva (gum)
(mandibular or maxillary periosteum)

Periodontium
(alveolar periosteum)

Papilla

Cement (cementum)

Root (central) canals
containing vessels and nerves

Bone

Apical foramina

© Novartis

Left upper
permanent
teeth:
labiobuccal
view

Left lower
permanent
teeth:
labiobuccal
view

Central      Lateral

Incisors

Canines
(cuspids)

1          2

Premolars

1          2          3

Molars

# Tongue

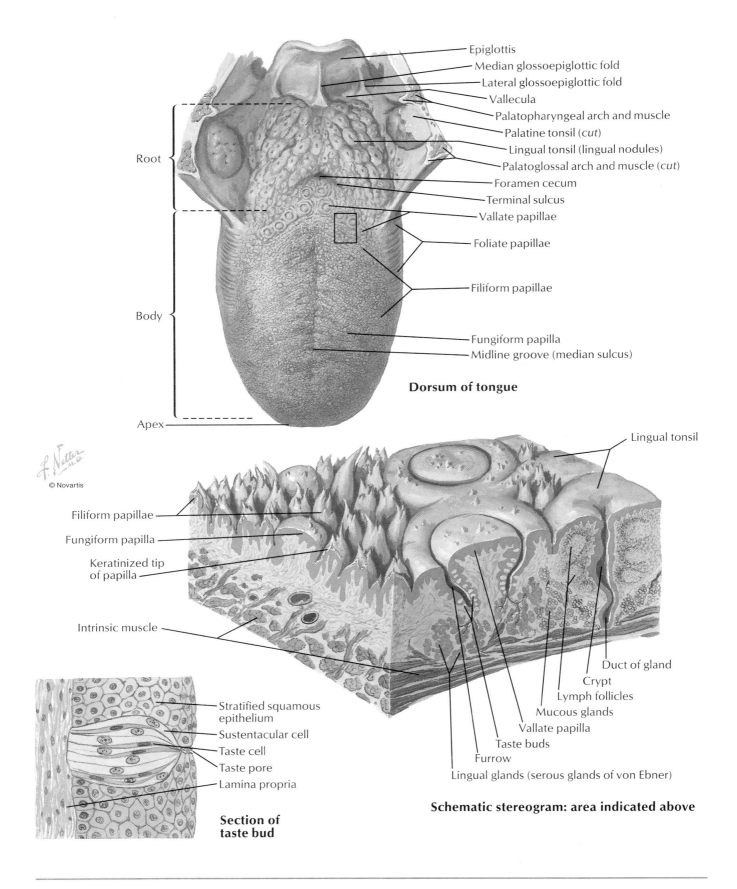

Epiglottis
Median glossoepiglottic fold
Lateral glossoepiglottic fold
Vallecula
Palatopharyngeal arch and muscle
Palatine tonsil (*cut*)
Lingual tonsil (lingual nodules)
Palatoglossal arch and muscle (*cut*)
Foramen cecum
Terminal sulcus
Vallate papillae
Foliate papillae
Filiform papillae
Fungiform papilla
Midline groove (median sulcus)

Root

Body

Apex

© Novartis

**Dorsum of tongue**

Lingual tonsil

Filiform papillae
Fungiform papilla
Keratinized tip of papilla

Intrinsic muscle

Duct of gland
Crypt
Lymph follicles
Mucous glands
Vallate papilla
Taste buds
Furrow
Lingual glands (serous glands of von Ebner)

**Schematic stereogram: area indicated above**

Stratified squamous epithelium
Sustentacular cell
Taste cell
Taste pore
Lamina propria

**Section of taste bud**

*PLATE 52*

**HEAD AND NECK**

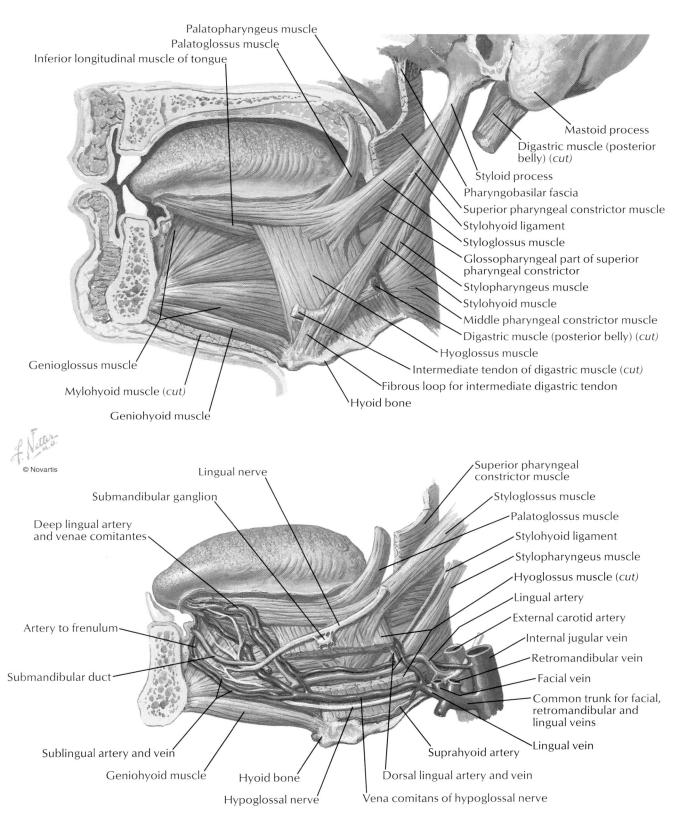

Palatopharyngeus muscle
Palatoglossus muscle
Inferior longitudinal muscle of tongue
Mastoid process
Digastric muscle (posterior belly) (*cut*)
Styloid process
Pharyngobasilar fascia
Superior pharyngeal constrictor muscle
Stylohyoid ligament
Styloglossus muscle
Glossopharyngeal part of superior pharyngeal constrictor
Stylopharyngeus muscle
Stylohyoid muscle
Middle pharyngeal constrictor muscle
Digastric muscle (posterior belly) (*cut*)
Hyoglossus muscle
Intermediate tendon of digastric muscle (*cut*)
Fibrous loop for intermediate digastric tendon
Hyoid bone
Geniohyoid muscle
Mylohyoid muscle (*cut*)
Genioglossus muscle

© Novartis

Lingual nerve
Submandibular ganglion
Deep lingual artery and venae comitantes
Superior pharyngeal constrictor muscle
Styloglossus muscle
Palatoglossus muscle
Stylohyoid ligament
Stylopharyngeus muscle
Hyoglossus muscle (*cut*)
Lingual artery
External carotid artery
Internal jugular vein
Retromandibular vein
Facial vein
Common trunk for facial, retromandibular and lingual veins
Lingual vein
Artery to frenulum
Submandibular duct
Sublingual artery and vein
Geniohyoid muscle
Hyoid bone
Hypoglossal nerve
Vena comitans of hypoglossal nerve
Dorsal lingual artery and vein
Suprahyoid artery

# Tongue and Salivary Glands: Sections

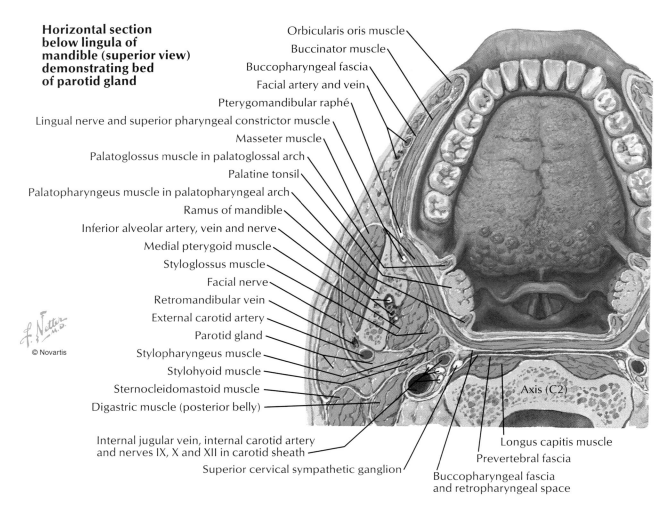

**Horizontal section below lingula of mandible (superior view) demonstrating bed of parotid gland**

Orbicularis oris muscle

Buccinator muscle

Buccopharyngeal fascia

Facial artery and vein

Pterygomandibular raphé

Lingual nerve and superior pharyngeal constrictor muscle

Masseter muscle

Palatoglossus muscle in palatoglossal arch

Palatine tonsil

Palatopharyngeus muscle in palatopharyngeal arch

Ramus of mandible

Inferior alveolar artery, vein and nerve

Medial pterygoid muscle

Styloglossus muscle

Facial nerve

Retromandibular vein

External carotid artery

Parotid gland

Stylopharyngeus muscle

Stylohyoid muscle

Sternocleidomastoid muscle

Digastric muscle (posterior belly)

Internal jugular vein, internal carotid artery and nerves IX, X and XII in carotid sheath

Superior cervical sympathetic ganglion

Axis (C2)

Longus capitis muscle

Prevertebral fascia

Buccopharyngeal fascia and retropharyngeal space

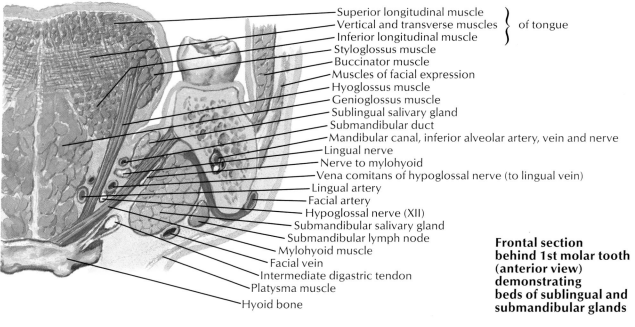

Superior longitudinal muscle

Vertical and transverse muscles } of tongue

Inferior longitudinal muscle

Styloglossus muscle

Buccinator muscle

Muscles of facial expression

Hyoglossus muscle

Genioglossus muscle

Sublingual salivary gland

Submandibular duct

Mandibular canal, inferior alveolar artery, vein and nerve

Lingual nerve

Nerve to mylohyoid

Vena comitans of hypoglossal nerve (to lingual vein)

Lingual artery

Facial artery

Hypoglossal nerve (XII)

Submandibular salivary gland

Submandibular lymph node

Mylohyoid muscle

Facial vein

Intermediate digastric tendon

Platysma muscle

Hyoid bone

**Frontal section behind 1st molar tooth (anterior view) demonstrating beds of sublingual and submandibular glands**

*PLATE 54*

**HEAD AND NECK**

SEE ALSO PLATES 19, 47, 127, 128, 153

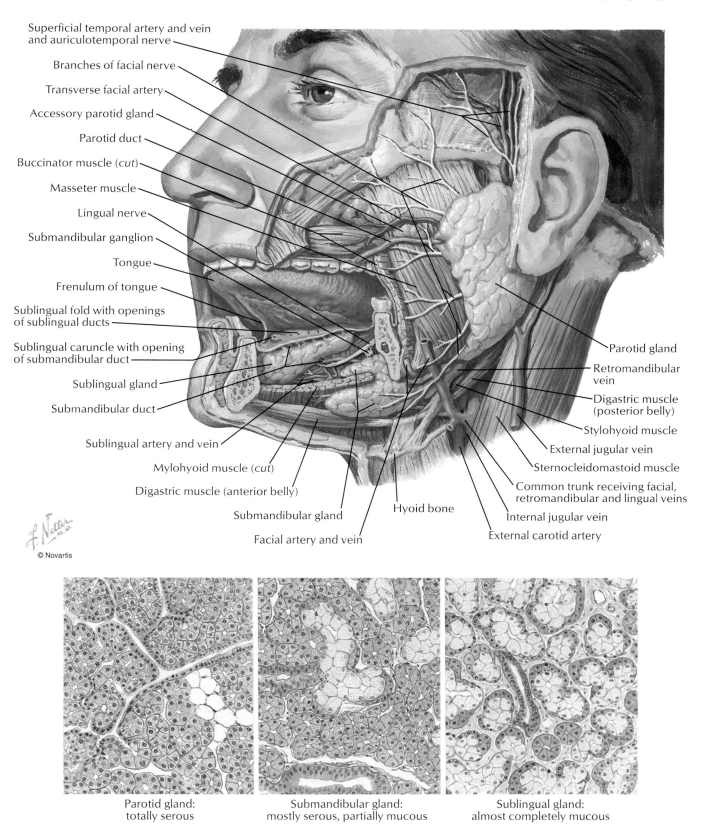

Superficial temporal artery and vein and auriculotemporal nerve

Branches of facial nerve

Transverse facial artery

Accessory parotid gland

Parotid duct

Buccinator muscle (cut)

Masseter muscle

Lingual nerve

Submandibular ganglion

Tongue

Frenulum of tongue

Sublingual fold with openings of sublingual ducts

Sublingual caruncle with opening of submandibular duct

Sublingual gland

Submandibular duct

Sublingual artery and vein

Mylohyoid muscle (cut)

Digastric muscle (anterior belly)

Submandibular gland

Facial artery and vein

Hyoid bone

Parotid gland

Retromandibular vein

Digastric muscle (posterior belly)

Stylohyoid muscle

External jugular vein

Sternocleidomastoid muscle

Common trunk receiving facial, retromandibular and lingual veins

Internal jugular vein

External carotid artery

© Novartis

Parotid gland:
totally serous

Submandibular gland:
mostly serous, partially mucous

Sublingual gland:
almost completely mucous

*SEE ALSO PLATES 41, 46, 53, 58, 116, 117, 119, 127, 129*

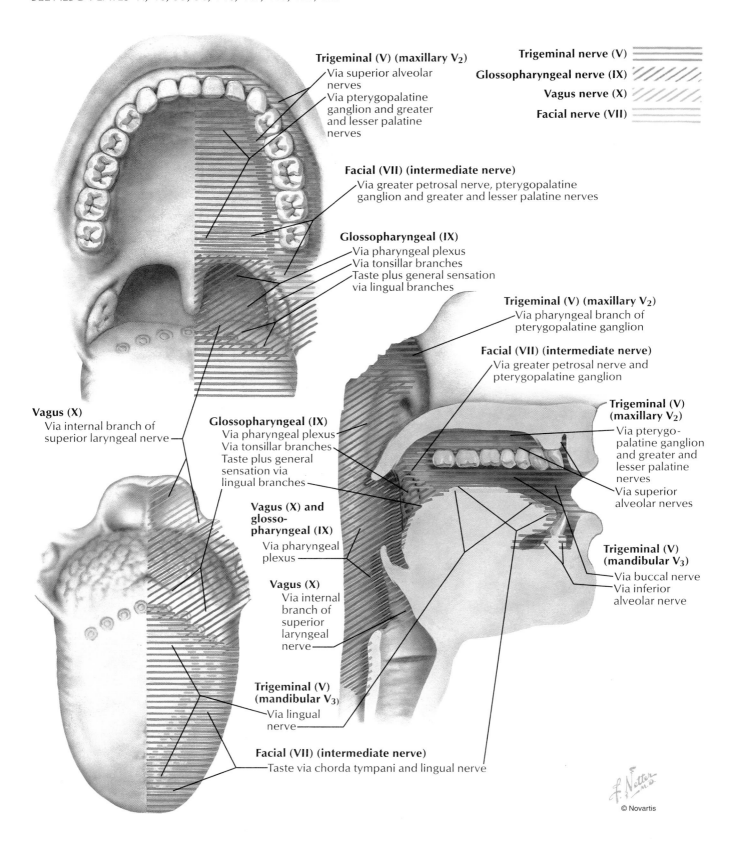

**Trigeminal (V) (maxillary V₂)**
Via superior alveolar nerves
Via pterygopalatine ganglion and greater and lesser palatine nerves

**Trigeminal nerve (V)**
**Glossopharyngeal nerve (IX)**
**Vagus nerve (X)**
**Facial nerve (VII)**

**Facial (VII) (intermediate nerve)**
Via greater petrosal nerve, pterygopalatine ganglion and greater and lesser palatine nerves

**Glossopharyngeal (IX)**
Via pharyngeal plexus
Via tonsillar branches
Taste plus general sensation via lingual branches

**Trigeminal (V) (maxillary V₂)**
Via pharyngeal branch of pterygopalatine ganglion

**Facial (VII) (intermediate nerve)**
Via greater petrosal nerve and pterygopalatine ganglion

**Trigeminal (V) (maxillary V₂)**
Via pterygo-palatine ganglion and greater and lesser palatine nerves
Via superior alveolar nerves

**Vagus (X)**
Via internal branch of superior laryngeal nerve

**Glossopharyngeal (IX)**
Via pharyngeal plexus
Via tonsillar branches
Taste plus general sensation via lingual branches

**Vagus (X) and glosso-pharyngeal (IX)**
Via pharyngeal plexus

**Vagus (X)**
Via internal branch of superior laryngeal nerve

**Trigeminal (V) (mandibular V₃)**
Via buccal nerve
Via inferior alveolar nerve

**Trigeminal (V) (mandibular V₃)**
Via lingual nerve

**Facial (VII) (intermediate nerve)**
Taste via chorda tympani and lingual nerve

© Novartis

**PLATE 56**

**HEAD AND NECK**

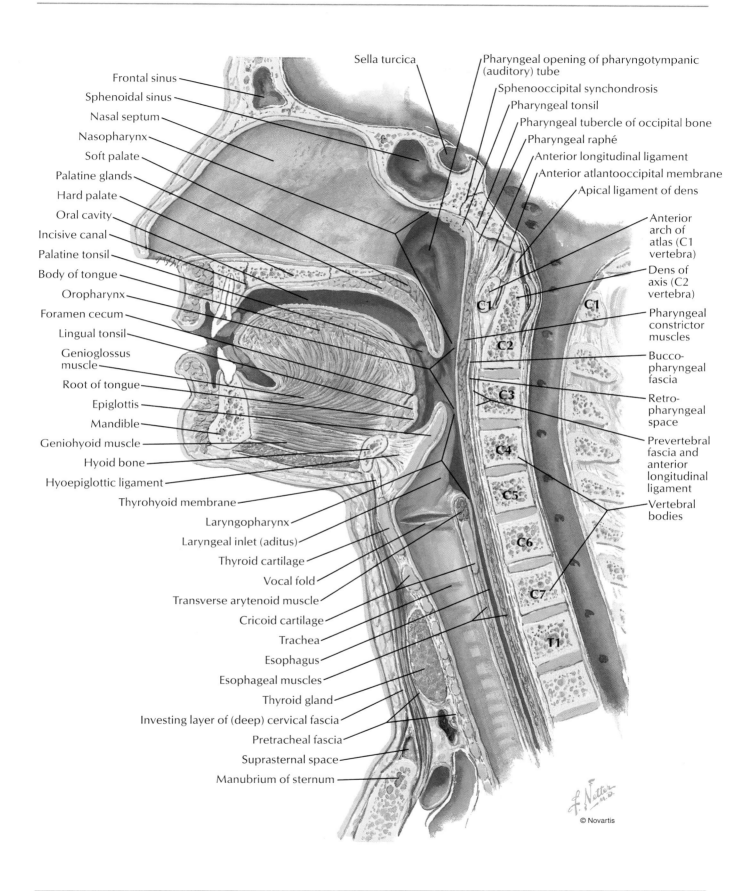

Frontal sinus

Sphenoidal sinus

Nasal septum

Nasopharynx

Soft palate

Palatine glands

Hard palate

Oral cavity

Incisive canal

Palatine tonsil

Body of tongue

Oropharynx

Foramen cecum

Lingual tonsil

Genioglossus muscle

Root of tongue

Epiglottis

Mandible

Geniohyoid muscle

Hyoid bone

Hyoepiglottic ligament

Thyrohyoid membrane

Laryngopharynx

Laryngeal inlet (aditus)

Thyroid cartilage

Vocal fold

Transverse arytenoid muscle

Cricoid cartilage

Trachea

Esophagus

Esophageal muscles

Thyroid gland

Investing layer of (deep) cervical fascia

Pretracheal fascia

Suprasternal space

Manubrium of sternum

Sella turcica

Pharyngeal opening of pharyngotympanic (auditory) tube

Sphenooccipital synchondrosis

Pharyngeal tonsil

Pharyngeal tubercle of occipital bone

Pharyngeal raphé

Anterior longitudinal ligament

Anterior atlantooccipital membrane

Apical ligament of dens

Anterior arch of atlas (C1 vertebra)

Dens of axis (C2 vertebra)

Pharyngeal constrictor muscles

Bucco-pharyngeal fascia

Retro-pharyngeal space

Prevertebral fascia and anterior longitudinal ligament

Vertebral bodies

C1

C2

C3

C4

C5

C6

C7

T1

C1

*f. Netter* m.d.

© Novartis

# *Fauces*

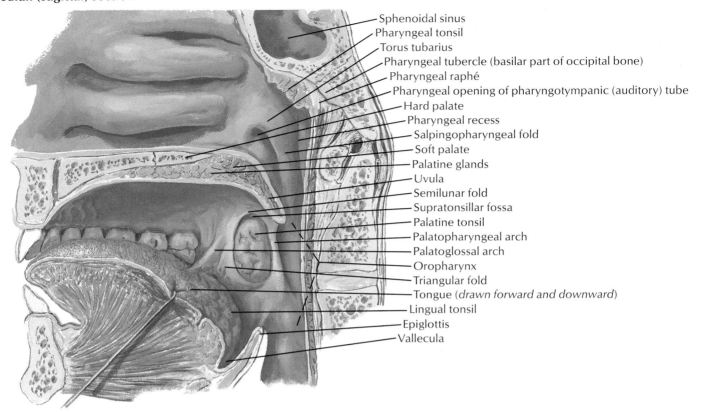

Sphenoidal sinus
Pharyngeal tonsil
Torus tubarius
Pharyngeal tubercle (basilar part of occipital bone)
Pharyngeal raphé
Pharyngeal opening of pharyngotympanic (auditory) tube
Hard palate
Pharyngeal recess
Salpingopharyngeal fold
Soft palate
Palatine glands
Uvula
Semilunar fold
Supratonsillar fossa
Palatine tonsil
Palatopharyngeal arch
Palatoglossal arch
Oropharynx
Triangular fold
Tongue (*drawn forward and downward*)
Lingual tonsil
Epiglottis
Vallecula

## Pharyngeal mucosa removed

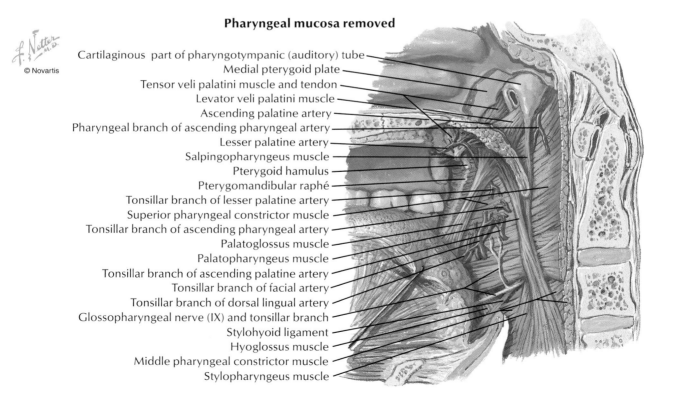

Cartilaginous part of pharyngotympanic (auditory) tube
Medial pterygoid plate
Tensor veli palatini muscle and tendon
Levator veli palatini muscle
Ascending palatine artery
Pharyngeal branch of ascending pharyngeal artery
Lesser palatine artery
Salpingopharyngeus muscle
Pterygoid hamulus
Pterygomandibular raphé
Tonsillar branch of lesser palatine artery
Superior pharyngeal constrictor muscle
Tonsillar branch of ascending pharyngeal artery
Palatoglossus muscle
Palatopharyngeus muscle
Tonsillar branch of ascending palatine artery
Tonsillar branch of facial artery
Tonsillar branch of dorsal lingual artery
Glossopharyngeal nerve (IX) and tonsillar branch
Stylohyoid ligament
Hyoglossus muscle
Middle pharyngeal constrictor muscle
Stylopharyngeus muscle

© Novartis

**PLATE 58**          **HEAD AND NECK**

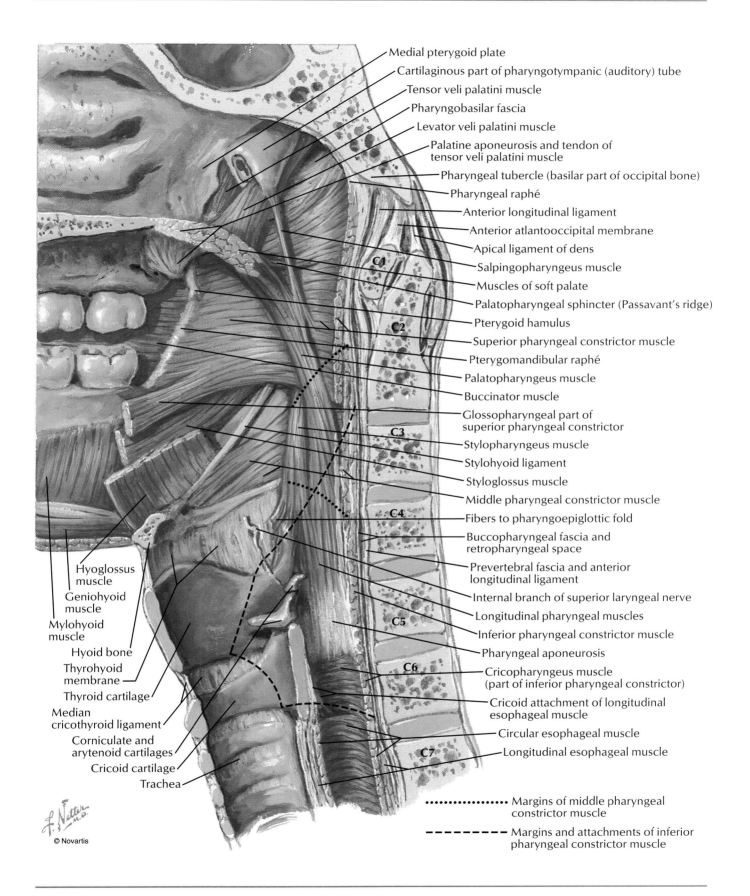

Medial pterygoid plate

Cartilaginous part of pharyngotympanic (auditory) tube

Tensor veli palatini muscle

Pharyngobasilar fascia

Levator veli palatini muscle

Palatine aponeurosis and tendon of tensor veli palatini muscle

Pharyngeal tubercle (basilar part of occipital bone)

Pharyngeal raphé

Anterior longitudinal ligament

Anterior atlantooccipital membrane

Apical ligament of dens

Salpingopharyngeus muscle

Muscles of soft palate

Palatopharyngeal sphincter (Passavant's ridge)

Pterygoid hamulus

Superior pharyngeal constrictor muscle

Pterygomandibular raphé

Palatopharyngeus muscle

Buccinator muscle

Glossopharyngeal part of superior pharyngeal constrictor

Stylopharyngeus muscle

Stylohyoid ligament

Styloglossus muscle

Middle pharyngeal constrictor muscle

Fibers to pharyngoepiglottic fold

Buccopharyngeal fascia and retropharyngeal space

Prevertebral fascia and anterior longitudinal ligament

Internal branch of superior laryngeal nerve

Longitudinal pharyngeal muscles

Inferior pharyngeal constrictor muscle

Pharyngeal aponeurosis

Cricopharyngeus muscle (part of inferior pharyngeal constrictor)

Cricoid attachment of longitudinal esophageal muscle

Circular esophageal muscle

Longitudinal esophageal muscle

C1
C2
C3
C4
C5
C6
C7

Hyoglossus muscle

Geniohyoid muscle

Mylohyoid muscle

Hyoid bone

Thyrohyoid membrane

Thyroid cartilage

Median cricothyroid ligament

Corniculate and arytenoid cartilages

Cricoid cartilage

Trachea

· · · · · · · · · · · Margins of middle pharyngeal constrictor muscle

– – – – – – – Margins and attachments of inferior pharyngeal constrictor muscle

© Novartis

**PHARYNX**

**PLATE 59**

# *Pharynx: Opened Posterior View*

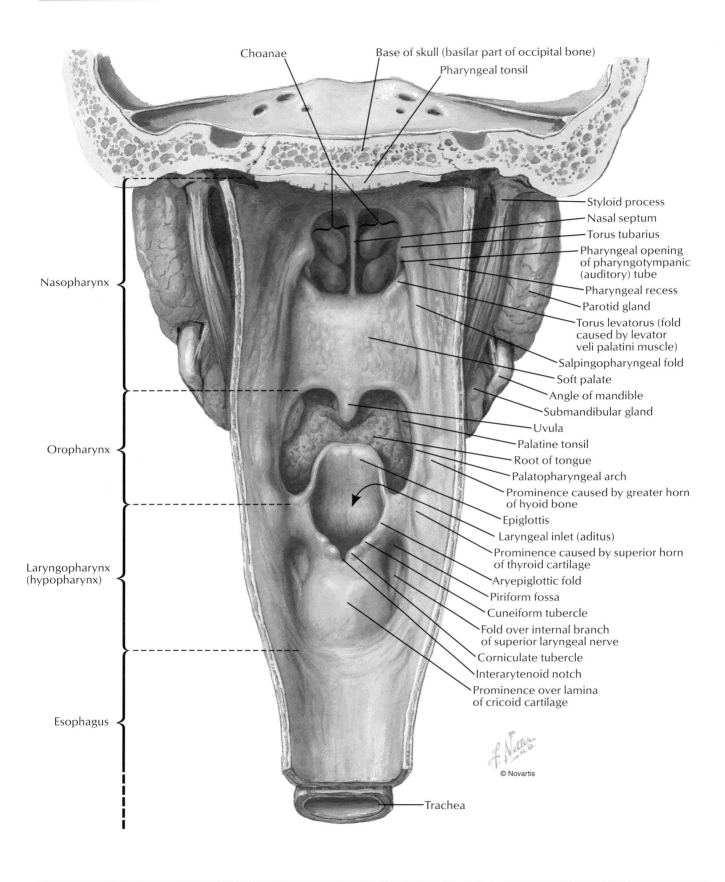

Choanae

Base of skull (basilar part of occipital bone)

Pharyngeal tonsil

Nasopharynx

Oropharynx

Laryngopharynx (hypopharynx)

Esophagus

Styloid process
Nasal septum
Torus tubarius
Pharyngeal opening of pharyngotympanic (auditory) tube
Pharyngeal recess
Parotid gland
Torus levatorus (fold caused by levator veli palatini muscle)
Salpingopharyngeal fold
Soft palate
Angle of mandible
Submandibular gland
Uvula
Palatine tonsil
Root of tongue
Palatopharyngeal arch
Prominence caused by greater horn of hyoid bone
Epiglottis
Laryngeal inlet (aditus)
Prominence caused by superior horn of thyroid cartilage
Aryepiglottic fold
Piriform fossa
Cuneiform tubercle
Fold over internal branch of superior laryngeal nerve
Corniculate tubercle
Interarytenoid notch
Prominence over lamina of cricoid cartilage

Trachea

© Novartis

**PLATE 60**

**HEAD AND NECK**

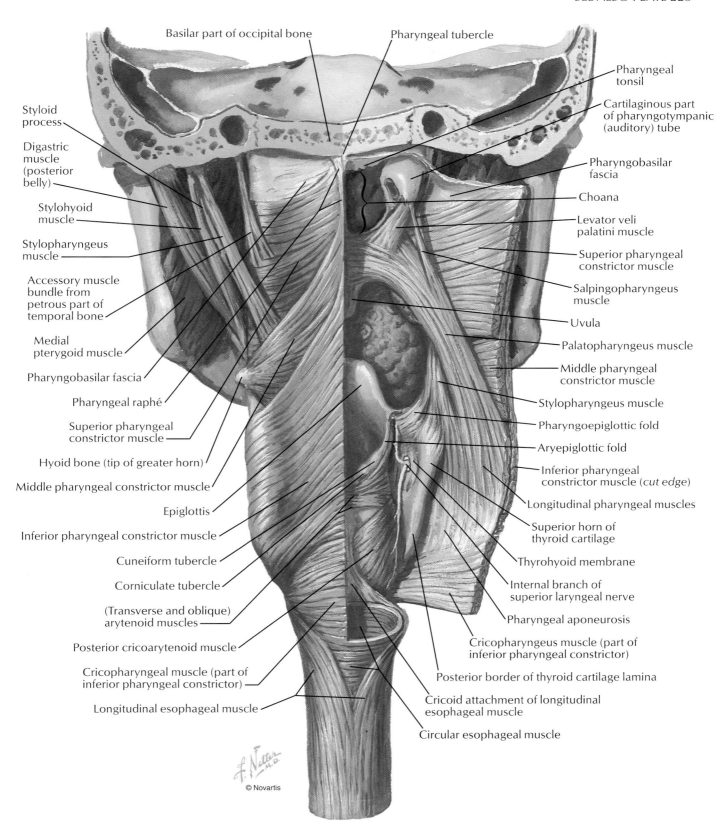

Basilar part of occipital bone

Pharyngeal tubercle

Pharyngeal tonsil

Styloid process

Digastric muscle (posterior belly)

Stylohyoid muscle

Stylopharyngeus muscle

Accessory muscle bundle from petrous part of temporal bone

Medial pterygoid muscle

Pharyngobasilar fascia

Pharyngeal raphé

Superior pharyngeal constrictor muscle

Hyoid bone (tip of greater horn)

Middle pharyngeal constrictor muscle

Epiglottis

Inferior pharyngeal constrictor muscle

Cuneiform tubercle

Corniculate tubercle

(Transverse and oblique) arytenoid muscles

Posterior cricoarytenoid muscle

Cricopharyngeal muscle (part of inferior pharyngeal constrictor)

Longitudinal esophageal muscle

Cartilaginous part of pharyngotympanic (auditory) tube

Pharyngobasilar fascia

Choana

Levator veli palatini muscle

Superior pharyngeal constrictor muscle

Salpingopharyngeus muscle

Uvula

Palatopharyngeus muscle

Middle pharyngeal constrictor muscle

Stylopharyngeus muscle

Pharyngoepiglottic fold

Aryepiglottic fold

Inferior pharyngeal constrictor muscle (*cut edge*)

Longitudinal pharyngeal muscles

Superior horn of thyroid cartilage

Thyrohyoid membrane

Internal branch of superior laryngeal nerve

Pharyngeal aponeurosis

Cricopharyngeus muscle (part of inferior pharyngeal constrictor)

Posterior border of thyroid cartilage lamina

Cricoid attachment of longitudinal esophageal muscle

Circular esophageal muscle

© Novartis

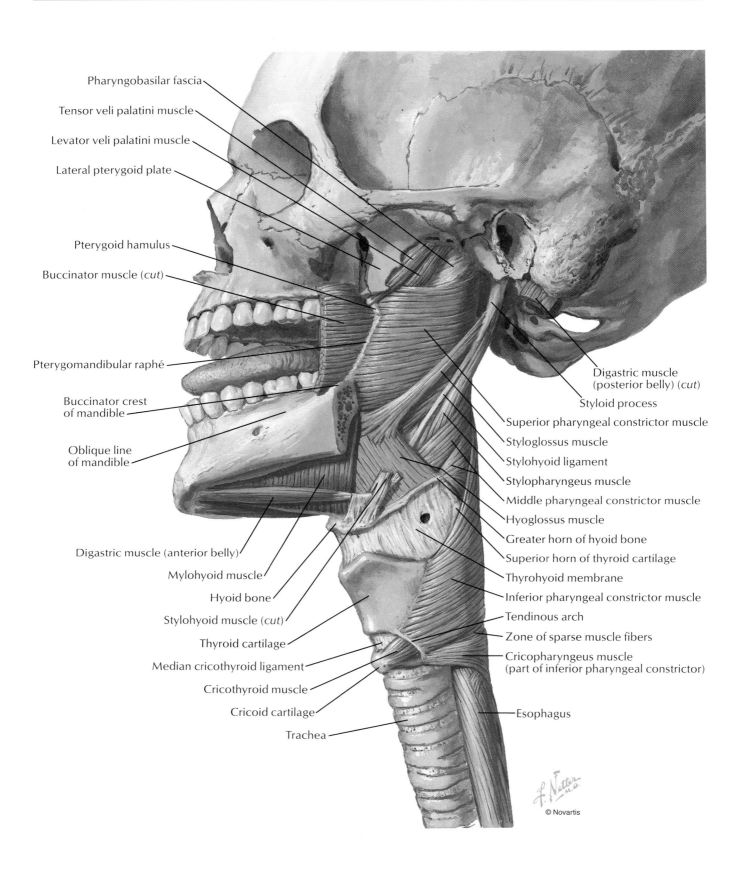

Pharyngobasilar fascia

Tensor veli palatini muscle

Levator veli palatini muscle

Lateral pterygoid plate

Pterygoid hamulus

Buccinator muscle (*cut*)

Pterygomandibular raphé

Buccinator crest
of mandible

Oblique line
of mandible

Digastric muscle (anterior belly)

Mylohyoid muscle

Hyoid bone

Stylohyoid muscle (*cut*)

Thyroid cartilage

Median cricothyroid ligament

Cricothyroid muscle

Cricoid cartilage

Trachea

Digastric muscle
(posterior belly) (*cut*)

Styloid process

Superior pharyngeal constrictor muscle

Styloglossus muscle

Stylohyoid ligament

Stylopharyngeus muscle

Middle pharyngeal constrictor muscle

Hyoglossus muscle

Greater horn of hyoid bone

Superior horn of thyroid cartilage

Thyrohyoid membrane

Inferior pharyngeal constrictor muscle

Tendinous arch

Zone of sparse muscle fibers

Cricopharyngeus muscle
(part of inferior pharyngeal constrictor)

Esophagus

© Novartis

*PLATE 62*

**HEAD AND NECK**

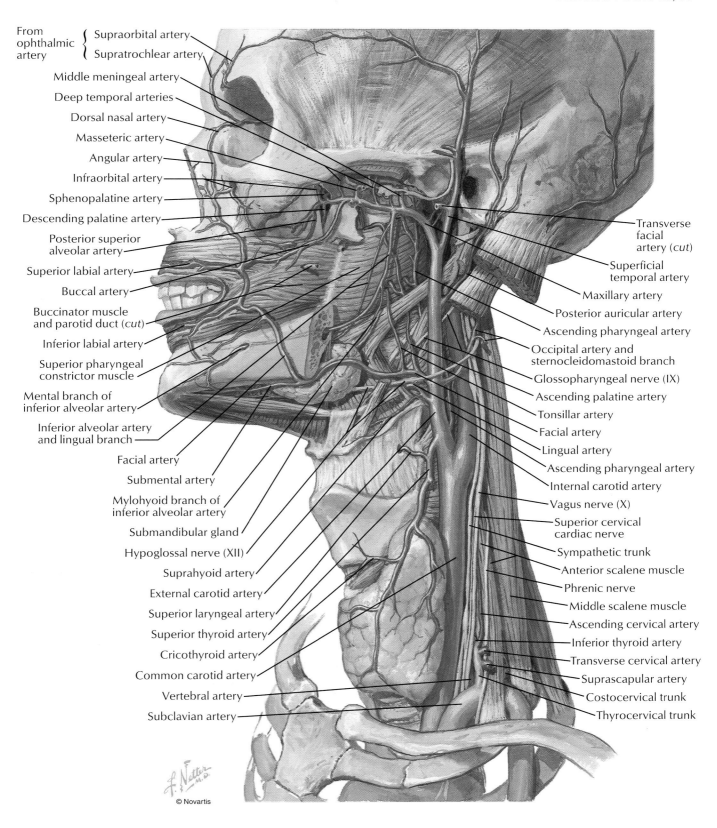

From ophthalmic artery {
Supraorbital artery
Supratrochlear artery

Middle meningeal artery

Deep temporal arteries

Dorsal nasal artery

Masseteric artery

Angular artery

Infraorbital artery

Sphenopalatine artery

Descending palatine artery

Posterior superior alveolar artery

Superior labial artery

Buccal artery

Buccinator muscle and parotid duct (cut)

Inferior labial artery

Superior pharyngeal constrictor muscle

Mental branch of inferior alveolar artery

Inferior alveolar artery and lingual branch

Facial artery

Submental artery

Mylohyoid branch of inferior alveolar artery

Submandibular gland

Hypoglossal nerve (XII)

Suprahyoid artery

External carotid artery

Superior laryngeal artery

Superior thyroid artery

Cricothyroid artery

Common carotid artery

Vertebral artery

Subclavian artery

Transverse facial artery (cut)

Superficial temporal artery

Maxillary artery

Posterior auricular artery

Ascending pharyngeal artery

Occipital artery and sternocleidomastoid branch

Glossopharyngeal nerve (IX)

Ascending palatine artery

Tonsillar artery

Facial artery

Lingual artery

Ascending pharyngeal artery

Internal carotid artery

Vagus nerve (X)

Superior cervical cardiac nerve

Sympathetic trunk

Anterior scalene muscle

Phrenic nerve

Middle scalene muscle

Ascending cervical artery

Inferior thyroid artery

Transverse cervical artery

Suprascapular artery

Costocervical trunk

Thyrocervical trunk

*f. Netter*

© Novartis

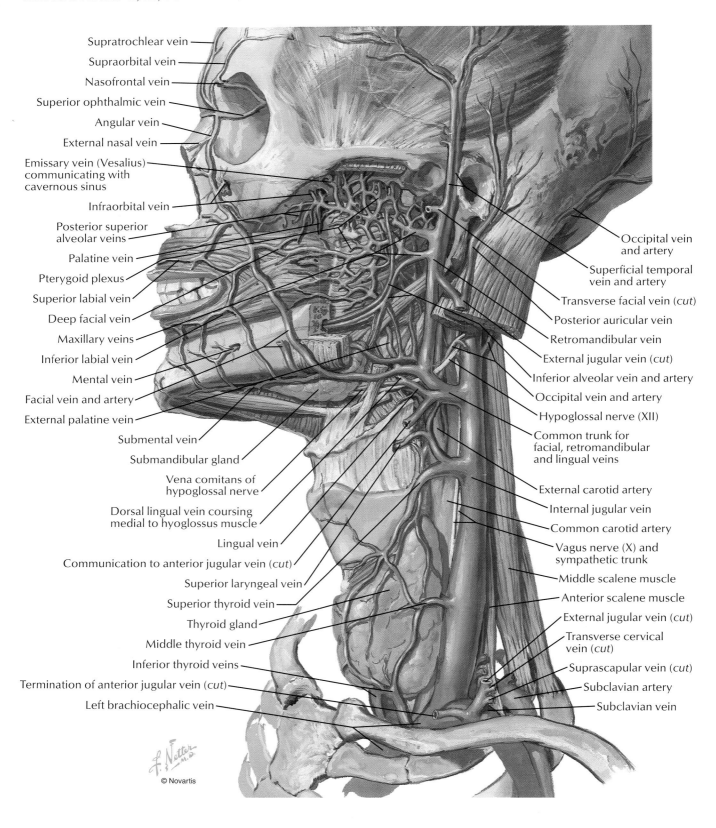

Supratrochlear vein

Supraorbital vein

Nasofrontal vein

Superior ophthalmic vein

Angular vein

External nasal vein

Emissary vein (Vesalius) communicating with cavernous sinus

Infraorbital vein

Posterior superior alveolar veins

Palatine vein

Pterygoid plexus

Superior labial vein

Deep facial vein

Maxillary veins

Inferior labial vein

Mental vein

Facial vein and artery

External palatine vein

Submental vein

Submandibular gland

Vena comitans of hypoglossal nerve

Dorsal lingual vein coursing medial to hyoglossus muscle

Lingual vein

Communication to anterior jugular vein (cut)

Superior laryngeal vein

Superior thyroid vein

Thyroid gland

Middle thyroid vein

Inferior thyroid veins

Termination of anterior jugular vein (cut)

Left brachiocephalic vein

Occipital vein and artery

Superficial temporal vein and artery

Transverse facial vein (cut)

Posterior auricular vein

Retromandibular vein

External jugular vein (cut)

Inferior alveolar vein and artery

Occipital vein and artery

Hypoglossal nerve (XII)

Common trunk for facial, retromandibular and lingual veins

External carotid artery

Internal jugular vein

Common carotid artery

Vagus nerve (X) and sympathetic trunk

Middle scalene muscle

Anterior scalene muscle

External jugular vein (cut)

Transverse cervical vein (cut)

Suprascapular vein (cut)

Subclavian artery

Subclavian vein

© Novartis

**PLATE 64**

**HEAD AND NECK**

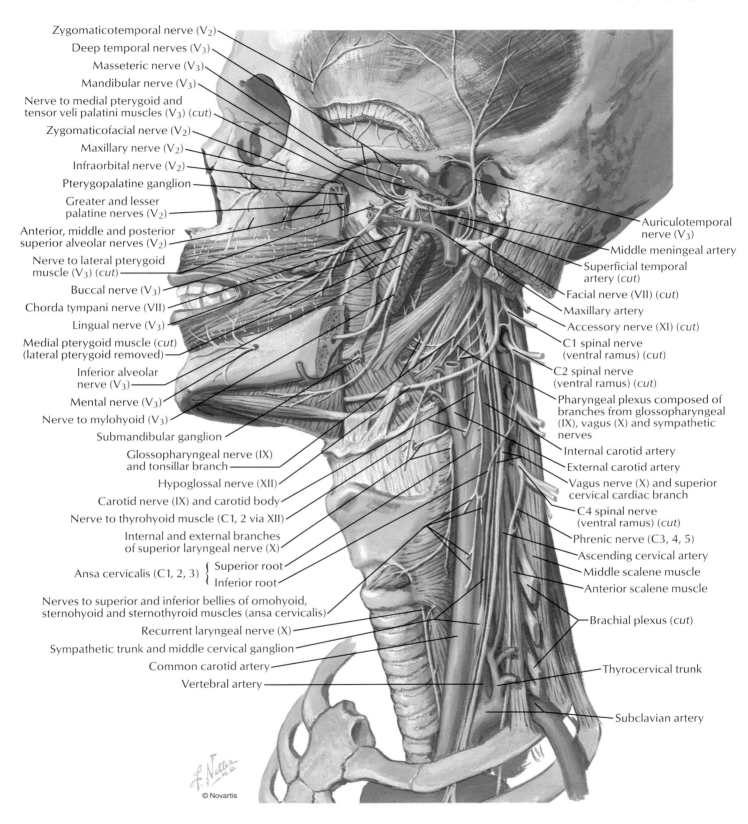

Zygomaticotemporal nerve (V₂)

Deep temporal nerves (V₃)

Masseteric nerve (V₃)

Mandibular nerve (V₃)

Nerve to medial pterygoid and tensor veli palatini muscles (V₃) (*cut*)

Zygomaticofacial nerve (V₂)

Maxillary nerve (V₂)

Infraorbital nerve (V₂)

Pterygopalatine ganglion

Greater and lesser palatine nerves (V₂)

Anterior, middle and posterior superior alveolar nerves (V₂)

Nerve to lateral pterygoid muscle (V₃) (*cut*)

Buccal nerve (V₃)

Chorda tympani nerve (VII)

Lingual nerve (V₃)

Medial pterygoid muscle (*cut*) (lateral pterygoid removed)

Inferior alveolar nerve (V₃)

Mental nerve (V₃)

Nerve to mylohyoid (V₃)

Submandibular ganglion

Glossopharyngeal nerve (IX) and tonsillar branch

Hypoglossal nerve (XII)

Carotid nerve (IX) and carotid body

Nerve to thyrohyoid muscle (C1, 2 via XII)

Internal and external branches of superior laryngeal nerve (X)

Ansa cervicalis (C1, 2, 3) { Superior root / Inferior root }

Nerves to superior and inferior bellies of omohyoid, sternohyoid and sternothyroid muscles (ansa cervicalis)

Recurrent laryngeal nerve (X)

Sympathetic trunk and middle cervical ganglion

Common carotid artery

Vertebral artery

Auriculotemporal nerve (V₃)

Middle meningeal artery

Superficial temporal artery (*cut*)

Facial nerve (VII) (*cut*)

Maxillary artery

Accessory nerve (XI) (*cut*)

C1 spinal nerve (ventral ramus) (*cut*)

C2 spinal nerve (ventral ramus) (*cut*)

Pharyngeal plexus composed of branches from glossopharyngeal (IX), vagus (X) and sympathetic nerves

Internal carotid artery

External carotid artery

Vagus nerve (X) and superior cervical cardiac branch

C4 spinal nerve (ventral ramus) (*cut*)

Phrenic nerve (C3, 4, 5)

Ascending cervical artery

Middle scalene muscle

Anterior scalene muscle

Brachial plexus (*cut*)

Thyrocervical trunk

Subclavian artery

© Novartis

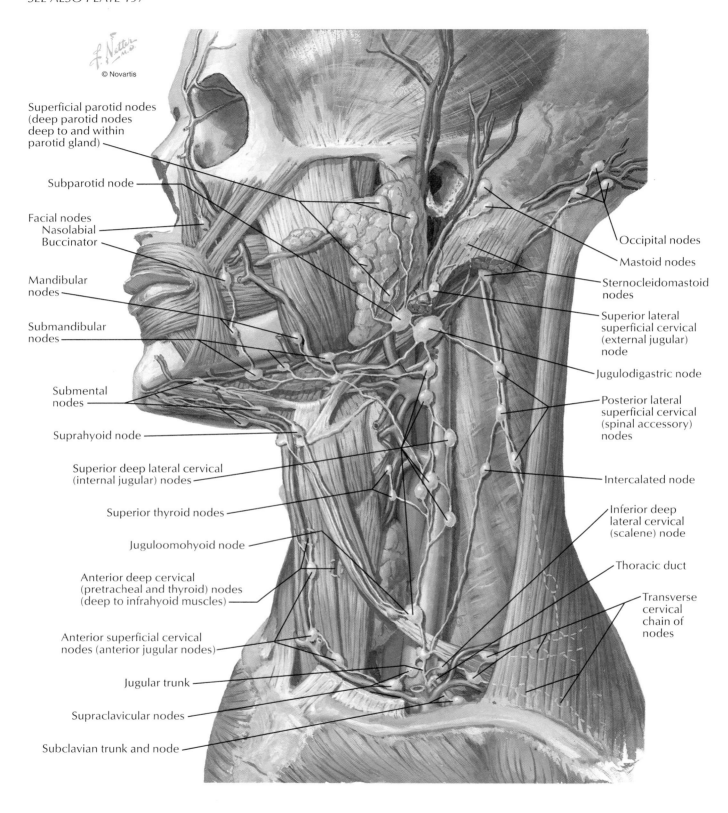

Superficial parotid nodes
(deep parotid nodes
deep to and within
parotid gland)

Subparotid node

Facial nodes
Nasolabial
Buccinator

Mandibular
nodes

Submandibular
nodes

Submental
nodes

Suprahyoid node

Superior deep lateral cervical
(internal jugular) nodes

Superior thyroid nodes

Juguloomohyoid node

Anterior deep cervical
(pretracheal and thyroid) nodes
(deep to infrahyoid muscles)

Anterior superficial cervical
nodes (anterior jugular nodes)

Jugular trunk

Supraclavicular nodes

Subclavian trunk and node

Occipital nodes

Mastoid nodes

Sternocleidomastoid
nodes

Superior lateral
superficial cervical
(external jugular)
node

Jugulodigastric node

Posterior lateral
superficial cervical
(spinal accessory)
nodes

Intercalated node

Inferior deep
lateral cervical
(scalene) node

Thoracic duct

Transverse
cervical
chain of
nodes

© Novartis

**PLATE 66**                                                                                          **HEAD AND NECK**

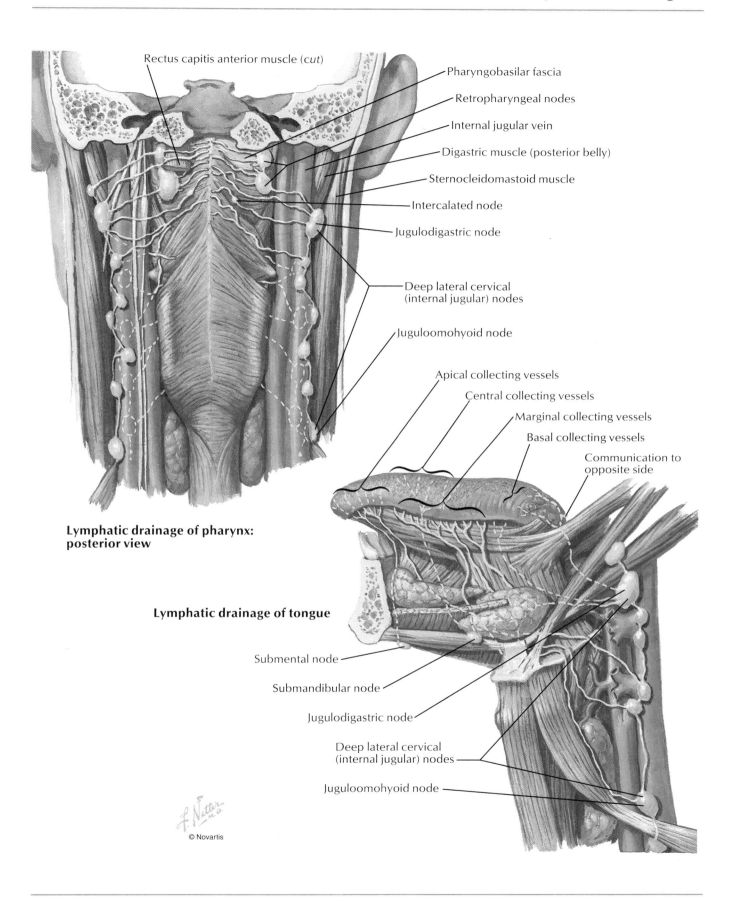

Rectus capitis anterior muscle (*cut*)

Pharyngobasilar fascia

Retropharyngeal nodes

Internal jugular vein

Digastric muscle (posterior belly)

Sternocleidomastoid muscle

Intercalated node

Jugulodigastric node

Deep lateral cervical (internal jugular) nodes

Juguloomohyoid node

**Lymphatic drainage of pharynx: posterior view**

Apical collecting vessels

Central collecting vessels

Marginal collecting vessels

Basal collecting vessels

Communication to opposite side

**Lymphatic drainage of tongue**

Submental node

Submandibular node

Jugulodigastric node

Deep lateral cervical (internal jugular) nodes

Juguloomohyoid node

© Novartis

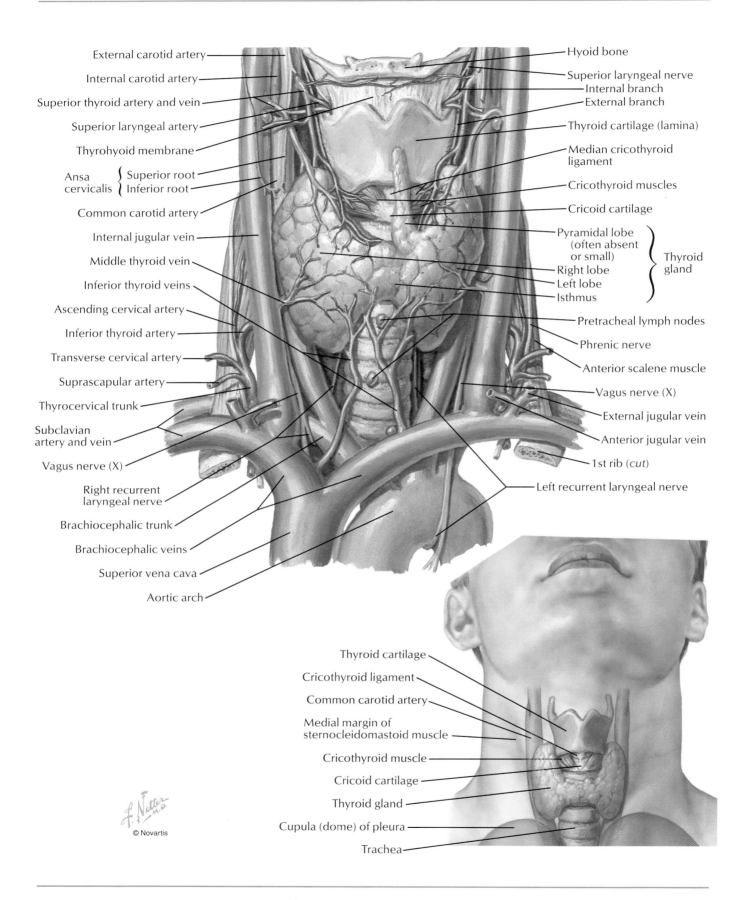

External carotid artery

Internal carotid artery

Superior thyroid artery and vein

Superior laryngeal artery

Thyrohyoid membrane

Ansa cervicalis { Superior root / Inferior root

Common carotid artery

Internal jugular vein

Middle thyroid vein

Inferior thyroid veins

Ascending cervical artery

Inferior thyroid artery

Transverse cervical artery

Suprascapular artery

Thyrocervical trunk

Subclavian artery and vein

Vagus nerve (X)

Right recurrent laryngeal nerve

Brachiocephalic trunk

Brachiocephalic veins

Superior vena cava

Aortic arch

Hyoid bone

Superior laryngeal nerve
Internal branch
External branch

Thyroid cartilage (lamina)

Median cricothyroid ligament

Cricothyroid muscles

Cricoid cartilage

Pyramidal lobe (often absent or small)
Right lobe
Left lobe } Thyroid gland
Isthmus

Pretracheal lymph nodes

Phrenic nerve

Anterior scalene muscle

Vagus nerve (X)

External jugular vein

Anterior jugular vein

1st rib (cut)

Left recurrent laryngeal nerve

Thyroid cartilage

Cricothyroid ligament

Common carotid artery

Medial margin of sternocleidomastoid muscle

Cricothyroid muscle

Cricoid cartilage

Thyroid gland

Cupula (dome) of pleura

Trachea

© Novartis

**PLATE 68**

**HEAD AND NECK**

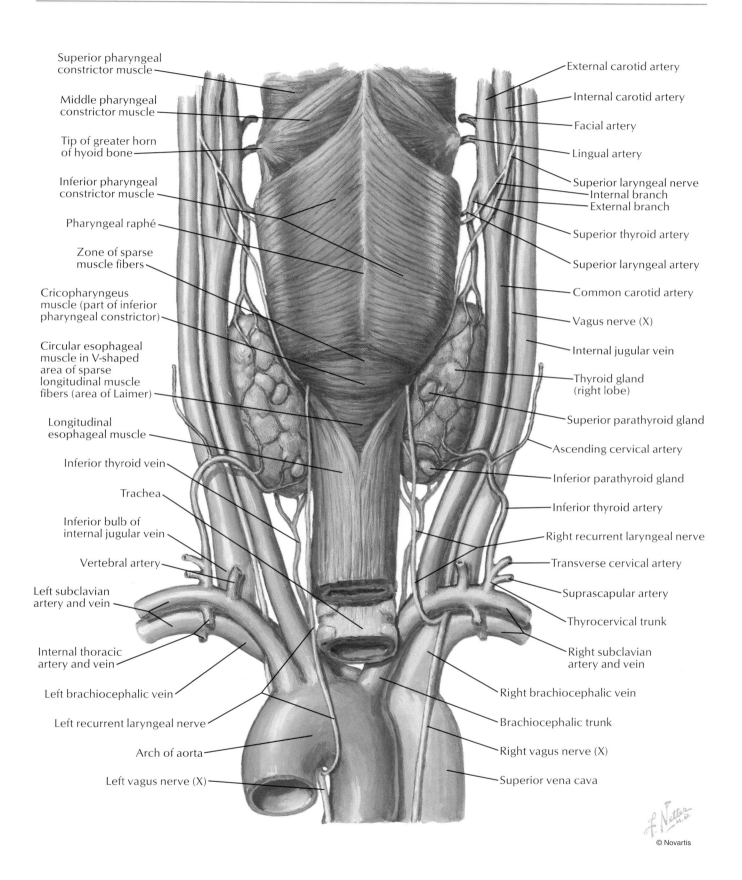

Superior pharyngeal constrictor muscle

Middle pharyngeal constrictor muscle

Tip of greater horn of hyoid bone

Inferior pharyngeal constrictor muscle

Pharyngeal raphé

Zone of sparse muscle fibers

Cricopharyngeus muscle (part of inferior pharyngeal constrictor)

Circular esophageal muscle in V-shaped area of sparse longitudinal muscle fibers (area of Laimer)

Longitudinal esophageal muscle

Inferior thyroid vein

Trachea

Inferior bulb of internal jugular vein

Vertebral artery

Left subclavian artery and vein

Internal thoracic artery and vein

Left brachiocephalic vein

Left recurrent laryngeal nerve

Arch of aorta

Left vagus nerve (X)

External carotid artery

Internal carotid artery

Facial artery

Lingual artery

Superior laryngeal nerve
Internal branch
External branch

Superior thyroid artery

Superior laryngeal artery

Common carotid artery

Vagus nerve (X)

Internal jugular vein

Thyroid gland (right lobe)

Superior parathyroid gland

Ascending cervical artery

Inferior parathyroid gland

Inferior thyroid artery

Right recurrent laryngeal nerve

Transverse cervical artery

Suprascapular artery

Thyrocervical trunk

Right subclavian artery and vein

Right brachiocephalic vein

Brachiocephalic trunk

Right vagus nerve (X)

Superior vena cava

© Novartis

# Parathyroid Glands

*SEE ALSO PLATE 74*

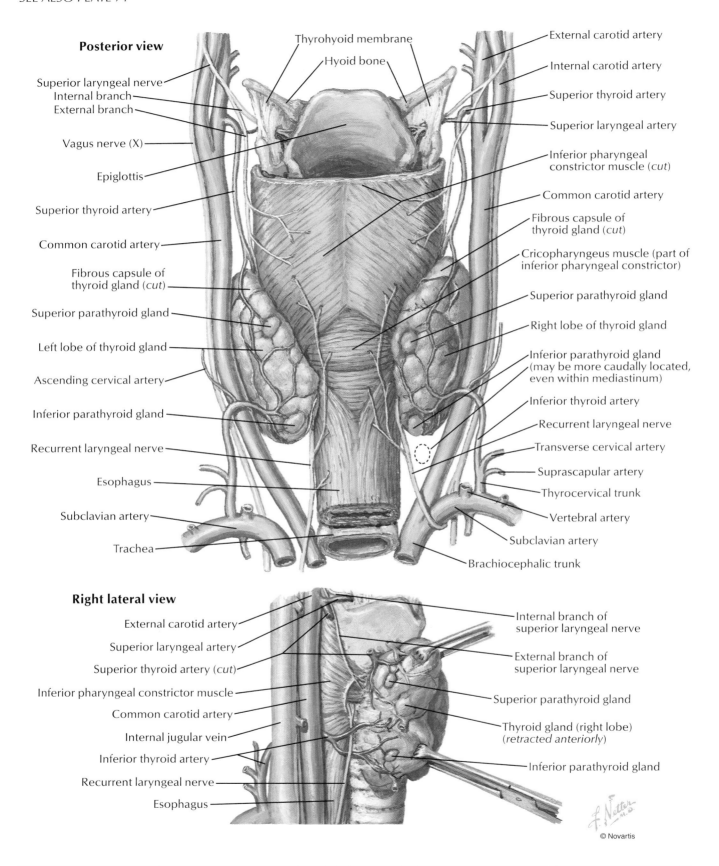

**Posterior view**

- Superior laryngeal nerve
- Internal branch
- External branch
- Vagus nerve (X)
- Epiglottis
- Superior thyroid artery
- Common carotid artery
- Fibrous capsule of thyroid gland (*cut*)
- Superior parathyroid gland
- Left lobe of thyroid gland
- Ascending cervical artery
- Inferior parathyroid gland
- Recurrent laryngeal nerve
- Esophagus
- Subclavian artery
- Trachea

- Thyrohyoid membrane
- Hyoid bone

- External carotid artery
- Internal carotid artery
- Superior thyroid artery
- Superior laryngeal artery
- Inferior pharyngeal constrictor muscle (*cut*)
- Common carotid artery
- Fibrous capsule of thyroid gland (*cut*)
- Cricopharyngeus muscle (part of inferior pharyngeal constrictor)
- Superior parathyroid gland
- Right lobe of thyroid gland
- Inferior parathyroid gland (may be more caudally located, even within mediastinum)
- Inferior thyroid artery
- Recurrent laryngeal nerve
- Transverse cervical artery
- Suprascapular artery
- Thyrocervical trunk
- Vertebral artery
- Subclavian artery
- Brachiocephalic trunk

**Right lateral view**

- External carotid artery
- Superior laryngeal artery
- Superior thyroid artery (*cut*)
- Inferior pharyngeal constrictor muscle
- Common carotid artery
- Internal jugular vein
- Inferior thyroid artery
- Recurrent laryngeal nerve
- Esophagus

- Internal branch of superior laryngeal nerve
- External branch of superior laryngeal nerve
- Superior parathyroid gland
- Thyroid gland (right lobe) (*retracted anteriorly*)
- Inferior parathyroid gland

*f. Netter*
© Novartis

**PLATE 70**                    **HEAD AND NECK**

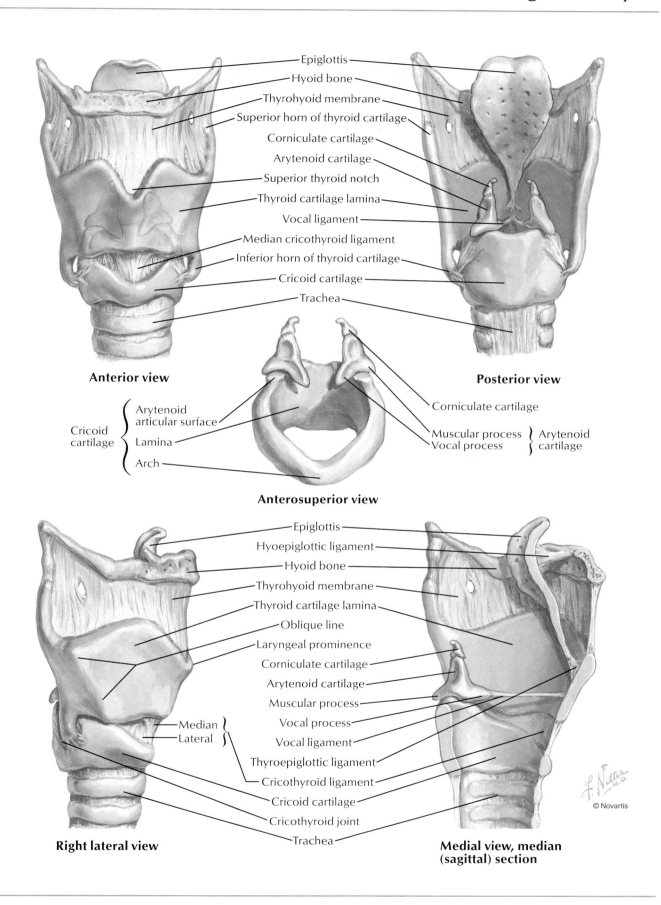

**Anterior view**

Epiglottis
Hyoid bone
Thyrohyoid membrane
Superior horn of thyroid cartilage
Corniculate cartilage
Arytenoid cartilage
Superior thyroid notch
Thyroid cartilage lamina
Vocal ligament
Median cricothyroid ligament
Inferior horn of thyroid cartilage
Cricoid cartilage
Trachea

**Posterior view**

Cricoid cartilage { Arytenoid articular surface
Lamina
Arch

Corniculate cartilage
Muscular process } Arytenoid cartilage
Vocal process

**Anterosuperior view**

**Right lateral view**

Epiglottis
Hyoepiglottic ligament
Hyoid bone
Thyrohyoid membrane
Thyroid cartilage lamina
Oblique line
Laryngeal prominence
Corniculate cartilage
Arytenoid cartilage
Muscular process
Vocal process
Vocal ligament
Thyroepiglottic ligament
Cricothyroid ligament
Cricoid cartilage
Cricothyroid joint
Trachea

Median }
Lateral }

**Medial view, median
(sagittal) section**

© Novartis

**THYROID GLAND AND LARYNX**

*PLATE 71*

# Intrinsic Muscles of Larynx

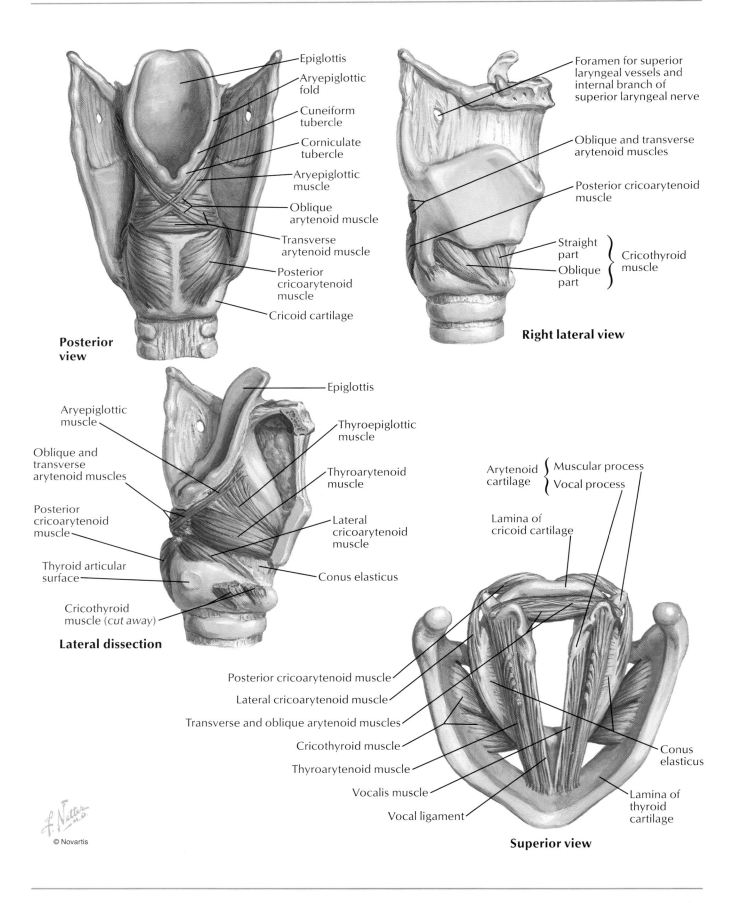

Epiglottis

Aryepiglottic fold

Cuneiform tubercle

Corniculate tubercle

Aryepiglottic muscle

Oblique arytenoid muscle

Transverse arytenoid muscle

Posterior cricoarytenoid muscle

Cricoid cartilage

**Posterior view**

Foramen for superior laryngeal vessels and internal branch of superior laryngeal nerve

Oblique and transverse arytenoid muscles

Posterior cricoarytenoid muscle

Straight part
Oblique part
} Cricothyroid muscle

**Right lateral view**

Aryepiglottic muscle

Oblique and transverse arytenoid muscles

Posterior cricoarytenoid muscle

Thyroid articular surface

Cricothyroid muscle (*cut away*)

**Lateral dissection**

Epiglottis

Thyroepiglottic muscle

Thyroarytenoid muscle

Lateral cricoarytenoid muscle

Conus elasticus

Arytenoid cartilage { Muscular process / Vocal process }

Lamina of cricoid cartilage

Posterior cricoarytenoid muscle

Lateral cricoarytenoid muscle

Transverse and oblique arytenoid muscles

Cricothyroid muscle

Thyroarytenoid muscle

Vocalis muscle

Vocal ligament

Conus elasticus

Lamina of thyroid cartilage

**Superior view**

© Novartis

**PLATE 72**

**HEAD AND NECK**

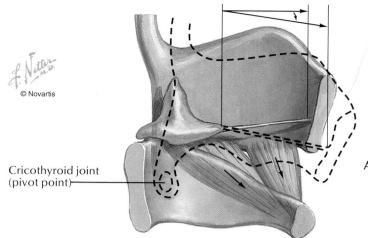

Cricothyroid joint
(pivot point)

**Action of cricothyroid muscles**
Lengthening (increasing tension)
of vocal ligaments

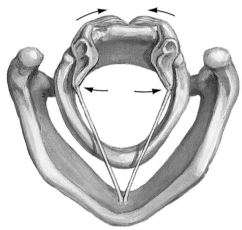

**Action of posterior cricoarytenoid muscles**
Abduction of vocal ligaments

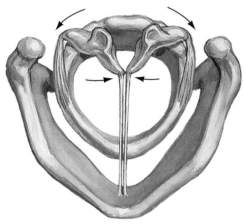

**Action of lateral cricoarytenoid muscles**
Adduction of vocal ligaments

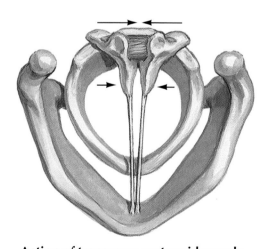

**Action of transverse arytenoid muscle**
Adduction of vocal ligaments

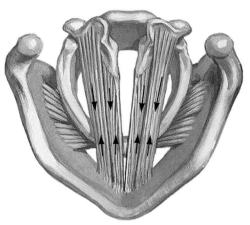

**Action of vocalis and thyroarytenoid muscles**
Shortening (relaxation) of vocal ligaments

# Nerves of Larynx

SEE ALSO PLATES 68, 69, 70, 223

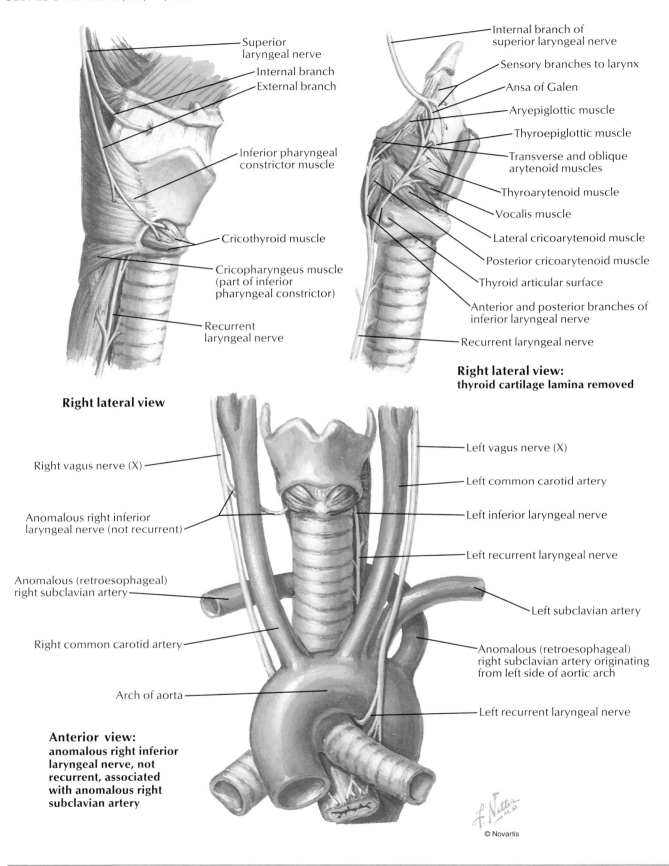

**Right lateral view**

Superior laryngeal nerve
Internal branch
External branch
Inferior pharyngeal constrictor muscle
Cricothyroid muscle
Cricopharyngeus muscle (part of inferior pharyngeal constrictor)
Recurrent laryngeal nerve

**Right lateral view: thyroid cartilage lamina removed**

Internal branch of superior laryngeal nerve
Sensory branches to larynx
Ansa of Galen
Aryepiglottic muscle
Thyroepiglottic muscle
Transverse and oblique arytenoid muscles
Thyroarytenoid muscle
Vocalis muscle
Lateral cricoarytenoid muscle
Posterior cricoarytenoid muscle
Thyroid articular surface
Anterior and posterior branches of inferior laryngeal nerve
Recurrent laryngeal nerve

**Anterior view: anomalous right inferior laryngeal nerve, not recurrent, associated with anomalous right subclavian artery**

Right vagus nerve (X)
Anomalous right inferior laryngeal nerve (not recurrent)
Anomalous (retroesophageal) right subclavian artery
Right common carotid artery
Arch of aorta

Left vagus nerve (X)
Left common carotid artery
Left inferior laryngeal nerve
Left recurrent laryngeal nerve
Left subclavian artery
Anomalous (retroesophageal) right subclavian artery originating from left side of aortic arch
Left recurrent laryngeal nerve

© Novartis

**PLATE 74**                                                    **HEAD AND NECK**

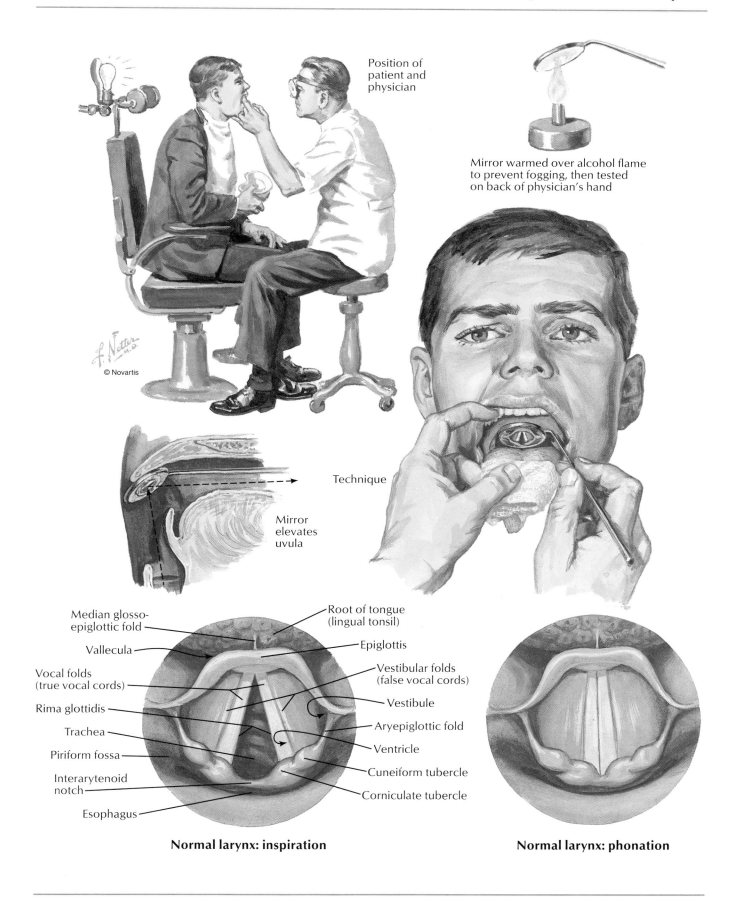

Position of patient and physician

Mirror warmed over alcohol flame to prevent fogging, then tested on back of physician's hand

Technique

Mirror elevates uvula

Median glosso-epiglottic fold

Vallecula

Vocal folds (true vocal cords)

Rima glottidis

Trachea

Piriform fossa

Interarytenoid notch

Esophagus

Root of tongue (lingual tonsil)

Epiglottis

Vestibular folds (false vocal cords)

Vestibule

Aryepiglottic fold

Ventricle

Cuneiform tubercle

Corniculate tubercle

**Normal larynx: inspiration**

**Normal larynx: phonation**

# Eyelids

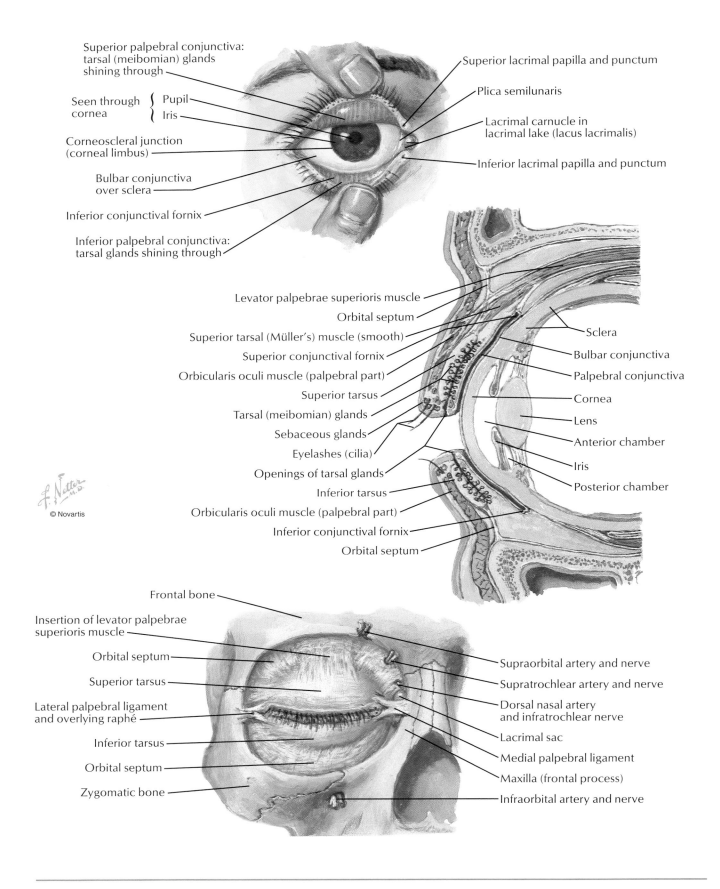

Superior palpebral conjunctiva: tarsal (meibomian) glands shining through

Seen through cornea { Pupil / Iris

Corneoscleral junction (corneal limbus)

Bulbar conjunctiva over sclera

Inferior conjunctival fornix

Inferior palpebral conjunctiva: tarsal glands shining through

Superior lacrimal papilla and punctum

Plica semilunaris

Lacrimal carnucle in lacrimal lake (lacus lacrimalis)

Inferior lacrimal papilla and punctum

Levator palpebrae superioris muscle

Orbital septum

Superior tarsal (Müller's) muscle (smooth)

Superior conjunctival fornix

Orbicularis oculi muscle (palpebral part)

Superior tarsus

Tarsal (meibomian) glands

Sebaceous glands

Eyelashes (cilia)

Openings of tarsal glands

Inferior tarsus

Orbicularis oculi muscle (palpebral part)

Inferior conjunctival fornix

Orbital septum

Sclera

Bulbar conjunctiva

Palpebral conjunctiva

Cornea

Lens

Anterior chamber

Iris

Posterior chamber

Frontal bone

Insertion of levator palpebrae superioris muscle

Orbital septum

Superior tarsus

Lateral palpebral ligament and overlying raphé

Inferior tarsus

Orbital septum

Zygomatic bone

Supraorbital artery and nerve

Supratrochlear artery and nerve

Dorsal nasal artery and infratrochlear nerve

Lacrimal sac

Medial palpebral ligament

Maxilla (frontal process)

Infraorbital artery and nerve

F. Netter M.D.

© Novartis

**PLATE 76**

**HEAD AND NECK**

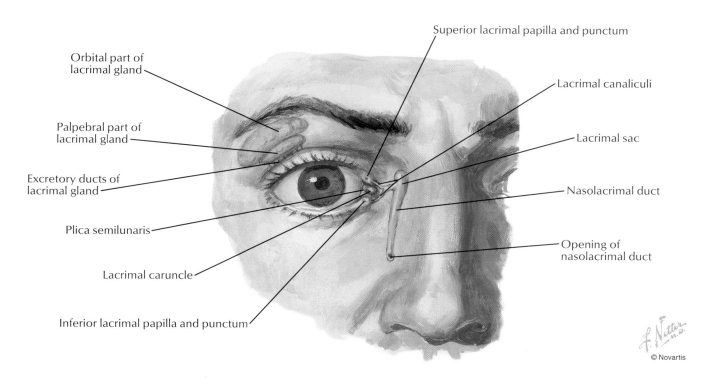

Superior lacrimal papilla and punctum

Orbital part of lacrimal gland

Lacrimal canaliculi

Palpebral part of lacrimal gland

Lacrimal sac

Excretory ducts of lacrimal gland

Nasolacrimal duct

Plica semilunaris

Opening of nasolacrimal duct

Lacrimal caruncle

Inferior lacrimal papilla and punctum

F. Netter M.D.
© Novartis

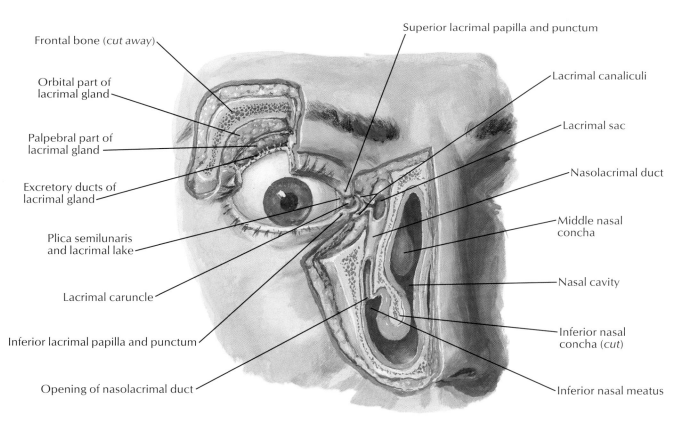

Superior lacrimal papilla and punctum

Frontal bone (*cut away*)

Orbital part of lacrimal gland

Lacrimal canaliculi

Palpebral part of lacrimal gland

Lacrimal sac

Excretory ducts of lacrimal gland

Nasolacrimal duct

Plica semilunaris and lacrimal lake

Middle nasal concha

Lacrimal caruncle

Nasal cavity

Inferior lacrimal papilla and punctum

Inferior nasal concha (*cut*)

Opening of nasolacrimal duct

Inferior nasal meatus

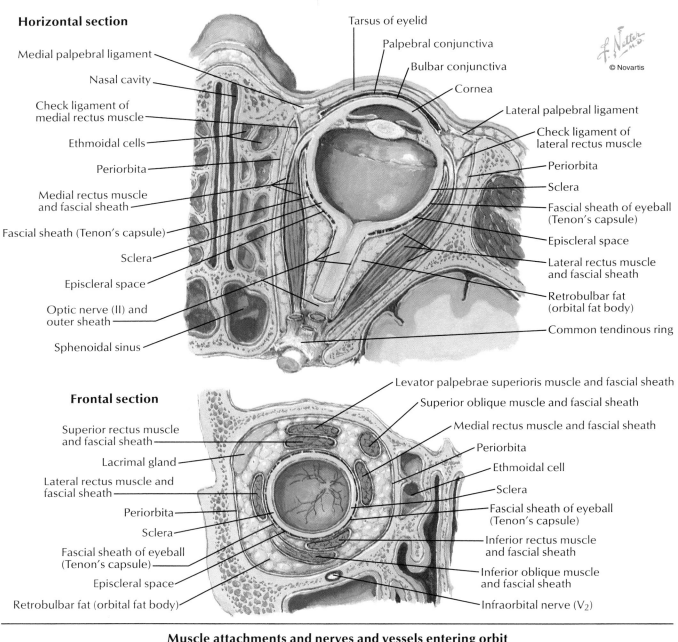

## Horizontal section

Medial palpebral ligament

Nasal cavity

Check ligament of medial rectus muscle

Ethmoidal cells

Periorbita

Medial rectus muscle and fascial sheath

Fascial sheath (Tenon's capsule)

Sclera

Episcleral space

Optic nerve (II) and outer sheath

Sphenoidal sinus

Tarsus of eyelid

Palpebral conjunctiva

Bulbar conjunctiva

Cornea

Lateral palpebral ligament

Check ligament of lateral rectus muscle

Periorbita

Sclera

Fascial sheath of eyeball (Tenon's capsule)

Episcleral space

Lateral rectus muscle and fascial sheath

Retrobulbar fat (orbital fat body)

Common tendinous ring

## Frontal section

Superior rectus muscle and fascial sheath

Lacrimal gland

Lateral rectus muscle and fascial sheath

Periorbita

Sclera

Fascial sheath of eyeball (Tenon's capsule)

Episcleral space

Retrobulbar fat (orbital fat body)

Levator palpebrae superioris muscle and fascial sheath

Superior oblique muscle and fascial sheath

Medial rectus muscle and fascial sheath

Periorbita

Ethmoidal cell

Sclera

Fascial sheath of eyeball (Tenon's capsule)

Inferior rectus muscle and fascial sheath

Inferior oblique muscle and fascial sheath

Infraorbital nerve ($V_2$)

## Muscle attachments and nerves and vessels entering orbit

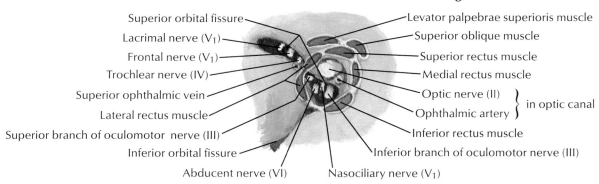

Superior orbital fissure

Lacrimal nerve ($V_1$)

Frontal nerve ($V_1$)

Trochlear nerve (IV)

Superior ophthalmic vein

Lateral rectus muscle

Superior branch of oculomotor nerve (III)

Inferior orbital fissure

Abducent nerve (VI)

Levator palpebrae superioris muscle

Superior oblique muscle

Superior rectus muscle

Medial rectus muscle

Optic nerve (II)

Ophthalmic artery } in optic canal

Inferior rectus muscle

Inferior branch of oculomotor nerve (III)

Nasociliary nerve ($V_1$)

**PLATE 78**                                                              **HEAD AND NECK**

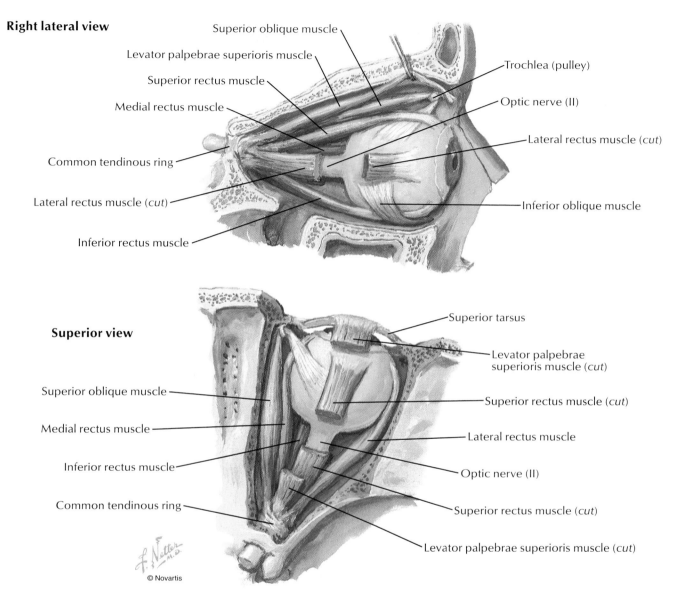

**Right lateral view**

Superior oblique muscle

Levator palpebrae superioris muscle

Superior rectus muscle

Medial rectus muscle

Common tendinous ring

Lateral rectus muscle (*cut*)

Inferior rectus muscle

Trochlea (pulley)

Optic nerve (II)

Lateral rectus muscle (*cut*)

Inferior oblique muscle

**Superior view**

Superior tarsus

Levator palpebrae superioris muscle (*cut*)

Superior oblique muscle

Medial rectus muscle

Inferior rectus muscle

Common tendinous ring

Superior rectus muscle (*cut*)

Lateral rectus muscle

Optic nerve (II)

Superior rectus muscle (*cut*)

Levator palpebrae superioris muscle (*cut*)

© Novartis

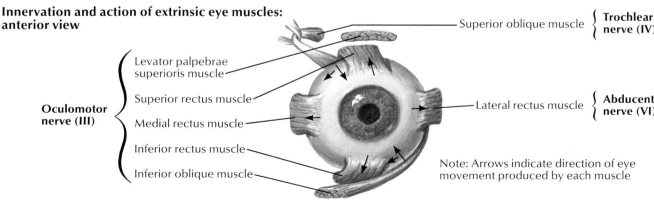

**Innervation and action of extrinsic eye muscles: anterior view**

Superior oblique muscle  } **Trochlear nerve (IV)**

Oculomotor nerve (III) {

Levator palpebrae superioris muscle

Superior rectus muscle

Medial rectus muscle

Inferior rectus muscle

Inferior oblique muscle

Lateral rectus muscle  } **Abducent nerve (VI)**

Note: Arrows indicate direction of eye movement produced by each muscle

# Arteries and Veins of Orbit and Eyelids

SEE ALSO PLATES 17, 98

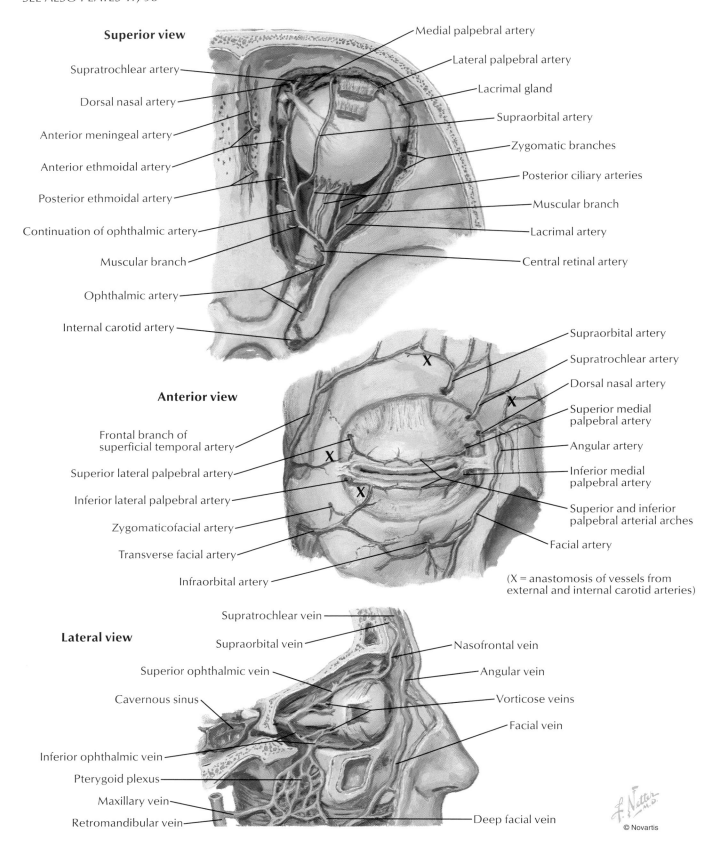

**Superior view**

Supratrochlear artery

Dorsal nasal artery

Anterior meningeal artery

Anterior ethmoidal artery

Posterior ethmoidal artery

Continuation of ophthalmic artery

Muscular branch

Ophthalmic artery

Internal carotid artery

Medial palpebral artery

Lateral palpebral artery

Lacrimal gland

Supraorbital artery

Zygomatic branches

Posterior ciliary arteries

Muscular branch

Lacrimal artery

Central retinal artery

**Anterior view**

Frontal branch of superficial temporal artery

Superior lateral palpebral artery

Inferior lateral palpebral artery

Zygomaticofacial artery

Transverse facial artery

Infraorbital artery

Supraorbital artery

Supratrochlear artery

Dorsal nasal artery

Superior medial palpebral artery

Angular artery

Inferior medial palpebral artery

Superior and inferior palpebral arterial arches

Facial artery

(X = anastomosis of vessels from external and internal carotid arteries)

**Lateral view**

Supratrochlear vein

Supraorbital vein

Superior ophthalmic vein

Cavernous sinus

Inferior ophthalmic vein

Pterygoid plexus

Maxillary vein

Retromandibular vein

Nasofrontal vein

Angular vein

Vorticose veins

Facial vein

Deep facial vein

© Novartis

**PLATE 80**                                                                 **HEAD AND NECK**

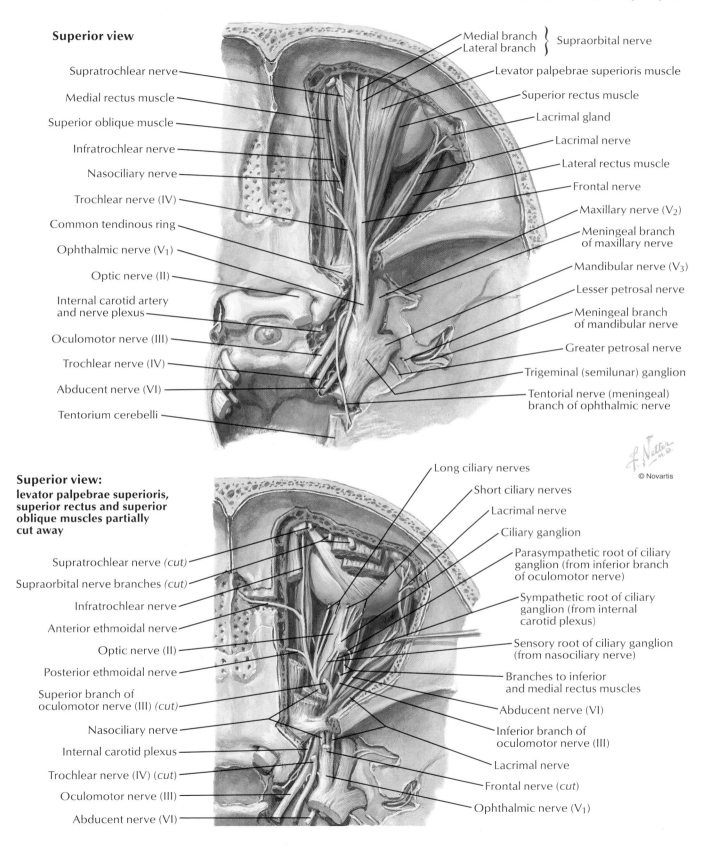

**Superior view**

Supratrochlear nerve

Medial rectus muscle

Superior oblique muscle

Infratrochlear nerve

Nasociliary nerve

Trochlear nerve (IV)

Common tendinous ring

Ophthalmic nerve (V₁)

Optic nerve (II)

Internal carotid artery and nerve plexus

Oculomotor nerve (III)

Trochlear nerve (IV)

Abducent nerve (VI)

Tentorium cerebelli

Medial branch
Lateral branch } Supraorbital nerve

Levator palpebrae superioris muscle

Superior rectus muscle

Lacrimal gland

Lacrimal nerve

Lateral rectus muscle

Frontal nerve

Maxillary nerve (V₂)

Meningeal branch of maxillary nerve

Mandibular nerve (V₃)

Lesser petrosal nerve

Meningeal branch of mandibular nerve

Greater petrosal nerve

Trigeminal (semilunar) ganglion

Tentorial nerve (meningeal) branch of ophthalmic nerve

**Superior view:**
**levator palpebrae superioris, superior rectus and superior oblique muscles partially cut away**

Supratrochlear nerve *(cut)*

Supraorbital nerve branches *(cut)*

Infratrochlear nerve

Anterior ethmoidal nerve

Optic nerve (II)

Posterior ethmoidal nerve

Superior branch of oculomotor nerve (III) *(cut)*

Nasociliary nerve

Internal carotid plexus

Trochlear nerve (IV) *(cut)*

Oculomotor nerve (III)

Abducent nerve (VI)

Long ciliary nerves

Short ciliary nerves

Lacrimal nerve

Ciliary ganglion

Parasympathetic root of ciliary ganglion (from inferior branch of oculomotor nerve)

Sympathetic root of ciliary ganglion (from internal carotid plexus)

Sensory root of ciliary ganglion (from nasociliary nerve)

Branches to inferior and medial rectus muscles

Abducent nerve (VI)

Inferior branch of oculomotor nerve (III)

Lacrimal nerve

Frontal nerve *(cut)*

Ophthalmic nerve (V₁)

© Novartis

# *Eyeball*

**Horizontal section**

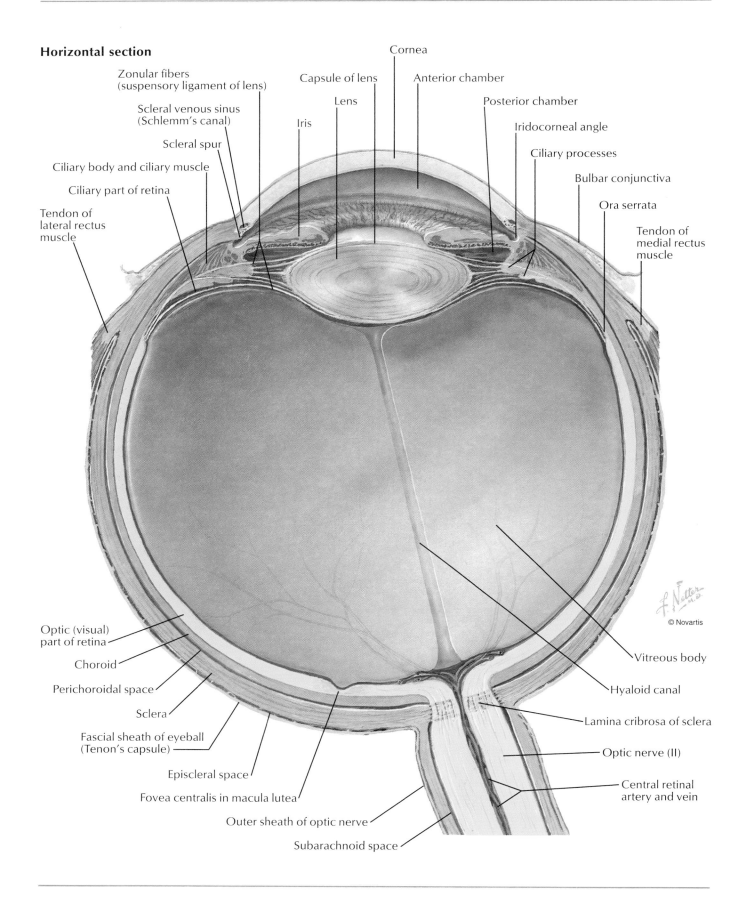

Zonular fibers
(suspensory ligament of lens)

Scleral venous sinus
(Schlemm's canal)

Scleral spur

Ciliary body and ciliary muscle

Ciliary part of retina

Tendon of
lateral rectus
muscle

Capsule of lens

Lens

Iris

Cornea

Anterior chamber

Posterior chamber

Iridocorneal angle

Ciliary processes

Bulbar conjunctiva

Ora serrata

Tendon of
medial rectus
muscle

Optic (visual)
part of retina

Choroid

Perichoroidal space

Sclera

Fascial sheath of eyeball
(Tenon's capsule)

Episcleral space

Fovea centralis in macula lutea

Outer sheath of optic nerve

Subarachnoid space

Vitreous body

Hyaloid canal

Lamina cribrosa of sclera

Optic nerve (II)

Central retinal
artery and vein

© Novartis

**PLATE 82**

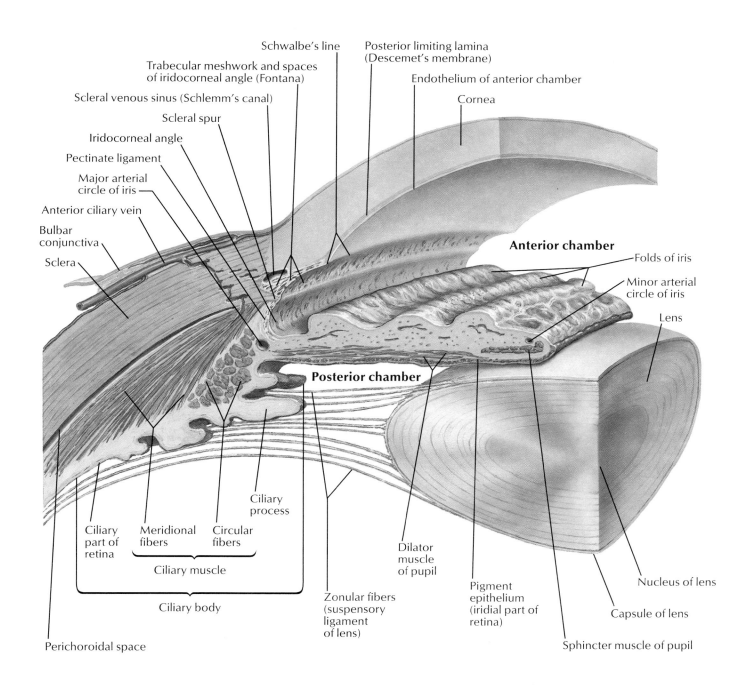

Schwalbe's line

Posterior limiting lamina (Descemet's membrane)

Trabecular meshwork and spaces of iridocorneal angle (Fontana)

Endothelium of anterior chamber

Scleral venous sinus (Schlemm's canal)

Cornea

Scleral spur

Iridocorneal angle

Pectinate ligament

Major arterial circle of iris

Anterior ciliary vein

Bulbar conjunctiva

Sclera

Anterior chamber

Folds of iris

Minor arterial circle of iris

Lens

Posterior chamber

Ciliary process

Ciliary part of retina

Meridional fibers

Circular fibers

Ciliary muscle

Dilator muscle of pupil

Ciliary body

Zonular fibers (suspensory ligament of lens)

Pigment epithelium (iridial part of retina)

Nucleus of lens

Capsule of lens

Perichoroidal space

Sphincter muscle of pupil

Note: For clarity, only single plane of zonular fibers shown; actually, fibers surround entire circumference of lens

© Novartis

# Iridocorneal Angle of Anterior Chamber of Eye

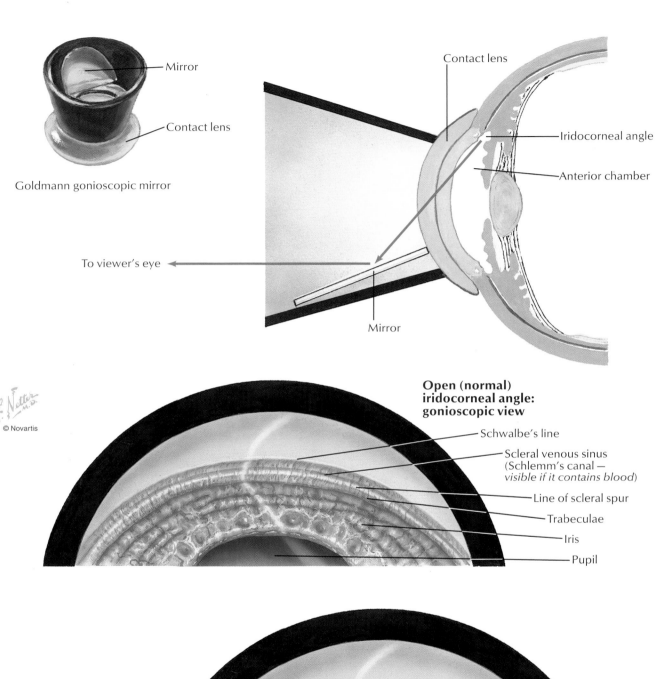

Mirror

Contact lens

Goldmann gonioscopic mirror

Contact lens

To viewer's eye

Mirror

Iridocorneal angle

Anterior chamber

© Novartis

**Open (normal)
iridocorneal angle:
gonioscopic view**

Schwalbe's line

Scleral venous sinus
(Schlemm's canal —
*visible if it contains blood*)

Line of scleral spur

Trabeculae

Iris

Pupil

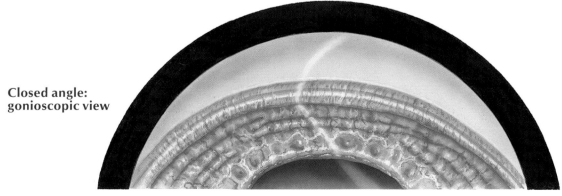

**Closed angle:
gonioscopic view**

**PLATE 84**

**HEAD AND NECK**

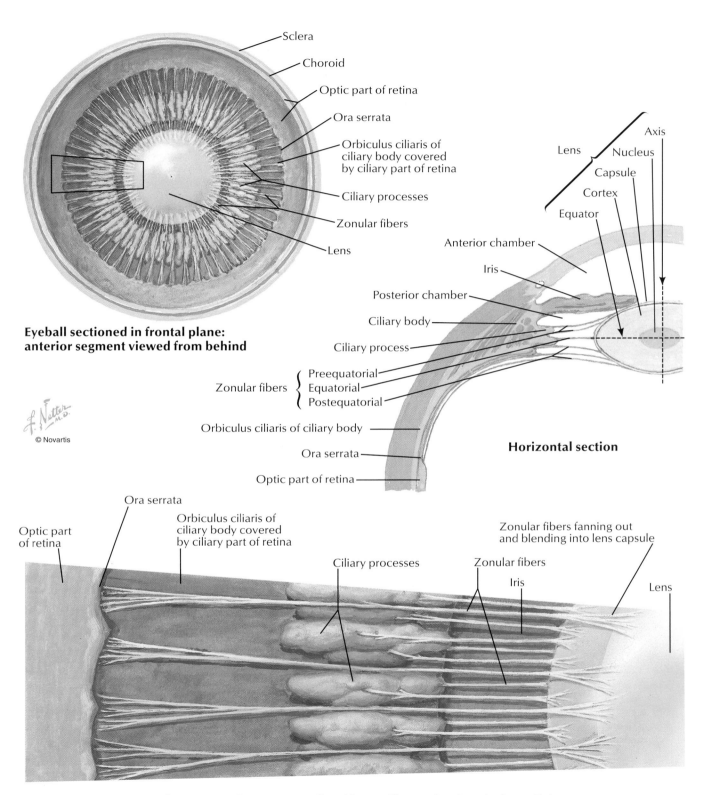

**Eyeball sectioned in frontal plane: anterior segment viewed from behind**

Sclera

Choroid

Optic part of retina

Ora serrata

Orbiculus ciliaris of ciliary body covered by ciliary part of retina

Ciliary processes

Zonular fibers

Lens

f. Netter M.D.

© Novartis

Axis

Lens

Nucleus

Capsule

Cortex

Equator

Anterior chamber

Iris

Posterior chamber

Ciliary body

Ciliary process

Zonular fibers { Preequatorial / Equatorial / Postequatorial

Orbiculus ciliaris of ciliary body

Ora serrata

Optic part of retina

**Horizontal section**

Ora serrata

Orbiculus ciliaris of ciliary body covered by ciliary part of retina

Optic part of retina

Ciliary processes

Zonular fibers fanning out and blending into lens capsule

Zonular fibers

Iris

Lens

**Enlargement of segment outlined in top illustration (semischematic)**

*SEE ALSO PLATE 80*

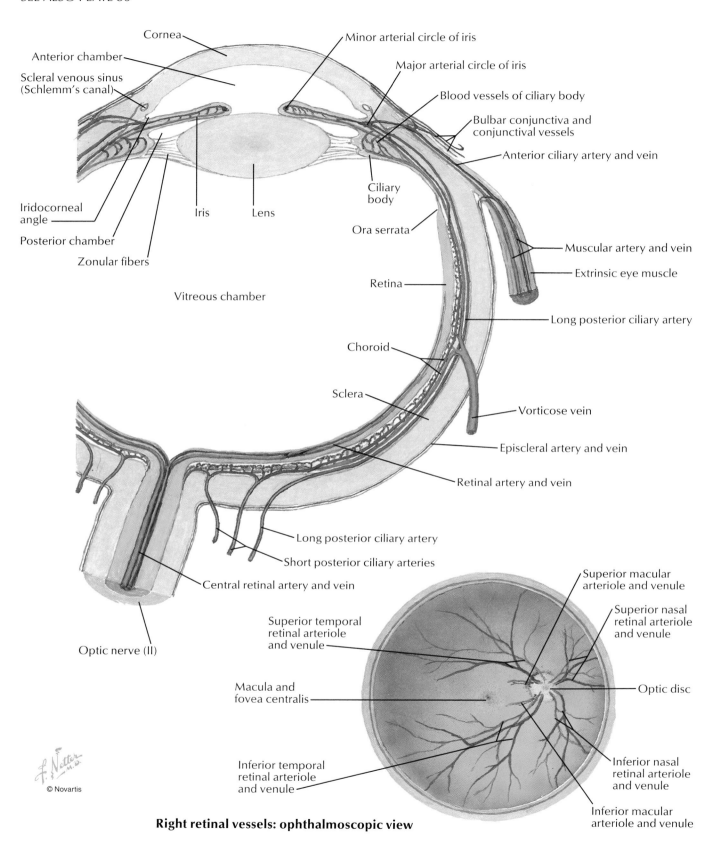

**Right retinal vessels: ophthalmoscopic view**

**PLATE 86**

**HEAD AND NECK**

**Frontal section**

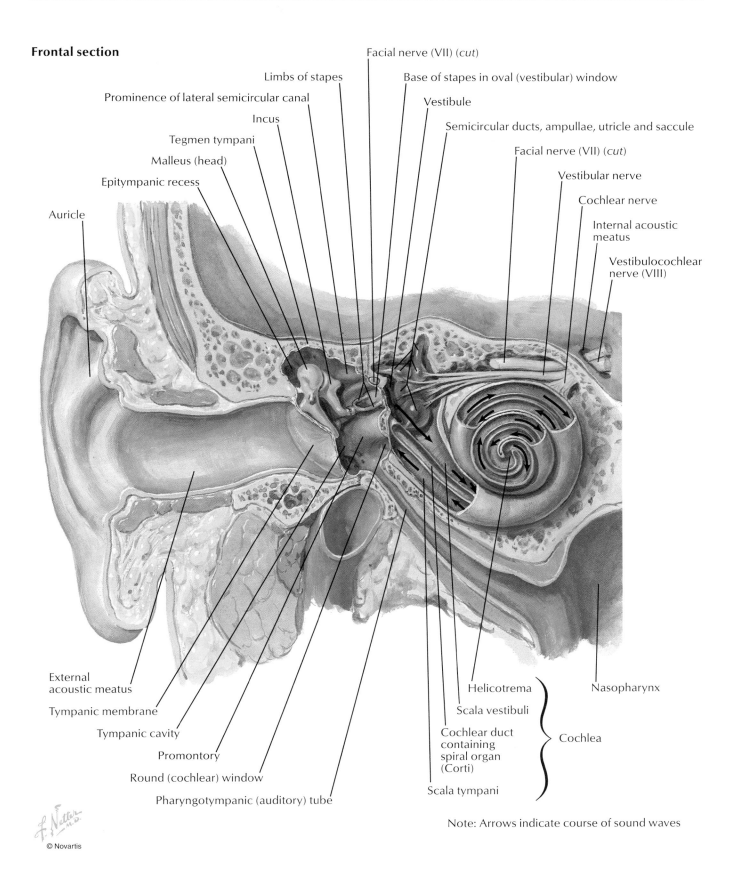

Facial nerve (VII) (*cut*)

Limbs of stapes

Base of stapes in oval (vestibular) window

Prominence of lateral semicircular canal

Vestibule

Incus

Semicircular ducts, ampullae, utricle and saccule

Tegmen tympani

Facial nerve (VII) (*cut*)

Malleus (head)

Vestibular nerve

Epitympanic recess

Cochlear nerve

Auricle

Internal acoustic meatus

Vestibulocochlear nerve (VIII)

External acoustic meatus

Tympanic membrane

Tympanic cavity

Promontory

Round (cochlear) window

Pharyngotympanic (auditory) tube

Helicotrema

Scala vestibuli

Cochlear duct containing spiral organ (Corti)

Scala tympani

Nasopharynx

Cochlea

Note: Arrows indicate course of sound waves

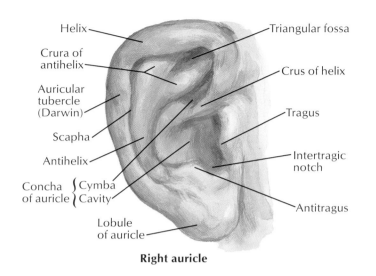

Helix

Crura of antihelix

Auricular tubercle (Darwin)

Scapha

Antihelix

Concha of auricle { Cymba { Cavity

Lobule of auricle

Triangular fossa

Crus of helix

Tragus

Intertragic notch

Antitragus

**Right auricle**

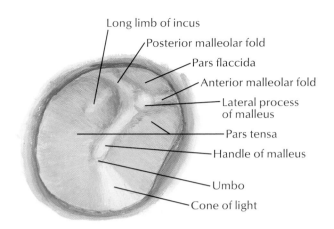

Long limb of incus

Posterior malleolar fold

Pars flaccida

Anterior malleolar fold

Lateral process of malleus

Pars tensa

Handle of malleus

Umbo

Cone of light

**Right tympanic membrane (eardrum) viewed through speculum**

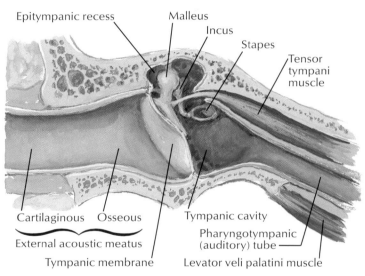

Epitympanic recess

Malleus

Incus

Stapes

Tensor tympani muscle

Cartilaginous  Osseous

External acoustic meatus

Tympanic membrane

Tympanic cavity

Pharyngotympanic (auditory) tube

Levator veli palatini muscle

**Coronal oblique section of external acoustic meatus and middle ear**

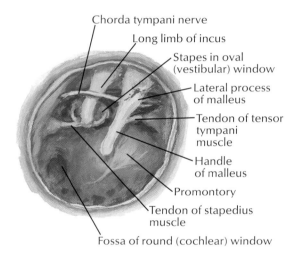

Chorda tympani nerve

Long limb of incus

Stapes in oval (vestibular) window

Lateral process of malleus

Tendon of tensor tympani muscle

Handle of malleus

Promontory

Tendon of stapedius muscle

Fossa of round (cochlear) window

**View into tympanic cavity after removal of tympanic membrane**

**Auditory ossicles**

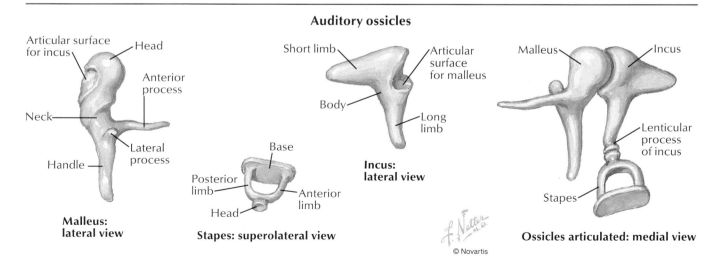

Articular surface for incus

Head

Anterior process

Neck

Handle

Lateral process

**Malleus: lateral view**

Base

Posterior limb

Anterior limb

Head

**Stapes: superolateral view**

Short limb

Body

Articular surface for malleus

Long limb

**Incus: lateral view**

Malleus

Incus

Lenticular process of incus

Stapes

**Ossicles articulated: medial view**

*f. Netter* M.D.

© Novartis

**PLATE 88**

**HEAD AND NECK**

## Lateral wall of tympanic cavity: medial (internal) view

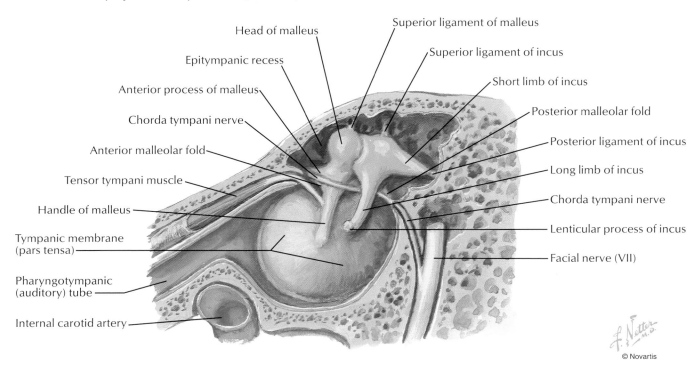

Head of malleus

Superior ligament of malleus

Epitympanic recess

Superior ligament of incus

Anterior process of malleus

Short limb of incus

Chorda tympani nerve

Posterior malleolar fold

Anterior malleolar fold

Posterior ligament of incus

Tensor tympani muscle

Long limb of incus

Handle of malleus

Chorda tympani nerve

Tympanic membrane (pars tensa)

Lenticular process of incus

Pharyngotympanic (auditory) tube

Facial nerve (VII)

Internal carotid artery

© Novartis

## Medial wall of tympanic cavity: lateral view

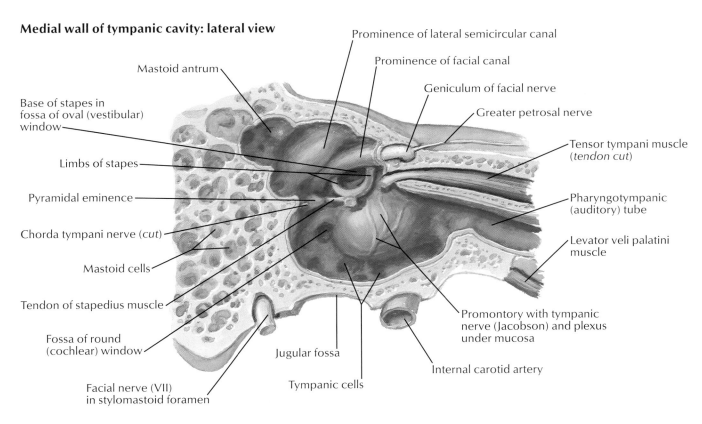

Prominence of lateral semicircular canal

Mastoid antrum

Prominence of facial canal

Geniculum of facial nerve

Base of stapes in fossa of oval (vestibular) window

Greater petrosal nerve

Limbs of stapes

Tensor tympani muscle (*tendon cut*)

Pyramidal eminence

Pharyngotympanic (auditory) tube

Chorda tympani nerve (*cut*)

Levator veli palatini muscle

Mastoid cells

Tendon of stapedius muscle

Promontory with tympanic nerve (Jacobson) and plexus under mucosa

Fossa of round (cochlear) window

Internal carotid artery

Facial nerve (VII) in stylomastoid foramen

Jugular fossa

Tympanic cells

# Bony and Membranous Labyrinths

SEE ALSO PLATE 118

**Right bony labyrinth (otic capsule), anterolateral view: surrounding cancellous bone removed**

**Dissected right bony labyrinth (otic capsule): membranous labyrinth removed**

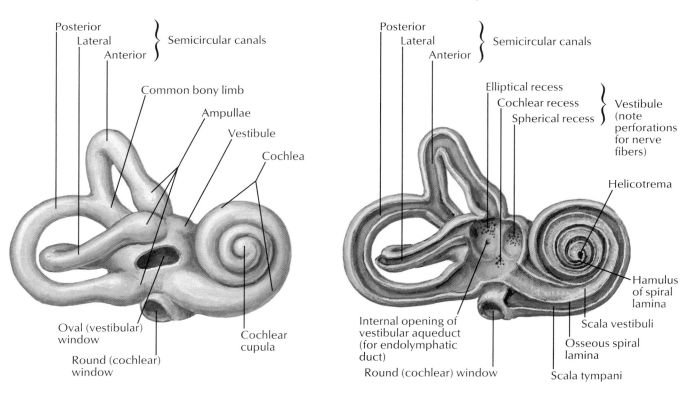

Posterior
Lateral
Anterior } Semicircular canals

Common bony limb

Ampullae

Vestibule

Cochlea

Oval (vestibular) window

Round (cochlear) window

Cochlear cupula

Posterior
Lateral
Anterior } Semicircular canals

Elliptical recess
Cochlear recess
Spherical recess } Vestibule (note perforations for nerve fibers)

Helicotrema

Hamulus of spiral lamina

Scala vestibuli

Osseous spiral lamina

Scala tympani

Internal opening of vestibular aqueduct (for endolymphatic duct)

Round (cochlear) window

**Right membranous labyrinth with nerves: posteromedial view**

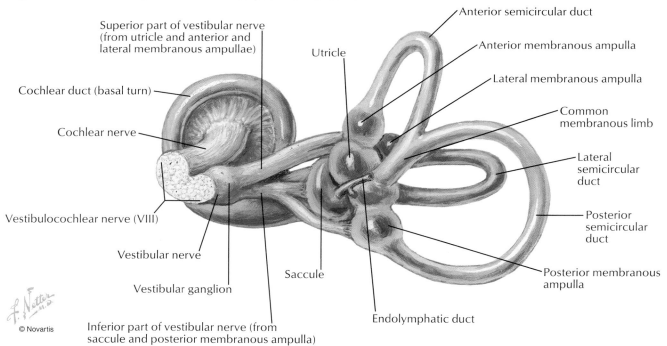

Superior part of vestibular nerve (from utricle and anterior and lateral membranous ampullae)

Utricle

Anterior semicircular duct

Anterior membranous ampulla

Lateral membranous ampulla

Cochlear duct (basal turn)

Common membranous limb

Cochlear nerve

Lateral semicircular duct

Vestibulocochlear nerve (VIII)

Posterior semicircular duct

Vestibular nerve

Saccule

Posterior membranous ampulla

Vestibular ganglion

Endolymphatic duct

Inferior part of vestibular nerve (from saccule and posterior membranous ampulla)

© Novartis

**PLATE 90**

**HEAD AND NECK**

## Bony and membranous labyrinths: schema

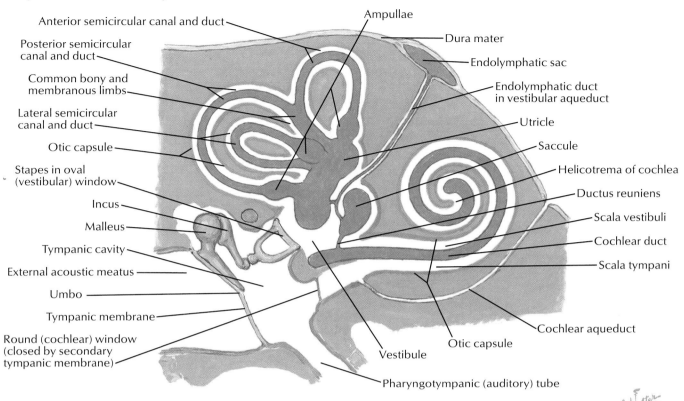

Anterior semicircular canal and duct
Posterior semicircular canal and duct
Common bony and membranous limbs
Lateral semicircular canal and duct
Otic capsule
Stapes in oval (vestibular) window
Incus
Malleus
Tympanic cavity
External acoustic meatus
Umbo
Tympanic membrane
Round (cochlear) window (closed by secondary tympanic membrane)

Ampullae
Dura mater
Endolymphatic sac
Endolymphatic duct in vestibular aqueduct
Utricle
Saccule
Helicotrema of cochlea
Ductus reuniens
Scala vestibuli
Cochlear duct
Scala tympani
Cochlear aqueduct
Otic capsule
Vestibule
Pharyngotympanic (auditory) tube

© Novartis

## Section through turn of cochlea

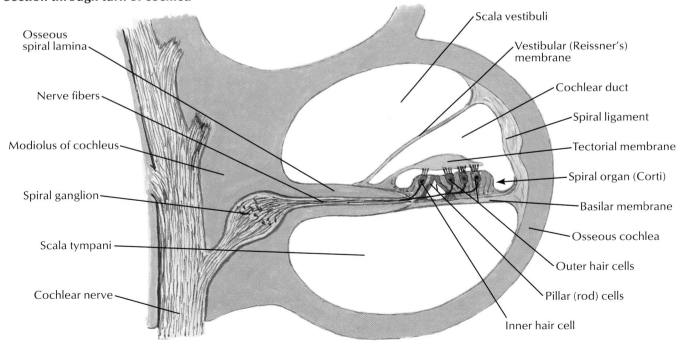

Osseous spiral lamina
Nerve fibers
Modiolus of cochleus
Spiral ganglion
Scala tympani
Cochlear nerve

Scala vestibuli
Vestibular (Reissner's) membrane
Cochlear duct
Spiral ligament
Tectorial membrane
Spiral organ (Corti)
Basilar membrane
Osseous cochlea
Outer hair cells
Pillar (rod) cells
Inner hair cell

# *Orientation of Labyrinth in Skull*

**Superior projection of right bony labyrinth on floor of skull**

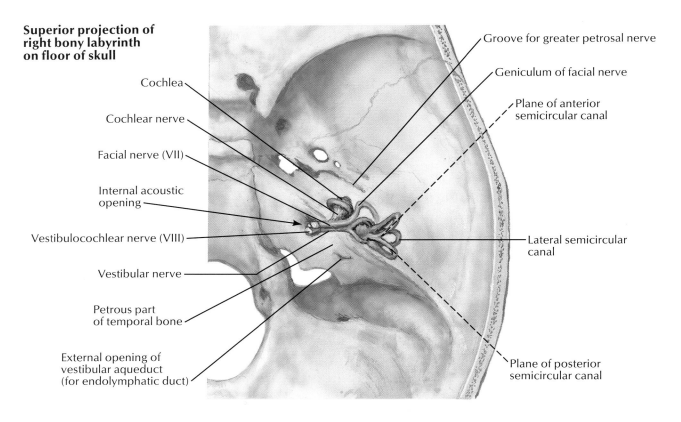

Cochlea

Cochlear nerve

Facial nerve (VII)

Internal acoustic opening

Vestibulocochlear nerve (VIII)

Vestibular nerve

Petrous part of temporal bone

External opening of vestibular aqueduct (for endolymphatic duct)

Groove for greater petrosal nerve

Geniculum of facial nerve

Plane of anterior semicircular canal

Lateral semicircular canal

Plane of posterior semicircular canal

## Lateral projection of right membranous labyrinth

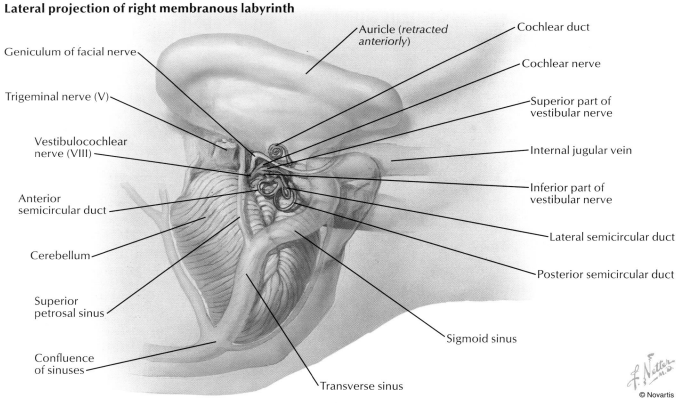

Geniculum of facial nerve

Trigeminal nerve (V)

Vestibulocochlear nerve (VIII)

Anterior semicircular duct

Cerebellum

Superior petrosal sinus

Confluence of sinuses

Auricle (*retracted anteriorly*)

Cochlear duct

Cochlear nerve

Superior part of vestibular nerve

Internal jugular vein

Inferior part of vestibular nerve

Lateral semicircular duct

Posterior semicircular duct

Sigmoid sinus

Transverse sinus

© Novartis

**PLATE 92**

**HEAD AND NECK**

**Cartilaginous part of pharyngotympanic (auditory) tube at base of skull: inferior view**

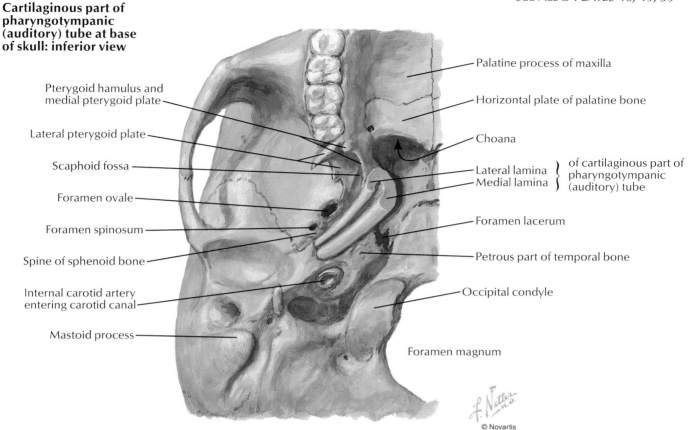

Pterygoid hamulus and medial pterygoid plate

Lateral pterygoid plate

Scaphoid fossa

Foramen ovale

Foramen spinosum

Spine of sphenoid bone

Internal carotid artery entering carotid canal

Mastoid process

Palatine process of maxilla

Horizontal plate of palatine bone

Choana

Lateral lamina
Medial lamina
} of cartilaginous part of pharyngotympanic (auditory) tube

Foramen lacerum

Petrous part of temporal bone

Occipital condyle

Foramen magnum

© Novartis

**Section through cartilaginous part of pharyngotympanic (auditory) tube, with tube closed**

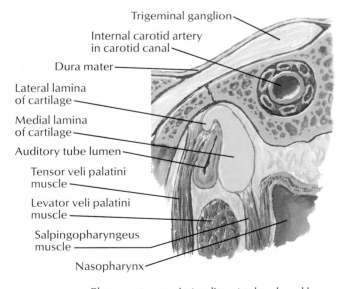

Trigeminal ganglion

Internal carotid artery in carotid canal

Dura mater

Lateral lamina of cartilage

Medial lamina of cartilage

Auditory tube lumen

Tensor veli palatini muscle

Levator veli palatini muscle

Salpingopharyngeus muscle

Nasopharynx

Pharyngotympanic (auditory) tube closed by elastic recoil of cartilage, tissue turgidity and tension of salpingopharyngeus muscles

**Section through cartilaginous part of pharyngotympanic (auditory) tube, with tube open**

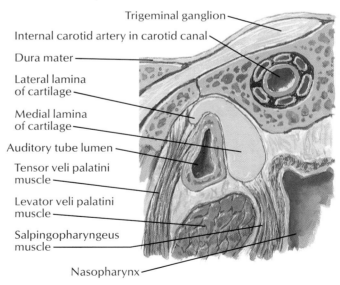

Trigeminal ganglion

Internal carotid artery in carotid canal

Dura mater

Lateral lamina of cartilage

Medial lamina of cartilage

Auditory tube lumen

Tensor veli palatini muscle

Levator veli palatini muscle

Salpingopharyngeus muscle

Nasopharynx

Lumen opened chiefly when attachment of tensor veli palatini muscle pulls wall of tube laterally during swallowing

# Meninges and Diploic Veins

SEE ALSO PLATE 17

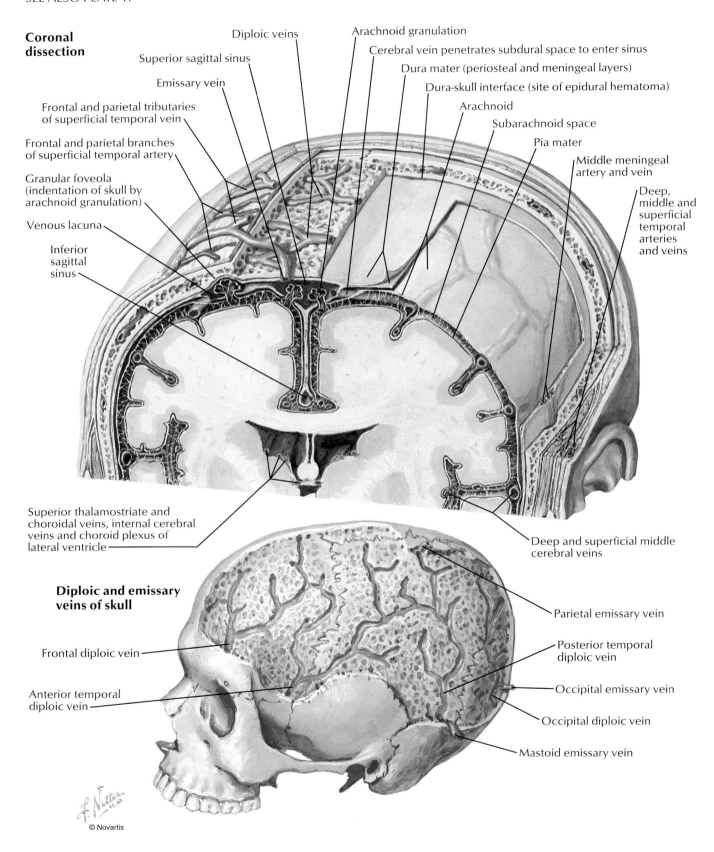

**Coronal dissection**

Diploic veins

Arachnoid granulation

Cerebral vein penetrates subdural space to enter sinus

Superior sagittal sinus

Dura mater (periosteal and meningeal layers)

Emissary vein

Dura-skull interface (site of epidural hematoma)

Frontal and parietal tributaries of superficial temporal vein

Arachnoid

Subarachnoid space

Frontal and parietal branches of superficial temporal artery

Pia mater

Middle meningeal artery and vein

Granular foveola (indentation of skull by arachnoid granulation)

Deep, middle and superficial temporal arteries and veins

Venous lacuna

Inferior sagittal sinus

Superior thalamostriate and choroidal veins, internal cerebral veins and choroid plexus of lateral ventricle

Deep and superficial middle cerebral veins

**Diploic and emissary veins of skull**

Frontal diploic vein

Parietal emissary vein

Posterior temporal diploic vein

Anterior temporal diploic vein

Occipital emissary vein

Occipital diploic vein

Mastoid emissary vein

**PLATE 94**                                                                                   **HEAD AND NECK**

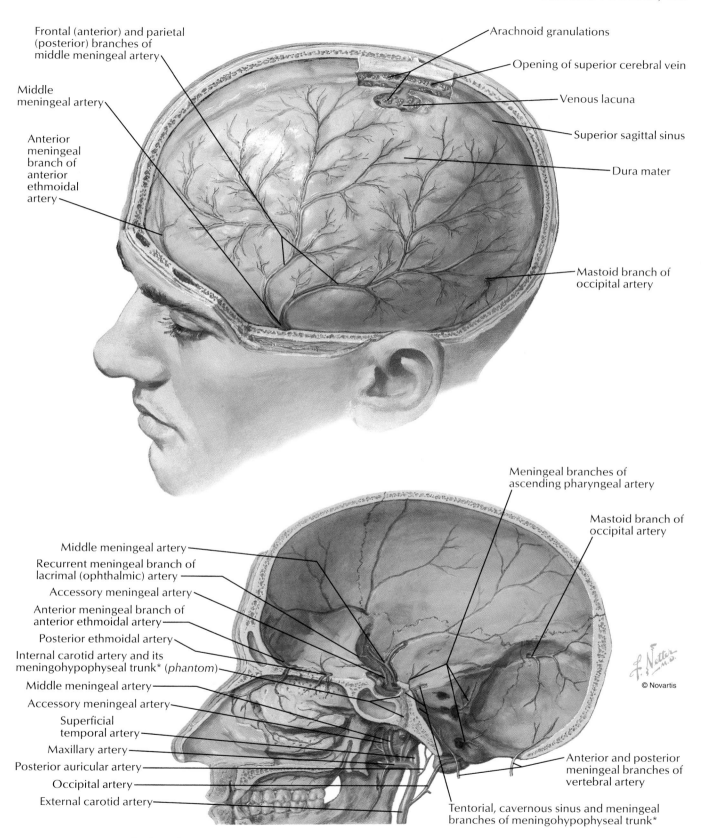

Frontal (anterior) and parietal (posterior) branches of middle meningeal artery

Middle meningeal artery

Anterior meningeal branch of anterior ethmoidal artery

Arachnoid granulations

Opening of superior cerebral vein

Venous lacuna

Superior sagittal sinus

Dura mater

Mastoid branch of occipital artery

Meningeal branches of ascending pharyngeal artery

Mastoid branch of occipital artery

Middle meningeal artery

Recurrent meningeal branch of lacrimal (ophthalmic) artery

Accessory meningeal artery

Anterior meningeal branch of anterior ethmoidal artery

Posterior ethmoidal artery

Internal carotid artery and its meningohypophyseal trunk* (*phantom*)

Middle meningeal artery

Accessory meningeal artery

Superficial temporal artery

Maxillary artery

Posterior auricular artery

Occipital artery

External carotid artery

Anterior and posterior meningeal branches of vertebral artery

Tentorial, cavernous sinus and meningeal branches of meningohypophyseal trunk*

© Novartis

*Variant; most commonly, these branches arise directly from internal carotid artery

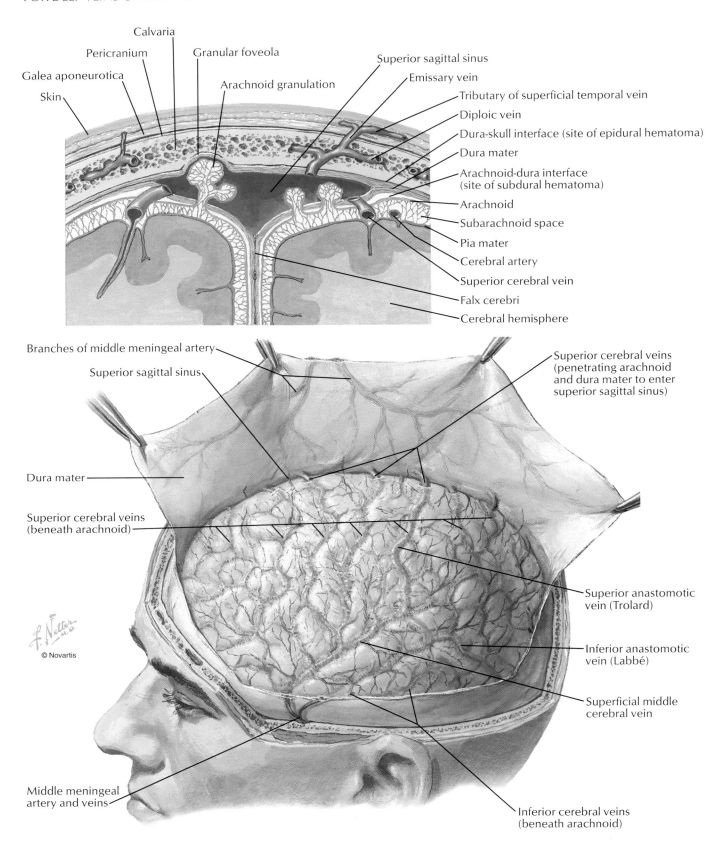

Calvaria

Pericranium

Galea aponeurotica

Granular foveola

Skin

Arachnoid granulation

Superior sagittal sinus

Emissary vein

Tributary of superficial temporal vein

Diploic vein

Dura-skull interface (site of epidural hematoma)

Dura mater

Arachnoid-dura interface (site of subdural hematoma)

Arachnoid

Subarachnoid space

Pia mater

Cerebral artery

Superior cerebral vein

Falx cerebri

Cerebral hemisphere

Branches of middle meningeal artery

Superior sagittal sinus

Superior cerebral veins (penetrating arachnoid and dura mater to enter superior sagittal sinus)

Dura mater

Superior cerebral veins (beneath arachnoid)

Superior anastomotic vein (Trolard)

Inferior anastomotic vein (Labbé)

Superficial middle cerebral vein

Middle meningeal artery and veins

Inferior cerebral veins (beneath arachnoid)

© Novartis

**PLATE 96**

**HEAD AND NECK**

**Sagittal section**

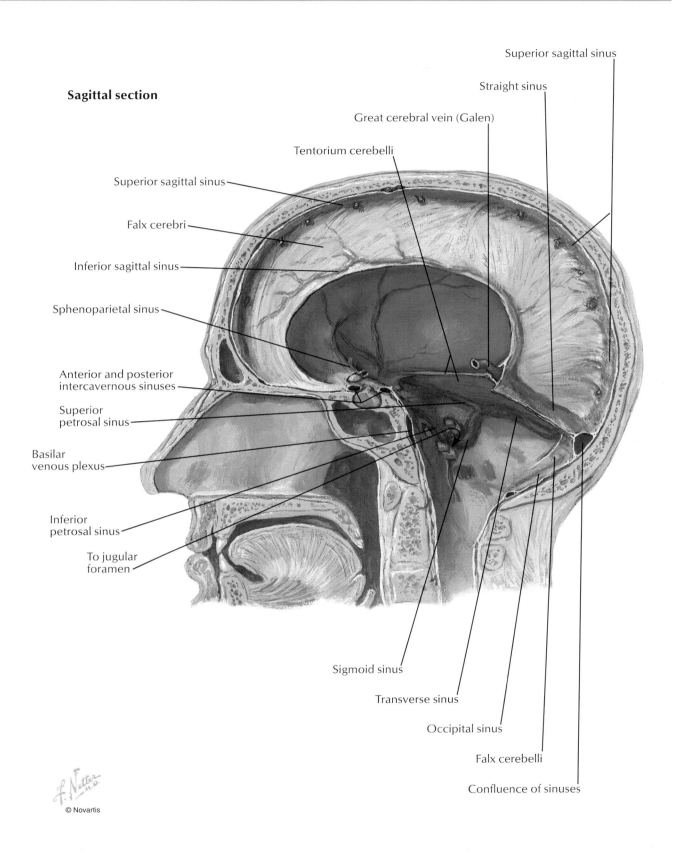

Superior sagittal sinus

Straight sinus

Great cerebral vein (Galen)

Tentorium cerebelli

Superior sagittal sinus

Falx cerebri

Inferior sagittal sinus

Sphenoparietal sinus

Anterior and posterior intercavernous sinuses

Superior petrosal sinus

Basilar venous plexus

Inferior petrosal sinus

To jugular foramen

Sigmoid sinus

Transverse sinus

Occipital sinus

Falx cerebelli

Confluence of sinuses

© Novartis

# *Dural Venous Sinuses (continued)*

*SEE ALSO PLATE 80*

**Skull sectioned horizontally: superior view**

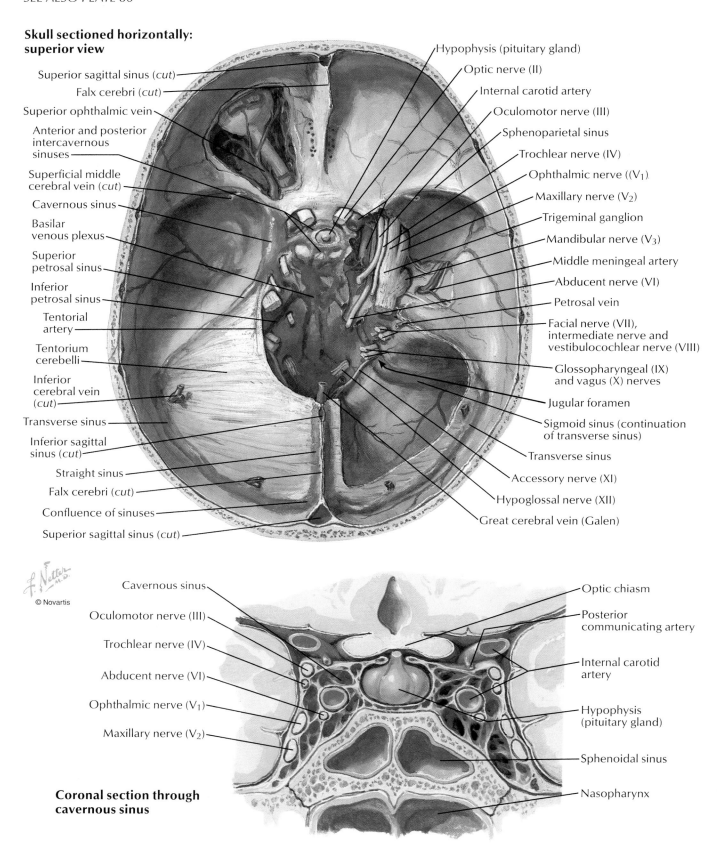

Superior sagittal sinus (*cut*)

Falx cerebri (*cut*)

Superior ophthalmic vein

Anterior and posterior intercavernous sinuses

Superficial middle cerebral vein (*cut*)

Cavernous sinus

Basilar venous plexus

Superior petrosal sinus

Inferior petrosal sinus

Tentorial artery

Tentorium cerebelli

Inferior cerebral vein (*cut*)

Transverse sinus

Inferior sagittal sinus (*cut*)

Straight sinus

Falx cerebri (*cut*)

Confluence of sinuses

Superior sagittal sinus (*cut*)

Hypophysis (pituitary gland)

Optic nerve (II)

Internal carotid artery

Oculomotor nerve (III)

Sphenoparietal sinus

Trochlear nerve (IV)

Ophthalmic nerve ((V₁)

Maxillary nerve (V₂)

Trigeminal ganglion

Mandibular nerve (V₃)

Middle meningeal artery

Abducent nerve (VI)

Petrosal vein

Facial nerve (VII), intermediate nerve and vestibulocochlear nerve (VIII)

Glossopharyngeal (IX) and vagus (X) nerves

Jugular foramen

Sigmoid sinus (continuation of transverse sinus)

Transverse sinus

Accessory nerve (XI)

Hypoglossal nerve (XII)

Great cerebral vein (Galen)

© Novartis

Cavernous sinus

Oculomotor nerve (III)

Trochlear nerve (IV)

Abducent nerve (VI)

Ophthalmic nerve (V₁)

Maxillary nerve (V₂)

**Coronal section through cavernous sinus**

Optic chiasm

Posterior communicating artery

Internal carotid artery

Hypophysis (pituitary gland)

Sphenoidal sinus

Nasopharynx

*PLATE 98*

**HEAD AND NECK**

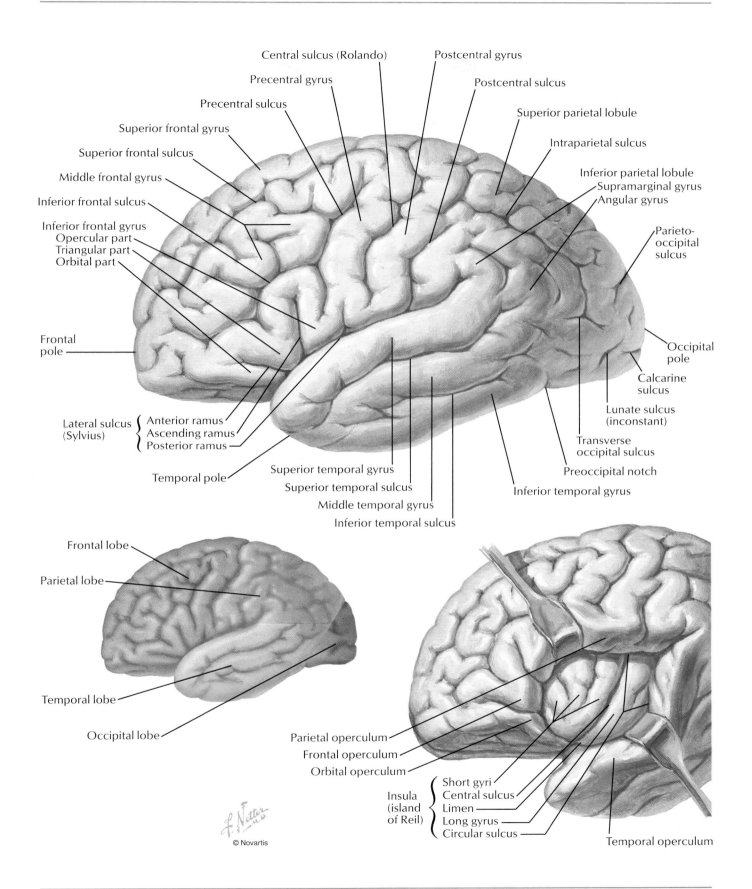

Central sulcus (Rolando)

Postcentral gyrus

Precentral gyrus

Postcentral sulcus

Precentral sulcus

Superior parietal lobule

Superior frontal gyrus

Intraparietal sulcus

Superior frontal sulcus

Inferior parietal lobule
Supramarginal gyrus
Angular gyrus

Middle frontal gyrus

Inferior frontal sulcus

Inferior frontal gyrus
Opercular part
Triangular part
Orbital part

Parieto-occipital sulcus

Frontal pole

Occipital pole

Calcarine sulcus

Lunate sulcus (inconstant)

Lateral sulcus (Sylvius) { Anterior ramus
Ascending ramus
Posterior ramus

Transverse occipital sulcus

Temporal pole

Preoccipital notch

Superior temporal gyrus

Inferior temporal gyrus

Superior temporal sulcus

Middle temporal gyrus

Inferior temporal sulcus

Frontal lobe

Parietal lobe

Temporal lobe

Occipital lobe

Parietal operculum

Frontal operculum

Orbital operculum

Insula (island of Reil) { Short gyri
Central sulcus
Limen
Long gyrus
Circular sulcus

Temporal operculum

© Novartis

*FOR HYPOPHYSIS SEE PLATE 140*

**Sagittal section of brain in situ**

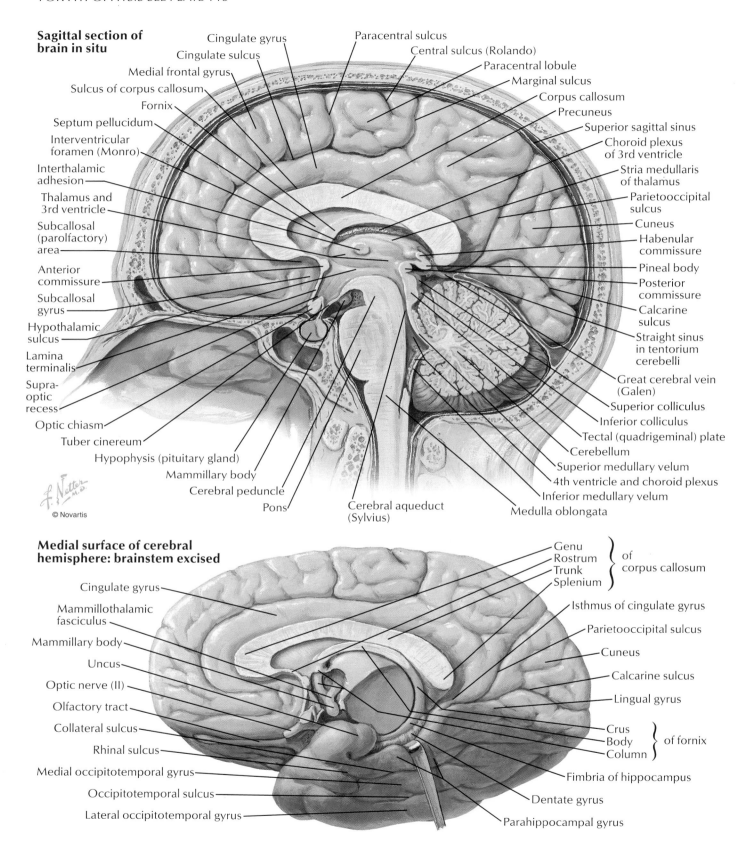

Cingulate gyrus
Paracentral sulcus
Central sulcus (Rolando)
Cingulate sulcus
Paracentral lobule
Medial frontal gyrus
Marginal sulcus
Sulcus of corpus callosum
Corpus callosum
Fornix
Precuneus
Septum pellucidum
Superior sagittal sinus
Interventricular foramen (Monro)
Choroid plexus of 3rd ventricle
Interthalamic adhesion
Stria medullaris of thalamus
Thalamus and 3rd ventricle
Parietooccipital sulcus
Subcallosal (parolfactory) area
Cuneus
Anterior commissure
Habenular commissure
Subcallosal gyrus
Pineal body
Posterior commissure
Hypothalamic sulcus
Calcarine sulcus
Lamina terminalis
Straight sinus in tentorium cerebelli
Supra-optic recess
Great cerebral vein (Galen)
Optic chiasm
Superior colliculus
Tuber cinereum
Inferior colliculus
Tectal (quadrigeminal) plate
Hypophysis (pituitary gland)
Cerebellum
Mammillary body
Superior medullary velum
Cerebral peduncle
4th ventricle and choroid plexus
Pons
Inferior medullary velum
Cerebral aqueduct (Sylvius)
Medulla oblongata

*f. Netter M.D.*

© Novartis

**Medial surface of cerebral hemisphere: brainstem excised**

Genu
Rostrum
Trunk
Splenium
} of corpus callosum

Cingulate gyrus
Mammillothalamic fasciculus
Isthmus of cingulate gyrus
Mammillary body
Parietooccipital sulcus
Uncus
Cuneus
Optic nerve (II)
Calcarine sulcus
Olfactory tract
Lingual gyrus
Collateral sulcus
Crus
Body
Column
} of fornix
Rhinal sulcus
Medial occipitotemporal gyrus
Fimbria of hippocampus
Occipitotemporal sulcus
Dentate gyrus
Lateral occipitotemporal gyrus
Parahippocampal gyrus

**PLATE 100**

**HEAD AND NECK**

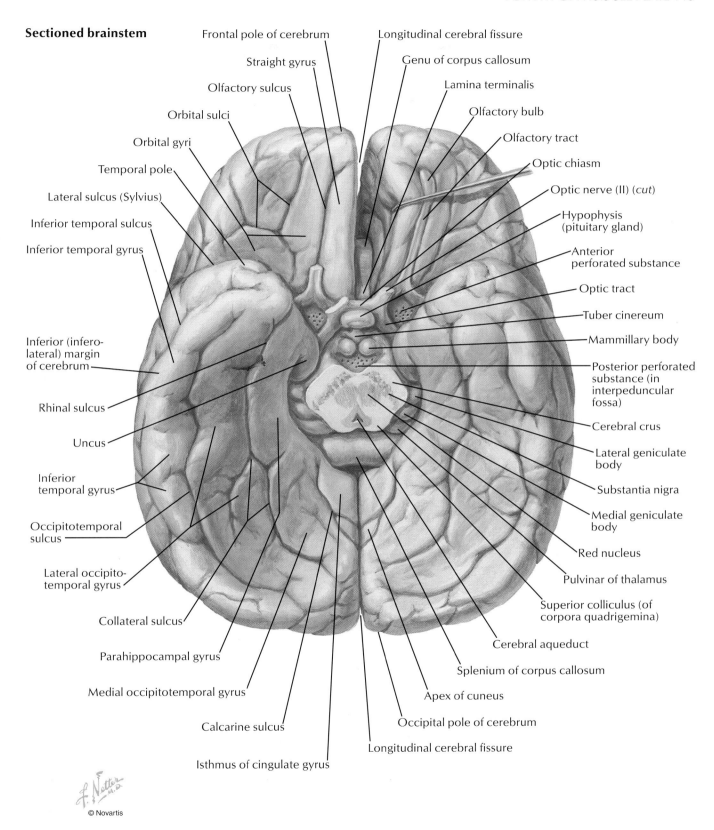

Sectioned brainstem

Frontal pole of cerebrum

Straight gyrus

Olfactory sulcus

Orbital sulci

Orbital gyri

Temporal pole

Lateral sulcus (Sylvius)

Inferior temporal sulcus

Inferior temporal gyrus

Inferior (infero-lateral) margin of cerebrum

Rhinal sulcus

Uncus

Inferior temporal gyrus

Occipitotemporal sulcus

Lateral occipito-temporal gyrus

Collateral sulcus

Parahippocampal gyrus

Medial occipitotemporal gyrus

Calcarine sulcus

Isthmus of cingulate gyrus

Longitudinal cerebral fissure

Genu of corpus callosum

Lamina terminalis

Olfactory bulb

Olfactory tract

Optic chiasm

Optic nerve (II) (cut)

Hypophysis (pituitary gland)

Anterior perforated substance

Optic tract

Tuber cinereum

Mammillary body

Posterior perforated substance (in interpeduncular fossa)

Cerebral crus

Lateral geniculate body

Substantia nigra

Medial geniculate body

Red nucleus

Pulvinar of thalamus

Superior colliculus (of corpora quadrigemina)

Cerebral aqueduct

Splenium of corpus callosum

Apex of cuneus

Occipital pole of cerebrum

Longitudinal cerebral fissure

© Novartis

# *Ventricles of Brain*

**Left lateral phantom view**

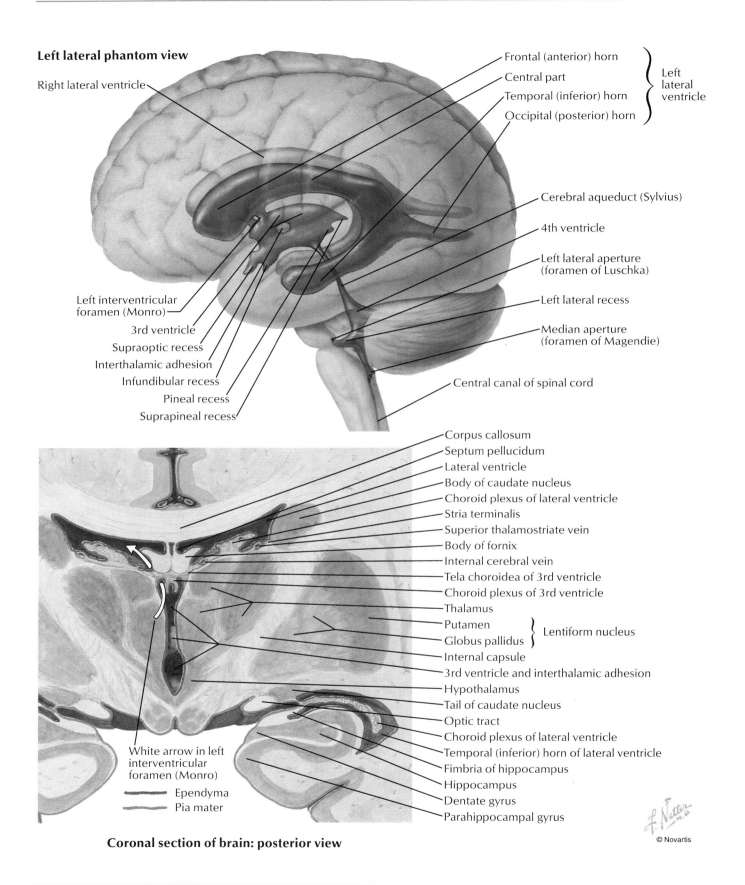

Right lateral ventricle

Frontal (anterior) horn
Central part
Temporal (inferior) horn
Occipital (posterior) horn

Left lateral ventricle

Cerebral aqueduct (Sylvius)

4th ventricle

Left lateral aperture (foramen of Luschka)

Left lateral recess

Median aperture (foramen of Magendie)

Central canal of spinal cord

Left interventricular foramen (Monro)
3rd ventricle
Supraoptic recess
Interthalamic adhesion
Infundibular recess
Pineal recess
Suprapineal recess

Corpus callosum
Septum pellucidum
Lateral ventricle
Body of caudate nucleus
Choroid plexus of lateral ventricle
Stria terminalis
Superior thalamostriate vein
Body of fornix
Internal cerebral vein
Tela choroidea of 3rd ventricle
Choroid plexus of 3rd ventricle
Thalamus
Putamen
Globus pallidus

Lentiform nucleus

Internal capsule
3rd ventricle and interthalamic adhesion
Hypothalamus
Tail of caudate nucleus
Optic tract
Choroid plexus of lateral ventricle
Temporal (inferior) horn of lateral ventricle
Fimbria of hippocampus
Hippocampus
Dentate gyrus
Parahippocampal gyrus

White arrow in left interventricular foramen (Monro)

Ependyma
Pia mater

**Coronal section of brain: posterior view**

© Novartis

*PLATE 102*

**HEAD AND NECK**

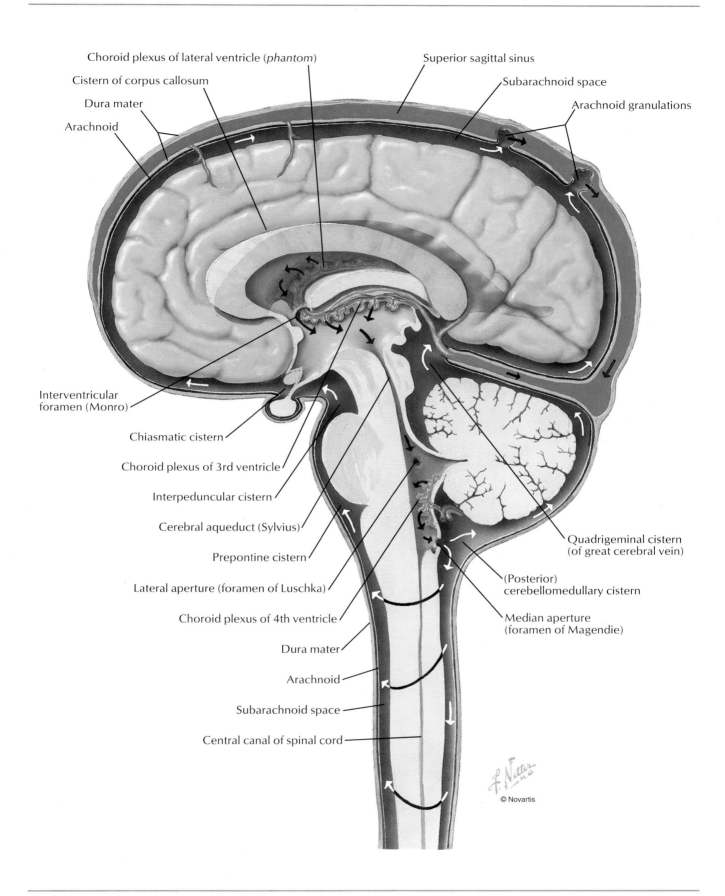

Choroid plexus of lateral ventricle (*phantom*)

Cistern of corpus callosum

Dura mater

Arachnoid

Superior sagittal sinus

Subarachnoid space

Arachnoid granulations

Interventricular foramen (Monro)

Chiasmatic cistern

Choroid plexus of 3rd ventricle

Interpeduncular cistern

Cerebral aqueduct (Sylvius)

Prepontine cistern

Lateral aperture (foramen of Luschka)

Choroid plexus of 4th ventricle

Dura mater

Arachnoid

Subarachnoid space

Central canal of spinal cord

Quadrigeminal cistern (of great cerebral vein)

(Posterior) cerebellomedullary cistern

Median aperture (foramen of Magendie)

© Novartis

# Basal Nuclei (Ganglia)

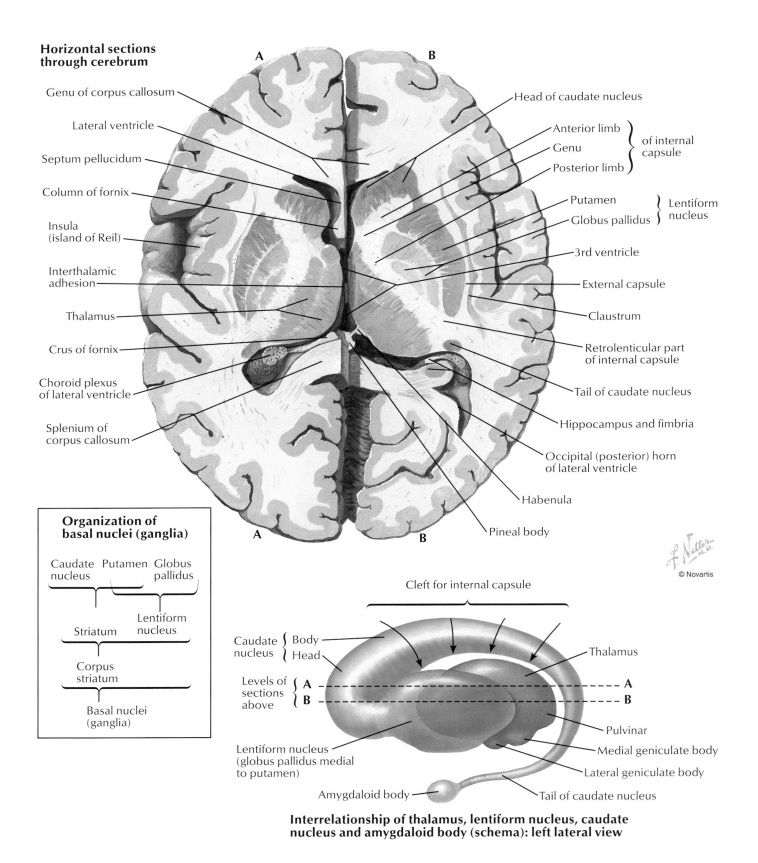

**Horizontal sections through cerebrum**

A  B

Genu of corpus callosum

Lateral ventricle

Septum pellucidum

Column of fornix

Insula (island of Reil)

Interthalamic adhesion

Thalamus

Crus of fornix

Choroid plexus of lateral ventricle

Splenium of corpus callosum

Head of caudate nucleus

Anterior limb
Genu
Posterior limb } of internal capsule

Putamen
Globus pallidus } Lentiform nucleus

3rd ventricle

External capsule

Claustrum

Retrolenticular part of internal capsule

Tail of caudate nucleus

Hippocampus and fimbria

Occipital (posterior) horn of lateral ventricle

Habenula

Pineal body

A  B

© Novartis

**Organization of basal nuclei (ganglia)**

Caudate nucleus   Putamen   Globus pallidus

Lentiform nucleus

Striatum

Corpus striatum

Basal nuclei (ganglia)

Cleft for internal capsule

Caudate nucleus { Body
Head

Thalamus

Levels of sections above { A
B

A
B

Pulvinar

Medial geniculate body

Lateral geniculate body

Lentiform nucleus (globus pallidus medial to putamen)

Amygdaloid body

Tail of caudate nucleus

**Interrelationship of thalamus, lentiform nucleus, caudate nucleus and amygdaloid body (schema): left lateral view**

PLATE 104

HEAD AND NECK

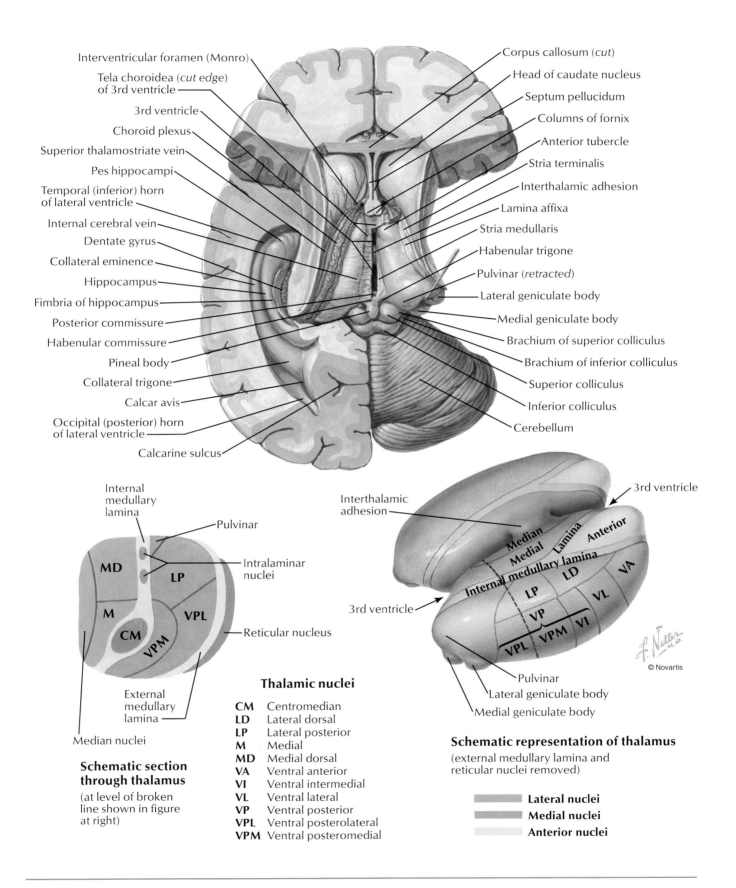

Interventricular foramen (Monro)

Tela choroidea (*cut edge*) of 3rd ventricle

3rd ventricle

Choroid plexus

Superior thalamostriate vein

Pes hippocampi

Temporal (inferior) horn of lateral ventricle

Internal cerebral vein

Dentate gyrus

Collateral eminence

Hippocampus

Fimbria of hippocampus

Posterior commissure

Habenular commissure

Pineal body

Collateral trigone

Calcar avis

Occipital (posterior) horn of lateral ventricle

Calcarine sulcus

Corpus callosum (*cut*)

Head of caudate nucleus

Septum pellucidum

Columns of fornix

Anterior tubercle

Stria terminalis

Interthalamic adhesion

Lamina affixa

Stria medullaris

Habenular trigone

Pulvinar (*retracted*)

Lateral geniculate body

Medial geniculate body

Brachium of superior colliculus

Brachium of inferior colliculus

Superior colliculus

Inferior colliculus

Cerebellum

Internal medullary lamina

Pulvinar

Intralaminar nuclei

Reticular nucleus

MD

LP

M

VPL

CM

VPM

External medullary lamina

Median nuclei

Interthalamic adhesion

3rd ventricle

Median

Medial

Anterior

Lamina

Internal medullary lamina

LD

VA

LP

VL

VP

VPM

VI

VPL

3rd ventricle

Pulvinar

Lateral geniculate body

Medial geniculate body

**Thalamic nuclei**

| | |
|---|---|
| **CM** | Centromedian |
| **LD** | Lateral dorsal |
| **LP** | Lateral posterior |
| **M** | Medial |
| **MD** | Medial dorsal |
| **VA** | Ventral anterior |
| **VI** | Ventral intermedial |
| **VL** | Ventral lateral |
| **VP** | Ventral posterior |
| **VPL** | Ventral posterolateral |
| **VPM** | Ventral posteromedial |

**Schematic section through thalamus**

(at level of broken line shown in figure at right)

**Schematic representation of thalamus**

(external medullary lamina and reticular nuclei removed)

Lateral nuclei

Medial nuclei

Anterior nuclei

© Novartis

**MENINGES AND BRAIN**

**PLATE 105**

# Hippocampus and Fornix

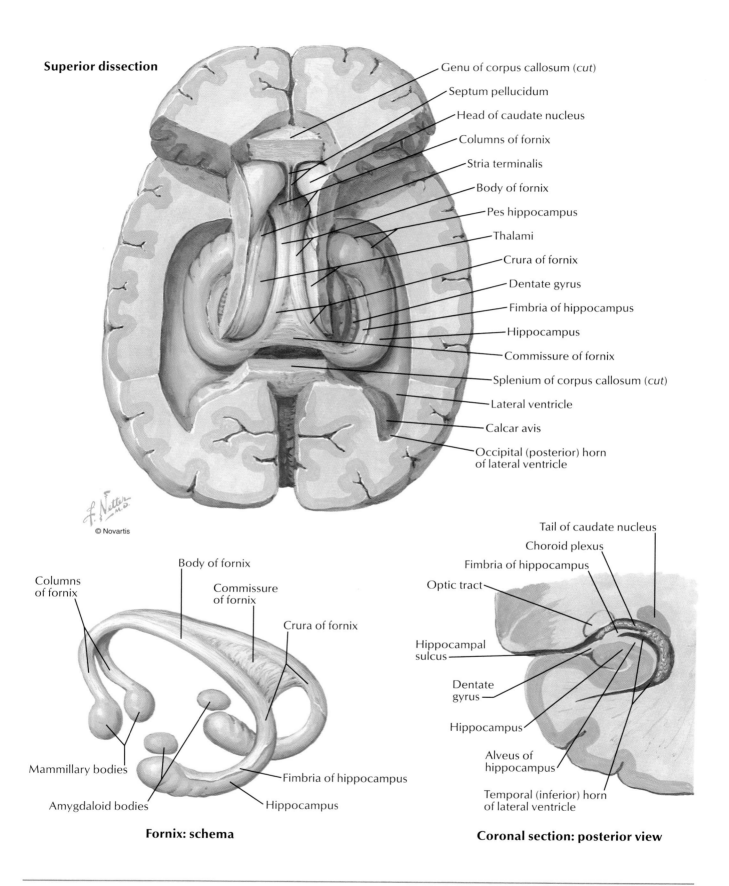

**Superior dissection**

Genu of corpus callosum (*cut*)

Septum pellucidum

Head of caudate nucleus

Columns of fornix

Stria terminalis

Body of fornix

Pes hippocampus

Thalami

Crura of fornix

Dentate gyrus

Fimbria of hippocampus

Hippocampus

Commissure of fornix

Splenium of corpus callosum (*cut*)

Lateral ventricle

Calcar avis

Occipital (posterior) horn
of lateral ventricle

© Novartis

Columns
of fornix

Body of fornix

Commissure
of fornix

Crura of fornix

Mammillary bodies

Amygdaloid bodies

Fimbria of hippocampus

Hippocampus

**Fornix: schema**

Tail of caudate nucleus

Choroid plexus

Fimbria of hippocampus

Optic tract

Hippocampal
sulcus

Dentate
gyrus

Hippocampus

Alveus of
hippocampus

Temporal (inferior) horn
of lateral ventricle

**Coronal section: posterior view**

**PLATE 106**

**HEAD AND NECK**

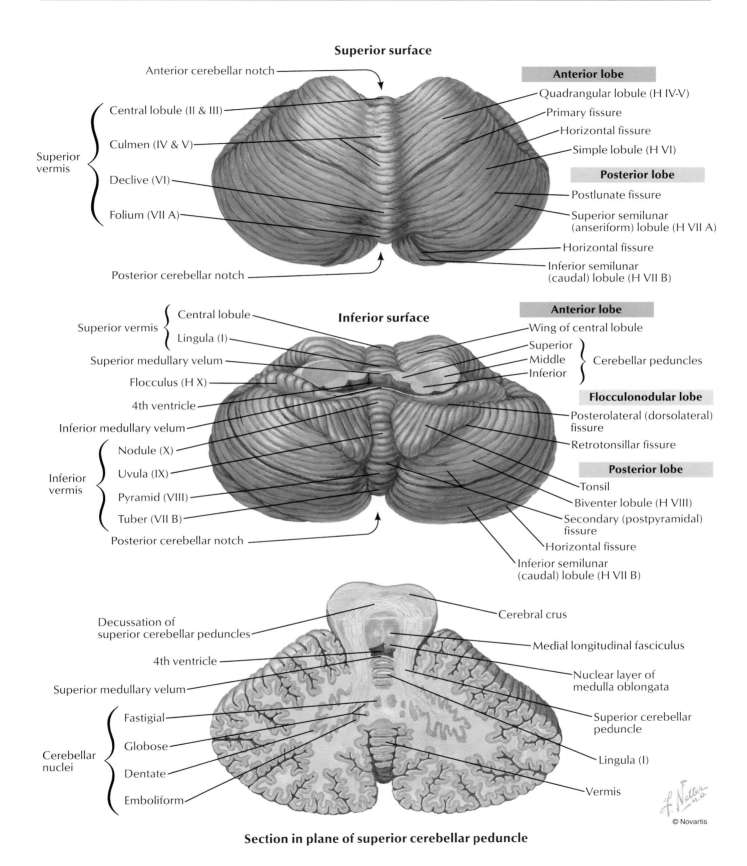

**Superior surface**

Anterior cerebellar notch

**Anterior lobe**

Central lobule (II & III)

Quadrangular lobule (H IV-V)

Culmen (IV & V)

Primary fissure

Superior vermis

Horizontal fissure

Declive (VI)

Simple lobule (H VI)

Folium (VII A)

**Posterior lobe**

Postlunate fissure

Superior semilunar (anseriform) lobule (H VII A)

Posterior cerebellar notch

Horizontal fissure

Inferior semilunar (caudal) lobule (H VII B)

**Inferior surface**

**Anterior lobe**

Superior vermis — Central lobule

Wing of central lobule

Lingula (I)

Superior

Superior medullary velum

Middle — Cerebellar peduncles

Flocculus (H X)

Inferior

4th ventricle

**Flocculonodular lobe**

Inferior medullary velum

Posterolateral (dorsolateral) fissure

Nodule (X)

Retrotonsillar fissure

Inferior vermis — Uvula (IX)

**Posterior lobe**

Pyramid (VIII)

Tonsil

Tuber (VII B)

Biventer lobule (H VIII)

Posterior cerebellar notch

Secondary (postpyramidal) fissure

Horizontal fissure

Inferior semilunar (caudal) lobule (H VII B)

Decussation of superior cerebellar peduncles

Cerebral crus

4th ventricle

Medial longitudinal fasciculus

Superior medullary velum

Nuclear layer of medulla oblongata

Cerebellar nuclei — Fastigial

Globose

Superior cerebellar peduncle

Dentate

Lingula (I)

Emboliform

Vermis

**Section in plane of superior cerebellar peduncle**

# *Brainstem*

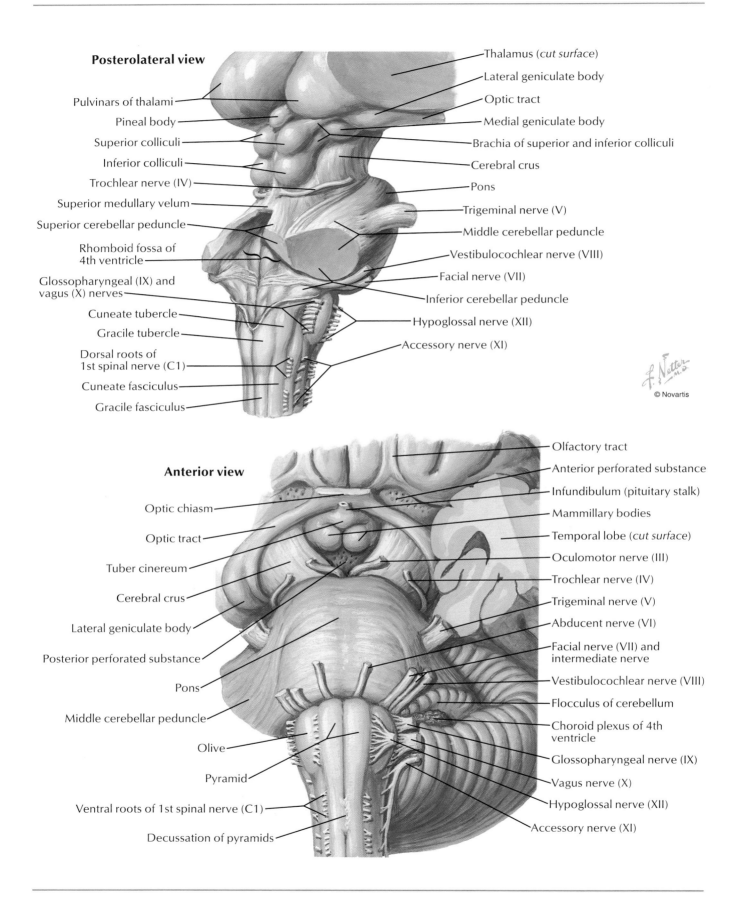

**Posterolateral view**

Pulvinars of thalami

Pineal body

Superior colliculi

Inferior colliculi

Trochlear nerve (IV)

Superior medullary velum

Superior cerebellar peduncle

Rhomboid fossa of 4th ventricle

Glossopharyngeal (IX) and vagus (X) nerves

Cuneate tubercle

Gracile tubercle

Dorsal roots of 1st spinal nerve (C1)

Cuneate fasciculus

Gracile fasciculus

Thalamus (*cut surface*)

Lateral geniculate body

Optic tract

Medial geniculate body

Brachia of superior and inferior colliculi

Cerebral crus

Pons

Trigeminal nerve (V)

Middle cerebellar peduncle

Vestibulocochlear nerve (VIII)

Facial nerve (VII)

Inferior cerebellar peduncle

Hypoglossal nerve (XII)

Accessory nerve (XI)

**Anterior view**

Optic chiasm

Optic tract

Tuber cinereum

Cerebral crus

Lateral geniculate body

Posterior perforated substance

Pons

Middle cerebellar peduncle

Olive

Pyramid

Ventral roots of 1st spinal nerve (C1)

Decussation of pyramids

Olfactory tract

Anterior perforated substance

Infundibulum (pituitary stalk)

Mammillary bodies

Temporal lobe (*cut surface*)

Oculomotor nerve (III)

Trochlear nerve (IV)

Trigeminal nerve (V)

Abducent nerve (VI)

Facial nerve (VII) and intermediate nerve

Vestibulocochlear nerve (VIII)

Flocculus of cerebellum

Choroid plexus of 4th ventricle

Glossopharyngeal nerve (IX)

Vagus nerve (X)

Hypoglossal nerve (XII)

Accessory nerve (XI)

*f. Netter M.D.*

© Novartis

*PLATE 108*

**HEAD AND NECK**

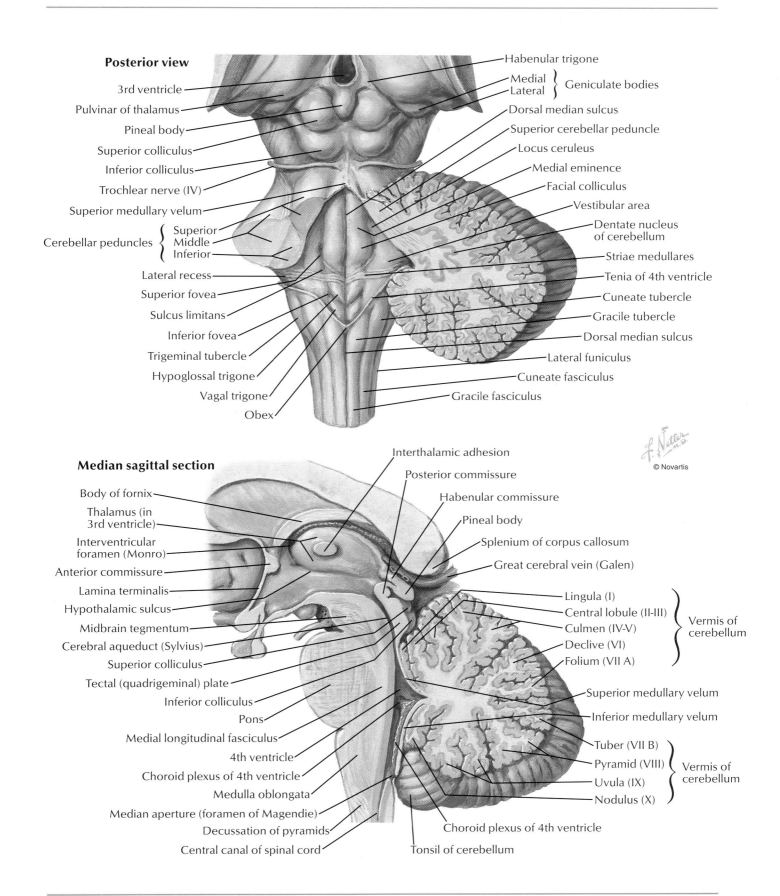

**Posterior view**

- Habenular trigone
- Medial } Geniculate bodies
- Lateral }
- 3rd ventricle
- Pulvinar of thalamus
- Pineal body
- Superior colliculus
- Inferior colliculus
- Trochlear nerve (IV)
- Superior medullary velum
- Cerebellar peduncles { Superior / Middle / Inferior
- Lateral recess
- Superior fovea
- Sulcus limitans
- Inferior fovea
- Trigeminal tubercle
- Hypoglossal trigone
- Vagal trigone
- Obex
- Dorsal median sulcus
- Superior cerebellar peduncle
- Locus ceruleus
- Medial eminence
- Facial colliculus
- Vestibular area
- Dentate nucleus of cerebellum
- Striae medullares
- Tenia of 4th ventricle
- Cuneate tubercle
- Gracile tubercle
- Dorsal median sulcus
- Lateral funiculus
- Cuneate fasciculus
- Gracile fasciculus

*F. Netter M.D.*
© Novartis

**Median sagittal section**

- Interthalamic adhesion
- Posterior commissure
- Habenular commissure
- Pineal body
- Splenium of corpus callosum
- Great cerebral vein (Galen)
- Body of fornix
- Thalamus (in 3rd ventricle)
- Interventricular foramen (Monro)
- Anterior commissure
- Lamina terminalis
- Hypothalamic sulcus
- Midbrain tegmentum
- Cerebral aqueduct (Sylvius)
- Superior colliculus
- Tectal (quadrigeminal) plate
- Inferior colliculus
- Pons
- Medial longitudinal fasciculus
- 4th ventricle
- Choroid plexus of 4th ventricle
- Medulla oblongata
- Median aperture (foramen of Magendie)
- Decussation of pyramids
- Central canal of spinal cord
- Lingula (I)
- Central lobule (II-III)
- Culmen (IV-V) } Vermis of cerebellum
- Declive (VI)
- Folium (VII A)
- Superior medullary velum
- Inferior medullary velum
- Tuber (VII B)
- Pyramid (VIII) } Vermis of cerebellum
- Uvula (IX)
- Nodulus (X)
- Choroid plexus of 4th ventricle
- Tonsil of cerebellum

# Cranial Nerve Nuclei in Brainstem: Schema

**Posterior phantom view**

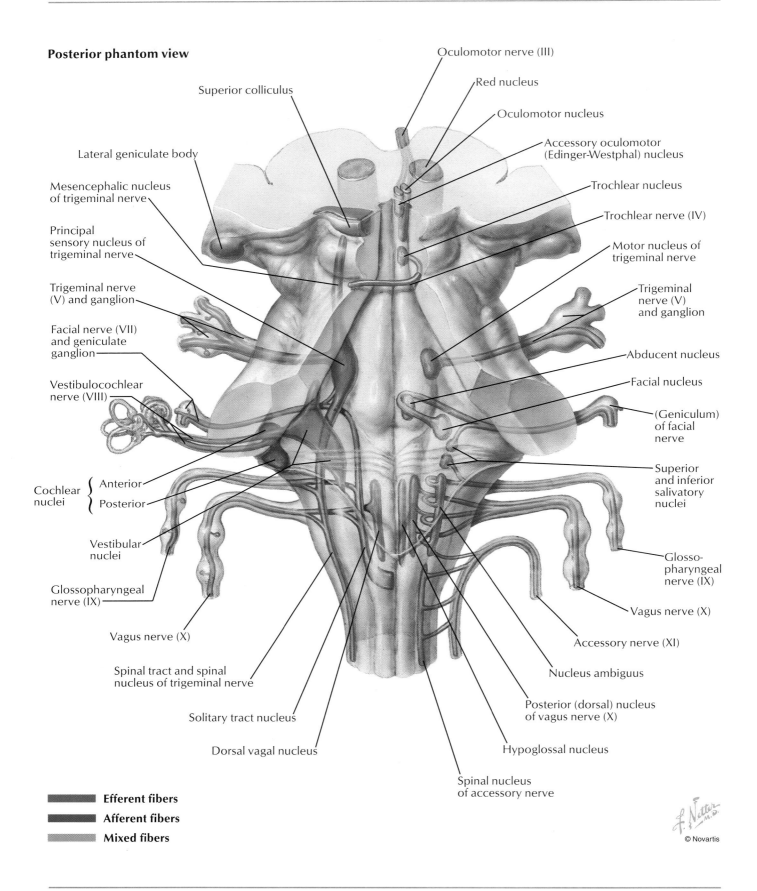

Oculomotor nerve (III)

Red nucleus

Oculomotor nucleus

Superior colliculus

Accessory oculomotor
(Edinger-Westphal) nucleus

Lateral geniculate body

Trochlear nucleus

Mesencephalic nucleus
of trigeminal nerve

Trochlear nerve (IV)

Principal
sensory nucleus of
trigeminal nerve

Motor nucleus of
trigeminal nerve

Trigeminal nerve
(V) and ganglion

Trigeminal
nerve (V)
and ganglion

Facial nerve (VII)
and geniculate
ganglion

Abducent nucleus

Facial nucleus

Vestibulocochlear
nerve (VIII)

(Geniculum)
of facial
nerve

Cochlear { Anterior
nuclei { Posterior

Superior
and inferior
salivatory
nuclei

Vestibular
nuclei

Glosso-
pharyngeal
nerve (IX)

Glossopharyngeal
nerve (IX)

Vagus nerve (X)

Vagus nerve (X)

Accessory nerve (XI)

Spinal tract and spinal
nucleus of trigeminal nerve

Nucleus ambiguus

Posterior (dorsal) nucleus
of vagus nerve (X)

Solitary tract nucleus

Hypoglossal nucleus

Dorsal vagal nucleus

Spinal nucleus
of accessory nerve

▬▬ **Efferent fibers**
▬▬ **Afferent fibers**
▬▬ **Mixed fibers**

© Novartis

**PLATE 110**

**HEAD AND NECK**

**Medial dissection**

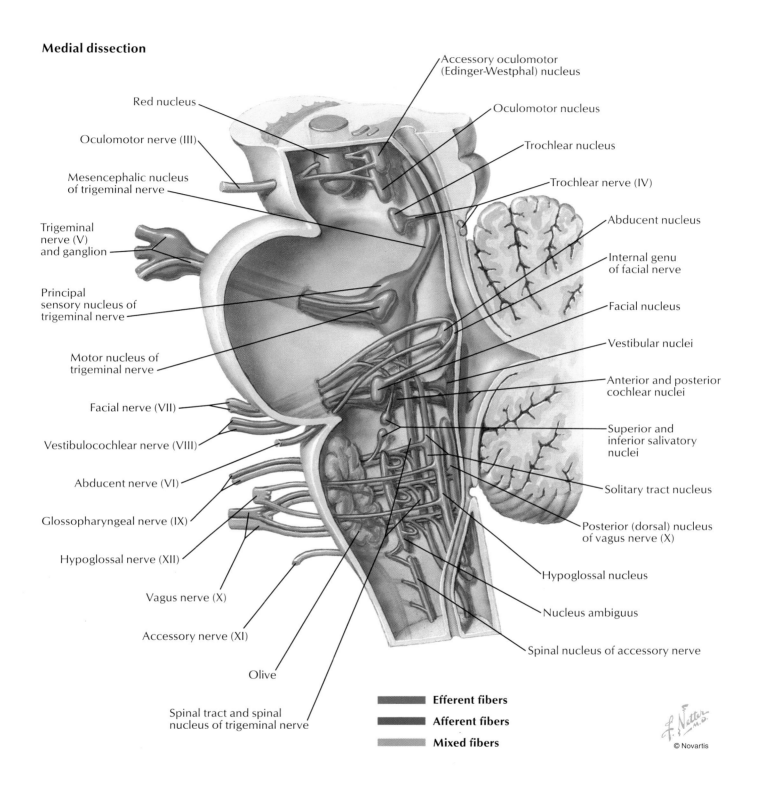

Accessory oculomotor (Edinger-Westphal) nucleus

Red nucleus

Oculomotor nucleus

Oculomotor nerve (III)

Trochlear nucleus

Mesencephalic nucleus of trigeminal nerve

Trochlear nerve (IV)

Trigeminal nerve (V) and ganglion

Abducent nucleus

Internal genu of facial nerve

Principal sensory nucleus of trigeminal nerve

Facial nucleus

Vestibular nuclei

Motor nucleus of trigeminal nerve

Anterior and posterior cochlear nuclei

Facial nerve (VII)

Superior and inferior salivatory nuclei

Vestibulocochlear nerve (VIII)

Abducent nerve (VI)

Solitary tract nucleus

Glossopharyngeal nerve (IX)

Posterior (dorsal) nucleus of vagus nerve (X)

Hypoglossal nerve (XII)

Hypoglossal nucleus

Vagus nerve (X)

Nucleus ambiguus

Accessory nerve (XI)

Spinal nucleus of accessory nerve

Olive

Efferent fibers

Afferent fibers

Spinal tract and spinal nucleus of trigeminal nerve

Mixed fibers

© Novartis

# Cranial Nerves (Motor and Sensory Distribution): Schema

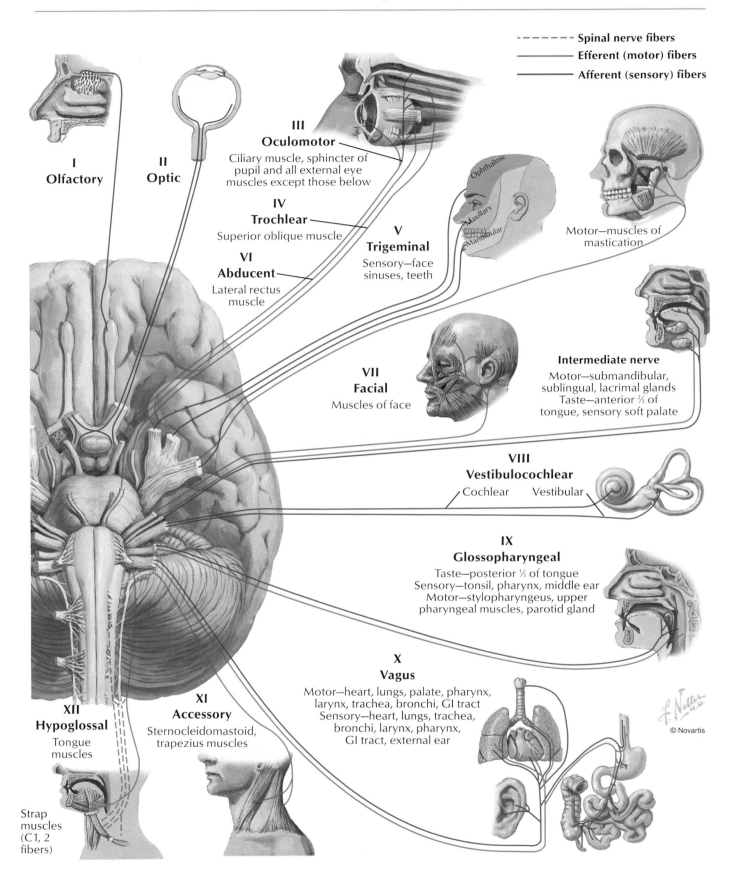

Spinal nerve fibers
Efferent (motor) fibers
Afferent (sensory) fibers

**I**
**Olfactory**

**II**
**Optic**

**III**
**Oculomotor**
Ciliary muscle, sphincter of pupil and all external eye muscles except those below

**IV**
**Trochlear**
Superior oblique muscle

**VI**
**Abducent**
Lateral rectus muscle

Ophthalmic
Maxillary
Mandibular

**V**
**Trigeminal**
Sensory—face sinuses, teeth

Motor—muscles of mastication

**VII**
**Facial**
Muscles of face

**Intermediate nerve**
Motor—submandibular, sublingual, lacrimal glands
Taste—anterior ⅔ of tongue, sensory soft palate

**VIII**
**Vestibulocochlear**
Cochlear    Vestibular

**IX**
**Glossopharyngeal**
Taste—posterior ⅓ of tongue
Sensory—tonsil, pharynx, middle ear
Motor—stylopharyngeus, upper pharyngeal muscles, parotid gland

**X**
**Vagus**
Motor—heart, lungs, palate, pharynx, larynx, trachea, bronchi, GI tract
Sensory—heart, lungs, trachea, bronchi, larynx, pharynx, GI tract, external ear

**XII**
**Hypoglossal**
Tongue muscles

Strap muscles (C1, 2 fibers)

**XI**
**Accessory**
Sternocleidomastoid, trapezius muscles

© Novartis

**PLATE 112**

**HEAD AND NECK**

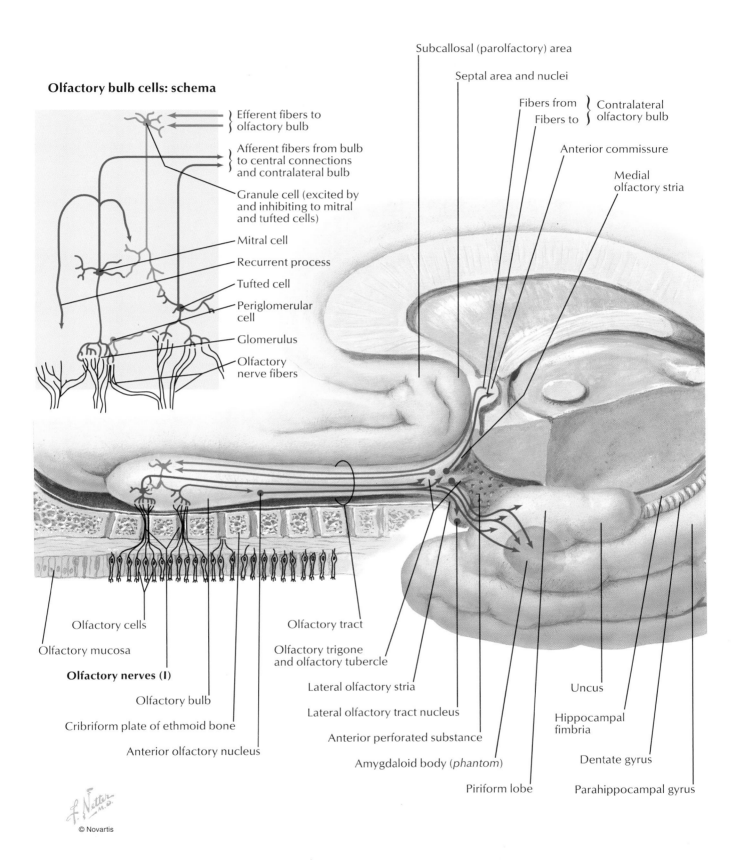

**Olfactory bulb cells: schema**

Efferent fibers to olfactory bulb

Afferent fibers from bulb to central connections and contralateral bulb

Granule cell (excited by and inhibiting to mitral and tufted cells)

Mitral cell

Recurrent process

Tufted cell

Periglomerular cell

Glomerulus

Olfactory nerve fibers

Subcallosal (parolfactory) area

Septal area and nuclei

Fibers from } Contralateral
Fibers to } olfactory bulb

Anterior commissure

Medial olfactory stria

Olfactory cells

Olfactory mucosa

**Olfactory nerves (I)**

Olfactory bulb

Cribriform plate of ethmoid bone

Anterior olfactory nucleus

Olfactory tract

Olfactory trigone and olfactory tubercle

Lateral olfactory stria

Lateral olfactory tract nucleus

Anterior perforated substance

Amygdaloid body (*phantom*)

Piriform lobe

Uncus

Hippocampal fimbria

Dentate gyrus

Parahippocampal gyrus

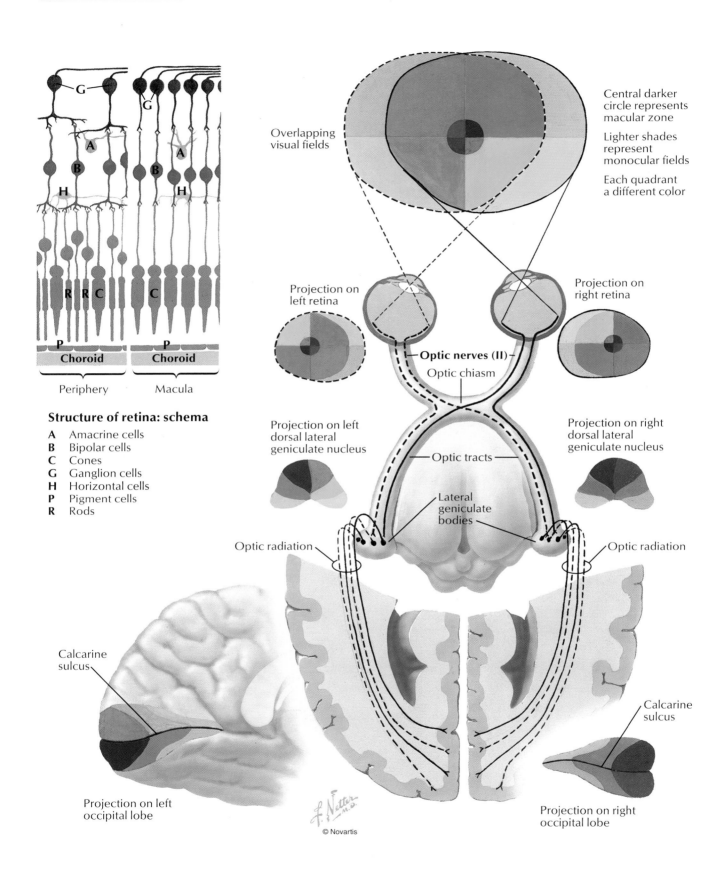

Structure of retina: schema

A  Amacrine cells
B  Bipolar cells
C  Cones
G  Ganglion cells
H  Horizontal cells
P  Pigment cells
R  Rods

Periphery    Macula

Choroid    Choroid

Central darker circle represents macular zone

Lighter shades represent monocular fields

Each quadrant a different color

Overlapping visual fields

Projection on left retina    Projection on right retina

Optic nerves (II)
Optic chiasm

Projection on left dorsal lateral geniculate nucleus    Projection on right dorsal lateral geniculate nucleus

Optic tracts

Lateral geniculate bodies

Optic radiation    Optic radiation

Calcarine sulcus    Calcarine sulcus

Projection on left occipital lobe    Projection on right occipital lobe

© Novartis

**PLATE 114**    **HEAD AND NECK**

# Oculomotor (III), Trochlear (IV) and Abducent (VI) Nerves: Schema

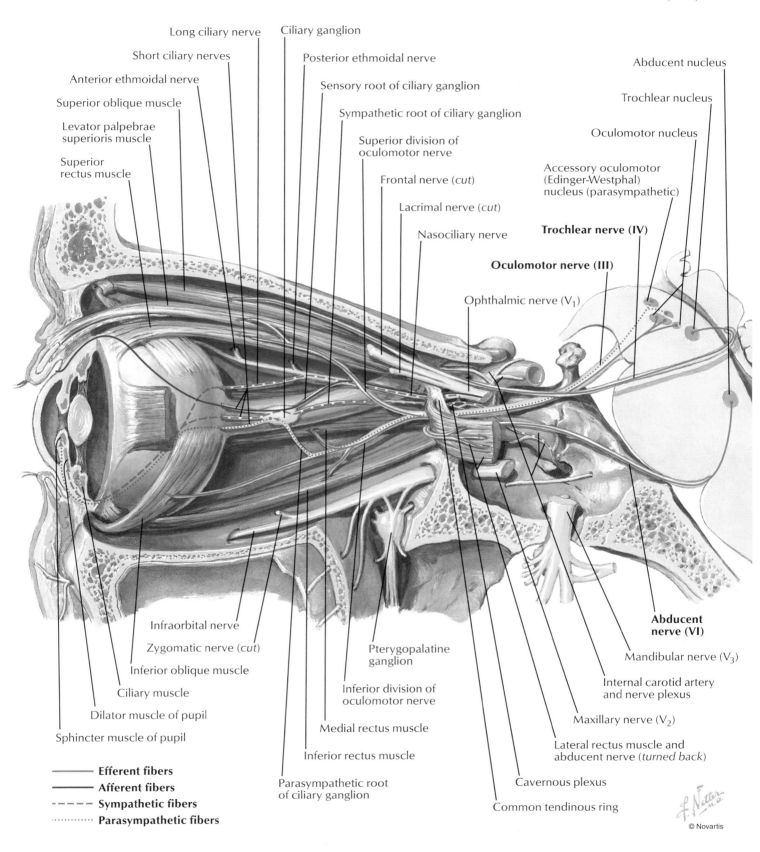

Long ciliary nerve

Short ciliary nerves

Anterior ethmoidal nerve

Superior oblique muscle

Levator palpebrae superioris muscle

Superior rectus muscle

Ciliary ganglion

Posterior ethmoidal nerve

Sensory root of ciliary ganglion

Sympathetic root of ciliary ganglion

Superior division of oculomotor nerve

Frontal nerve (*cut*)

Lacrimal nerve (*cut*)

Nasociliary nerve

Abducent nucleus

Trochlear nucleus

Oculomotor nucleus

Accessory oculomotor (Edinger-Westphal) nucleus (parasympathetic)

**Trochlear nerve (IV)**

**Oculomotor nerve (III)**

Ophthalmic nerve ($V_1$)

Infraorbital nerve

Zygomatic nerve (*cut*)

Inferior oblique muscle

Ciliary muscle

Dilator muscle of pupil

Sphincter muscle of pupil

Pterygopalatine ganglion

Inferior division of oculomotor nerve

Medial rectus muscle

Inferior rectus muscle

Parasympathetic root of ciliary ganglion

**Abducent nerve (VI)**

Mandibular nerve ($V_3$)

Internal carotid artery and nerve plexus

Maxillary nerve ($V_2$)

Lateral rectus muscle and abducent nerve (*turned back*)

Cavernous plexus

Common tendinous ring

——— **Efferent fibers**

——— **Afferent fibers**

– – – **Sympathetic fibers**

·········· **Parasympathetic fibers**

*f. Netter*
M.D.

© Novartis

**CRANIAL AND CERVICAL NERVES**

*PLATE 115*

# Trigeminal Nerve (V): Schema

SEE ALSO PLATES 18, 37, 38, 40, 41, 153

—— Efferent fibers
—— Afferent fibers
······· Proprioceptive fibers
········ Parasympathetic fibers
----- Sympathetic fibers

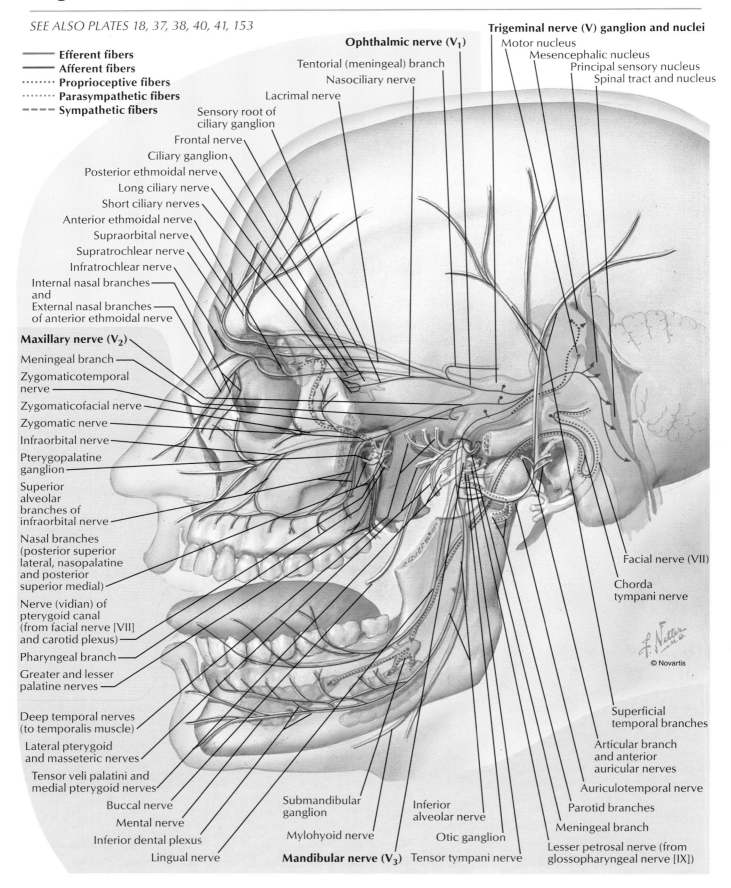

**Trigeminal nerve (V) ganglion and nuclei**
Motor nucleus
Mesencephalic nucleus
Principal sensory nucleus
Spinal tract and nucleus

**Ophthalmic nerve (V₁)**
Tentorial (meningeal) branch
Nasociliary nerve
Lacrimal nerve
Sensory root of ciliary ganglion
Frontal nerve
Ciliary ganglion
Posterior ethmoidal nerve
Long ciliary nerve
Short ciliary nerves
Anterior ethmoidal nerve
Supraorbital nerve
Supratrochlear nerve
Infratrochlear nerve
Internal nasal branches and
External nasal branches of anterior ethmoidal nerve

**Maxillary nerve (V₂)**
Meningeal branch
Zygomaticotemporal nerve
Zygomaticofacial nerve
Zygomatic nerve
Infraorbital nerve
Pterygopalatine ganglion
Superior alveolar branches of infraorbital nerve
Nasal branches (posterior superior lateral, nasopalatine and posterior superior medial)
Nerve (vidian) of pterygoid canal (from facial nerve [VII] and carotid plexus)
Pharyngeal branch
Greater and lesser palatine nerves
Deep temporal nerves (to temporalis muscle)
Lateral pterygoid and masseteric nerves
Tensor veli palatini and medial pterygoid nerves
Buccal nerve
Mental nerve
Inferior dental plexus
Lingual nerve

Submandibular ganglion
Mylohyoid nerve
**Mandibular nerve (V₃)**

Inferior alveolar nerve
Otic ganglion
Tensor tympani nerve

Facial nerve (VII)
Chorda tympani nerve

Superficial temporal branches
Articular branch and anterior auricular nerves
Auriculotemporal nerve
Parotid branches
Meningeal branch
Lesser petrosal nerve (from glossopharyngeal nerve [IX])

*f. Netter M.D.*
© Novartis

**PLATE 116**                    **HEAD AND NECK**

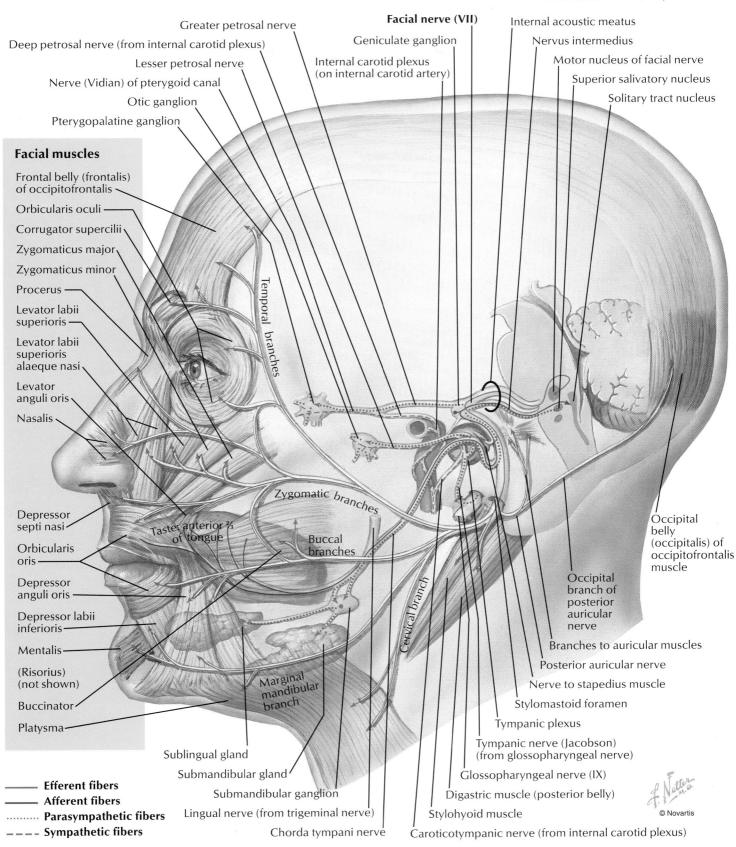

Greater petrosal nerve

Deep petrosal nerve (from internal carotid plexus)

Lesser petrosal nerve

Nerve (Vidian) of pterygoid canal

Otic ganglion

Pterygopalatine ganglion

**Facial nerve (VII)**

Geniculate ganglion

Internal carotid plexus (on internal carotid artery)

Internal acoustic meatus

Nervus intermedius

Motor nucleus of facial nerve

Superior salivatory nucleus

Solitary tract nucleus

**Facial muscles**

Frontal belly (frontalis) of occipitofrontalis

Orbicularis oculi

Corrugator supercilii

Zygomaticus major

Zygomaticus minor

Procerus

Levator labii superioris

Levator labii superioris alaeque nasi

Levator anguli oris

Nasalis

Depressor septi nasi

Orbicularis oris

Depressor anguli oris

Depressor labii inferioris

Mentalis

(Risorius) (not shown)

Buccinator

Platysma

Temporal branches

Zygomatic branches

Taste anterior ⅔ of tongue

Buccal branches

Cervical branch

Marginal mandibular branch

Sublingual gland

Submandibular gland

Submandibular ganglion

Lingual nerve (from trigeminal nerve)

Chorda tympani nerve

Occipital belly (occipitalis) of occipitofrontalis muscle

Occipital branch of posterior auricular nerve

Branches to auricular muscles

Posterior auricular nerve

Nerve to stapedius muscle

Stylomastoid foramen

Tympanic plexus

Tympanic nerve (Jacobson) (from glossopharyngeal nerve)

Glossopharyngeal nerve (IX)

Digastric muscle (posterior belly)

Stylohyoid muscle

Caroticotympanic nerve (from internal carotid plexus)

——— **Efferent fibers**

——— **Afferent fibers**

········· **Parasympathetic fibers**

– – – **Sympathetic fibers**

© Novartis

# Vestibulocochlear Nerve (VIII): Schema

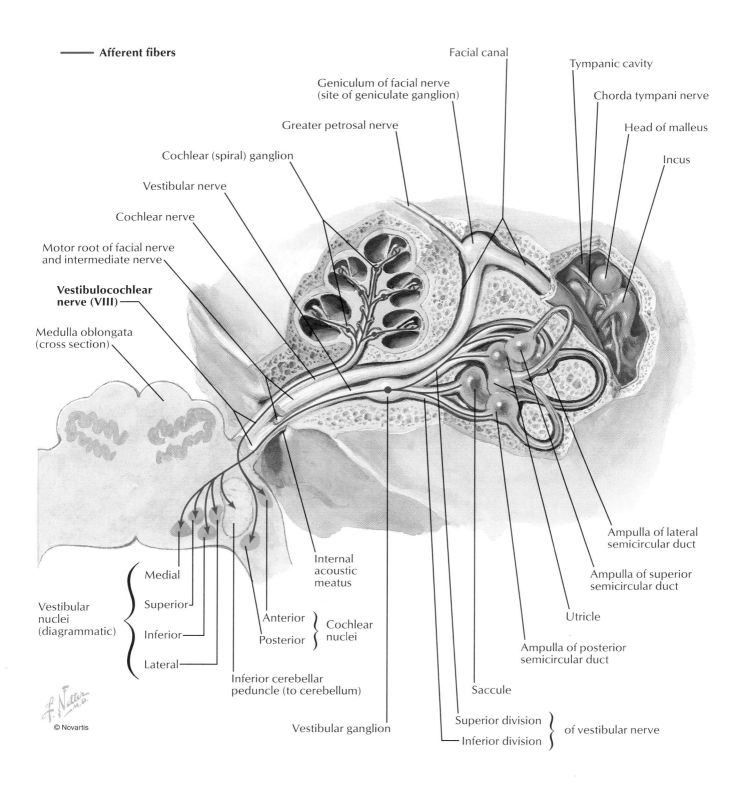

Afferent fibers

Facial canal

Geniculum of facial nerve
(site of geniculate ganglion)

Greater petrosal nerve

Tympanic cavity

Chorda tympani nerve

Head of malleus

Incus

Cochlear (spiral) ganglion

Vestibular nerve

Cochlear nerve

Motor root of facial nerve
and intermediate nerve

**Vestibulocochlear
nerve (VIII)**

Medulla oblongata
(cross section)

Internal
acoustic
meatus

Ampulla of lateral
semicircular duct

Ampulla of superior
semicircular duct

Utricle

Ampulla of posterior
semicircular duct

Saccule

Vestibular
nuclei
(diagrammatic) { Medial, Superior, Inferior, Lateral }

Anterior
Posterior } Cochlear
nuclei

Inferior cerebellar
peduncle (to cerebellum)

Vestibular ganglion

Superior division
Inferior division } of vestibular nerve

© Novartis

**PLATE 118**

**HEAD AND NECK**

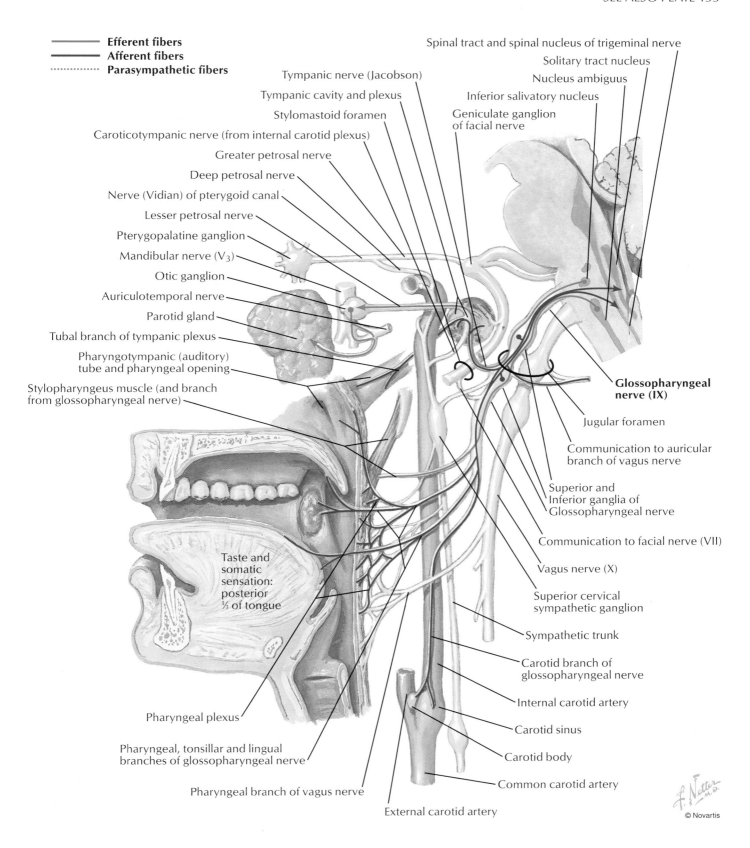

Efferent fibers
Afferent fibers
Parasympathetic fibers

Spinal tract and spinal nucleus of trigeminal nerve
Solitary tract nucleus
Nucleus ambiguus
Inferior salivatory nucleus
Geniculate ganglion of facial nerve

Tympanic nerve (Jacobson)
Tympanic cavity and plexus
Stylomastoid foramen
Caroticotympanic nerve (from internal carotid plexus)
Greater petrosal nerve
Deep petrosal nerve
Nerve (Vidian) of pterygoid canal
Lesser petrosal nerve
Pterygopalatine ganglion
Mandibular nerve (V₃)
Otic ganglion
Auriculotemporal nerve
Parotid gland
Tubal branch of tympanic plexus
Pharyngotympanic (auditory) tube and pharyngeal opening
Stylopharyngeus muscle (and branch from glossopharyngeal nerve)

Glossopharyngeal nerve (IX)
Jugular foramen
Communication to auricular branch of vagus nerve
Superior and Inferior ganglia of Glossopharyngeal nerve
Communication to facial nerve (VII)
Vagus nerve (X)
Superior cervical sympathetic ganglion
Sympathetic trunk
Carotid branch of glossopharyngeal nerve
Internal carotid artery
Carotid sinus
Carotid body
Common carotid artery

Taste and somatic sensation: posterior ⅓ of tongue

Pharyngeal plexus
Pharyngeal, tonsillar and lingual branches of glossopharyngeal nerve
Pharyngeal branch of vagus nerve
External carotid artery

# Vagus Nerve (X): Schema

SEE ALSO PLATE 153

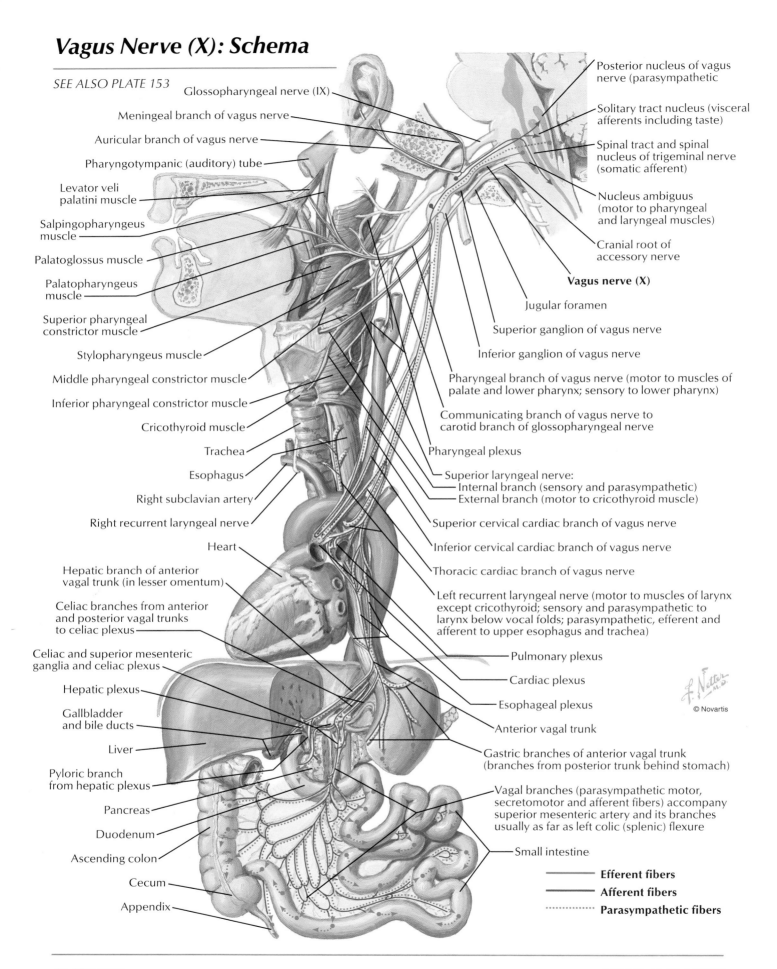

Glossopharyngeal nerve (IX)

Meningeal branch of vagus nerve

Auricular branch of vagus nerve

Pharyngotympanic (auditory) tube

Levator veli palatini muscle

Salpingopharyngeus muscle

Palatoglossus muscle

Palatopharyngeus muscle

Superior pharyngeal constrictor muscle

Stylopharyngeus muscle

Middle pharyngeal constrictor muscle

Inferior pharyngeal constrictor muscle

Cricothyroid muscle

Trachea

Esophagus

Right subclavian artery

Right recurrent laryngeal nerve

Heart

Hepatic branch of anterior vagal trunk (in lesser omentum)

Celiac branches from anterior and posterior vagal trunks to celiac plexus

Celiac and superior mesenteric ganglia and celiac plexus

Hepatic plexus

Gallbladder and bile ducts

Liver

Pyloric branch from hepatic plexus

Pancreas

Duodenum

Ascending colon

Cecum

Appendix

Posterior nucleus of vagus nerve (parasympathetic

Solitary tract nucleus (visceral afferents including taste)

Spinal tract and spinal nucleus of trigeminal nerve (somatic afferent)

Nucleus ambiguus (motor to pharyngeal and laryngeal muscles)

Cranial root of accessory nerve

**Vagus nerve (X)**

Jugular foramen

Superior ganglion of vagus nerve

Inferior ganglion of vagus nerve

Pharyngeal branch of vagus nerve (motor to muscles of palate and lower pharynx; sensory to lower pharynx)

Communicating branch of vagus nerve to carotid branch of glossopharyngeal nerve

Pharyngeal plexus

Superior laryngeal nerve:
Internal branch (sensory and parasympathetic)
External branch (motor to cricothyroid muscle)

Superior cervical cardiac branch of vagus nerve

Inferior cervical cardiac branch of vagus nerve

Thoracic cardiac branch of vagus nerve

Left recurrent laryngeal nerve (motor to muscles of larynx except cricothyroid; sensory and parasympathetic to larynx below vocal folds; parasympathetic, efferent and afferent to upper esophagus and trachea)

Pulmonary plexus

Cardiac plexus

Esophageal plexus

Anterior vagal trunk

Gastric branches of anterior vagal trunk (branches from posterior trunk behind stomach)

Vagal branches (parasympathetic motor, secretomotor and afferent fibers) accompany superior mesenteric artery and its branches usually as far as left colic (splenic) flexure

Small intestine

———— **Efferent fibers**

———— **Afferent fibers**

·········· **Parasympathetic fibers**

*F. Netter M.D.*
© Novartis

**PLATE 120**                    **HEAD AND NECK**

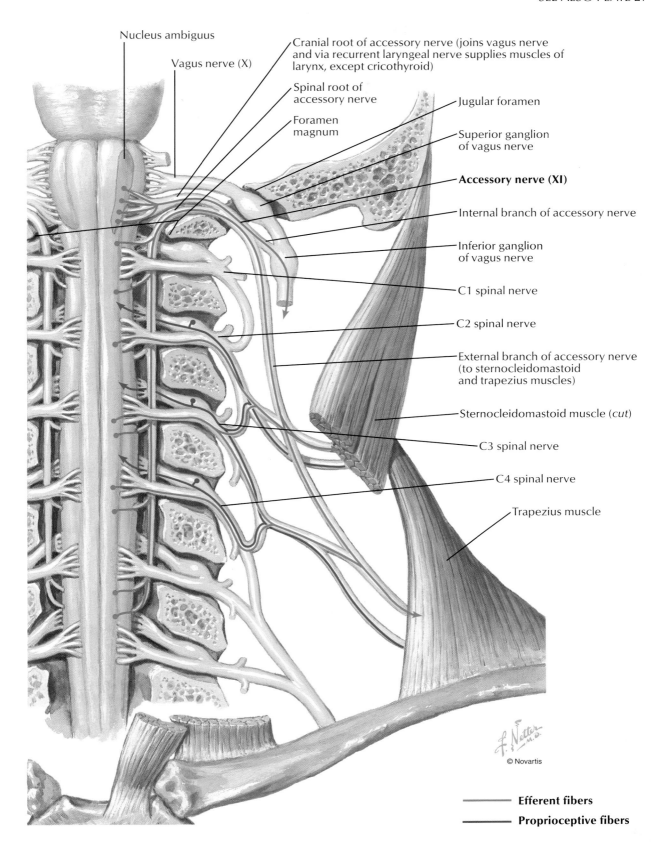

Nucleus ambiguus

Vagus nerve (X)

Cranial root of accessory nerve (joins vagus nerve and via recurrent laryngeal nerve supplies muscles of larynx, except cricothyroid)

Spinal root of accessory nerve

Foramen magnum

Jugular foramen

Superior ganglion of vagus nerve

**Accessory nerve (XI)**

Internal branch of accessory nerve

Inferior ganglion of vagus nerve

C1 spinal nerve

C2 spinal nerve

External branch of accessory nerve (to sternocleidomastoid and trapezius muscles)

Sternocleidomastoid muscle (*cut*)

C3 spinal nerve

C4 spinal nerve

Trapezius muscle

© Novartis

—— **Efferent fibers**

—— **Proprioceptive fibers**

# Hypoglossal Nerve (XII): Schema

SEE ALSO PLATE 27

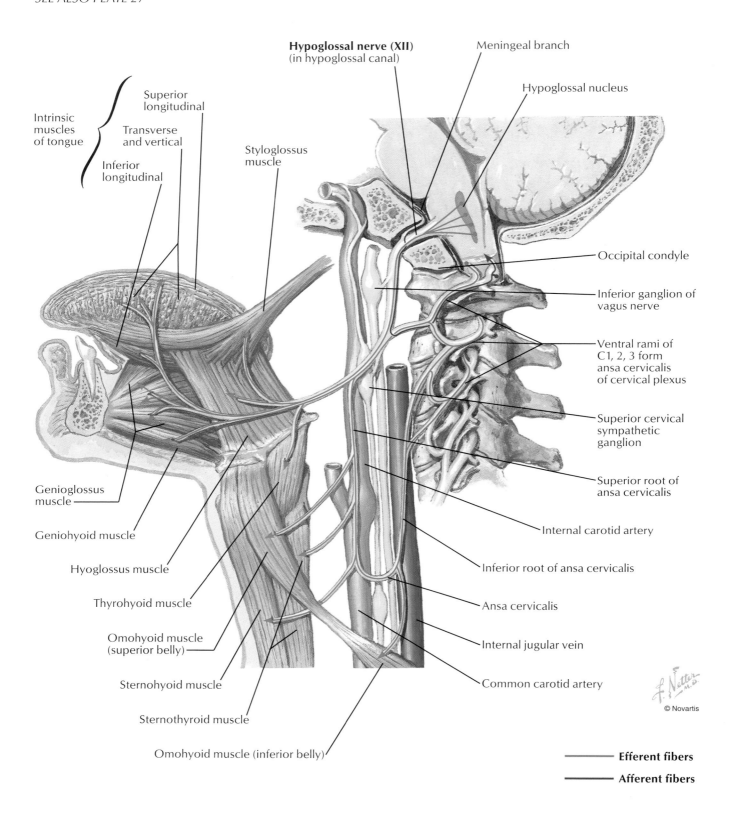

Intrinsic muscles of tongue
- Superior longitudinal
- Transverse and vertical
- Inferior longitudinal

Styloglossus muscle

**Hypoglossal nerve (XII)** (in hypoglossal canal)

Meningeal branch

Hypoglossal nucleus

Occipital condyle

Inferior ganglion of vagus nerve

Ventral rami of C1, 2, 3 form ansa cervicalis of cervical plexus

Superior cervical sympathetic ganglion

Superior root of ansa cervicalis

Internal carotid artery

Inferior root of ansa cervicalis

Ansa cervicalis

Internal jugular vein

Common carotid artery

Genioglossus muscle

Geniohyoid muscle

Hyoglossus muscle

Thyrohyoid muscle

Omohyoid muscle (superior belly)

Sternohyoid muscle

Sternothyroid muscle

Omohyoid muscle (inferior belly)

———— **Efferent fibers**

———— **Afferent fibers**

© Novartis

*PLATE 122*

**HEAD AND NECK**

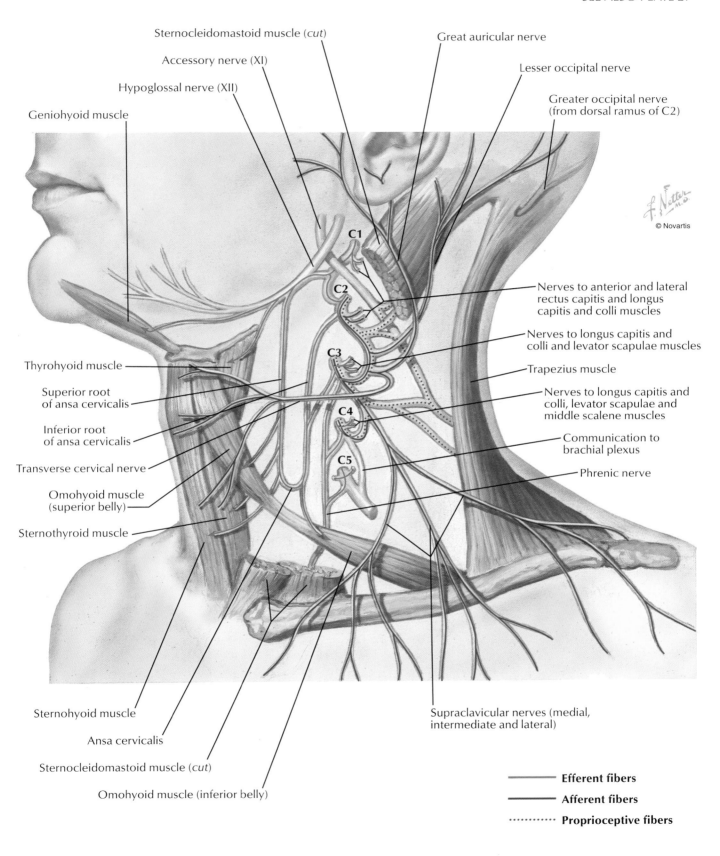

Sternocleidomastoid muscle (*cut*)

Accessory nerve (XI)

Hypoglossal nerve (XII)

Geniohyoid muscle

Great auricular nerve

Lesser occipital nerve

Greater occipital nerve (from dorsal ramus of C2)

C1

C2

C3

C4

C5

Nerves to anterior and lateral rectus capitis and longus capitis and colli muscles

Nerves to longus capitis and colli and levator scapulae muscles

Trapezius muscle

Nerves to longus capitis and colli, levator scapulae and middle scalene muscles

Communication to brachial plexus

Phrenic nerve

Thyrohyoid muscle

Superior root of ansa cervicalis

Inferior root of ansa cervicalis

Transverse cervical nerve

Omohyoid muscle (superior belly)

Sternothyroid muscle

Sternohyoid muscle

Ansa cervicalis

Sternocleidomastoid muscle (*cut*)

Omohyoid muscle (inferior belly)

Supraclavicular nerves (medial, intermediate and lateral)

Efferent fibers

Afferent fibers

Proprioceptive fibers

© Novartis

*SEE ALSO PLATES 65, 119, 120, 152, 198, 214, 228, 300*

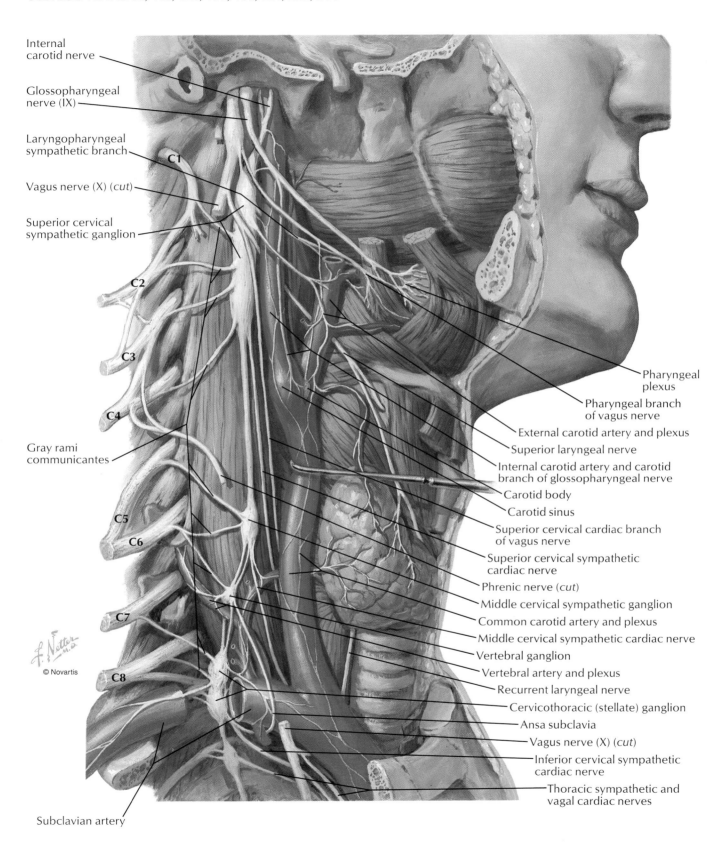

Internal
carotid nerve

Glossopharyngeal
nerve (IX)

Laryngopharyngeal
sympathetic branch

Vagus nerve (X) (*cut*)

Superior cervical
sympathetic ganglion

C1

C2

C3

C4

Gray rami
communicantes

C5

C6

C7

© Novartis

C8

Subclavian artery

Pharyngeal
plexus

Pharyngeal branch
of vagus nerve

External carotid artery and plexus

Superior laryngeal nerve

Internal carotid artery and carotid
branch of glossopharyngeal nerve

Carotid body

Carotid sinus

Superior cervical cardiac branch
of vagus nerve

Superior cervical sympathetic
cardiac nerve

Phrenic nerve (*cut*)

Middle cervical sympathetic ganglion

Common carotid artery and plexus

Middle cervical sympathetic cardiac nerve

Vertebral ganglion

Vertebral artery and plexus

Recurrent laryngeal nerve

Cervicothoracic (stellate) ganglion

Ansa subclavia

Vagus nerve (X) (*cut*)

Inferior cervical sympathetic
cardiac nerve

Thoracic sympathetic and
vagal cardiac nerves

**PLATE 124**

**HEAD AND NECK**

SEE ALSO PLATES 39, 40, 41, 81, 115, 126, 127, 128, 152

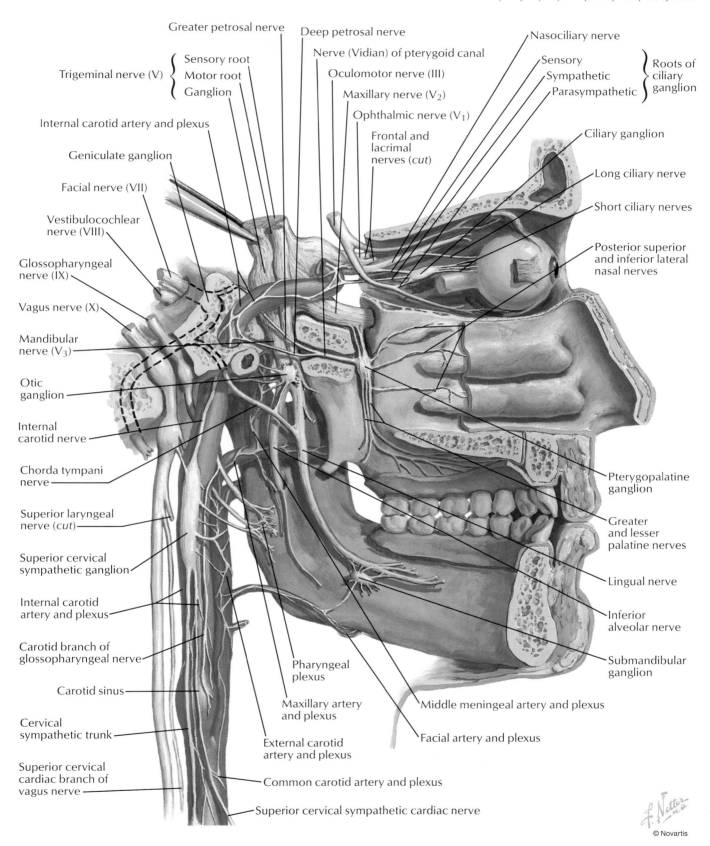

Greater petrosal nerve

Deep petrosal nerve

Nasociliary nerve

Trigeminal nerve (V) { Sensory root / Motor root / Ganglion }

Nerve (Vidian) of pterygoid canal

Sensory
Sympathetic
Parasympathetic } Roots of ciliary ganglion

Oculomotor nerve (III)

Internal carotid artery and plexus

Maxillary nerve (V₂)

Ciliary ganglion

Geniculate ganglion

Ophthalmic nerve (V₁)

Long ciliary nerve

Facial nerve (VII)

Frontal and lacrimal nerves (cut)

Short ciliary nerves

Vestibulocochlear nerve (VIII)

Posterior superior and inferior lateral nasal nerves

Glossopharyngeal nerve (IX)

Vagus nerve (X)

Mandibular nerve (V₃)

Otic ganglion

Internal carotid nerve

Chorda tympani nerve

Pterygopalatine ganglion

Superior laryngeal nerve (cut)

Greater and lesser palatine nerves

Superior cervical sympathetic ganglion

Lingual nerve

Internal carotid artery and plexus

Inferior alveolar nerve

Carotid branch of glossopharyngeal nerve

Submandibular ganglion

Carotid sinus

Pharyngeal plexus

Cervical sympathetic trunk

Maxillary artery and plexus

Middle meningeal artery and plexus

Superior cervical cardiac branch of vagus nerve

External carotid artery and plexus

Facial artery and plexus

Common carotid artery and plexus

Superior cervical sympathetic cardiac nerve

f. Netter
© Novartis

# Ciliary Ganglion: Schema

*SEE ALSO PLATE 153*

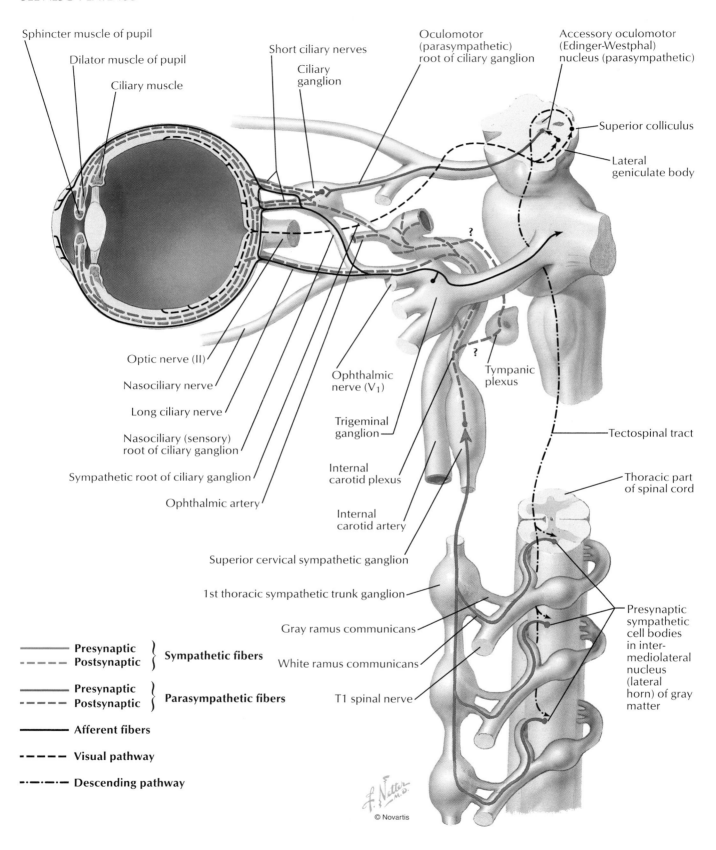

Sphincter muscle of pupil

Dilator muscle of pupil

Ciliary muscle

Short ciliary nerves

Ciliary ganglion

Oculomotor (parasympathetic) root of ciliary ganglion

Accessory oculomotor (Edinger-Westphal) nucleus (parasympathetic)

Superior colliculus

Lateral geniculate body

Optic nerve (II)

Nasociliary nerve

Long ciliary nerve

Nasociliary (sensory) root of ciliary ganglion

Sympathetic root of ciliary ganglion

Ophthalmic artery

Ophthalmic nerve (V$_1$)

Trigeminal ganglion

Internal carotid plexus

Internal carotid artery

Tympanic plexus

Tectospinal tract

Thoracic part of spinal cord

Superior cervical sympathetic ganglion

1st thoracic sympathetic trunk ganglion

Gray ramus communicans

White ramus communicans

T1 spinal nerve

Presynaptic sympathetic cell bodies in inter-mediolateral nucleus (lateral horn) of gray matter

——— **Presynaptic**
‐ ‐ ‐ **Postsynaptic**  } **Sympathetic fibers**

——— **Presynaptic**
‐ ‐ ‐ **Postsynaptic**  } **Parasympathetic fibers**

——— **Afferent fibers**

‐ ‐ ‐ **Visual pathway**

‐·‐·‐ **Descending pathway**

*F. Netter M.D.*

© Novartis

*PLATE 126*

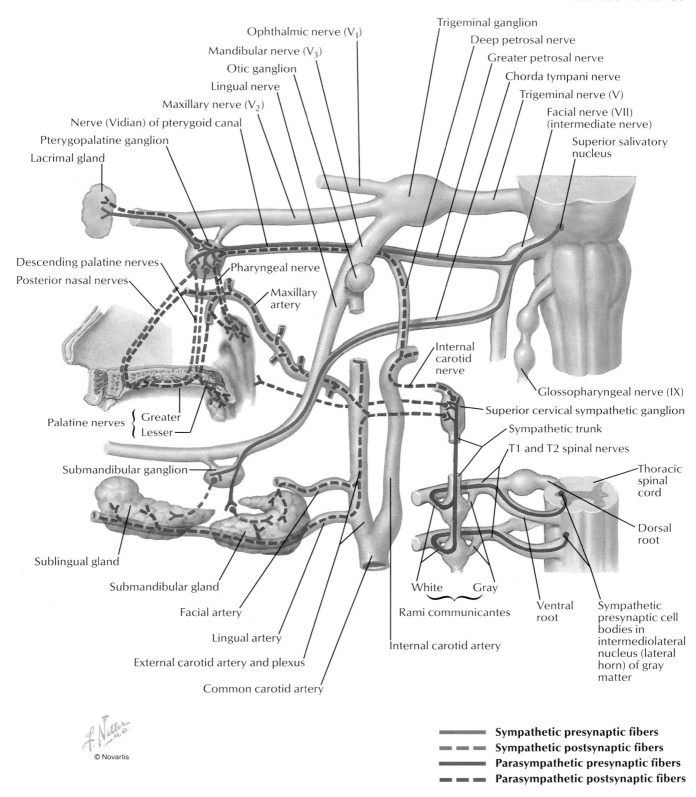

Ophthalmic nerve (V₁)

Mandibular nerve (V₃)

Otic ganglion

Lingual nerve

Maxillary nerve (V₂)

Nerve (Vidian) of pterygoid canal

Pterygopalatine ganglion

Lacrimal gland

Trigeminal ganglion

Deep petrosal nerve

Greater petrosal nerve

Chorda tympani nerve

Trigeminal nerve (V)

Facial nerve (VII) (intermediate nerve)

Superior salivatory nucleus

Descending palatine nerves

Posterior nasal nerves

Pharyngeal nerve

Maxillary artery

Internal carotid nerve

Glossopharyngeal nerve (IX)

Superior cervical sympathetic ganglion

Sympathetic trunk

T1 and T2 spinal nerves

Palatine nerves { Greater / Lesser }

Submandibular ganglion

Thoracic spinal cord

Dorsal root

Sublingual gland

Submandibular gland

Facial artery

Lingual artery

External carotid artery and plexus

Common carotid artery

White    Gray

Rami communicantes

Internal carotid artery

Ventral root

Sympathetic presynaptic cell bodies in intermediolateral nucleus (lateral horn) of gray matter

*f. Netter* m.d.

© Novartis

— Sympathetic presynaptic fibers
--- Sympathetic postsynaptic fibers
— Parasympathetic presynaptic fibers
--- Parasympathetic postsynaptic fibers

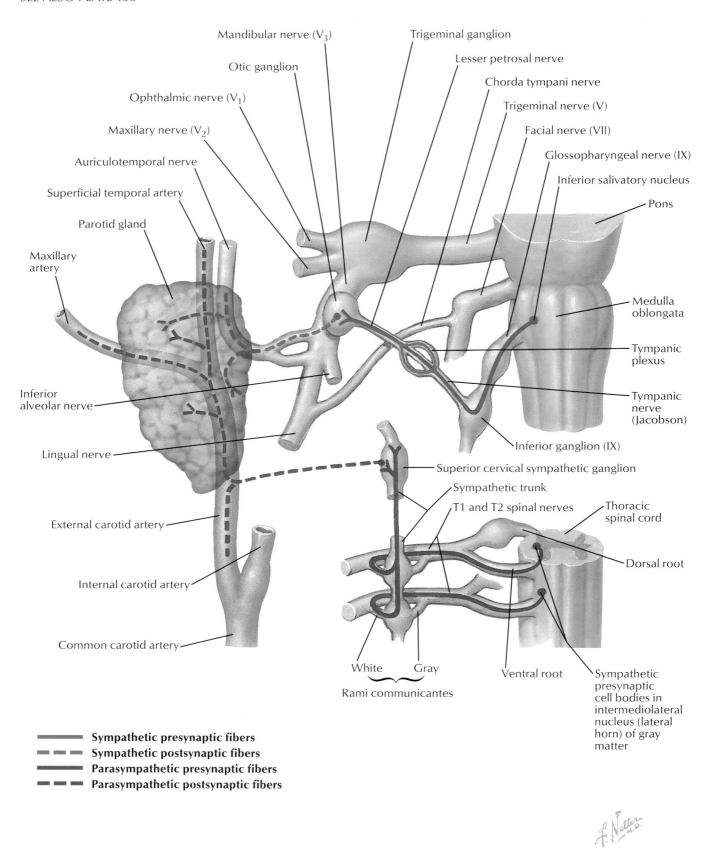

Mandibular nerve (V₃)

Otic ganglion

Ophthalmic nerve (V₁)

Maxillary nerve (V₂)

Auriculotemporal nerve

Superficial temporal artery

Parotid gland

Maxillary artery

Inferior alveolar nerve

Lingual nerve

External carotid artery

Internal carotid artery

Common carotid artery

Trigeminal ganglion

Lesser petrosal nerve

Chorda tympani nerve

Trigeminal nerve (V)

Facial nerve (VII)

Glossopharyngeal nerve (IX)

Inferior salivatory nucleus

Pons

Medulla oblongata

Tympanic plexus

Tympanic nerve (Jacobson)

Inferior ganglion (IX)

Superior cervical sympathetic ganglion

Sympathetic trunk

T1 and T2 spinal nerves

Thoracic spinal cord

Dorsal root

Ventral root

Sympathetic presynaptic cell bodies in intermediolateral nucleus (lateral horn) of gray matter

White    Gray

Rami communicantes

━━━━━ **Sympathetic presynaptic fibers**
╍╍╍╍ **Sympathetic postsynaptic fibers**
━━━━━ **Parasympathetic presynaptic fibers**
╍╍╍╍ **Parasympathetic postsynaptic fibers**

© Novartis

**PLATE 128**                                    **HEAD AND NECK**

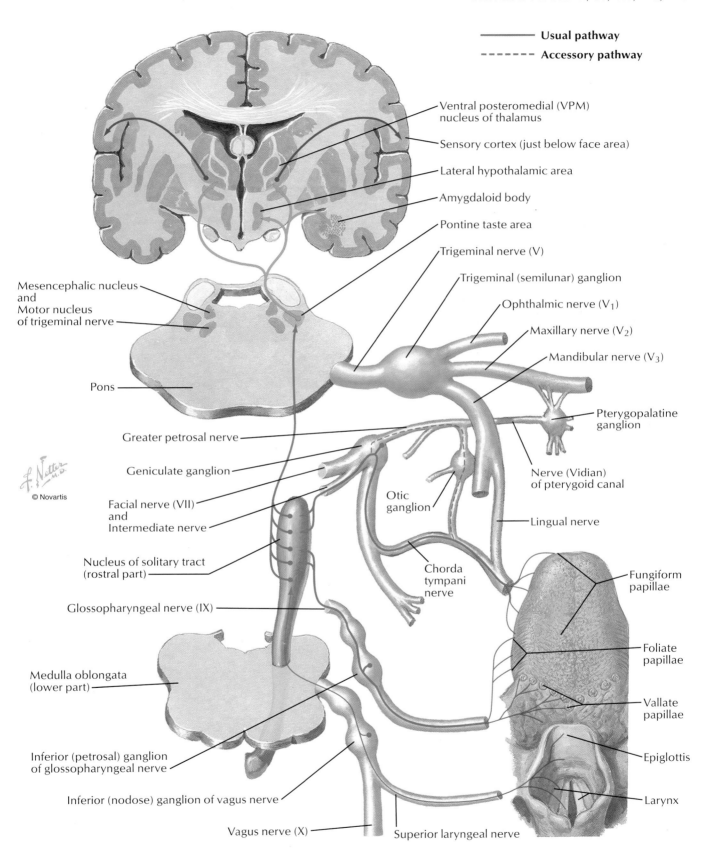

Usual pathway
------- Accessory pathway

Ventral posteromedial (VPM) nucleus of thalamus

Sensory cortex (just below face area)

Lateral hypothalamic area

Amygdaloid body

Pontine taste area

Trigeminal nerve (V)

Trigeminal (semilunar) ganglion

Ophthalmic nerve (V₁)

Maxillary nerve (V₂)

Mandibular nerve (V₃)

Pterygopalatine ganglion

Nerve (Vidian) of pterygoid canal

Lingual nerve

Fungiform papillae

Foliate papillae

Vallate papillae

Epiglottis

Larynx

Mesencephalic nucleus and Motor nucleus of trigeminal nerve

Pons

Greater petrosal nerve

Geniculate ganglion

Facial nerve (VII) and Intermediate nerve

Nucleus of solitary tract (rostral part)

Glossopharyngeal nerve (IX)

Medulla oblongata (lower part)

Inferior (petrosal) ganglion of glossopharyngeal nerve

Inferior (nodose) ganglion of vagus nerve

Vagus nerve (X)

Otic ganglion

Chorda tympani nerve

Superior laryngeal nerve

© Novartis

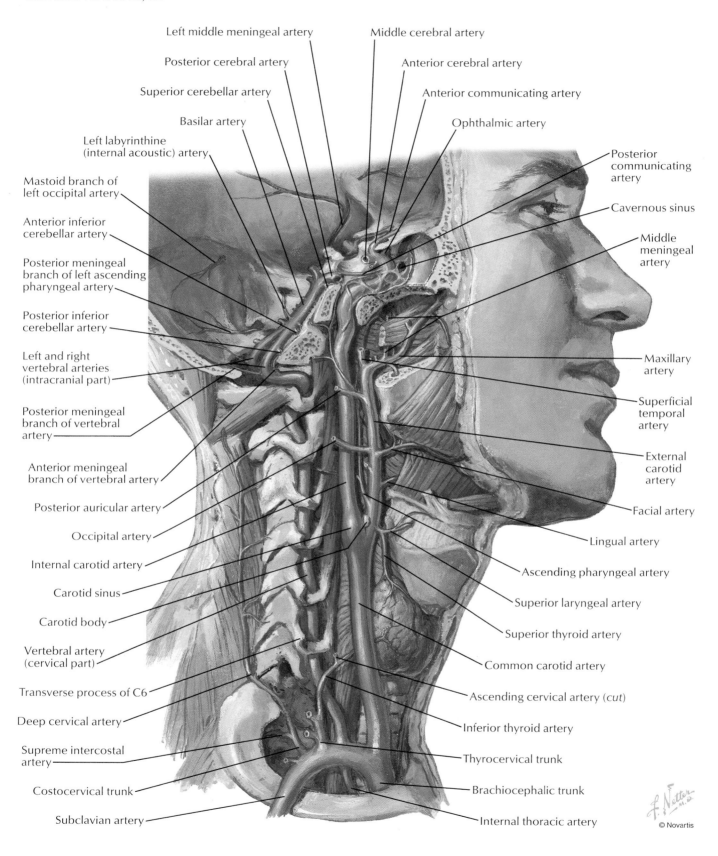

Left middle meningeal artery

Posterior cerebral artery

Superior cerebellar artery

Basilar artery

Left labyrinthine (internal acoustic) artery

Mastoid branch of left occipital artery

Anterior inferior cerebellar artery

Posterior meningeal branch of left ascending pharyngeal artery

Posterior inferior cerebellar artery

Left and right vertebral arteries (intracranial part)

Posterior meningeal branch of vertebral artery

Anterior meningeal branch of vertebral artery

Posterior auricular artery

Occipital artery

Internal carotid artery

Carotid sinus

Carotid body

Vertebral artery (cervical part)

Transverse process of C6

Deep cervical artery

Supreme intercostal artery

Costocervical trunk

Subclavian artery

Middle cerebral artery

Anterior cerebral artery

Anterior communicating artery

Ophthalmic artery

Posterior communicating artery

Cavernous sinus

Middle meningeal artery

Maxillary artery

Superficial temporal artery

External carotid artery

Facial artery

Lingual artery

Ascending pharyngeal artery

Superior laryngeal artery

Superior thyroid artery

Common carotid artery

Ascending cervical artery (*cut*)

Inferior thyroid artery

Thyrocervical trunk

Brachiocephalic trunk

Internal thoracic artery

© Novartis

**PLATE 130**

**HEAD AND NECK**

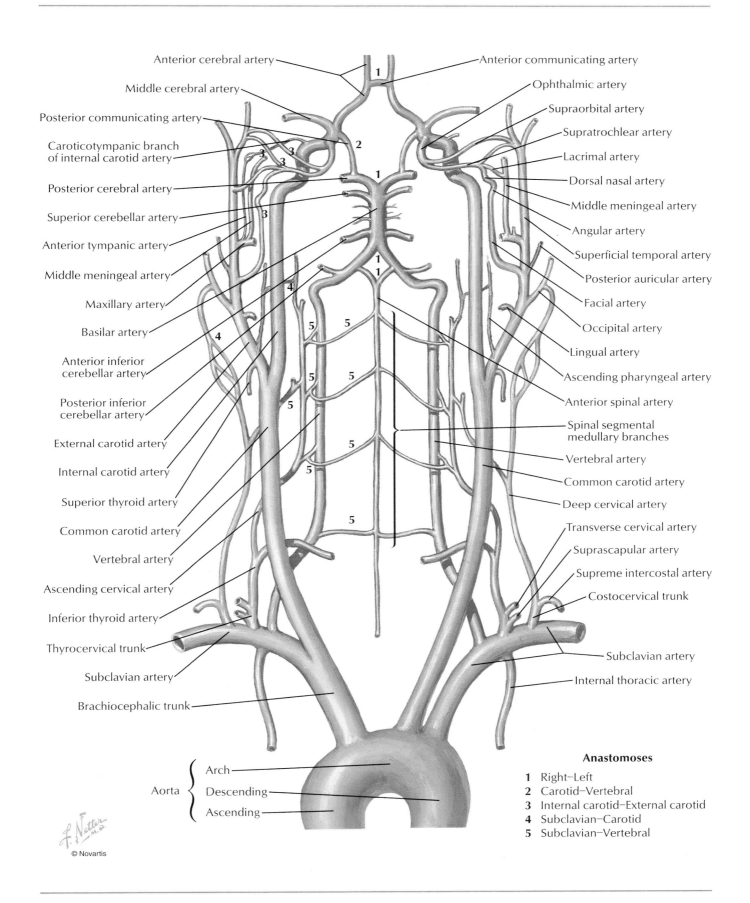

Anterior cerebral artery

Middle cerebral artery

Posterior communicating artery

Caroticotympanic branch of internal carotid artery

Posterior cerebral artery

Superior cerebellar artery

Anterior tympanic artery

Middle meningeal artery

Maxillary artery

Basilar artery

Anterior inferior cerebellar artery

Posterior inferior cerebellar artery

External carotid artery

Internal carotid artery

Superior thyroid artery

Common carotid artery

Vertebral artery

Ascending cervical artery

Inferior thyroid artery

Thyrocervical trunk

Subclavian artery

Brachiocephalic trunk

Anterior communicating artery

Ophthalmic artery

Supraorbital artery

Supratrochlear artery

Lacrimal artery

Dorsal nasal artery

Middle meningeal artery

Angular artery

Superficial temporal artery

Posterior auricular artery

Facial artery

Occipital artery

Lingual artery

Ascending pharyngeal artery

Anterior spinal artery

Spinal segmental medullary branches

Vertebral artery

Common carotid artery

Deep cervical artery

Transverse cervical artery

Suprascapular artery

Supreme intercostal artery

Costocervical trunk

Subclavian artery

Internal thoracic artery

Aorta { Arch, Descending, Ascending }

**Anastomoses**

1  Right–Left
2  Carotid–Vertebral
3  Internal carotid–External carotid
4  Subclavian–Carotid
5  Subclavian–Vertebral

© Novartis

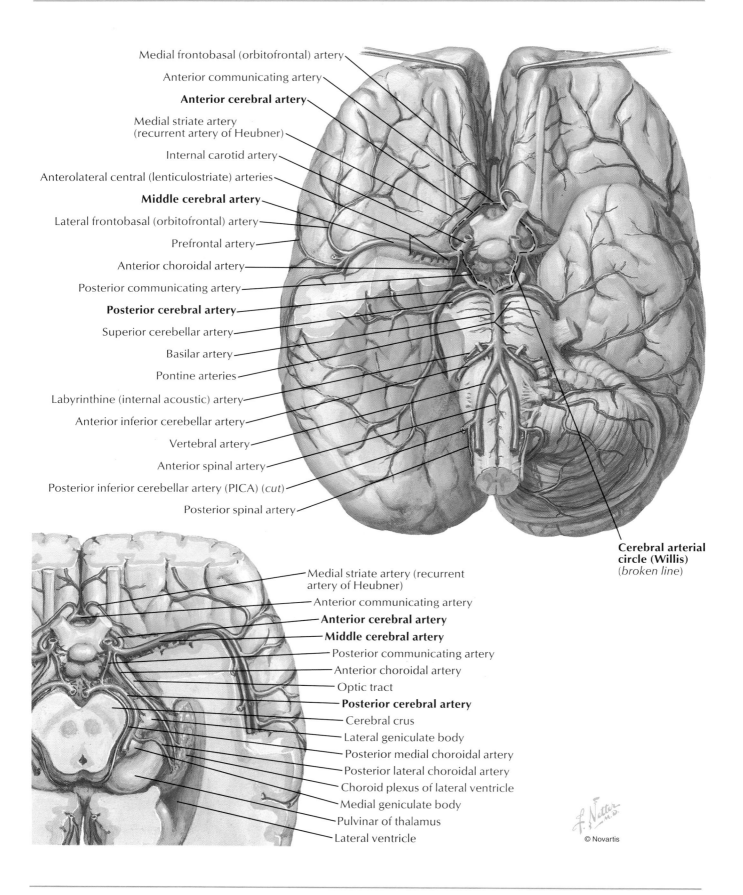

Medial frontobasal (orbitofrontal) artery

Anterior communicating artery

**Anterior cerebral artery**

Medial striate artery
(recurrent artery of Heubner)

Internal carotid artery

Anterolateral central (lenticulostriate) arteries

**Middle cerebral artery**

Lateral frontobasal (orbitofrontal) artery

Prefrontal artery

Anterior choroidal artery

Posterior communicating artery

**Posterior cerebral artery**

Superior cerebellar artery

Basilar artery

Pontine arteries

Labyrinthine (internal acoustic) artery

Anterior inferior cerebellar artery

Vertebral artery

Anterior spinal artery

Posterior inferior cerebellar artery (PICA) (cut)

Posterior spinal artery

**Cerebral arterial
circle (Willis)**
(broken line)

Medial striate artery (recurrent
artery of Heubner)

Anterior communicating artery

**Anterior cerebral artery**

**Middle cerebral artery**

Posterior communicating artery

Anterior choroidal artery

Optic tract

**Posterior cerebral artery**

Cerebral crus

Lateral geniculate body

Posterior medial choroidal artery

Posterior lateral choroidal artery

Choroid plexus of lateral ventricle

Medial geniculate body

Pulvinar of thalamus

Lateral ventricle

© Novartis

**PLATE 132**

**HEAD AND NECK**

**Vessels dissected out: inferior view**

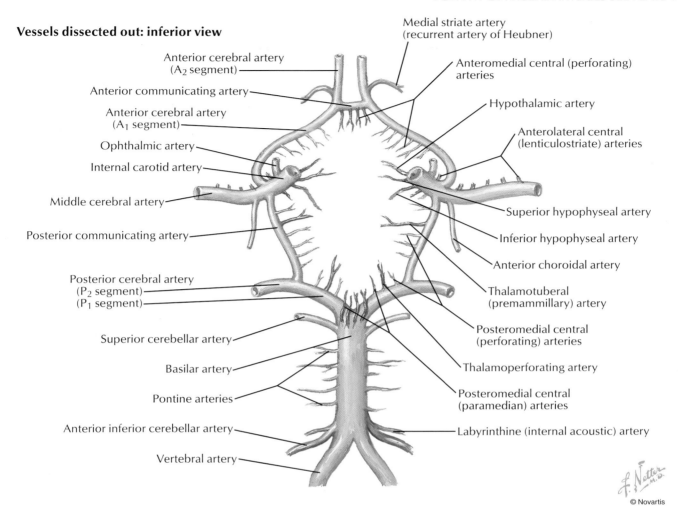

Anterior cerebral artery ($A_2$ segment)

Anterior communicating artery

Anterior cerebral artery ($A_1$ segment)

Ophthalmic artery

Internal carotid artery

Middle cerebral artery

Posterior communicating artery

Posterior cerebral artery ($P_2$ segment) ($P_1$ segment)

Superior cerebellar artery

Basilar artery

Pontine arteries

Anterior inferior cerebellar artery

Vertebral artery

Medial striate artery (recurrent artery of Heubner)

Anteromedial central (perforating) arteries

Hypothalamic artery

Anterolateral central (lenticulostriate) arteries

Superior hypophyseal artery

Inferior hypophyseal artery

Anterior choroidal artery

Thalamotuberal (premammillary) artery

Posteromedial central (perforating) arteries

Thalamoperforating artery

Posteromedial central (paramedian) arteries

Labyrinthine (internal acoustic) artery

© Novartis

**Vessels in situ: inferior view**

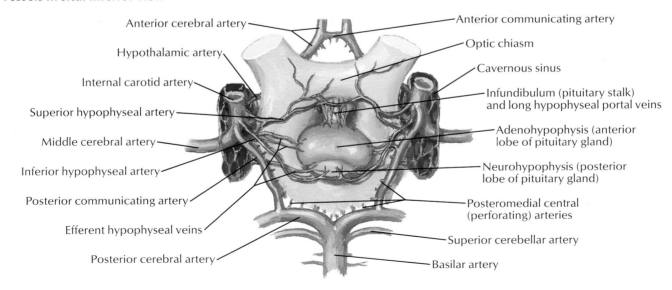

Anterior cerebral artery

Hypothalamic artery

Internal carotid artery

Superior hypophyseal artery

Middle cerebral artery

Inferior hypophyseal artery

Posterior communicating artery

Efferent hypophyseal veins

Posterior cerebral artery

Anterior communicating artery

Optic chiasm

Cavernous sinus

Infundibulum (pituitary stalk) and long hypophyseal portal veins

Adenohypophysis (anterior lobe of pituitary gland)

Neurohypophysis (posterior lobe of pituitary gland)

Posteromedial central (perforating) arteries

Superior cerebellar artery

Basilar artery

# Arteries of Brain: Frontal View and Section

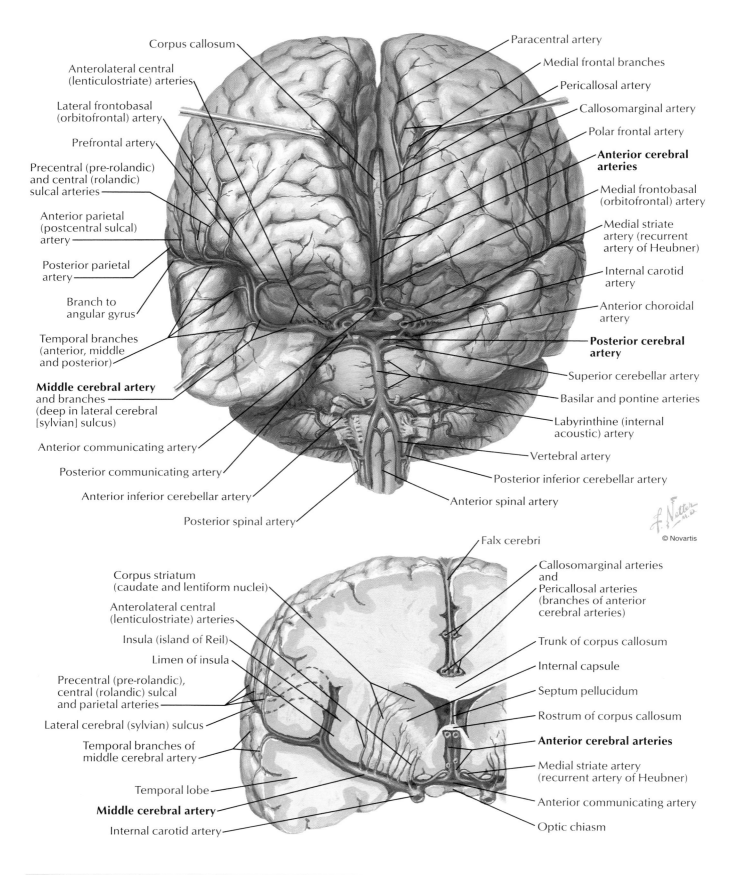

Corpus callosum

Anterolateral central (lenticulostriate) arteries

Lateral frontobasal (orbitofrontal) artery

Prefrontal artery

Precentral (pre-rolandic) and central (rolandic) sulcal arteries

Anterior parietal (postcentral sulcal) artery

Posterior parietal artery

Branch to angular gyrus

Temporal branches (anterior, middle and posterior)

**Middle cerebral artery** and branches (deep in lateral cerebral [sylvian] sulcus)

Anterior communicating artery

Posterior communicating artery

Anterior inferior cerebellar artery

Posterior spinal artery

Paracentral artery

Medial frontal branches

Pericallosal artery

Callosomarginal artery

Polar frontal artery

**Anterior cerebral arteries**

Medial frontobasal (orbitofrontal) artery

Medial striate artery (recurrent artery of Heubner)

Internal carotid artery

Anterior choroidal artery

**Posterior cerebral artery**

Superior cerebellar artery

Basilar and pontine arteries

Labyrinthine (internal acoustic) artery

Vertebral artery

Posterior inferior cerebellar artery

Anterior spinal artery

© Novartis

Corpus striatum (caudate and lentiform nuclei)

Anterolateral central (lenticulostriate) arteries

Insula (island of Reil)

Limen of insula

Precentral (pre-rolandic), central (rolandic) sulcal and parietal arteries

Lateral cerebral (sylvian) sulcus

Temporal branches of middle cerebral artery

Temporal lobe

**Middle cerebral artery**

Internal carotid artery

Falx cerebri

Callosomarginal arteries and Pericallosal arteries (branches of anterior cerebral arteries)

Trunk of corpus callosum

Internal capsule

Septum pellucidum

Rostrum of corpus callosum

**Anterior cerebral arteries**

Medial striate artery (recurrent artery of Heubner)

Anterior communicating artery

Optic chiasm

**PLATE 134**

**HEAD AND NECK**

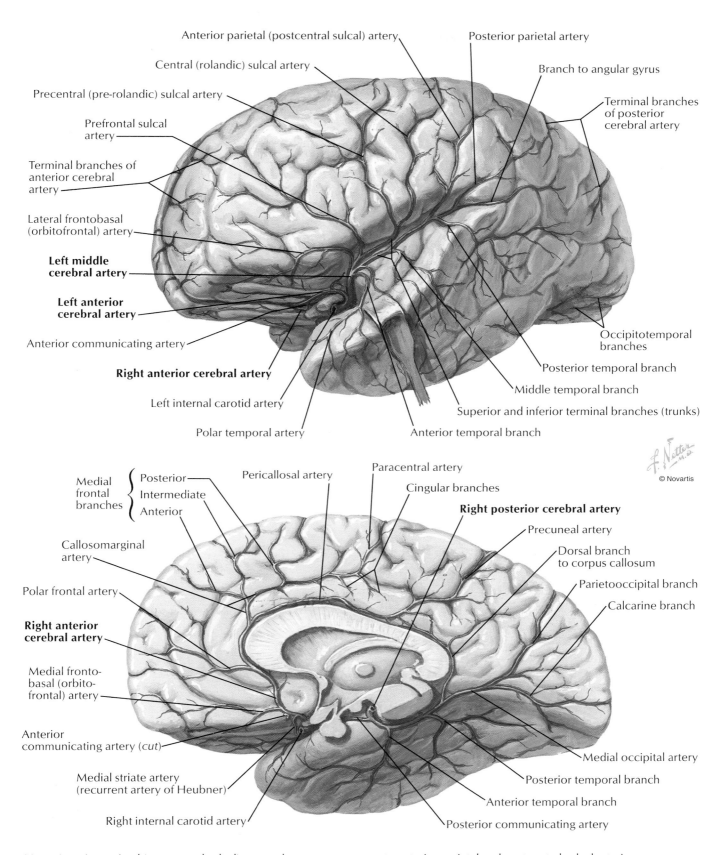

Anterior parietal (postcentral sulcal) artery

Central (rolandic) sulcal artery

Precentral (pre-rolandic) sulcal artery

Prefrontal sulcal artery

Terminal branches of anterior cerebral artery

Lateral frontobasal (orbitofrontal) artery

**Left middle cerebral artery**

**Left anterior cerebral artery**

Anterior communicating artery

**Right anterior cerebral artery**

Left internal carotid artery

Polar temporal artery

Posterior parietal artery

Branch to angular gyrus

Terminal branches of posterior cerebral artery

Occipitotemporal branches

Posterior temporal branch

Middle temporal branch

Superior and inferior terminal branches (trunks)

Anterior temporal branch

Medial frontal branches { Posterior — Intermediate — Anterior

Pericallosal artery

Paracentral artery

Cingular branches

**Right posterior cerebral artery**

Precuneal artery

Dorsal branch to corpus callosum

Parietooccipital branch

Calcarine branch

Callosomarginal artery

Polar frontal artery

**Right anterior cerebral artery**

Medial fronto-basal (orbito-frontal) artery

Anterior communicating artery (*cut*)

Medial striate artery (recurrent artery of Heubner)

Right internal carotid artery

Medial occipital artery

Posterior temporal branch

Anterior temporal branch

Posterior communicating artery

Note: Anterior parietal (postcentral sulcal) artery also occurs as separate anterior parietal and postcentral sulcal arteries

© Novartis

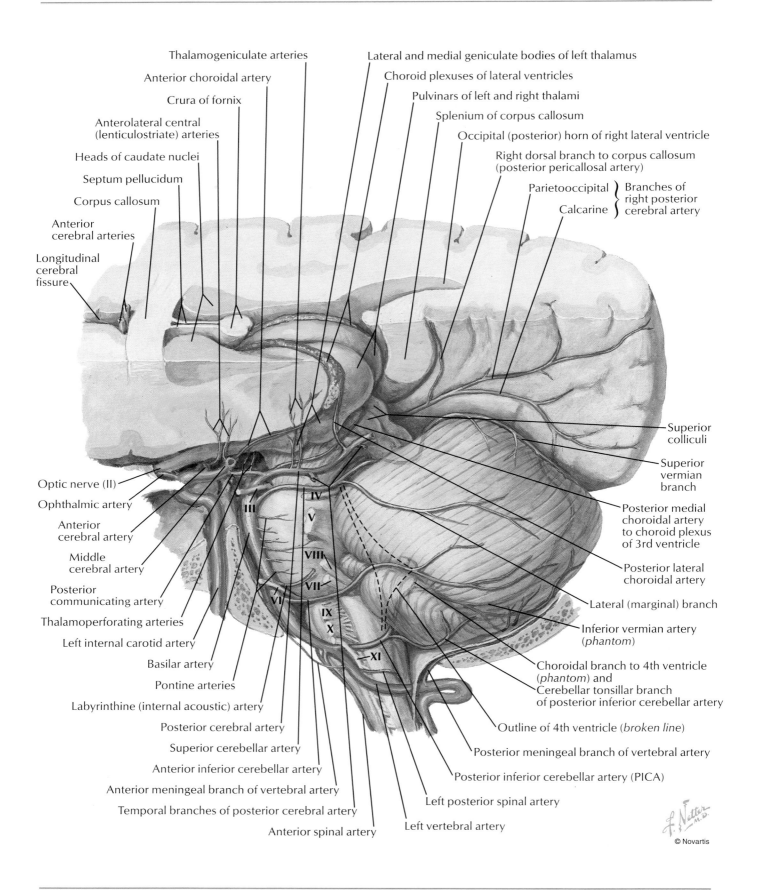

Thalamogeniculate arteries

Anterior choroidal artery

Crura of fornix

Anterolateral central (lenticulostriate) arteries

Heads of caudate nuclei

Septum pellucidum

Corpus callosum

Anterior cerebral arteries

Longitudinal cerebral fissure

Lateral and medial geniculate bodies of left thalamus

Choroid plexuses of lateral ventricles

Pulvinars of left and right thalami

Splenium of corpus callosum

Occipital (posterior) horn of right lateral ventricle

Right dorsal branch to corpus callosum (posterior pericallosal artery)

Parietooccipital ⎱ Branches of
Calcarine ⎰ right posterior cerebral artery

Superior colliculi

Superior vermian branch

Posterior medial choroidal artery to choroid plexus of 3rd ventricle

Posterior lateral choroidal artery

Lateral (marginal) branch

Inferior vermian artery (*phantom*)

Choroidal branch to 4th ventricle (*phantom*) and Cerebellar tonsillar branch of posterior inferior cerebellar artery

Outline of 4th ventricle (*broken line*)

Posterior meningeal branch of vertebral artery

Posterior inferior cerebellar artery (PICA)

Left posterior spinal artery

Left vertebral artery

Optic nerve (II)

Ophthalmic artery

Anterior cerebral artery

Middle cerebral artery

Posterior communicating artery

Thalamoperforating arteries

Left internal carotid artery

Basilar artery

Pontine arteries

Labyrinthine (internal acoustic) artery

Posterior cerebral artery

Superior cerebellar artery

Anterior inferior cerebellar artery

Anterior meningeal branch of vertebral artery

Temporal branches of posterior cerebral artery

Anterior spinal artery

III

IV

V

VIII

VII

VI

IX

X

XI

**PLATE 136**

**HEAD AND NECK**

© Novartis

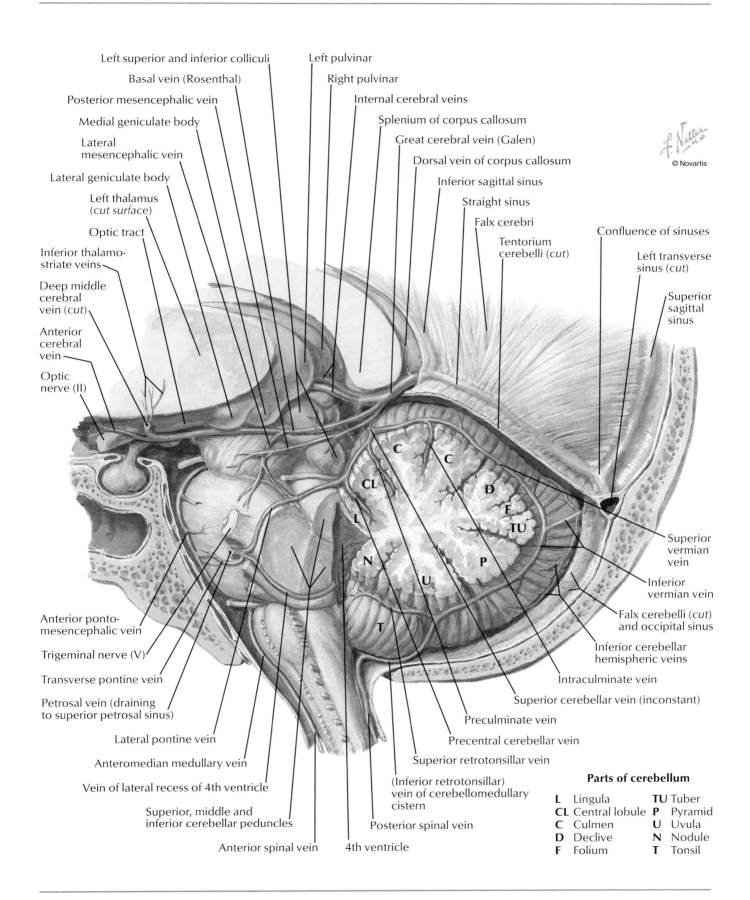

Left superior and inferior colliculi

Basal vein (Rosenthal)

Posterior mesencephalic vein

Medial geniculate body

Lateral mesencephalic vein

Lateral geniculate body

Left thalamus (*cut surface*)

Optic tract

Inferior thalamo-striate veins

Deep middle cerebral vein (*cut*)

Anterior cerebral vein

Optic nerve (II)

Left pulvinar

Right pulvinar

Internal cerebral veins

Splenium of corpus callosum

Great cerebral vein (Galen)

Dorsal vein of corpus callosum

Inferior sagittal sinus

Straight sinus

Falx cerebri

Tentorium cerebelli (*cut*)

Confluence of sinuses

Left transverse sinus (*cut*)

Superior sagittal sinus

Superior vermian vein

Inferior vermian vein

Falx cerebelli (*cut*) and occipital sinus

Inferior cerebellar hemispheric veins

Intraculminate vein

Superior cerebellar vein (inconstant)

Precentral cerebellar vein

Preculminate vein

Superior retrotonsillar vein

(Inferior retrotonsillar) vein of cerebellomedullary cistern

Posterior spinal vein

4th ventricle

Anterior spinal vein

Superior, middle and inferior cerebellar peduncles

Vein of lateral recess of 4th ventricle

Anteromedian medullary vein

Lateral pontine vein

Petrosal vein (draining to superior petrosal sinus)

Transverse pontine vein

Trigeminal nerve (V)

Anterior ponto-mesencephalic vein

f. Netter
M.D.
© Novartis

**Parts of cerebellum**

| | | | |
|---|---|---|---|
| **L** | Lingula | **TU** | Tuber |
| **CL** | Central lobule | **P** | Pyramid |
| **C** | Culmen | **U** | Uvula |
| **D** | Declive | **N** | Nodule |
| **F** | Folium | **T** | Tonsil |

# Deep Veins of Brain

*FOR SUPERFICIAL VEINS OF BRAIN SEE PLATE 96*

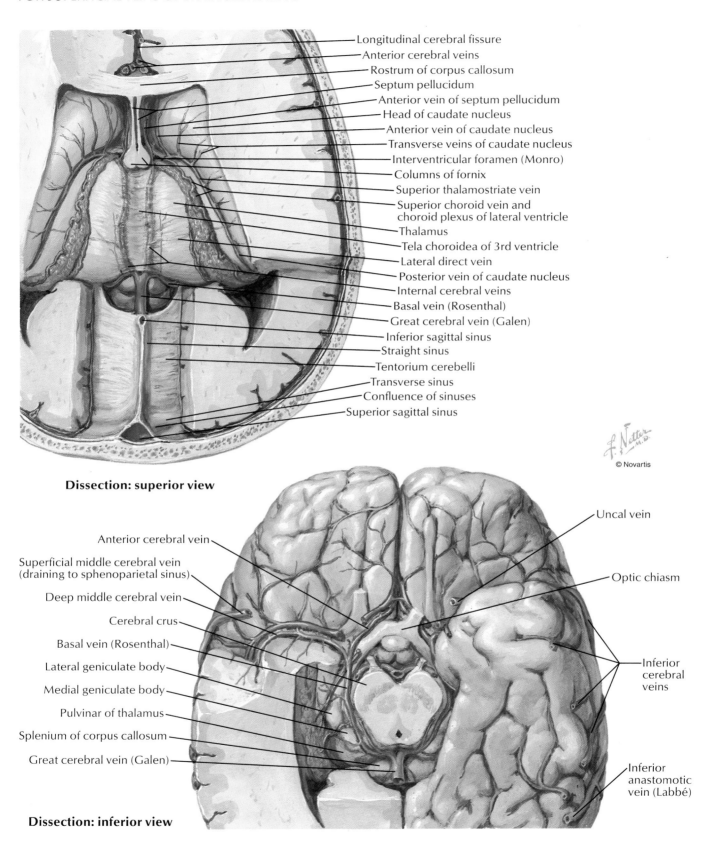

Longitudinal cerebral fissure
Anterior cerebral veins
Rostrum of corpus callosum
Septum pellucidum
Anterior vein of septum pellucidum
Head of caudate nucleus
Anterior vein of caudate nucleus
Transverse veins of caudate nucleus
Interventricular foramen (Monro)
Columns of fornix
Superior thalamostriate vein
Superior choroid vein and choroid plexus of lateral ventricle
Thalamus
Tela choroidea of 3rd ventricle
Lateral direct vein
Posterior vein of caudate nucleus
Internal cerebral veins
Basal vein (Rosenthal)
Great cerebral vein (Galen)
Inferior sagittal sinus
Straight sinus
Tentorium cerebelli
Transverse sinus
Confluence of sinuses
Superior sagittal sinus

**Dissection: superior view**

© Novartis

Anterior cerebral vein
Superficial middle cerebral vein (draining to sphenoparietal sinus)
Deep middle cerebral vein
Cerebral crus
Basal vein (Rosenthal)
Lateral geniculate body
Medial geniculate body
Pulvinar of thalamus
Splenium of corpus callosum
Great cerebral vein (Galen)

Uncal vein
Optic chiasm
Inferior cerebral veins
Inferior anastomotic vein (Labbé)

**Dissection: inferior view**

*PLATE 138*

**HEAD AND NECK**

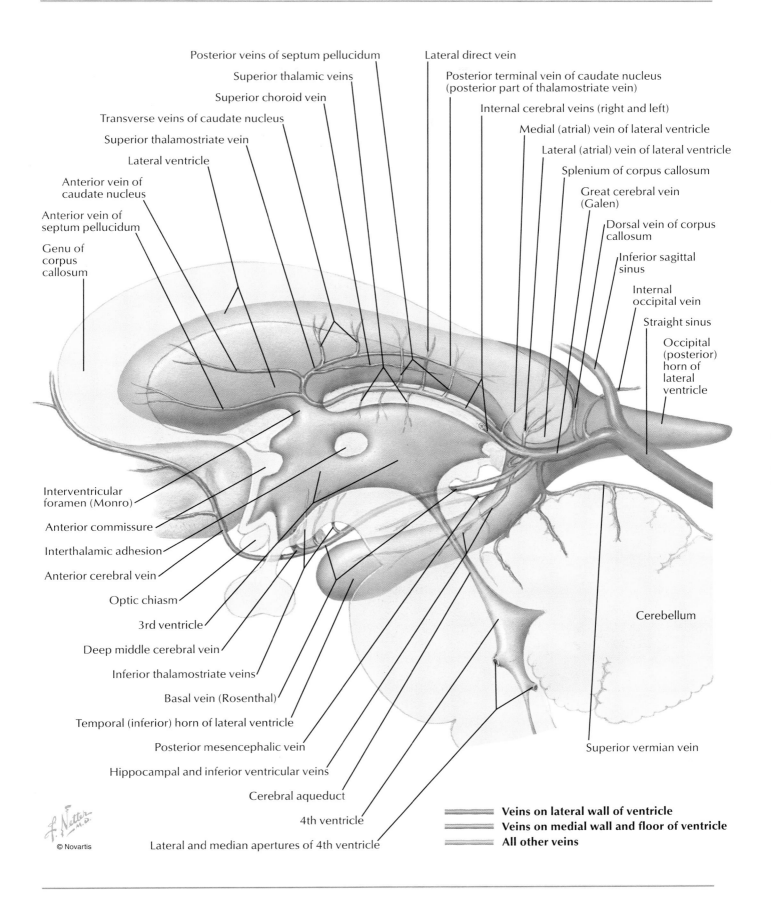

Posterior veins of septum pellucidum

Superior thalamic veins

Superior choroid vein

Transverse veins of caudate nucleus

Superior thalamostriate vein

Lateral ventricle

Anterior vein of caudate nucleus

Anterior vein of septum pellucidum

Genu of corpus callosum

Lateral direct vein

Posterior terminal vein of caudate nucleus (posterior part of thalamostriate vein)

Internal cerebral veins (right and left)

Medial (atrial) vein of lateral ventricle

Lateral (atrial) vein of lateral ventricle

Splenium of corpus callosum

Great cerebral vein (Galen)

Dorsal vein of corpus callosum

Inferior sagittal sinus

Internal occipital vein

Straight sinus

Occipital (posterior) horn of lateral ventricle

Interventricular foramen (Monro)

Anterior commissure

Interthalamic adhesion

Anterior cerebral vein

Optic chiasm

3rd ventricle

Deep middle cerebral vein

Inferior thalamostriate veins

Basal vein (Rosenthal)

Temporal (inferior) horn of lateral ventricle

Posterior mesencephalic vein

Hippocampal and inferior ventricular veins

Cerebral aqueduct

4th ventricle

Lateral and median apertures of 4th ventricle

Cerebellum

Superior vermian vein

Veins on lateral wall of ventricle

Veins on medial wall and floor of ventricle

All other veins

*f. Netter M.D.*

© Novartis

# Hypothalamus and Hypophysis

*SEE ALSO PLATES 100, 101*

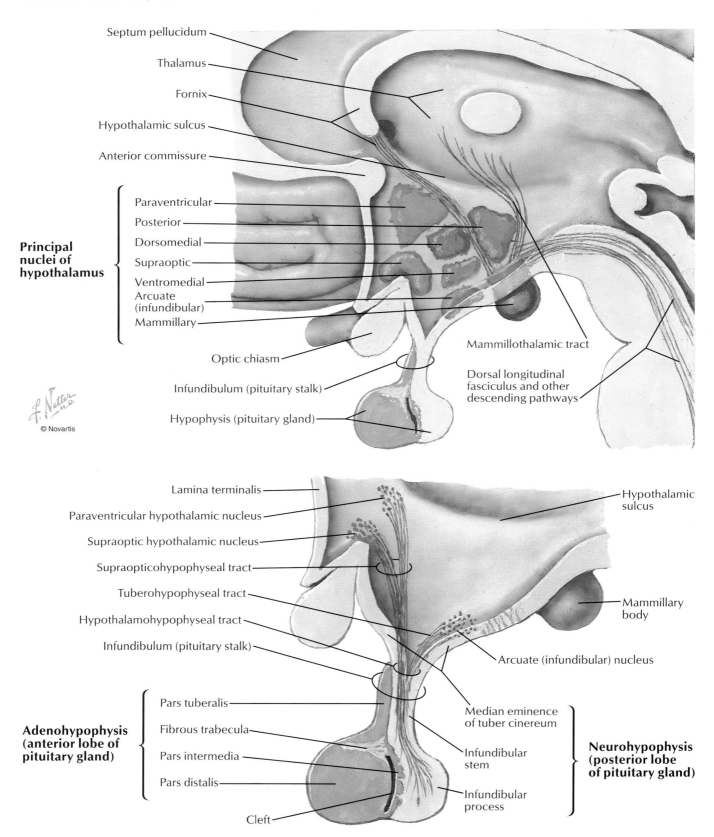

Septum pellucidum

Thalamus

Fornix

Hypothalamic sulcus

Anterior commissure

**Principal nuclei of hypothalamus**

Paraventricular

Posterior

Dorsomedial

Supraoptic

Ventromedial

Arcuate (infundibular)

Mammillary

Optic chiasm

Infundibulum (pituitary stalk)

Hypophysis (pituitary gland)

Mammillothalamic tract

Dorsal longitudinal fasciculus and other descending pathways

Lamina terminalis

Paraventricular hypothalamic nucleus

Supraoptic hypothalamic nucleus

Supraopticohypophyseal tract

Tuberohypophyseal tract

Hypothalamohypophyseal tract

Infundibulum (pituitary stalk)

Hypothalamic sulcus

Mammillary body

Arcuate (infundibular) nucleus

**Adenohypophysis (anterior lobe of pituitary gland)**

Pars tuberalis

Fibrous trabecula

Pars intermedia

Pars distalis

Cleft

Median eminence of tuber cinereum

Infundibular stem

Infundibular process

**Neurohypophysis (posterior lobe of pituitary gland)**

*F. Netter* M.D.

© Novartis

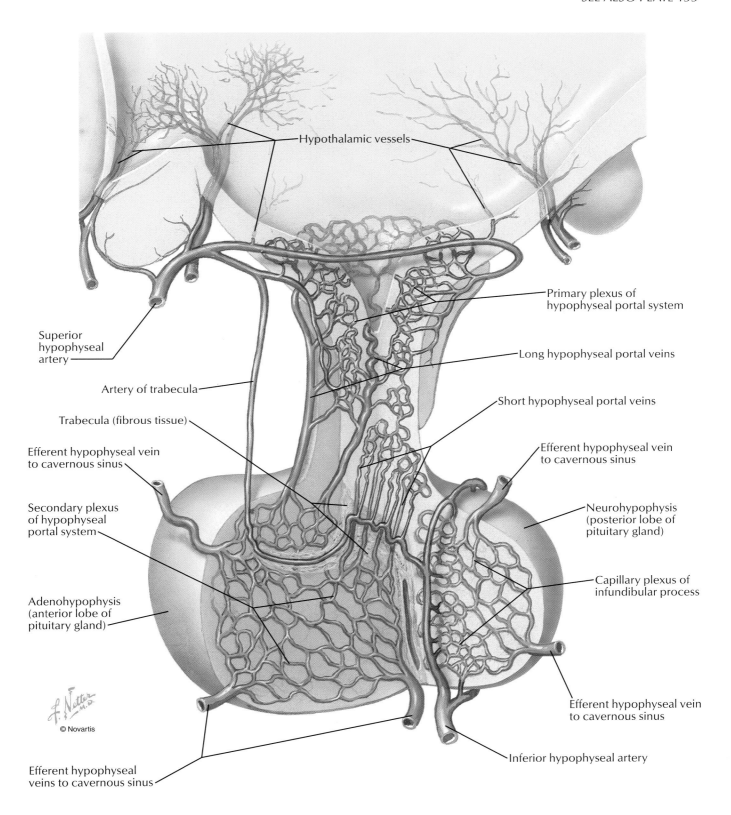

Hypothalamic vessels

Primary plexus of hypophyseal portal system

Superior hypophyseal artery

Long hypophyseal portal veins

Artery of trabecula

Short hypophyseal portal veins

Trabecula (fibrous tissue)

Efferent hypophyseal vein to cavernous sinus

Efferent hypophyseal vein to cavernous sinus

Secondary plexus of hypophyseal portal system

Neurohypophysis (posterior lobe of pituitary gland)

Capillary plexus of infundibular process

Adenohypophysis (anterior lobe of pituitary gland)

© Novartis

Efferent hypophyseal vein to cavernous sinus

Inferior hypophyseal artery

Efferent hypophyseal veins to cavernous sinus

# Section II
# BACK AND SPINAL CORD

**BONES AND LIGAMENTS**
*Plates 142 – 147*

142. Vertebral Column
143. Thoracic Vertebrae
144. Lumbar Vertebrae
145. Sacrum and Coccyx
146. Vertebral Ligaments:
     Lumbar Region
147. Vertebral Ligaments:
     Lumbosacral Region

**SPINAL CORD**
*Plates 148 – 159*

148. Spinal Cord In Situ
149. Relation of Spinal Nerve Roots
     to Vertebrae
150. Dermatomes
151. Spinal Cord Cross Sections:
     Fiber Tracts

152. Autonomic Nervous System:
     General Topography
153. Autonomic Nervous System:
     Schema
154. Cholinergic and Adrenergic Synapses:
     Schema
155. Spinal Membranes and Nerve Roots
156. Spinal Nerve Origin: Cross Sections
157. Arteries of Spinal Cord: Schema
158. Arteries of Spinal Cord: Intrinsic
     Distribution
159. Veins of Spinal Cord and
     Vertebral Column

**MUSCLES AND NERVES**
*Plates 160 – 166*

160. Muscles of Back: Superficial Layers
161. Muscles of Back: Intermediate Layers
162. Muscles of Back: Deep Layers

163. Nerves of Back
164. Suboccipital Triangle
165. Lumbar Region of Back: Cross
     Section (Superior View)
166. Typical Thoracic Spinal Nerve

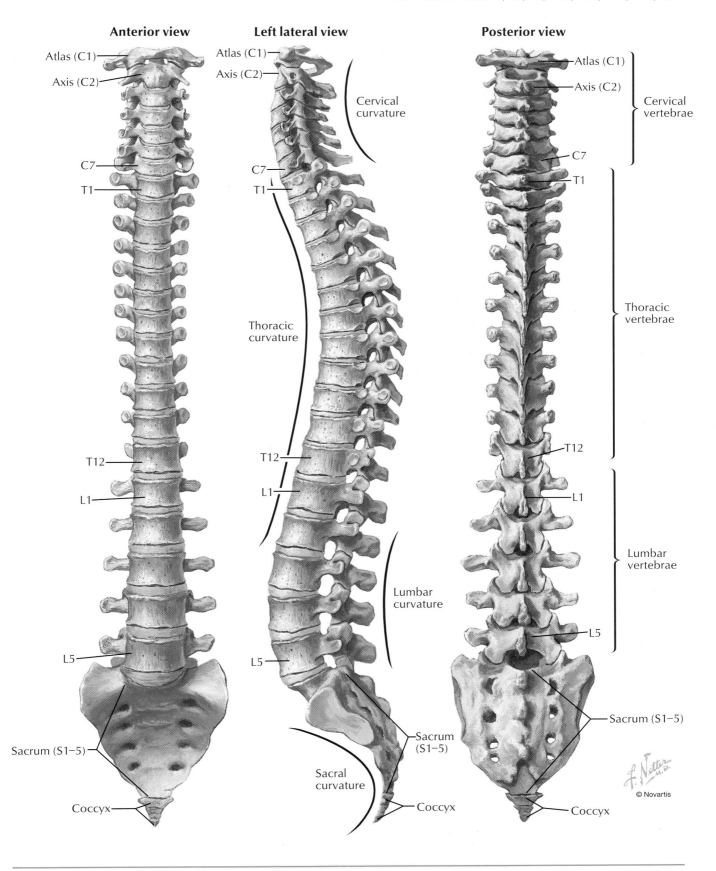

**Anterior view**

Atlas (C1)
Axis (C2)
C7
T1
T12
L1
L5
Sacrum (S1–5)
Coccyx

**Left lateral view**

Atlas (C1)
Axis (C2)
Cervical curvature
C7
T1
Thoracic curvature
T12
L1
Lumbar curvature
L5
Sacrum (S1–5)
Sacral curvature
Coccyx

**Posterior view**

Atlas (C1)
Axis (C2)
Cervical vertebrae
C7
T1
Thoracic vertebrae
T12
L1
Lumbar vertebrae
L5
Sacrum (S1–5)
Coccyx

© Novartis

# Thoracic Vertebrae

SEE ALSO PLATE 172

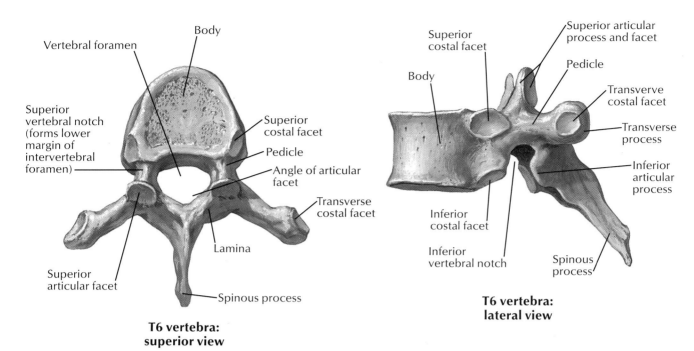

**T6 vertebra:
superior view**

Vertebral foramen

Body

Superior
vertebral notch
(forms lower
margin of
intervertebral
foramen)

Superior
costal facet

Pedicle

Angle of articular
facet

Transverse
costal facet

Lamina

Superior
articular facet

Spinous process

Superior
costal facet

Body

Superior articular
process and facet

Pedicle

Transverve
costal facet

Transverse
process

Inferior
articular
process

Inferior
costal facet

Inferior
vertebral notch

Spinous
process

**T6 vertebra:
lateral view**

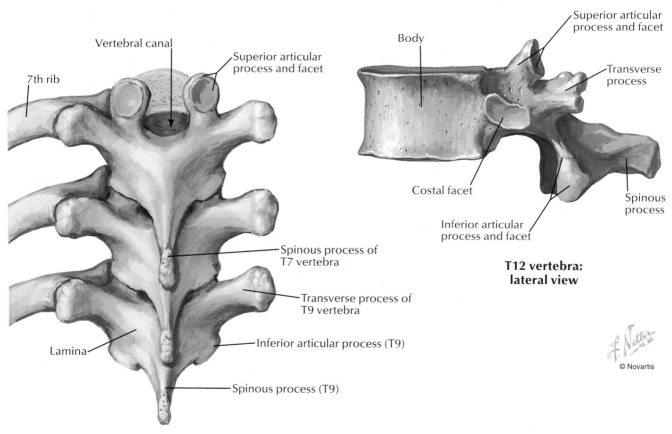

Vertebral canal

7th rib

Superior articular
process and facet

Spinous process of
T7 vertebra

Transverse process of
T9 vertebra

Inferior articular process (T9)

Lamina

Spinous process (T9)

**T7, T8 and T9 vertebrae:
posterior view**

Body

Superior articular
process and facet

Transverse
process

Costal facet

Inferior articular
process and facet

Spinous
process

**T12 vertebra:
lateral view**

© Novartis

**PLATE 143**

**BACK AND SPINAL CORD**

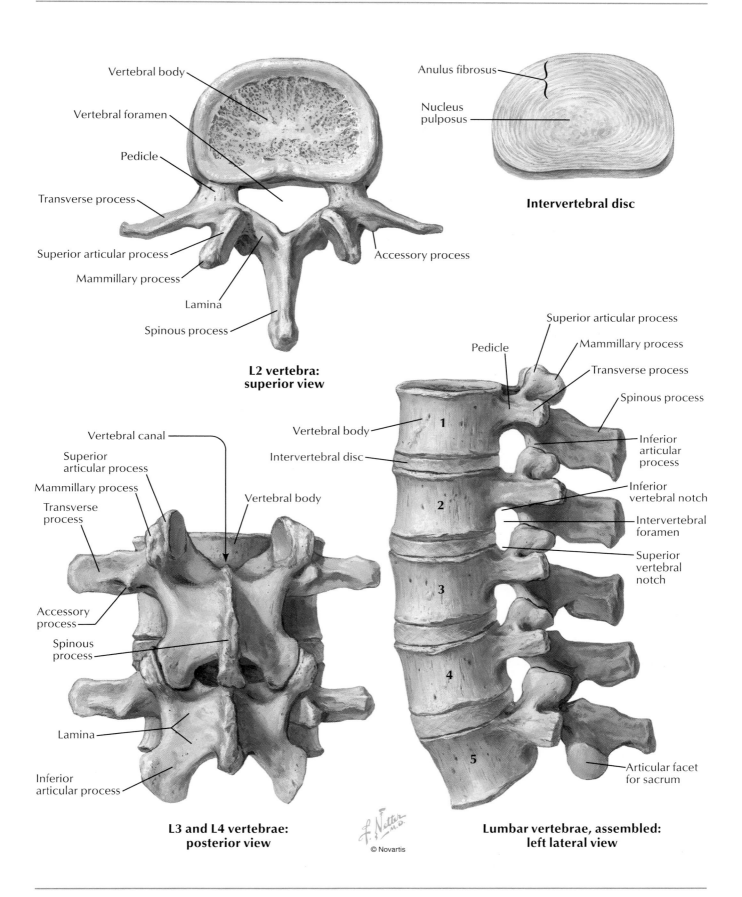

**L2 vertebra:
superior view**

**Intervertebral disc**

**L3 and L4 vertebrae:
posterior view**

**Lumbar vertebrae, assembled:
left lateral view**

# Sacrum and Coccyx

SEE ALSO PLATES 142, 147, 231, 330, 331, 332

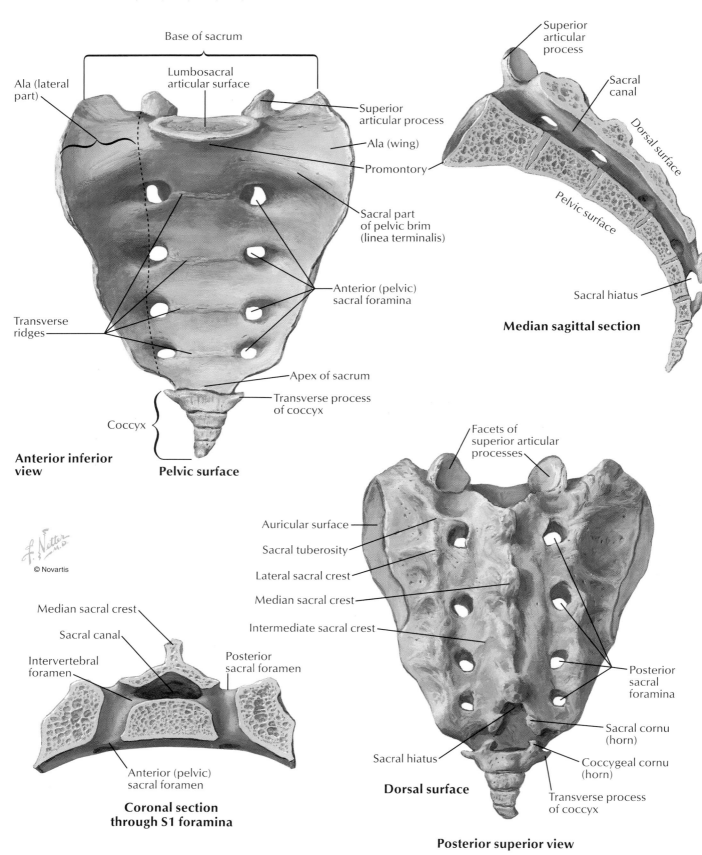

**Anterior inferior view**

Base of sacrum

Lumbosacral articular surface

Ala (lateral part)

Superior articular process

Ala (wing)

Promontory

Sacral part of pelvic brim (linea terminalis)

Anterior (pelvic) sacral foramina

Transverse ridges

Apex of sacrum

Transverse process of coccyx

Coccyx

**Pelvic surface**

**Median sagittal section**

Superior articular process

Sacral canal

Dorsal surface

Pelvic surface

Sacral hiatus

**Coronal section through S1 foramina**

Median sacral crest

Sacral canal

Intervertebral foramen

Posterior sacral foramen

Anterior (pelvic) sacral foramen

**Posterior superior view**

Facets of superior articular processes

Auricular surface

Sacral tuberosity

Lateral sacral crest

Median sacral crest

Intermediate sacral crest

Posterior sacral foramina

Sacral cornu (horn)

Coccygeal cornu (horn)

Transverse process of coccyx

Sacral hiatus

**Dorsal surface**

© Novartis

**PLATE 145**                    **BACK AND SPINAL CORD**

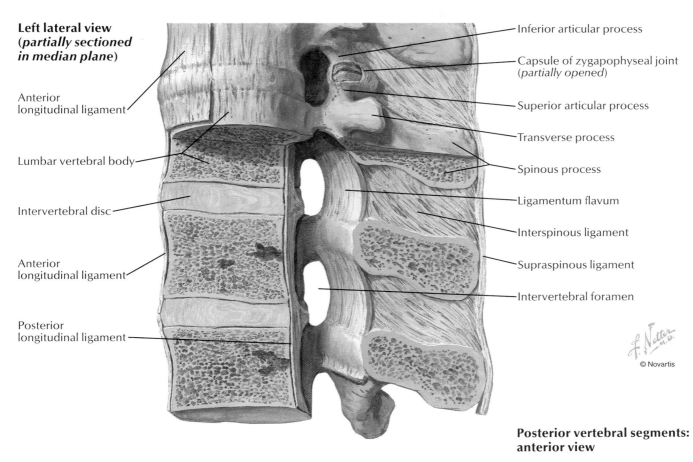

**Left lateral view** (*partially sectioned in median plane*)

Anterior longitudinal ligament

Lumbar vertebral body

Intervertebral disc

Anterior longitudinal ligament

Posterior longitudinal ligament

Inferior articular process

Capsule of zygapophyseal joint (*partially opened*)

Superior articular process

Transverse process

Spinous process

Ligamentum flavum

Interspinous ligament

Supraspinous ligament

Intervertebral foramen

© Novartis

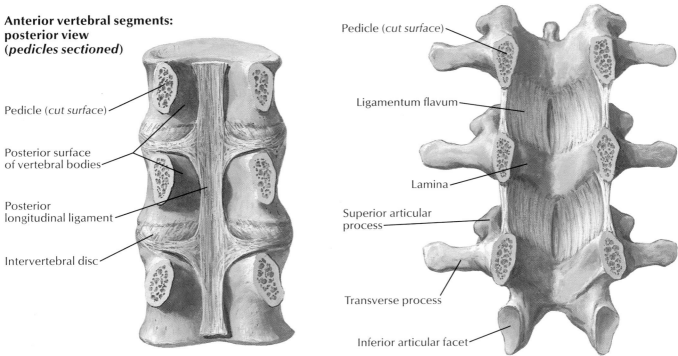

**Anterior vertebral segments: posterior view** (*pedicles sectioned*)

Pedicle (*cut surface*)

Posterior surface of vertebral bodies

Posterior longitudinal ligament

Intervertebral disc

**Posterior vertebral segments: anterior view**

Pedicle (*cut surface*)

Ligamentum flavum

Lamina

Superior articular process

Transverse process

Inferior articular facet

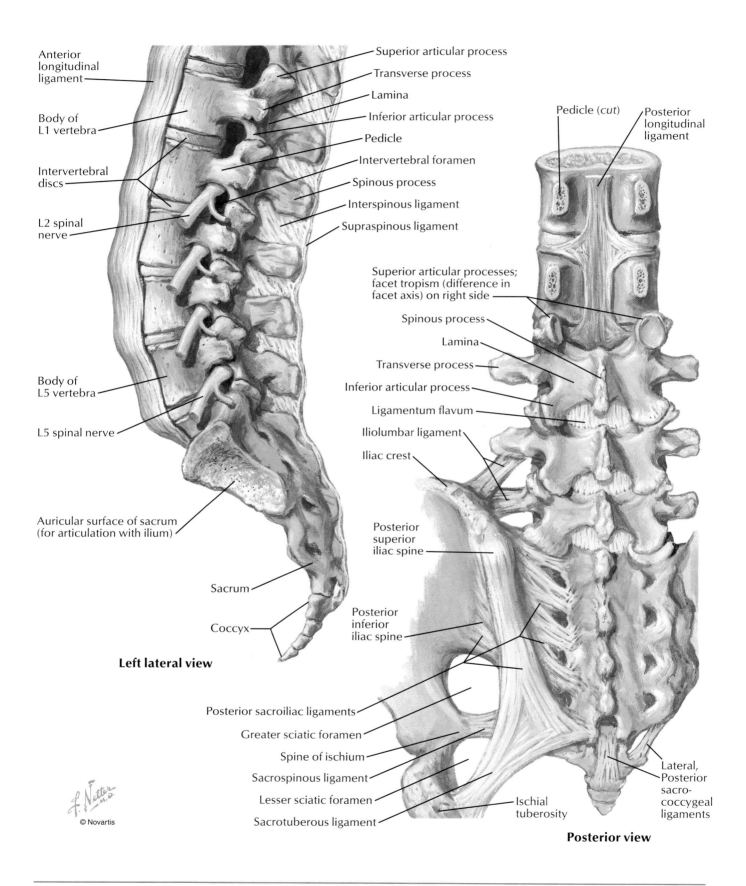

Anterior longitudinal ligament

Body of L1 vertebra

Intervertebral discs

L2 spinal nerve

Superior articular process

Transverse process

Lamina

Inferior articular process

Pedicle

Intervertebral foramen

Spinous process

Interspinous ligament

Supraspinous ligament

Pedicle (*cut*)

Posterior longitudinal ligament

Superior articular processes; facet tropism (difference in facet axis) on right side

Spinous process

Lamina

Transverse process

Inferior articular process

Ligamentum flavum

Iliolumbar ligament

Iliac crest

Body of L5 vertebra

L5 spinal nerve

Auricular surface of sacrum (for articulation with ilium)

Sacrum

Coccyx

Posterior superior iliac spine

Posterior inferior iliac spine

Posterior sacroiliac ligaments

Greater sciatic foramen

Spine of ischium

Sacrospinous ligament

Lesser sciatic foramen

Sacrotuberous ligament

Ischial tuberosity

Lateral, Posterior sacro-coccygeal ligaments

**Left lateral view**

**Posterior view**

*PLATE 147*

**BACK AND SPINAL CORD**

© Novartis

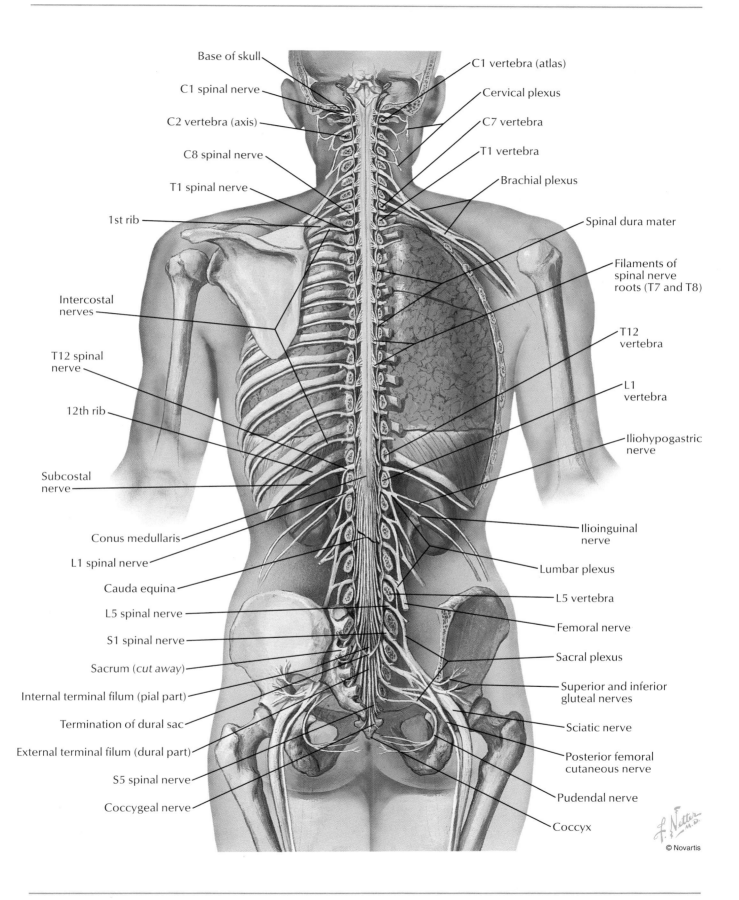

Base of skull

C1 spinal nerve

C2 vertebra (axis)

C8 spinal nerve

T1 spinal nerve

1st rib

Intercostal nerves

T12 spinal nerve

12th rib

Subcostal nerve

Conus medullaris

L1 spinal nerve

Cauda equina

L5 spinal nerve

S1 spinal nerve

Sacrum (*cut away*)

Internal terminal filum (pial part)

Termination of dural sac

External terminal filum (dural part)

S5 spinal nerve

Coccygeal nerve

C1 vertebra (atlas)

Cervical plexus

C7 vertebra

T1 vertebra

Brachial plexus

Spinal dura mater

Filaments of spinal nerve roots (T7 and T8)

T12 vertebra

L1 vertebra

Iliohypogastric nerve

Ilioinguinal nerve

Lumbar plexus

L5 vertebra

Femoral nerve

Sacral plexus

Superior and inferior gluteal nerves

Sciatic nerve

Posterior femoral cutaneous nerve

Pudendal nerve

Coccyx

*f. Netter m.d.*

© Novartis

# Relation of Spinal Nerve Roots to Vertebrae

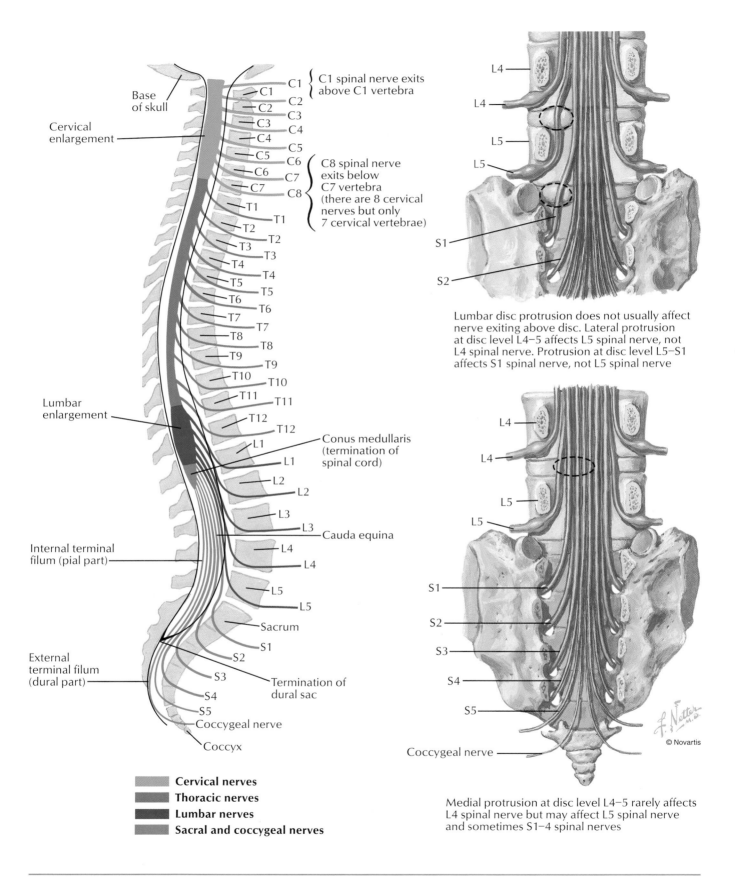

Base of skull

Cervical enlargement

C1
C1
C2
C2
C3
C3
C4
C4
C5
C5
C6
C6
C7
C7
C8

{ C1 spinal nerve exits above C1 vertebra

{ C8 spinal nerve exits below C7 vertebra (there are 8 cervical nerves but only 7 cervical vertebrae)

T1
T1
T2
T2
T3
T3
T4
T4
T5
T5
T6
T6
T7
T7
T8
T8
T9
T9
T10
T10
T11
T11

Lumbar enlargement

T12
T12
L1
L1
L2
L2
L3
L3
L4
L4
L5
L5

Conus medullaris (termination of spinal cord)

Internal terminal filum (pial part)

Cauda equina

Sacrum
S1
S2
S3
S4
S5

Termination of dural sac

External terminal filum (dural part)

Coccygeal nerve

Coccyx

Cervical nerves
Thoracic nerves
Lumbar nerves
Sacral and coccygeal nerves

L4
L4
L5
L5
S1
S2

Lumbar disc protrusion does not usually affect nerve exiting above disc. Lateral protrusion at disc level L4−5 affects L5 spinal nerve, not L4 spinal nerve. Protrusion at disc level L5−S1 affects S1 spinal nerve, not L5 spinal nerve

L4
L4
L5
L5
S1
S2
S3
S4
S5

Coccygeal nerve

© Novartis

Medial protrusion at disc level L4−5 rarely affects L4 spinal nerve but may affect L5 spinal nerve and sometimes S1−4 spinal nerves

PLATE 149

**BACK AND SPINAL CORD**

*SEE ALSO PLATES 451, 507; FOR MAPS OF CUTANEOUS NERVES SEE PLATES 18, 441, 443, 444, 445, 447, 450, 502–506*

Schematic demarcation of dermatomes
shown as distinct segments. There
is actually considerable overlap
between any two adjacent dermatomes

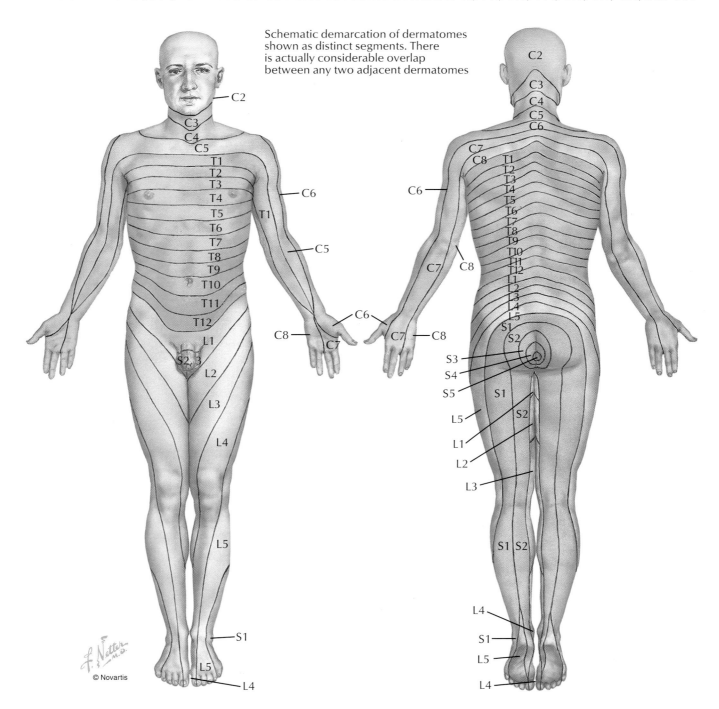

© Novartis

### Levels of principal dermatomes

| | |
|---|---|
| **C5** | Clavicles |
| **C5, 6, 7** | Lateral parts of upper limbs |
| **C8, T1** | Medial sides of upper limbs |
| **C6** | Thumb |
| **C6, 7, 8** | Hand |
| **C8** | Ring and little fingers |
| **T4** | Level of nipples |
| **T10** | Level of umbilicus |
| **T12** | Inguinal or groin regions |
| **L1, 2, 3, 4** | Anterior and inner surfaces of lower limbs |
| **L4, 5, S1** | Foot |
| **L4** | Medial side of great toe |
| **S1, 2, L5** | Posterior and outer surfaces of lower limbs |
| **S1** | Lateral margin of foot and little toe |
| **S2, 3, 4** | Perineum |

# Spinal Cord Cross Sections: Fiber Tracts

## Sections through spinal cord at various levels

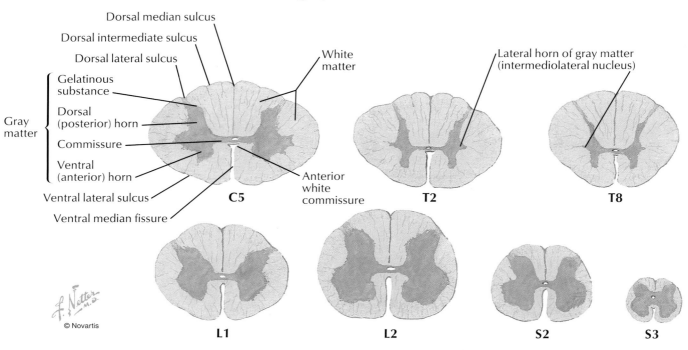

Dorsal median sulcus
Dorsal intermediate sulcus
Dorsal lateral sulcus

Gelatinous substance
Dorsal (posterior) horn
Commissure
Ventral (anterior) horn

Gray matter

Ventral lateral sulcus
Ventral median fissure

White matter

Anterior white commissure

**C5**

Lateral horn of gray matter (intermediolateral nucleus)

**T2**

**T8**

**L1**

**L2**

**S2**

**S3**

*f. Netter*
© Novartis

---

### Principal fiber tracts of spinal cord

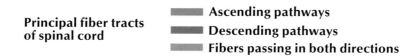

**Ascending pathways**
**Descending pathways**
**Fibers passing in both directions**

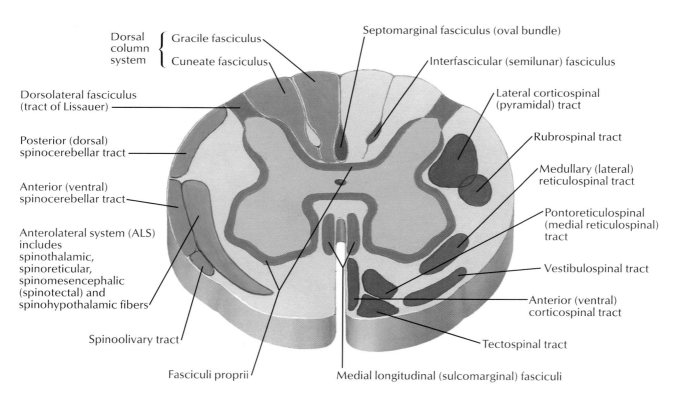

Dorsal column system
{ Gracile fasciculus
Cuneate fasciculus

Septomarginal fasciculus (oval bundle)

Interfascicular (semilunar) fasciculus

Dorsolateral fasciculus (tract of Lissauer)

Lateral corticospinal (pyramidal) tract

Posterior (dorsal) spinocerebellar tract

Rubrospinal tract

Anterior (ventral) spinocerebellar tract

Medullary (lateral) reticulospinal tract

Anterolateral system (ALS) includes spinothalamic, spinoreticular, spinomesencephalic (spinotectal) and spinohypothalamic fibers

Pontoreticulospinal (medial reticulospinal) tract

Vestibulospinal tract

Spinoolivary tract

Anterior (ventral) corticospinal tract

Fasciculi proprii

Tectospinal tract

Medial longitudinal (sulcomarginal) fasciculi

**PLATE 151**

**BACK AND SPINAL CORD**

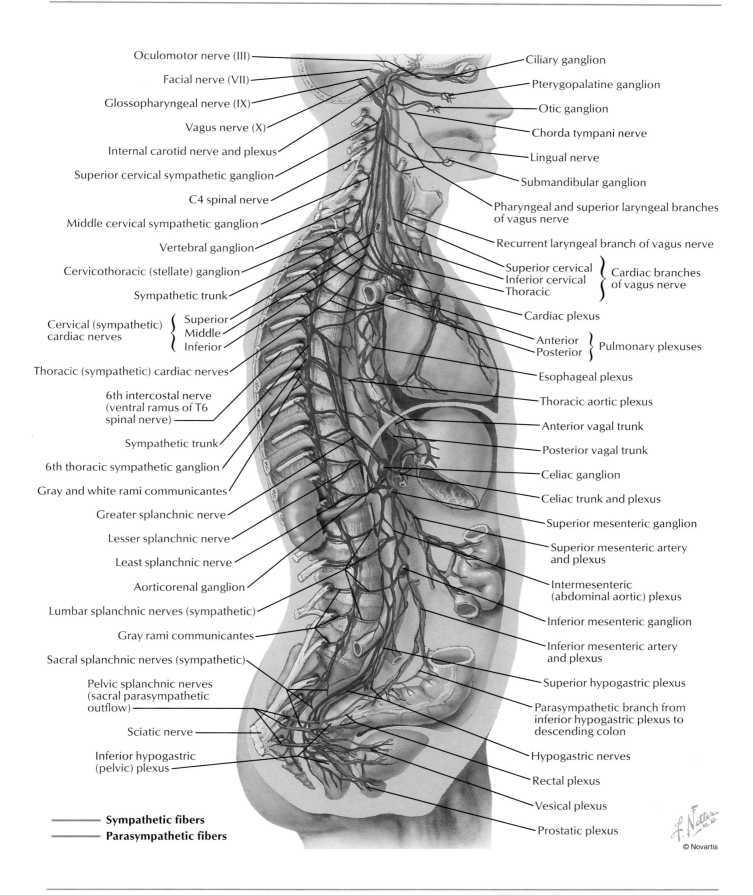

Oculomotor nerve (III)
Facial nerve (VII)
Glossopharyngeal nerve (IX)
Vagus nerve (X)
Internal carotid nerve and plexus
Superior cervical sympathetic ganglion
C4 spinal nerve
Middle cervical sympathetic ganglion
Vertebral ganglion
Cervicothoracic (stellate) ganglion
Sympathetic trunk
Cervical (sympathetic) cardiac nerves {
  Superior
  Middle
  Inferior
}
Thoracic (sympathetic) cardiac nerves
6th intercostal nerve (ventral ramus of T6 spinal nerve)
Sympathetic trunk
6th thoracic sympathetic ganglion
Gray and white rami communicantes
Greater splanchnic nerve
Lesser splanchnic nerve
Least splanchnic nerve
Aorticorenal ganglion
Lumbar splanchnic nerves (sympathetic)
Gray rami communicantes
Sacral splanchnic nerves (sympathetic)
Pelvic splanchnic nerves (sacral parasympathetic outflow)
Sciatic nerve
Inferior hypogastric (pelvic) plexus

Ciliary ganglion
Pterygopalatine ganglion
Otic ganglion
Chorda tympani nerve
Lingual nerve
Submandibular ganglion
Pharyngeal and superior laryngeal branches of vagus nerve
Recurrent laryngeal branch of vagus nerve
Superior cervical
Inferior cervical } Cardiac branches of vagus nerve
Thoracic
Cardiac plexus
Anterior
Posterior } Pulmonary plexuses
Esophageal plexus
Thoracic aortic plexus
Anterior vagal trunk
Posterior vagal trunk
Celiac ganglion
Celiac trunk and plexus
Superior mesenteric ganglion
Superior mesenteric artery and plexus
Intermesenteric (abdominal aortic) plexus
Inferior mesenteric ganglion
Inferior mesenteric artery and plexus
Superior hypogastric plexus
Parasympathetic branch from inferior hypogastric plexus to descending colon
Hypogastric nerves
Rectal plexus
Vesical plexus
Prostatic plexus

—— **Sympathetic fibers**
—— **Parasympathetic fibers**

© Novartis

# Autonomic Nervous System: Schema

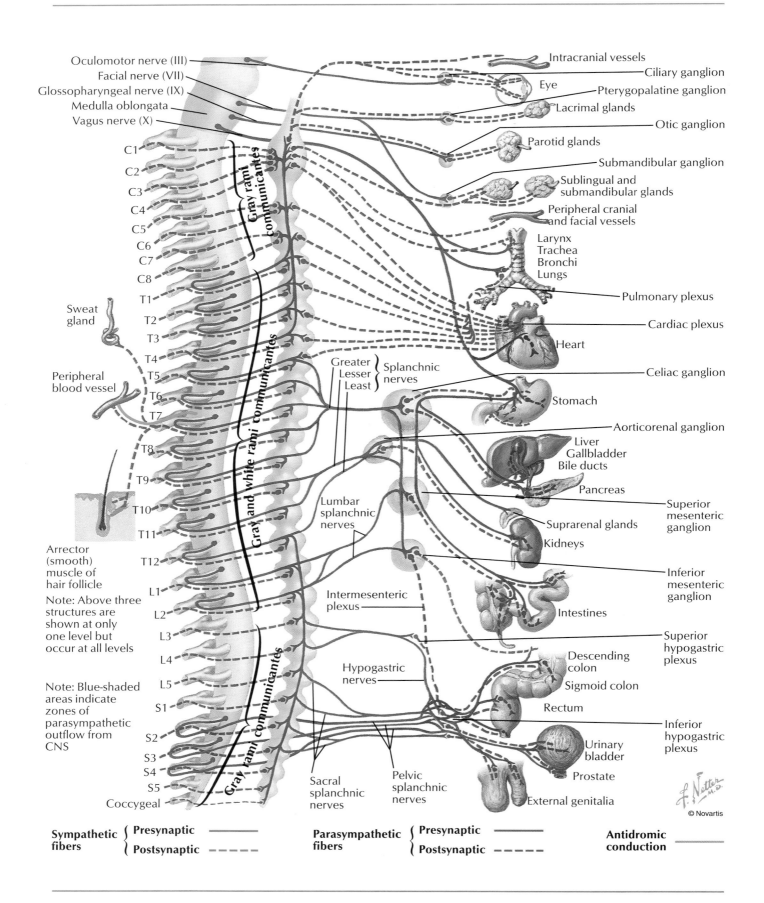

Oculomotor nerve (III)
Facial nerve (VII)
Glossopharyngeal nerve (IX)
Medulla oblongata
Vagus nerve (X)

Intracranial vessels
Ciliary ganglion
Eye
Pterygopalatine ganglion
Lacrimal glands
Otic ganglion
Parotid glands
Submandibular ganglion
Sublingual and submandibular glands
Peripheral cranial and facial vessels

C1
C2
C3
C4
C5
C6
C7
C8

Gray rami communicantes

Larynx
Trachea
Bronchi
Lungs
Pulmonary plexus

T1
T2
T3
T4
T5
T6
T7
T8
T9
T10
T11
T12

Cardiac plexus
Heart
Celiac ganglion
Stomach
Aorticorenal ganglion
Liver
Gallbladder
Bile ducts
Pancreas
Superior mesenteric ganglion
Suprarenal glands
Kidneys
Inferior mesenteric ganglion

Sweat gland

Peripheral blood vessel

Gray and white rami communicantes

Greater
Lesser
Least

Splanchnic nerves

Lumbar splanchnic nerves

L1
L2
L3
L4
L5

Arrector (smooth) muscle of hair follicle

Note: Above three structures are shown at only one level but occur at all levels

Intermesenteric plexus

Intestines

Superior hypogastric plexus

Descending colon
Sigmoid colon
Rectum

Note: Blue-shaded areas indicate zones of parasympathetic outflow from CNS

S1
S2
S3
S4
S5
Coccygeal

Gray rami communicantes

Hypogastric nerves

Sacral splanchnic nerves

Pelvic splanchnic nerves

Inferior hypogastric plexus

Urinary bladder
Prostate
External genitalia

f. Netter M.D.
© Novartis

| Sympathetic fibers | Presynaptic | —————— | Parasympathetic fibers | Presynaptic | —————— | Antidromic conduction | ————— |
| | Postsynaptic | - - - - - | | Postsynaptic | - - - - - | | |

**PLATE 153**

**BACK AND SPINAL CORD**

# Cholinergic and Adrenergic Synapses: Schema

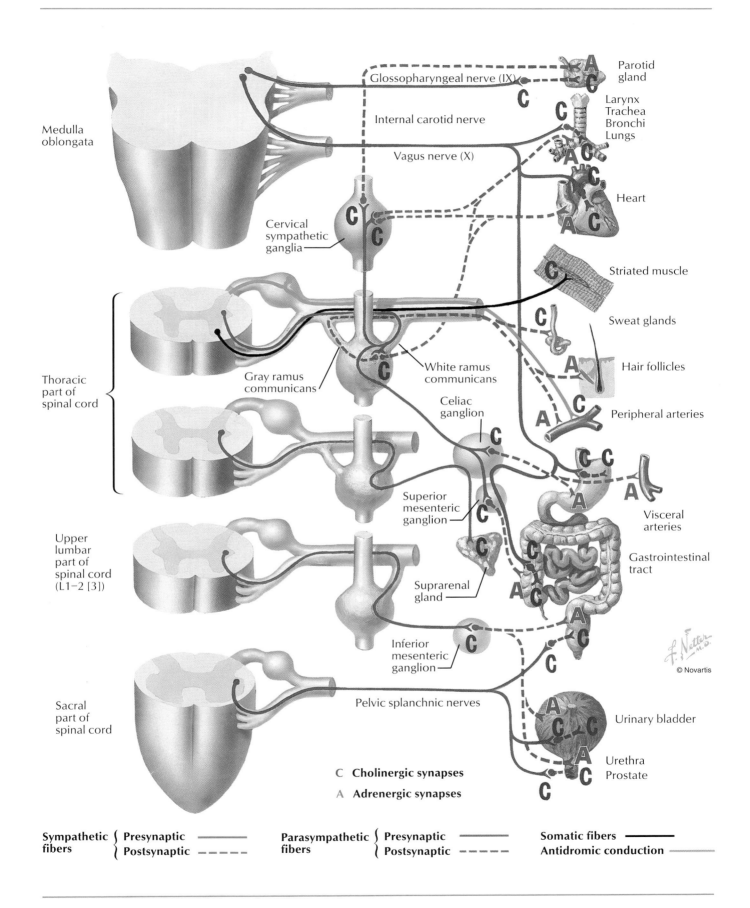

Medulla oblongata

Glossopharyngeal nerve (IX)

Internal carotid nerve

Vagus nerve (X)

Parotid gland

Larynx Trachea Bronchi Lungs

Heart

Cervical sympathetic ganglia

Striated muscle

Thoracic part of spinal cord

Gray ramus communicans

White ramus communicans

Sweat glands

Hair follicles

Celiac ganglion

Peripheral arteries

Superior mesenteric ganglion

Upper lumbar part of spinal cord (L1–2 [3])

Suprarenal gland

Visceral arteries

Gastrointestinal tract

Inferior mesenteric ganglion

Sacral part of spinal cord

Pelvic splanchnic nerves

Urinary bladder

Urethra Prostate

C  Cholinergic synapses

A  Adrenergic synapses

Sympathetic fibers { Presynaptic ——— Postsynaptic – – –

Parasympathetic fibers { Presynaptic ——— Postsynaptic – – –

Somatic fibers ——— Antidromic conduction ———

© Novartis

# Spinal Membranes and Nerve Roots

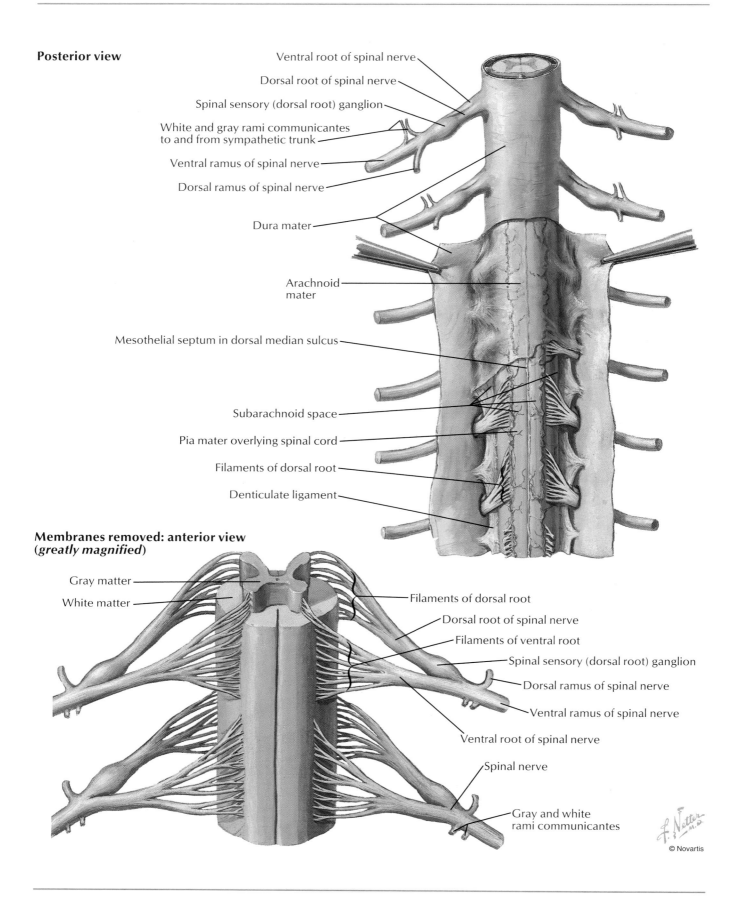

**Posterior view**

Ventral root of spinal nerve

Dorsal root of spinal nerve

Spinal sensory (dorsal root) ganglion

White and gray rami communicantes to and from sympathetic trunk

Ventral ramus of spinal nerve

Dorsal ramus of spinal nerve

Dura mater

Arachnoid mater

Mesothelial septum in dorsal median sulcus

Subarachnoid space

Pia mater overlying spinal cord

Filaments of dorsal root

Denticulate ligament

**Membranes removed: anterior view**
(*greatly magnified*)

Gray matter

White matter

Filaments of dorsal root

Dorsal root of spinal nerve

Filaments of ventral root

Spinal sensory (dorsal root) ganglion

Dorsal ramus of spinal nerve

Ventral ramus of spinal nerve

Ventral root of spinal nerve

Spinal nerve

Gray and white rami communicantes

© Novartis

**PLATE 155**

**BACK AND SPINAL CORD**

**Section through thoracic vertebra**

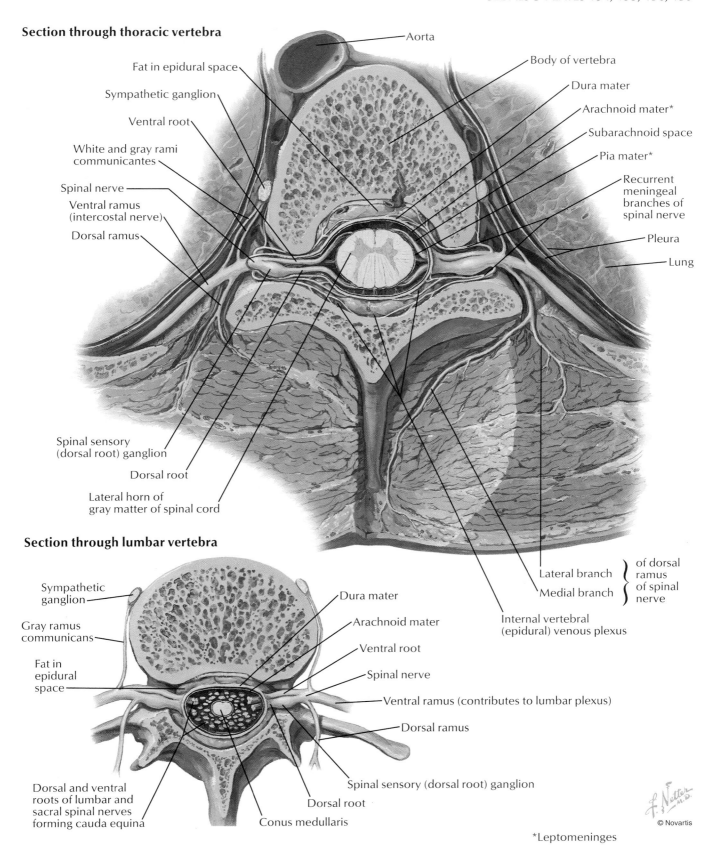

Aorta

Body of vertebra

Dura mater

Arachnoid mater*

Subarachnoid space

Pia mater*

Recurrent meningeal branches of spinal nerve

Pleura

Lung

Fat in epidural space

Sympathetic ganglion

Ventral root

White and gray rami communicantes

Spinal nerve

Ventral ramus (intercostal nerve)

Dorsal ramus

Spinal sensory (dorsal root) ganglion

Dorsal root

Lateral horn of gray matter of spinal cord

Lateral branch } of dorsal ramus
Medial branch } of spinal nerve

Internal vertebral (epidural) venous plexus

**Section through lumbar vertebra**

Sympathetic ganglion

Gray ramus communicans

Fat in epidural space

Dorsal and ventral roots of lumbar and sacral spinal nerves forming cauda equina

Conus medullaris

Dorsal root

Dura mater

Arachnoid mater

Ventral root

Spinal nerve

Ventral ramus (contributes to lumbar plexus)

Dorsal ramus

Spinal sensory (dorsal root) ganglion

*Leptomeninges

© Novartis

**SPINAL CORD**

**PLATE 156**

*SEE ALSO PLATE 131*

**Anterior view**

**Posterior view**

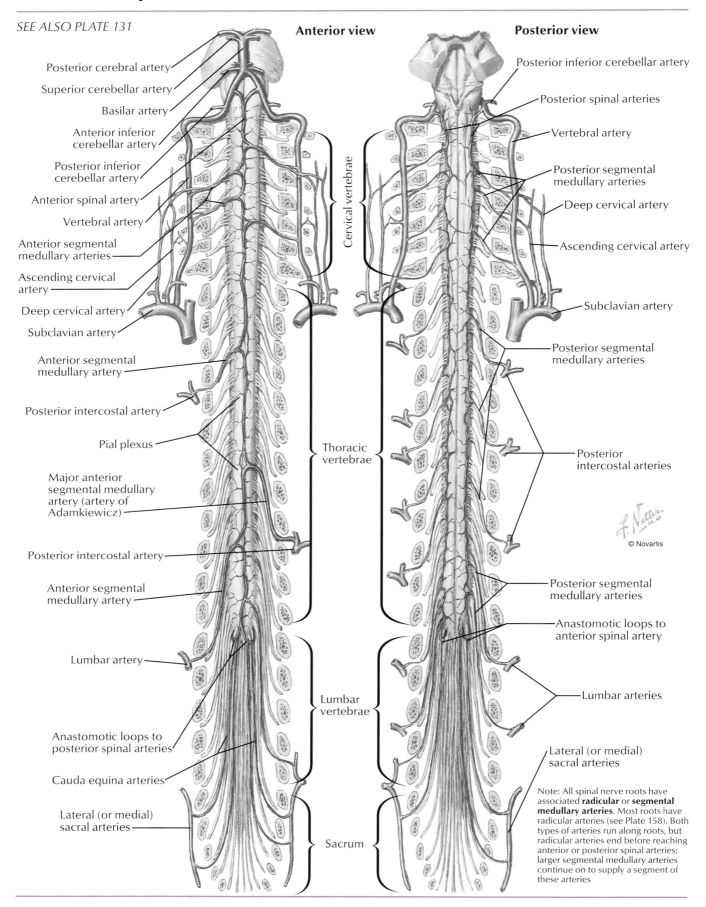

Posterior cerebral artery

Superior cerebellar artery

Basilar artery

Anterior inferior cerebellar artery

Posterior inferior cerebellar artery

Anterior spinal artery

Vertebral artery

Anterior segmental medullary arteries

Ascending cervical artery

Deep cervical artery

Subclavian artery

Anterior segmental medullary artery

Posterior intercostal artery

Pial plexus

Major anterior segmental medullary artery (artery of Adamkiewicz)

Posterior intercostal artery

Anterior segmental medullary artery

Lumbar artery

Anastomotic loops to posterior spinal arteries

Cauda equina arteries

Lateral (or medial) sacral arteries

Cervical vertebrae

Thoracic vertebrae

Lumbar vertebrae

Sacrum

Posterior inferior cerebellar artery

Posterior spinal arteries

Vertebral artery

Posterior segmental medullary arteries

Deep cervical artery

Ascending cervical artery

Subclavian artery

Posterior segmental medullary arteries

Posterior intercostal arteries

Posterior segmental medullary arteries

Anastomotic loops to anterior spinal artery

Lumbar arteries

Lateral (or medial) sacral arteries

Note: All spinal nerve roots have associated **radicular** or **segmental medullary arteries**. Most roots have radicular arteries (see Plate 158). Both types of arteries run along roots, but radicular arteries end before reaching anterior or posterior spinal arteries; larger segmental medullary arteries continue on to supply a segment of these arteries

*F. Netter M.D.*

© Novartis

**PLATE 157**

**BACK AND SPINAL CORD**

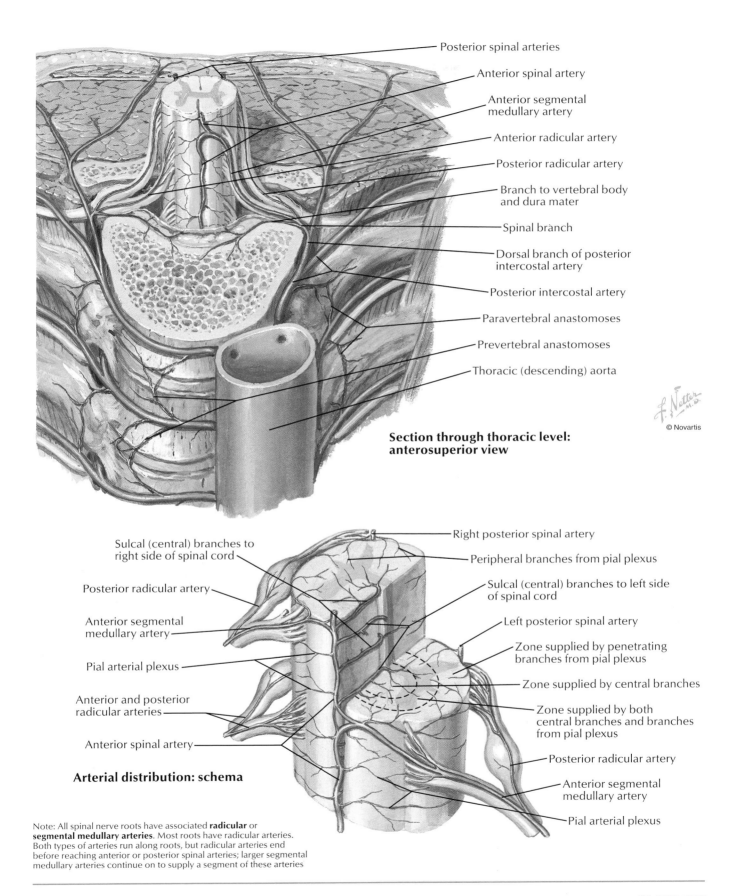

Posterior spinal arteries

Anterior spinal artery

Anterior segmental medullary artery

Anterior radicular artery

Posterior radicular artery

Branch to vertebral body and dura mater

Spinal branch

Dorsal branch of posterior intercostal artery

Posterior intercostal artery

Paravertebral anastomoses

Prevertebral anastomoses

Thoracic (descending) aorta

© Novartis

**Section through thoracic level: anterosuperior view**

Sulcal (central) branches to right side of spinal cord

Right posterior spinal artery

Peripheral branches from pial plexus

Posterior radicular artery

Sulcal (central) branches to left side of spinal cord

Anterior segmental medullary artery

Left posterior spinal artery

Pial arterial plexus

Zone supplied by penetrating branches from pial plexus

Anterior and posterior radicular arteries

Zone supplied by central branches

Zone supplied by both central branches and branches from pial plexus

Anterior spinal artery

Posterior radicular artery

**Arterial distribution: schema**

Anterior segmental medullary artery

Pial arterial plexus

Note: All spinal nerve roots have associated **radicular** or **segmental medullary arteries**. Most roots have radicular arteries. Both types of arteries run along roots, but radicular arteries end before reaching anterior or posterior spinal arteries; larger segmental medullary arteries continue on to supply a segment of these arteries

**SPINAL CORD**

**PLATE 158**

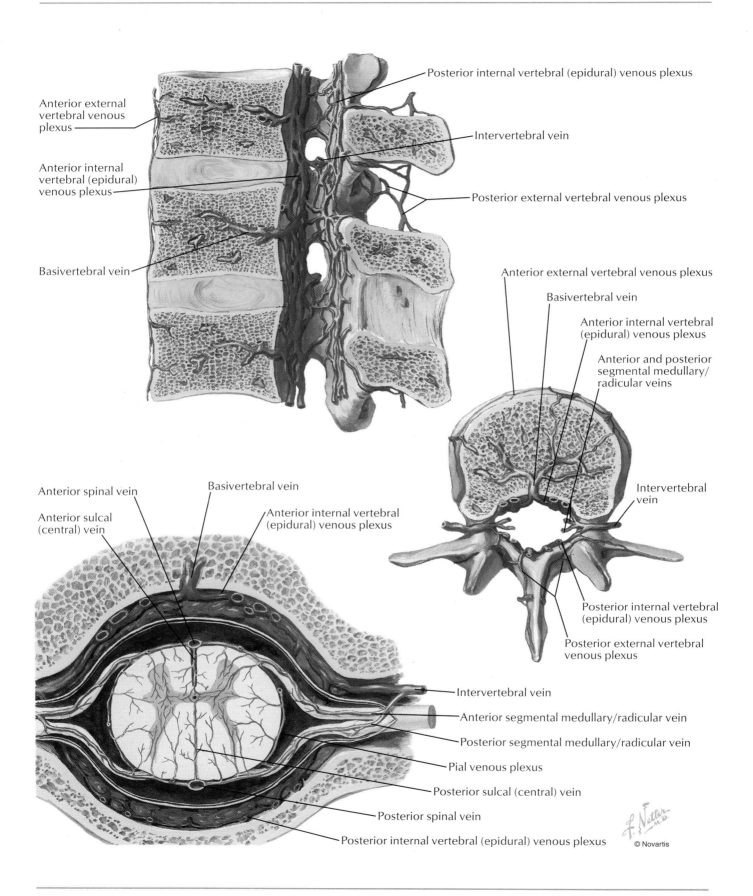

Posterior internal vertebral (epidural) venous plexus

Anterior external vertebral venous plexus

Intervertebral vein

Anterior internal vertebral (epidural) venous plexus

Posterior external vertebral venous plexus

Basivertebral vein

Anterior external vertebral venous plexus

Basivertebral vein

Anterior internal vertebral (epidural) venous plexus

Anterior and posterior segmental medullary/radicular veins

Anterior spinal vein

Basivertebral vein

Anterior sulcal (central) vein

Anterior internal vertebral (epidural) venous plexus

Intervertebral vein

Posterior internal vertebral (epidural) venous plexus

Posterior external vertebral venous plexus

Intervertebral vein

Anterior segmental medullary/radicular vein

Posterior segmental medullary/radicular vein

Pial venous plexus

Posterior sulcal (central) vein

Posterior spinal vein

Posterior internal vertebral (epidural) venous plexus

© Novartis

**PLATE 159**

**BACK AND SPINAL CORD**

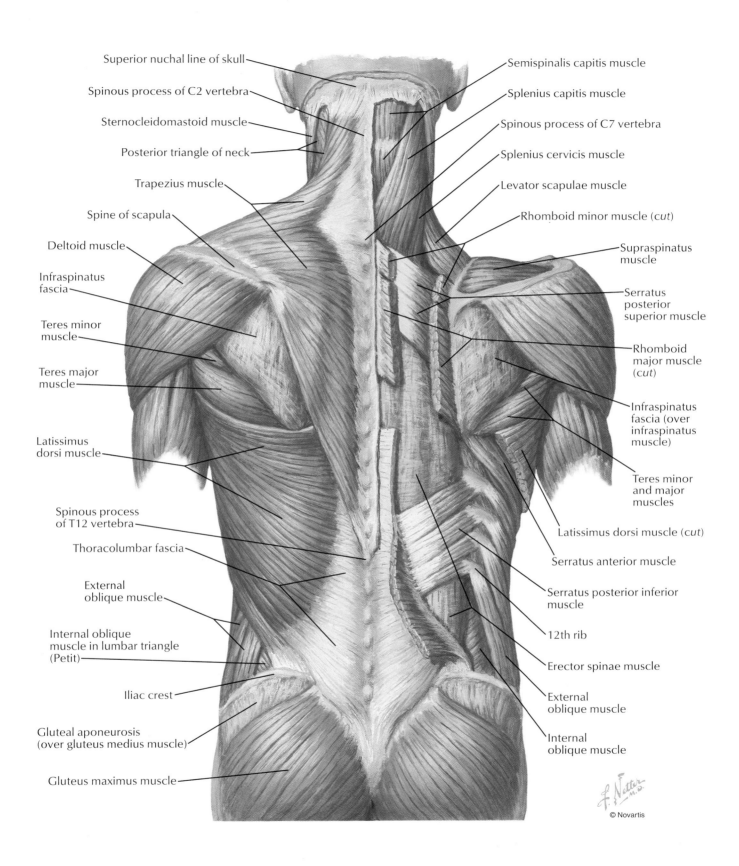

Superior nuchal line of skull

Spinous process of C2 vertebra

Sternocleidomastoid muscle

Posterior triangle of neck

Trapezius muscle

Spine of scapula

Deltoid muscle

Infraspinatus fascia

Teres minor muscle

Teres major muscle

Latissimus dorsi muscle

Spinous process of T12 vertebra

Thoracolumbar fascia

External oblique muscle

Internal oblique muscle in lumbar triangle (Petit)

Iliac crest

Gluteal aponeurosis (over gluteus medius muscle)

Gluteus maximus muscle

Semispinalis capitis muscle

Splenius capitis muscle

Spinous process of C7 vertebra

Splenius cervicis muscle

Levator scapulae muscle

Rhomboid minor muscle (*cut*)

Supraspinatus muscle

Serratus posterior superior muscle

Rhomboid major muscle (*cut*)

Infraspinatus fascia (over infraspinatus muscle)

Teres minor and major muscles

Latissimus dorsi muscle (*cut*)

Serratus anterior muscle

Serratus posterior inferior muscle

12th rib

Erector spinae muscle

External oblique muscle

Internal oblique muscle

© Novartis

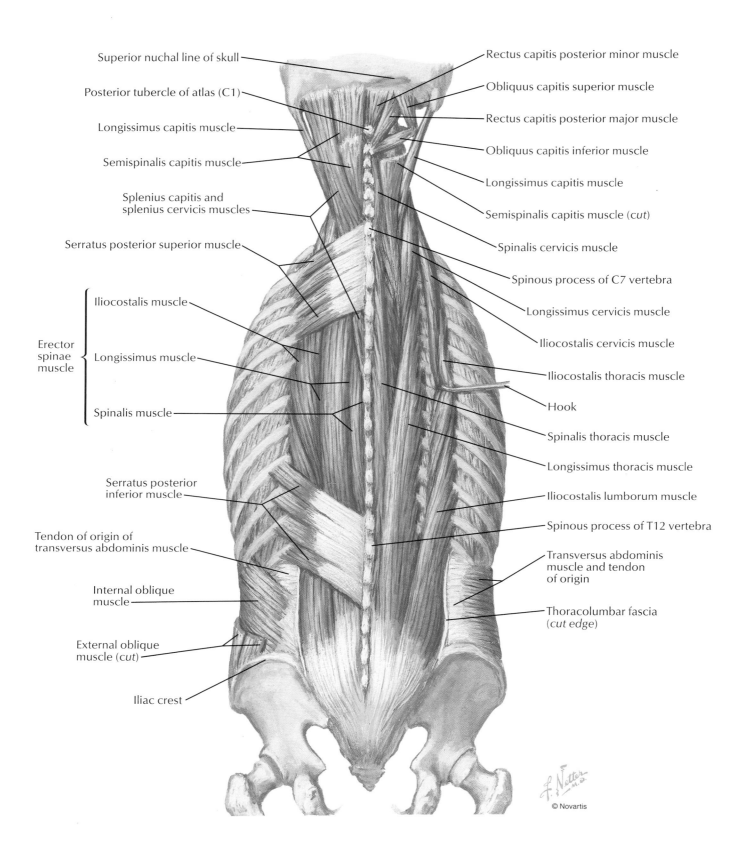

Superior nuchal line of skull

Posterior tubercle of atlas (C1)

Longissimus capitis muscle

Semispinalis capitis muscle

Splenius capitis and splenius cervicis muscles

Serratus posterior superior muscle

Erector spinae muscle
- Iliocostalis muscle
- Longissimus muscle
- Spinalis muscle

Serratus posterior inferior muscle

Tendon of origin of transversus abdominis muscle

Internal oblique muscle

External oblique muscle (cut)

Iliac crest

Rectus capitis posterior minor muscle

Obliquus capitis superior muscle

Rectus capitis posterior major muscle

Obliquus capitis inferior muscle

Longissimus capitis muscle

Semispinalis capitis muscle (cut)

Spinalis cervicis muscle

Spinous process of C7 vertebra

Longissimus cervicis muscle

Iliocostalis cervicis muscle

Iliocostalis thoracis muscle

Hook

Spinalis thoracis muscle

Longissimus thoracis muscle

Iliocostalis lumborum muscle

Spinous process of T12 vertebra

Transversus abdominis muscle and tendon of origin

Thoracolumbar fascia (cut edge)

**PLATE 161**

**BACK AND SPINAL CORD**

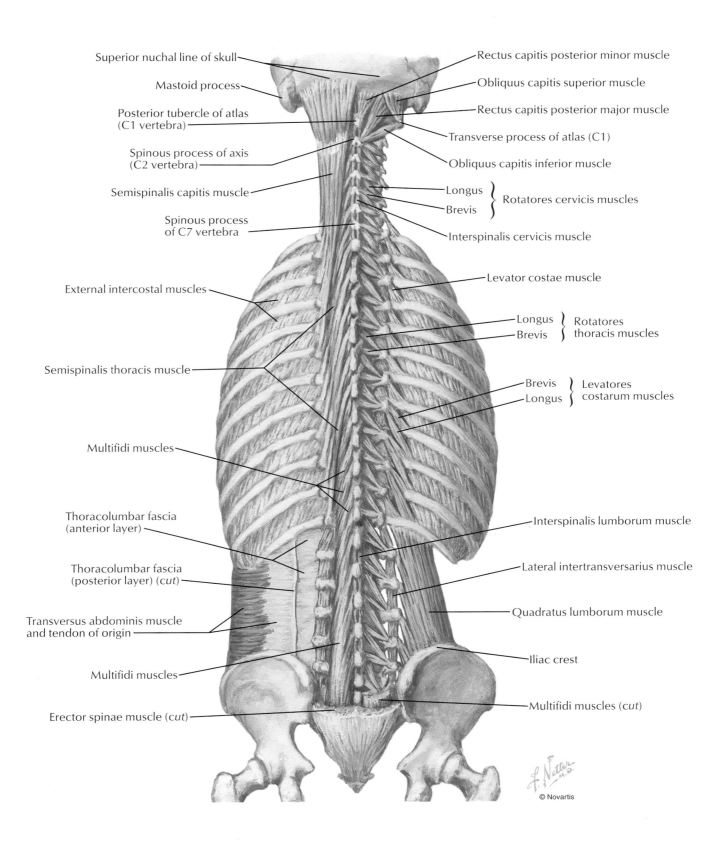

Superior nuchal line of skull

Mastoid process

Posterior tubercle of atlas
(C1 vertebra)

Spinous process of axis
(C2 vertebra)

Semispinalis capitis muscle

Spinous process
of C7 vertebra

External intercostal muscles

Semispinalis thoracis muscle

Multifidi muscles

Thoracolumbar fascia
(anterior layer)

Thoracolumbar fascia
(posterior layer) (cut)

Transversus abdominis muscle
and tendon of origin

Multifidi muscles

Erector spinae muscle (cut)

Rectus capitis posterior minor muscle

Obliquus capitis superior muscle

Rectus capitis posterior major muscle

Transverse process of atlas (C1)

Obliquus capitis inferior muscle

Longus
Brevis
} Rotatores cervicis muscles

Interspinalis cervicis muscle

Levator costae muscle

Longus
Brevis
} Rotatores
thoracis muscles

Brevis
Longus
} Levatores
costarum muscles

Interspinalis lumborum muscle

Lateral intertransversarius muscle

Quadratus lumborum muscle

Iliac crest

Multifidi muscles (cut)

© Novartis

SEE ALSO PLATES 166, 179, 237, 241

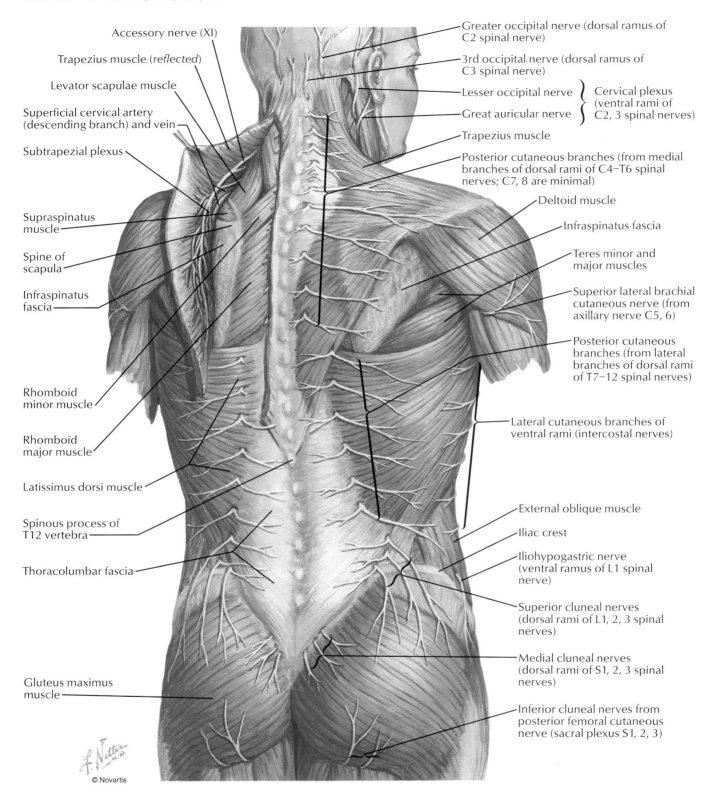

Accessory nerve (XI)

Trapezius muscle (*reflected*)

Levator scapulae muscle

Superficial cervical artery (descending branch) and vein

Subtrapezial plexus

Supraspinatus muscle

Spine of scapula

Infraspinatus fascia

Rhomboid minor muscle

Rhomboid major muscle

Latissimus dorsi muscle

Spinous process of T12 vertebra

Thoracolumbar fascia

Gluteus maximus muscle

Greater occipital nerve (dorsal ramus of C2 spinal nerve)

3rd occipital nerve (dorsal ramus of C3 spinal nerve)

Lesser occipital nerve ⎫ Cervical plexus
⎬ (ventral rami of
Great auricular nerve ⎭ C2, 3 spinal nerves)

Trapezius muscle

Posterior cutaneous branches (from medial branches of dorsal rami of C4–T6 spinal nerves; C7, 8 are minimal)

Deltoid muscle

Infraspinatus fascia

Teres minor and major muscles

Superior lateral brachial cutaneous nerve (from axillary nerve C5, 6)

Posterior cutaneous branches (from lateral branches of dorsal rami of T7–12 spinal nerves)

Lateral cutaneous branches of ventral rami (intercostal nerves)

External oblique muscle

Iliac crest

Iliohypogastric nerve (ventral ramus of L1 spinal nerve)

Superior cluneal nerves (dorsal rami of L1, 2, 3 spinal nerves)

Medial cluneal nerves (dorsal rami of S1, 2, 3 spinal nerves)

Inferior cluneal nerves from posterior femoral cutaneous nerve (sacral plexus S1, 2, 3)

© Novartis

**PLATE 163** **BACK AND SPINAL CORD**

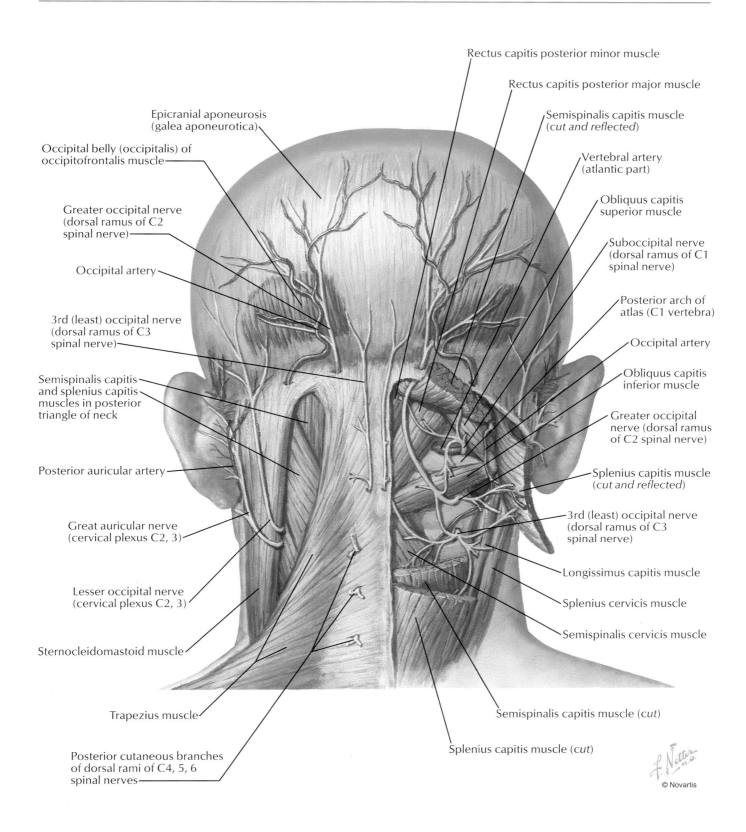

Rectus capitis posterior minor muscle

Rectus capitis posterior major muscle

Semispinalis capitis muscle (*cut and reflected*)

Vertebral artery (atlantic part)

Obliquus capitis superior muscle

Suboccipital nerve (dorsal ramus of C1 spinal nerve)

Posterior arch of atlas (C1 vertebra)

Occipital artery

Obliquus capitis inferior muscle

Greater occipital nerve (dorsal ramus of C2 spinal nerve)

Splenius capitis muscle (*cut and reflected*)

3rd (least) occipital nerve (dorsal ramus of C3 spinal nerve)

Longissimus capitis muscle

Splenius cervicis muscle

Semispinalis cervicis muscle

Semispinalis capitis muscle (*cut*)

Splenius capitis muscle (*cut*)

Epicranial aponeurosis (galea aponeurotica)

Occipital belly (occipitalis) of occipitofrontalis muscle

Greater occipital nerve (dorsal ramus of C2 spinal nerve)

Occipital artery

3rd (least) occipital nerve (dorsal ramus of C3 spinal nerve)

Semispinalis capitis and splenius capitis muscles in posterior triangle of neck

Posterior auricular artery

Great auricular nerve (cervical plexus C2, 3)

Lesser occipital nerve (cervical plexus C2, 3)

Sternocleidomastoid muscle

Trapezius muscle

Posterior cutaneous branches of dorsal rami of C4, 5, 6 spinal nerves

© Novartis

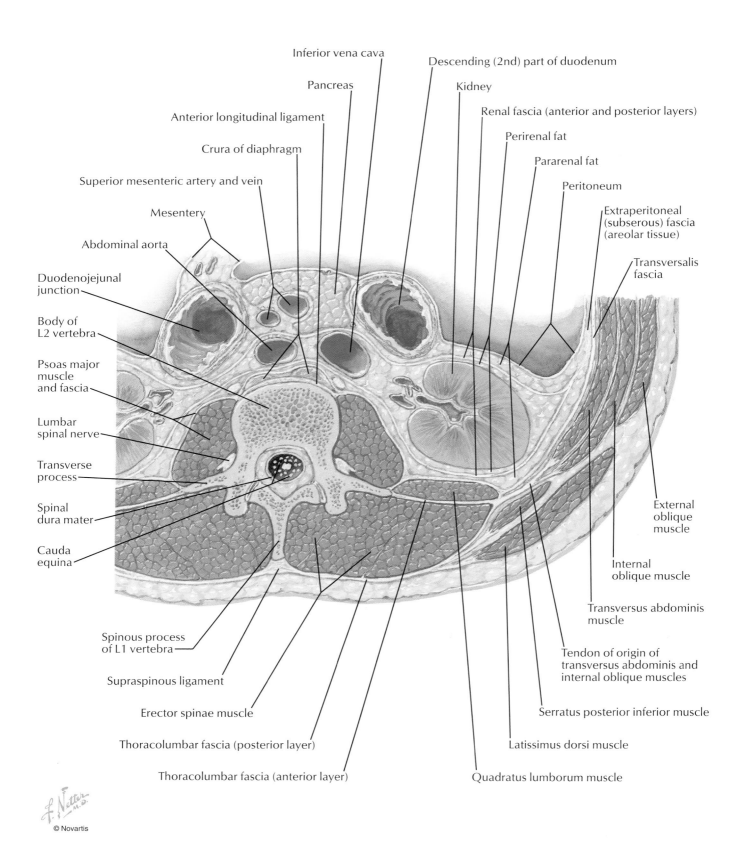

Inferior vena cava

Pancreas

Descending (2nd) part of duodenum

Kidney

Anterior longitudinal ligament

Renal fascia (anterior and posterior layers)

Crura of diaphragm

Perirenal fat

Superior mesenteric artery and vein

Pararenal fat

Mesentery

Peritoneum

Abdominal aorta

Extraperitoneal (subserous) fascia (areolar tissue)

Duodenojejunal junction

Transversalis fascia

Body of L2 vertebra

Psoas major muscle and fascia

Lumbar spinal nerve

Transverse process

External oblique muscle

Spinal dura mater

Cauda equina

Internal oblique muscle

Transversus abdominis muscle

Spinous process of L1 vertebra

Supraspinous ligament

Tendon of origin of transversus abdominis and internal oblique muscles

Erector spinae muscle

Serratus posterior inferior muscle

Thoracolumbar fascia (posterior layer)

Latissimus dorsi muscle

Thoracolumbar fascia (anterior layer)

Quadratus lumborum muscle

**PLATE 165**

**BACK AND SPINAL CORD**

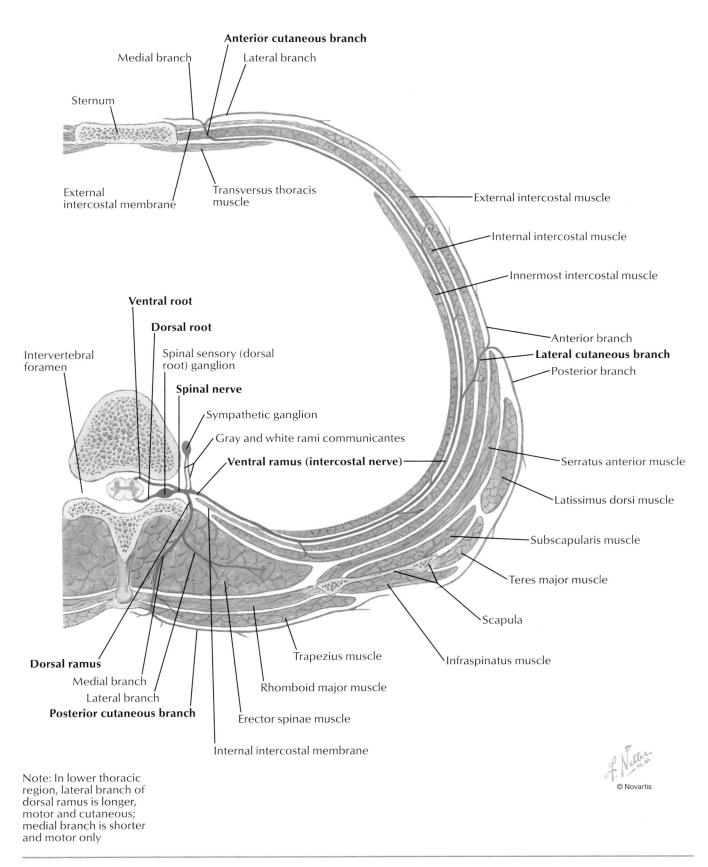

Medial branch
**Anterior cutaneous branch**
Lateral branch
Sternum
External intercostal membrane
Transversus thoracis muscle
External intercostal muscle
Internal intercostal muscle
Innermost intercostal muscle
**Ventral root**
**Dorsal root**
Spinal sensory (dorsal root) ganglion
Intervertebral foramen
**Spinal nerve**
Sympathetic ganglion
Gray and white rami communicantes
**Ventral ramus (intercostal nerve)**
Anterior branch
**Lateral cutaneous branch**
Posterior branch
Serratus anterior muscle
Latissimus dorsi muscle
Subscapularis muscle
Teres major muscle
Scapula
Infraspinatus muscle
**Dorsal ramus**
Medial branch
Lateral branch
**Posterior cutaneous branch**
Internal intercostal membrane
Erector spinae muscle
Rhomboid major muscle
Trapezius muscle

Note: In lower thoracic region, lateral branch of dorsal ramus is longer, motor and cutaneous; medial branch is shorter and motor only

# Section III
# THORAX

**MAMMARY GLAND**
*Plates 167 – 169*

167. Mammary Gland
168. Arteries of Mammary Gland
169. Lymph Vessels and Nodes of
     Mammary Gland

**BODY WALL**
*Plates 170 – 183*

170. Bony Framework of Thorax
171. Ribs and Sternocostal Joints
172. Costovertebral Joints
173. Cervical Ribs and Related Anomalies
174. Anterior Thoracic Wall
175. Anterior Thoracic Wall (*continued*)
176. Anterior Thoracic Wall: Internal View
177. Posterior and Lateral Thoracic Walls
178. Posterior Thoracic Wall
179. Intercostal Nerves and Arteries
180. Diaphragm: Thoracic Surface

181. Diaphragm: Abdominal Surface
182. Phrenic Nerve
183. Muscles of Respiration

**LUNGS**
*Plates 184 – 199*

184. Topography of Lungs: Anterior View
185. Topography of Lungs:
     Posterior View
186. Lungs In Situ: Anterior View
187. Lungs: Medial Views
188. Bronchopulmonary Segments
189. Bronchopulmonary Segments
     (*continued*)
190. Trachea and Major Bronchi
191. Nomenclature of Bronchi: Schema
192. Intrapulmonary Airways: Schema
193. Intrapulmonary Blood Circulation:
     Schema
194. Pulmonary Arteries and Veins

195. Great Vessels of Superior Mediastinum
196. Bronchial Arteries and Veins
197. Lymph Vessels and Nodes of Lung
198. Autonomic Nerves in Thorax
199. Innervation of Tracheobronchial Tree: Schema

**HEART**
*Plates 200 – 217*
200. Heart In Situ
201. Heart: Anterior Exposure
202. Heart: Base and Diaphragmatic Surfaces
203. Pericardial Sac
204. Coronary Arteries and Cardiac Veins
205. Coronary Arteries and Cardiac Veins: Variations
206. Coronary Arteries: Arteriographic Views
207. Coronary Arteries: Arteriographic Views (*continued*)
208. Right Atrium and Ventricle
209. Left Atrium and Ventricle
210. Valves and Fibrous Skeleton of Heart
211. Valves and Fibrous Skeleton of Heart (*continued*)

212. Atria, Ventricles and Interventricular Septum
213. Conducting System of Heart
214. Nerves of Heart
215. Innervation of Heart: Schema
216. Innervation of Blood Vessels: Schema
217. Prenatal and Postnatal Circulation

**MEDIASTINUM**
*Plates 218 – 230*
218. Mediastinum: Right Lateral View
219. Mediastinum: Left Lateral View
220. Esophagus In Situ
221. Topography and Constrictions of Esophagus
222. Musculature of Esophagus
223. Pharyngoesophageal Junction
224. Esophagogastric Junction
225. Arteries of Esophagus
226. Veins of Esophagus
227. Lymph Vessels and Nodes of Esophagus
228. Nerves of Esophagus
229. Intrinsic Nerves and Variations in Nerves of Esophagus
230. Mediastinum: Cross Section (Superior View)

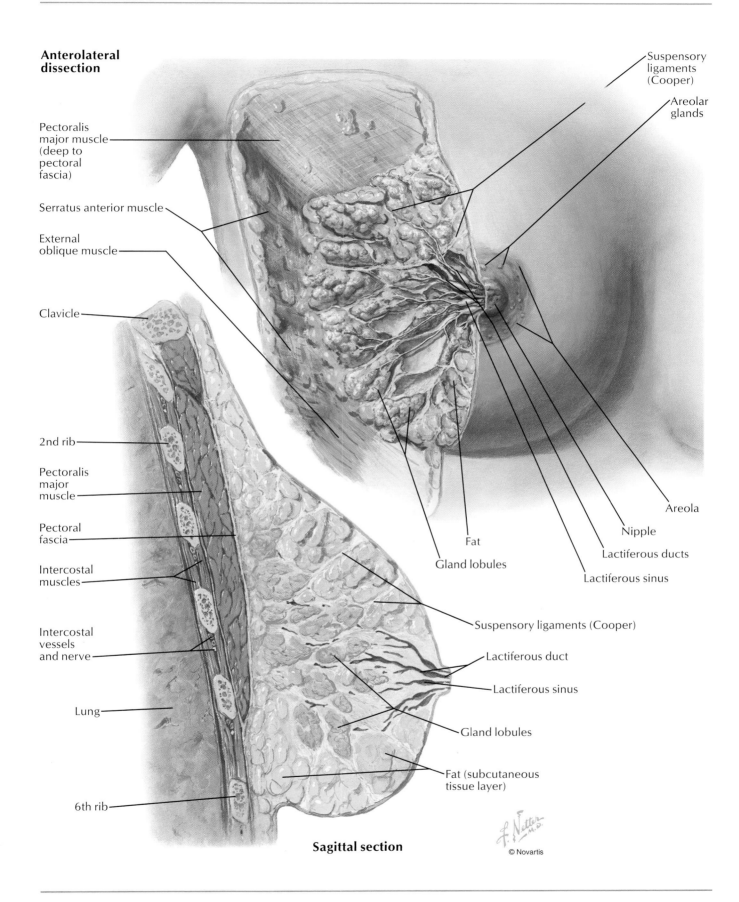

**Anterolateral dissection**

Suspensory ligaments (Cooper)

Areolar glands

Pectoralis major muscle (deep to pectoral fascia)

Serratus anterior muscle

External oblique muscle

Clavicle

2nd rib

Pectoralis major muscle

Pectoral fascia

Intercostal muscles

Intercostal vessels and nerve

Lung

6th rib

Areola

Nipple

Lactiferous ducts

Lactiferous sinus

Fat

Gland lobules

Suspensory ligaments (Cooper)

Lactiferous duct

Lactiferous sinus

Gland lobules

Fat (subcutaneous tissue layer)

**Sagittal section**

© Novartis

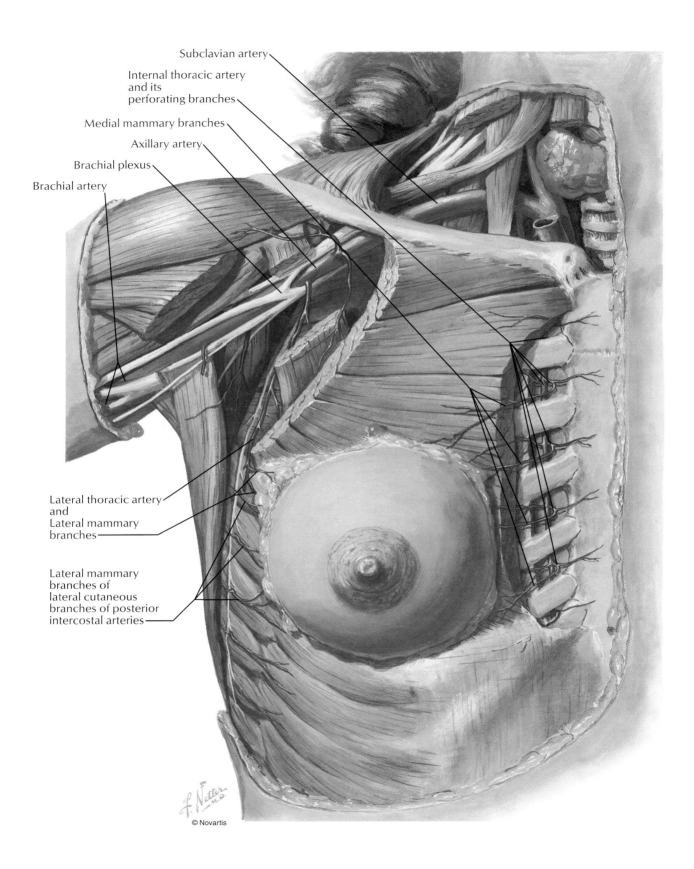

Subclavian artery

Internal thoracic artery
and its
perforating branches

Medial mammary branches

Axillary artery

Brachial plexus

Brachial artery

Lateral thoracic artery
and
Lateral mammary
branches

Lateral mammary
branches of
lateral cutaneous
branches of posterior
intercostal arteries

© Novartis

*PLATE 168*

**THORAX**

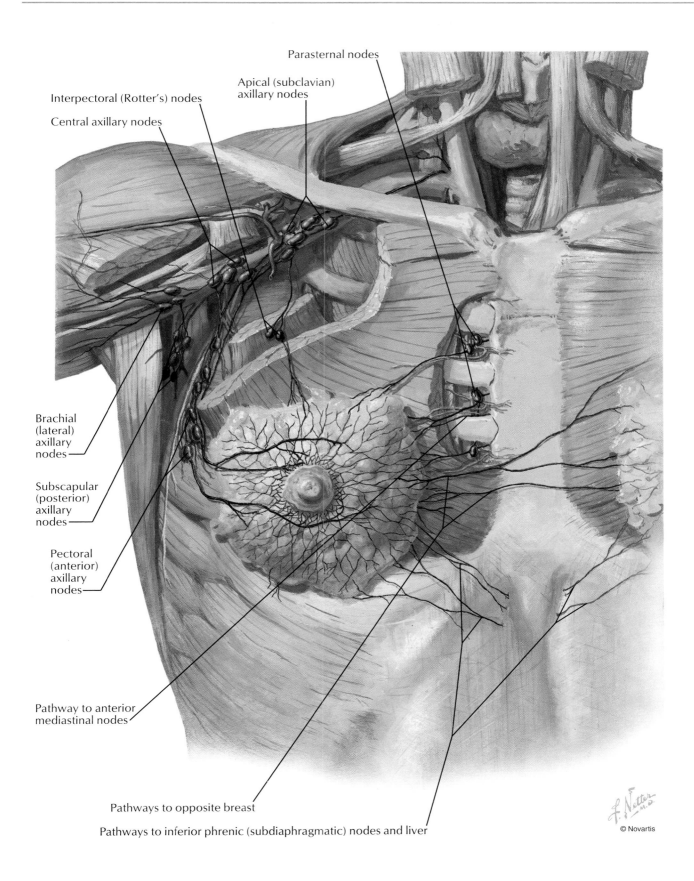

Parasternal nodes

Apical (subclavian) axillary nodes

Interpectoral (Rotter's) nodes

Central axillary nodes

Brachial (lateral) axillary nodes

Subscapular (posterior) axillary nodes

Pectoral (anterior) axillary nodes

Pathway to anterior mediastinal nodes

Pathways to opposite breast

Pathways to inferior phrenic (subdiaphragmatic) nodes and liver

© Novartis

*SEE ALSO PLATE 231*

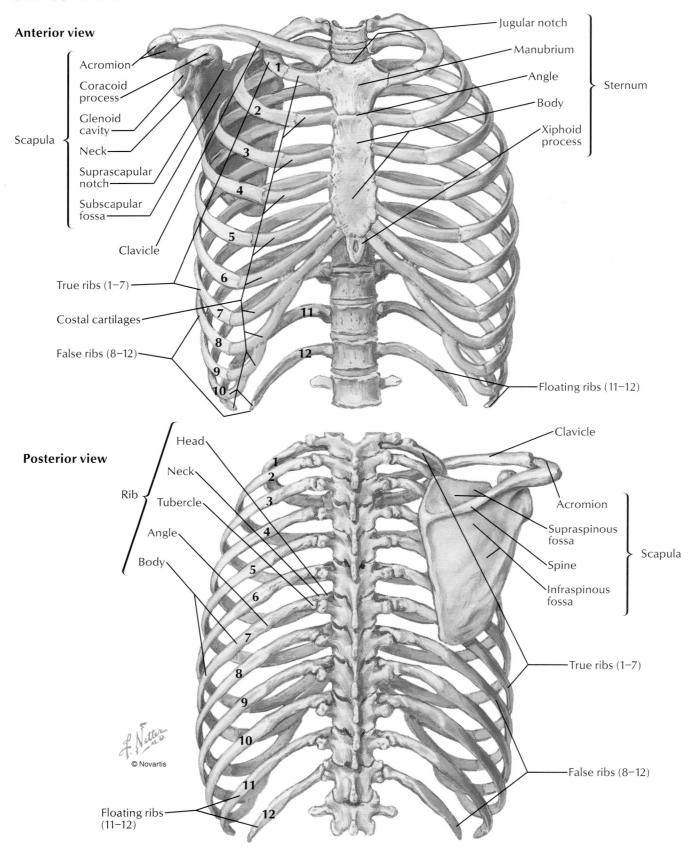

**Anterior view**

Acromion

Coracoid process

Glenoid cavity

Neck

Suprascapular notch

Subscapular fossa

Scapula

Clavicle

True ribs (1–7)

Costal cartilages

False ribs (8–12)

Jugular notch

Manubrium

Angle

Body

Xiphoid process

Sternum

Floating ribs (11–12)

**Posterior view**

Head

Neck

Tubercle

Angle

Body

Rib

Clavicle

Acromion

Supraspinous fossa

Spine

Infraspinous fossa

Scapula

True ribs (1–7)

False ribs (8–12)

Floating ribs (11–12)

© Novartis

**PLATE 170**

**THORAX**

# Ribs and Sternocostal Joints

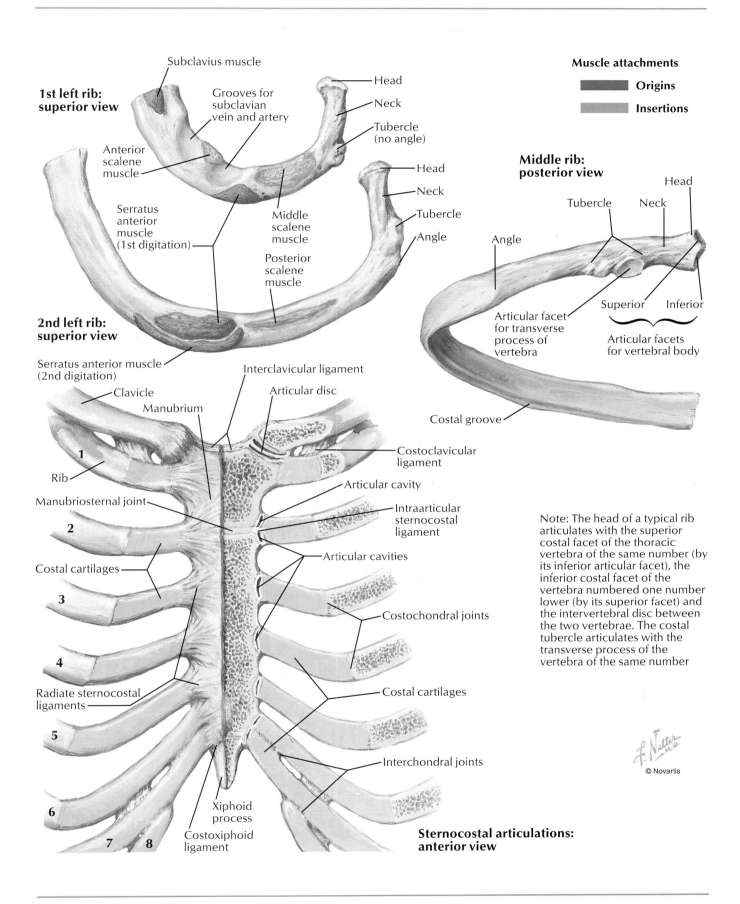

**1st left rib: superior view**

Subclavius muscle

Grooves for subclavian vein and artery

Anterior scalene muscle

Serratus anterior muscle (1st digitation)

Middle scalene muscle

Posterior scalene muscle

Head
Neck
Tubercle (no angle)

Head
Neck
Tubercle
Angle

**2nd left rib: superior view**

Serratus anterior muscle (2nd digitation)

Clavicle
Manubrium

Interclavicular ligament
Articular disc

Rib
Manubriosternal joint

Costal cartilages

Radiate sternocostal ligaments

Costoclavicular ligament
Articular cavity
Intraarticular sternocostal ligament
Articular cavities
Costochondral joints

Costal cartilages

Interchondral joints

Xiphoid process
Costoxiphoid ligament

**Sternocostal articulations: anterior view**

**Middle rib: posterior view**

Tubercle  Neck  Head
Angle
Angle
Articular facet for transverse process of vertebra
Superior  Inferior
Articular facets for vertebral body
Costal groove

Note: The head of a typical rib articulates with the superior costal facet of the thoracic vertebra of the same number (by its inferior articular facet), the inferior costal facet of the vertebra numbered one number lower (by its superior facet) and the intervertebral disc between the two vertebrae. The costal tubercle articulates with the transverse process of the vertebra of the same number

**Muscle attachments**
Origins
Insertions

© Novartis

SEE ALSO PLATE 143

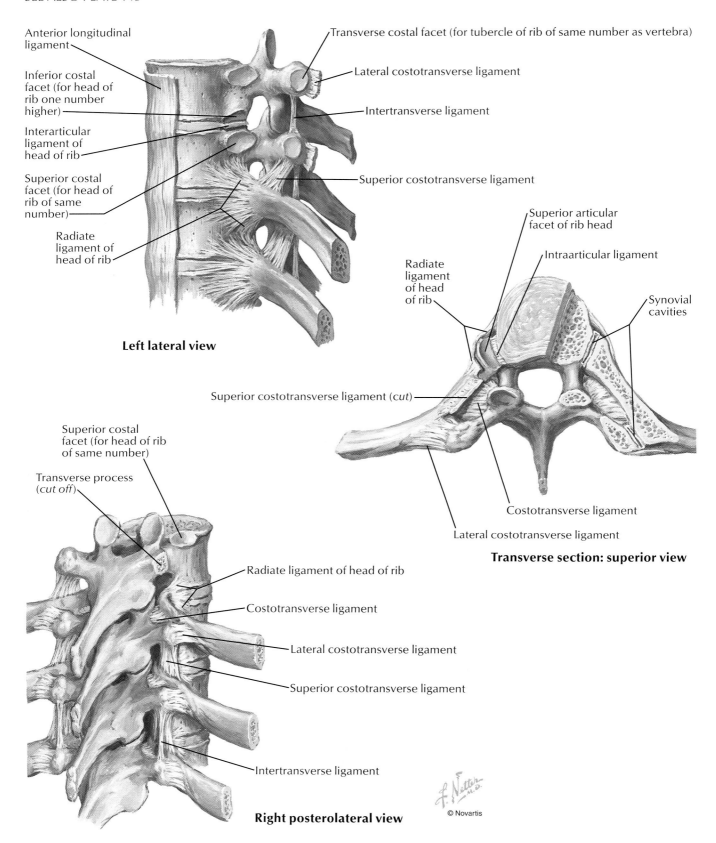

Anterior longitudinal ligament

Inferior costal facet (for head of rib one number higher)

Interarticular ligament of head of rib

Superior costal facet (for head of rib of same number)

Radiate ligament of head of rib

Transverse costal facet (for tubercle of rib of same number as vertebra)

Lateral costotransverse ligament

Intertransverse ligament

Superior costotransverse ligament

**Left lateral view**

Superior articular facet of rib head

Radiate ligament of head of rib

Intraarticular ligament

Synovial cavities

Superior costotransverse ligament (*cut*)

Costotransverse ligament

Lateral costotransverse ligament

**Transverse section: superior view**

Superior costal facet (for head of rib of same number)

Transverse process (*cut off*)

Radiate ligament of head of rib

Costotransverse ligament

Lateral costotransverse ligament

Superior costotransverse ligament

Intertransverse ligament

**Right posterolateral view**

© Novartis

**PLATE 172**

**THORAX**

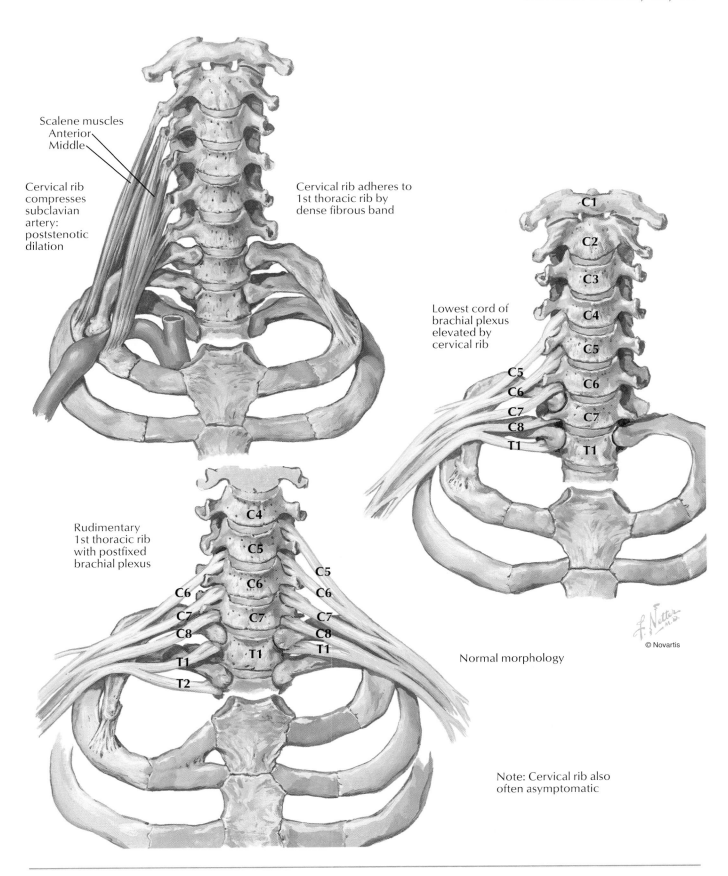

Scalene muscles
Anterior
Middle

Cervical rib compresses subclavian artery: poststenotic dilation

Cervical rib adheres to 1st thoracic rib by dense fibrous band

Lowest cord of brachial plexus elevated by cervical rib

C1
C2
C3
C4
C5
C6
C7
T1

C5
C6
C7
C8
T1

Normal morphology

Note: Cervical rib also often asymptomatic

Rudimentary 1st thoracic rib with postfixed brachial plexus

C4
C5
C6
C7
T1

C6
C7
C8
T1
T2

C5
C6
C7
C8
T1

© Novartis

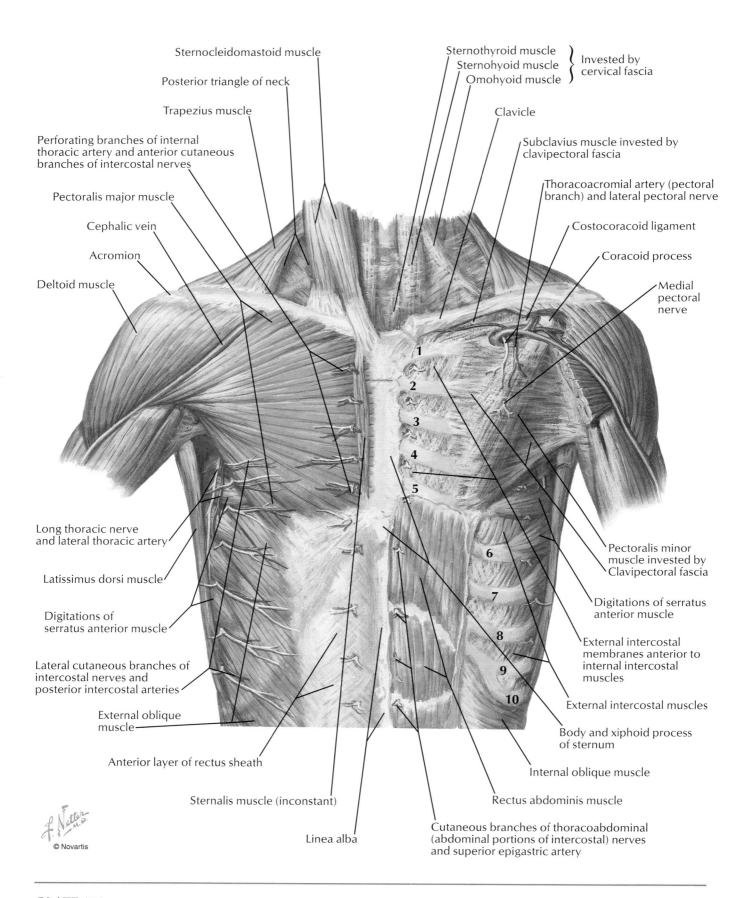

Sternocleidomastoid muscle

Posterior triangle of neck

Trapezius muscle

Perforating branches of internal
thoracic artery and anterior cutaneous
branches of intercostal nerves

Pectoralis major muscle

Cephalic vein

Acromion

Deltoid muscle

Long thoracic nerve
and lateral thoracic artery

Latissimus dorsi muscle

Digitations of
serratus anterior muscle

Lateral cutaneous branches of
intercostal nerves and
posterior intercostal arteries

External oblique
muscle

Anterior layer of rectus sheath

Sternalis muscle (inconstant)

Linea alba

Sternothyroid muscle
Sternohyoid muscle      } Invested by
Omohyoid muscle         } cervical fascia

Clavicle

Subclavius muscle invested by
clavipectoral fascia

Thoracoacromial artery (pectoral
branch) and lateral pectoral nerve

Costocoracoid ligament

Coracoid process

Medial
pectoral
nerve

Pectoralis minor
muscle invested by
Clavipectoral fascia

Digitations of serratus
anterior muscle

External intercostal
membranes anterior to
internal intercostal
muscles

External intercostal muscles

Body and xiphoid process
of sternum

Internal oblique muscle

Rectus abdominis muscle

Cutaneous branches of thoracoabdominal
(abdominal portions of intercostal) nerves
and superior epigastric artery

1
2
3
4
5
6
7
8
9
10

**PLATE 174**

**THORAX**

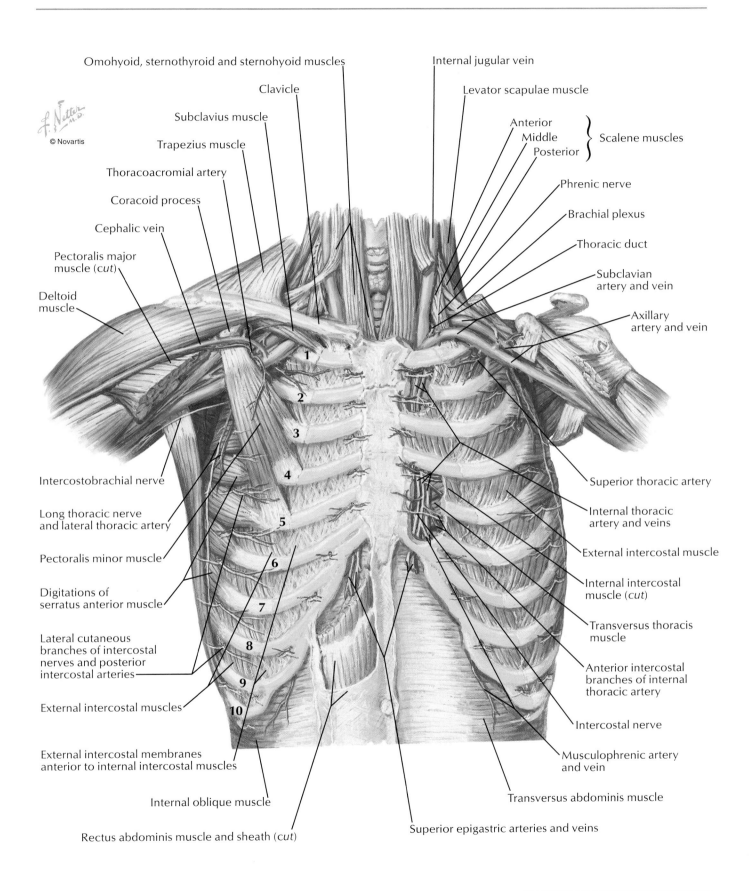

Omohyoid, sternothyroid and sternohyoid muscles

Clavicle

Subclavius muscle

Trapezius muscle

Thoracoacromial artery

Coracoid process

Cephalic vein

Pectoralis major muscle (cut)

Deltoid muscle

Intercostobrachial nerve

Long thoracic nerve and lateral thoracic artery

Pectoralis minor muscle

Digitations of serratus anterior muscle

Lateral cutaneous branches of intercostal nerves and posterior intercostal arteries

External intercostal muscles

External intercostal membranes anterior to internal intercostal muscles

Internal oblique muscle

Rectus abdominis muscle and sheath (cut)

Internal jugular vein

Levator scapulae muscle

Anterior
Middle
Posterior
} Scalene muscles

Phrenic nerve

Brachial plexus

Thoracic duct

Subclavian artery and vein

Axillary artery and vein

Superior thoracic artery

Internal thoracic artery and veins

External intercostal muscle

Internal intercostal muscle (cut)

Transversus thoracis muscle

Anterior intercostal branches of internal thoracic artery

Intercostal nerve

Musculophrenic artery and vein

Transversus abdominis muscle

Superior epigastric arteries and veins

1 2 3 4 5 6 7 8 9 10

© Novartis

*f. Netter*
M.D.

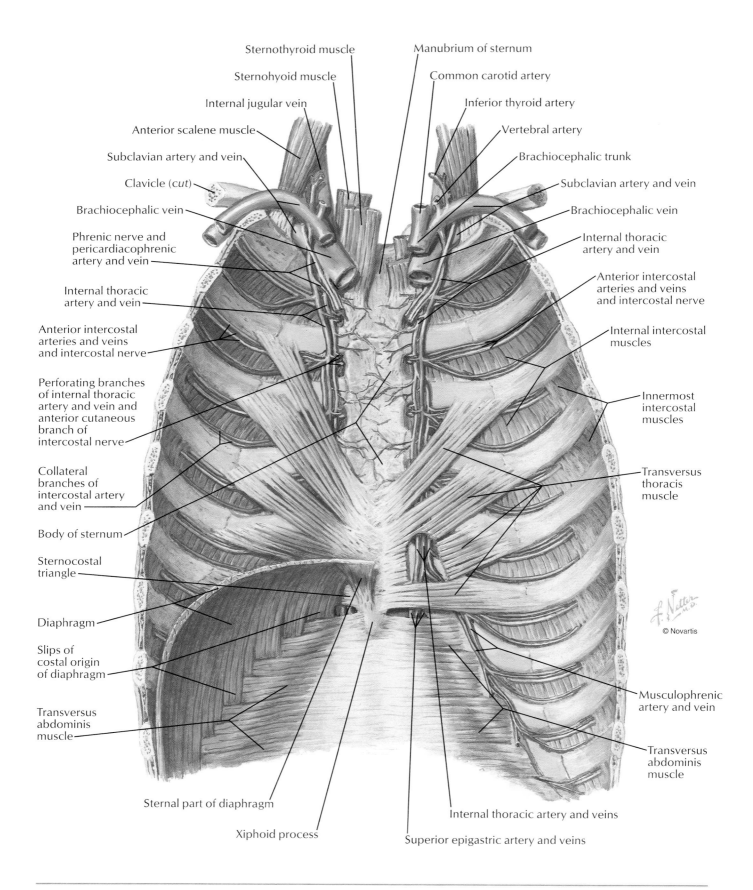

Sternothyroid muscle

Sternohyoid muscle

Internal jugular vein

Anterior scalene muscle

Subclavian artery and vein

Clavicle (*cut*)

Brachiocephalic vein

Phrenic nerve and pericardiacophrenic artery and vein

Internal thoracic artery and vein

Anterior intercostal arteries and veins and intercostal nerve

Perforating branches of internal thoracic artery and vein and anterior cutaneous branch of intercostal nerve

Collateral branches of intercostal artery and vein

Body of sternum

Sternocostal triangle

Diaphragm

Slips of costal origin of diaphragm

Transversus abdominis muscle

Manubrium of sternum

Common carotid artery

Inferior thyroid artery

Vertebral artery

Brachiocephalic trunk

Subclavian artery and vein

Brachiocephalic vein

Internal thoracic artery and vein

Anterior intercostal arteries and veins and intercostal nerve

Internal intercostal muscles

Innermost intercostal muscles

Transversus thoracis muscle

Musculophrenic artery and vein

Transversus abdominis muscle

Sternal part of diaphragm

Xiphoid process

Internal thoracic artery and veins

Superior epigastric artery and veins

**PLATE 176**

**THORAX**

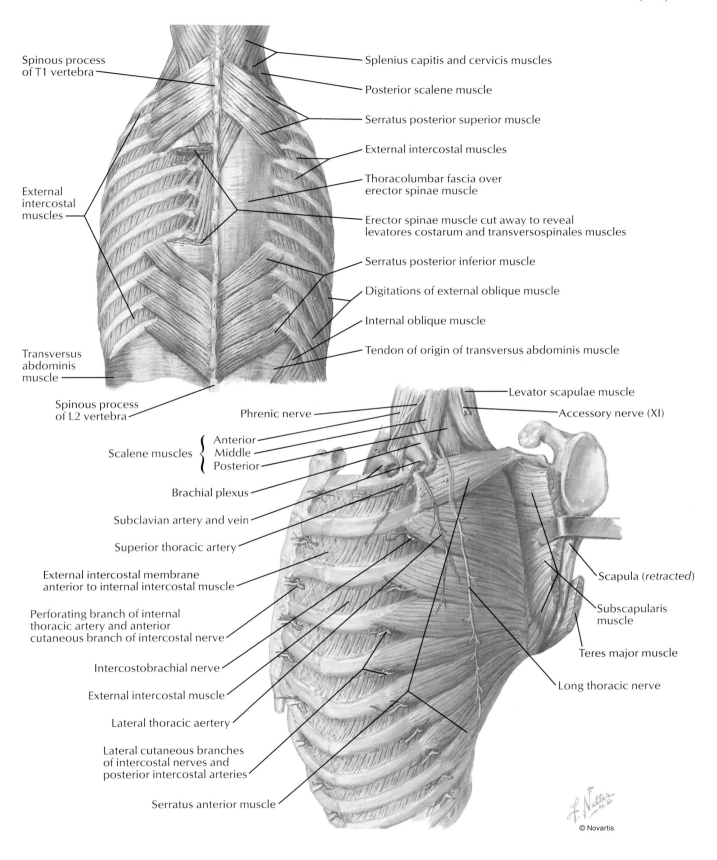

Spinous process of T1 vertebra

Splenius capitis and cervicis muscles

Posterior scalene muscle

Serratus posterior superior muscle

External intercostal muscles

Thoracolumbar fascia over erector spinae muscle

External intercostal muscles

Erector spinae muscle cut away to reveal levatores costarum and transversospinales muscles

Serratus posterior inferior muscle

Digitations of external oblique muscle

Internal oblique muscle

Tendon of origin of transversus abdominis muscle

Transversus abdominis muscle

Spinous process of L2 vertebra

Levator scapulae muscle

Phrenic nerve

Accessory nerve (XI)

Scalene muscles { Anterior / Middle / Posterior

Brachial plexus

Subclavian artery and vein

Superior thoracic artery

Scapula (*retracted*)

External intercostal membrane anterior to internal intercostal muscle

Subscapularis muscle

Perforating branch of internal thoracic artery and anterior cutaneous branch of intercostal nerve

Teres major muscle

Intercostobrachial nerve

Long thoracic nerve

External intercostal muscle

Lateral thoracic aertery

Lateral cutaneous branches of intercostal nerves and posterior intercostal arteries

Serratus anterior muscle

© Novartis

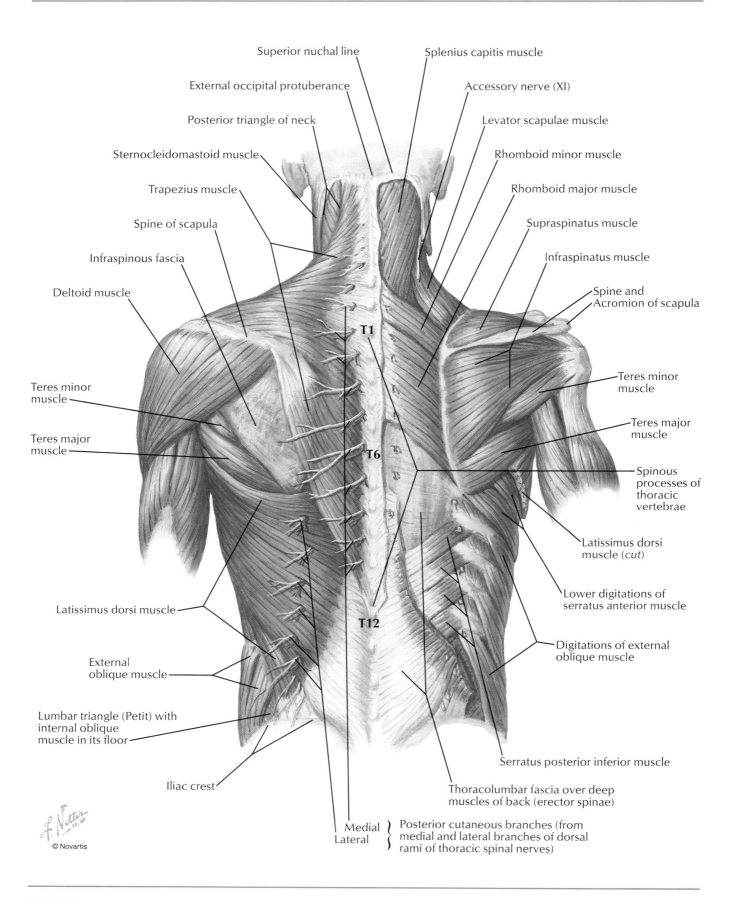

Superior nuchal line

Splenius capitis muscle

External occipital protuberance

Accessory nerve (XI)

Posterior triangle of neck

Levator scapulae muscle

Sternocleidomastoid muscle

Rhomboid minor muscle

Trapezius muscle

Rhomboid major muscle

Spine of scapula

Supraspinatus muscle

Infraspinous fascia

Infraspinatus muscle

Deltoid muscle

Spine and Acromion of scapula

T1

Teres minor muscle

Teres minor muscle

Teres major muscle

Teres major muscle

T6

Spinous processes of thoracic vertebrae

Latissimus dorsi muscle (cut)

T12

Lower digitations of serratus anterior muscle

Latissimus dorsi muscle

Digitations of external oblique muscle

External oblique muscle

Lumbar triangle (Petit) with internal oblique muscle in its floor

Serratus posterior inferior muscle

Iliac crest

Thoracolumbar fascia over deep muscles of back (erector spinae)

Medial
Lateral } Posterior cutaneous branches (from medial and lateral branches of dorsal rami of thoracic spinal nerves)

© Novartis

**PLATE 178**

**THORAX**

*SEE ALSO PLATES 166, 241*

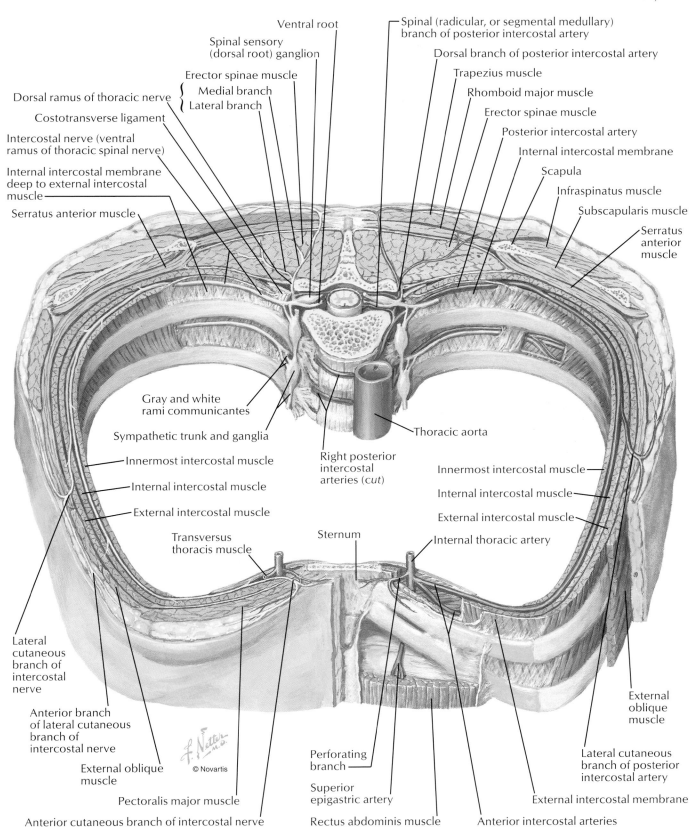

Ventral root

Spinal sensory
(dorsal root) ganglion

Erector spinae muscle
{ Medial branch
{ Lateral branch

Dorsal ramus of thoracic nerve

Costotransverse ligament

Intercostal nerve (ventral
ramus of thoracic spinal nerve)

Internal intercostal membrane
deep to external intercostal
muscle

Serratus anterior muscle

Spinal (radicular, or segmental medullary)
branch of posterior intercostal artery

Dorsal branch of posterior intercostal artery

Trapezius muscle

Rhomboid major muscle

Erector spinae muscle

Posterior intercostal artery

Internal intercostal membrane

Scapula

Infraspinatus muscle

Subscapularis muscle

Serratus
anterior
muscle

Gray and white
rami communicantes

Sympathetic trunk and ganglia

Innermost intercostal muscle

Internal intercostal muscle

External intercostal muscle

Transversus
thoracis muscle

Right posterior
intercostal
arteries (*cut*)

Thoracic aorta

Innermost intercostal muscle

Internal intercostal muscle

External intercostal muscle

Internal thoracic artery

Sternum

Lateral
cutaneous
branch of
intercostal
nerve

Anterior branch
of lateral cutaneous
branch of
intercostal nerve

External oblique
muscle

Pectoralis major muscle

Anterior cutaneous branch of intercostal nerve

Perforating
branch

Superior
epigastric artery

Rectus abdominis muscle

External
oblique
muscle

Lateral cutaneous
branch of posterior
intercostal artery

External intercostal membrane

Anterior intercostal arteries

© Novartis

**BODY WALL**

*PLATE 179*

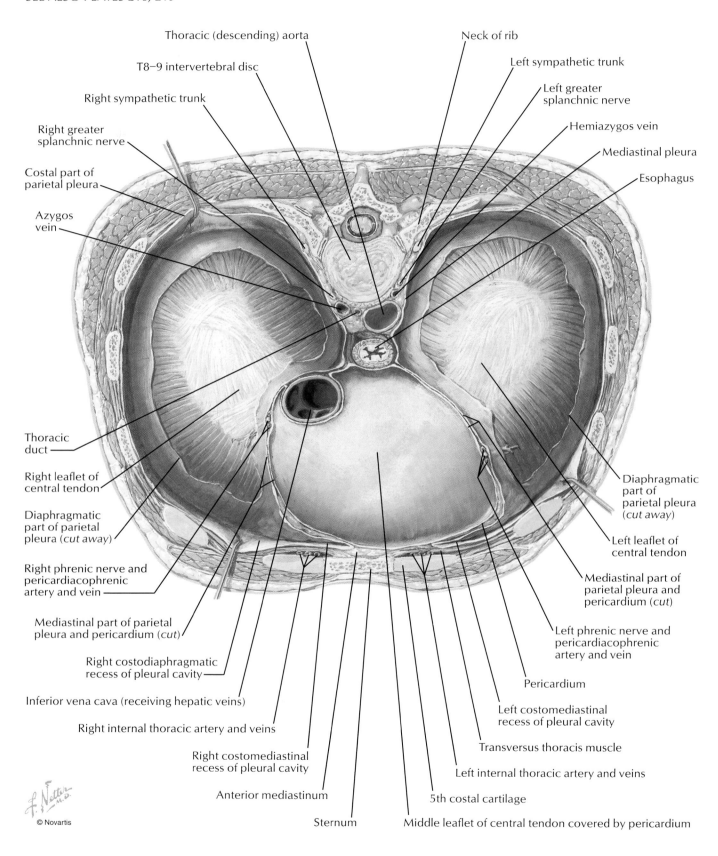

Thoracic (descending) aorta

T8–9 intervertebral disc

Right sympathetic trunk

Right greater splanchnic nerve

Costal part of parietal pleura

Azygos vein

Neck of rib

Left sympathetic trunk

Left greater splanchnic nerve

Hemiazygos vein

Mediastinal pleura

Esophagus

Thoracic duct

Right leaflet of central tendon

Diaphragmatic part of parietal pleura (cut away)

Right phrenic nerve and pericardiacophrenic artery and vein

Mediastinal part of parietal pleura and pericardium (cut)

Right costodiaphragmatic recess of pleural cavity

Inferior vena cava (receiving hepatic veins)

Right internal thoracic artery and veins

Right costomediastinal recess of pleural cavity

Anterior mediastinum

Sternum

Diaphragmatic part of parietal pleura (cut away)

Left leaflet of central tendon

Mediastinal part of parietal pleura and pericardium (cut)

Left phrenic nerve and pericardiacophrenic artery and vein

Pericardium

Left costomediastinal recess of pleural cavity

Transversus thoracis muscle

Left internal thoracic artery and veins

5th costal cartilage

Middle leaflet of central tendon covered by pericardium

f. Netter
© Novartis

**PLATE 180**

**THORAX**

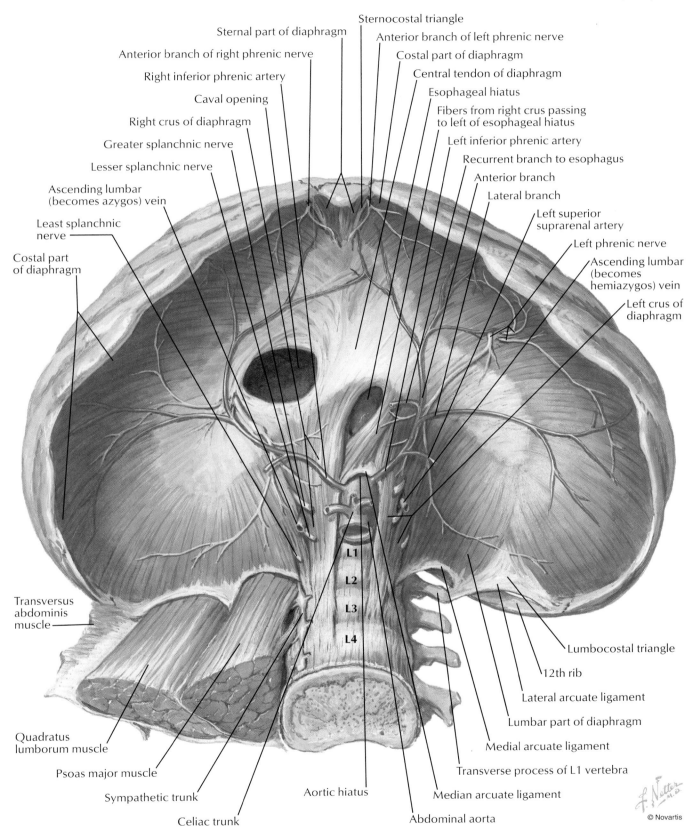

Sternal part of diaphragm

Sternocostal triangle

Anterior branch of left phrenic nerve

Anterior branch of right phrenic nerve

Costal part of diaphragm

Right inferior phrenic artery

Central tendon of diaphragm

Caval opening

Esophageal hiatus

Right crus of diaphragm

Fibers from right crus passing to left of esophageal hiatus

Greater splanchnic nerve

Left inferior phrenic artery

Lesser splanchnic nerve

Recurrent branch to esophagus

Ascending lumbar (becomes azygos) vein

Anterior branch

Lateral branch

Least splanchnic nerve

Left superior suprarenal artery

Costal part of diaphragm

Left phrenic nerve

Ascending lumbar (becomes hemiazygos) vein

Left crus of diaphragm

L1

L2

L3

L4

Transversus abdominis muscle

Lumbocostal triangle

12th rib

Lateral arcuate ligament

Lumbar part of diaphragm

Quadratus lumborum muscle

Medial arcuate ligament

Psoas major muscle

Transverse process of L1 vertebra

Sympathetic trunk

Median arcuate ligament

Celiac trunk

Aortic hiatus

Abdominal aorta

© Novartis

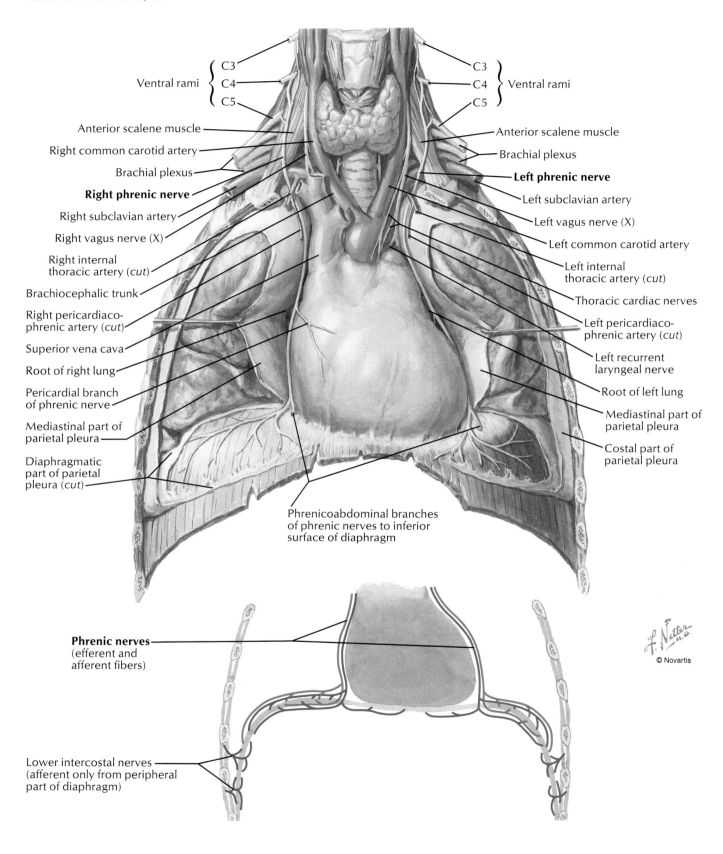

Ventral rami { C3 / C4 / C5

Anterior scalene muscle

Right common carotid artery

Brachial plexus

**Right phrenic nerve**

Right subclavian artery

Right vagus nerve (X)

Right internal thoracic artery (*cut*)

Brachiocephalic trunk

Right pericardiaco-phrenic artery (*cut*)

Superior vena cava

Root of right lung

Pericardial branch of phrenic nerve

Mediastinal part of parietal pleura

Diaphragmatic part of parietal pleura (*cut*)

C3 / C4 / C5 } Ventral rami

Anterior scalene muscle

Brachial plexus

**Left phrenic nerve**

Left subclavian artery

Left vagus nerve (X)

Left common carotid artery

Left internal thoracic artery (*cut*)

Thoracic cardiac nerves

Left pericardiaco-phrenic artery (*cut*)

Left recurrent laryngeal nerve

Root of left lung

Mediastinal part of parietal pleura

Costal part of parietal pleura

Phrenicoabdominal branches of phrenic nerves to inferior surface of diaphragm

**Phrenic nerves** (efferent and afferent fibers)

Lower intercostal nerves (afferent only from peripheral part of diaphragm)

© Novartis

**PLATE 182**

**THORAX**

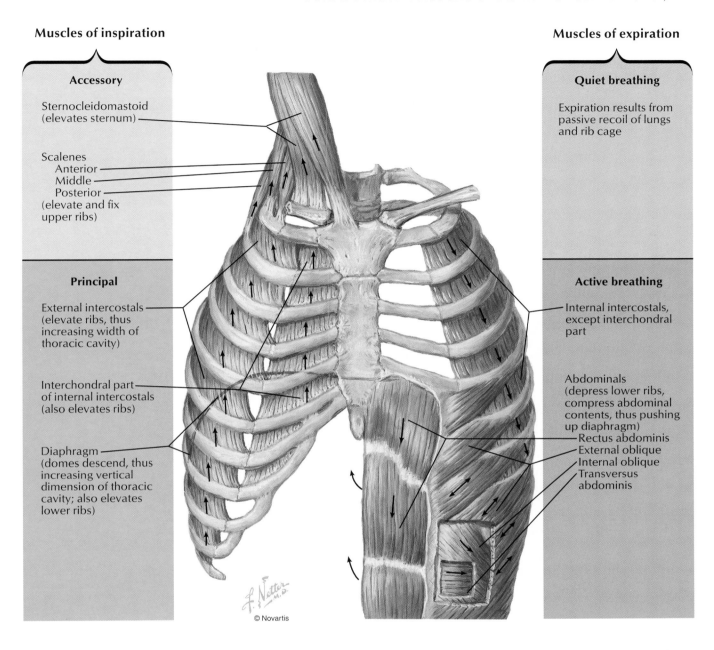

**Muscles of inspiration**

**Accessory**

Sternocleidomastoid
(elevates sternum)

Scalenes
   Anterior
   Middle
   Posterior
(elevate and fix
upper ribs)

**Principal**

External intercostals
(elevate ribs, thus
increasing width of
thoracic cavity)

Interchondral part
of internal intercostals
(also elevates ribs)

Diaphragm
(domes descend, thus
increasing vertical
dimension of thoracic
cavity; also elevates
lower ribs)

**Muscles of expiration**

**Quiet breathing**

Expiration results from
passive recoil of lungs
and rib cage

**Active breathing**

Internal intercostals,
except interchondral
part

Abdominals
(depress lower ribs,
compress abdominal
contents, thus pushing
up diaphragm)
   Rectus abdominis
   External oblique
   Internal oblique
   Transversus
   abdominis

© Novartis

# Topography of Lungs: Anterior View

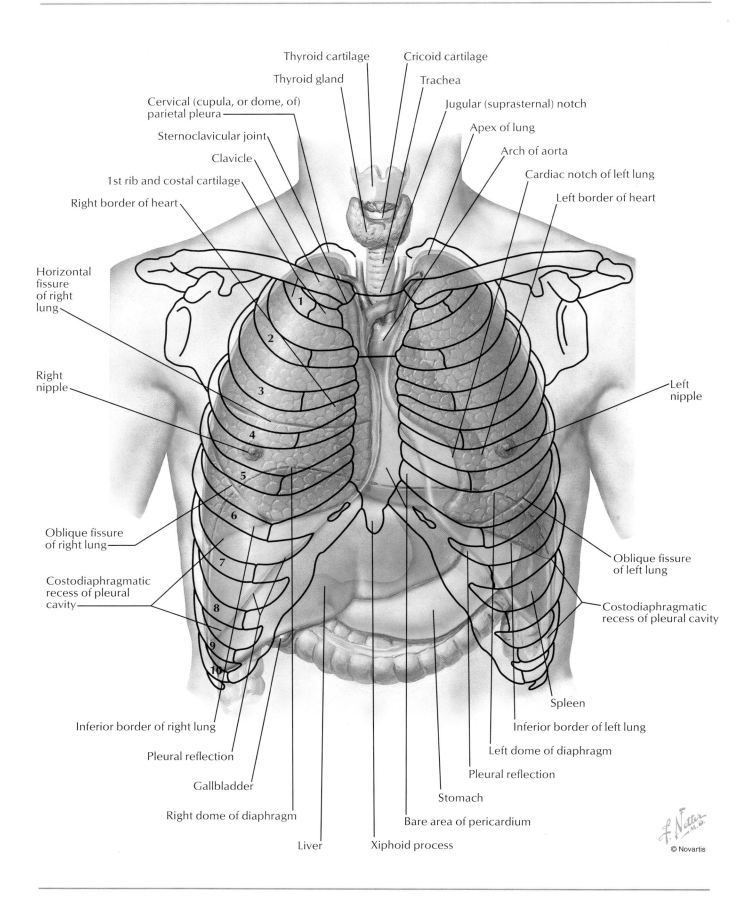

Thyroid cartilage

Cricoid cartilage

Thyroid gland

Trachea

Cervical (cupula, or dome, of) parietal pleura

Jugular (suprasternal) notch

Sternoclavicular joint

Apex of lung

Clavicle

Arch of aorta

1st rib and costal cartilage

Cardiac notch of left lung

Right border of heart

Left border of heart

Horizontal fissure of right lung

Right nipple

Left nipple

Oblique fissure of right lung

Oblique fissure of left lung

Costodiaphragmatic recess of pleural cavity

Costodiaphragmatic recess of pleural cavity

Spleen

Inferior border of right lung

Inferior border of left lung

Pleural reflection

Left dome of diaphragm

Gallbladder

Pleural reflection

Right dome of diaphragm

Stomach

Liver

Xiphoid process

Bare area of pericardium

**PLATE 184**

**THORAX**

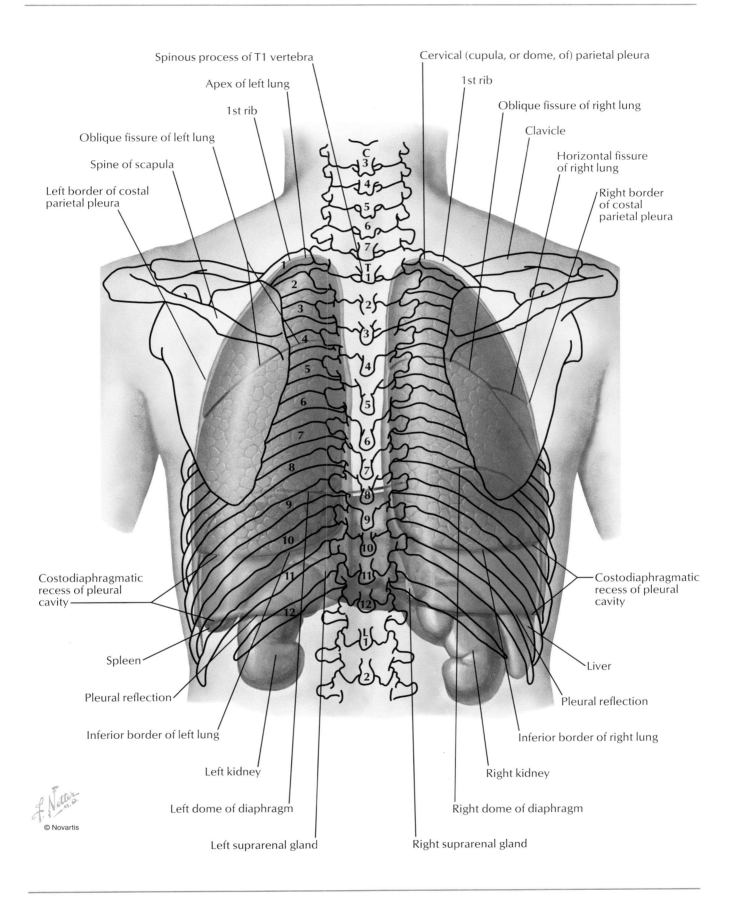

Spinous process of T1 vertebra

Apex of left lung

1st rib

Oblique fissure of left lung

Spine of scapula

Left border of costal parietal pleura

Cervical (cupula, or dome, of) parietal pleura

1st rib

Oblique fissure of right lung

Clavicle

Horizontal fissure of right lung

Right border of costal parietal pleura

Costodiaphragmatic recess of pleural cavity

Costodiaphragmatic recess of pleural cavity

Spleen

Pleural reflection

Inferior border of left lung

Left kidney

Left dome of diaphragm

Left suprarenal gland

Liver

Pleural reflection

Inferior border of right lung

Right kidney

Right dome of diaphragm

Right suprarenal gland

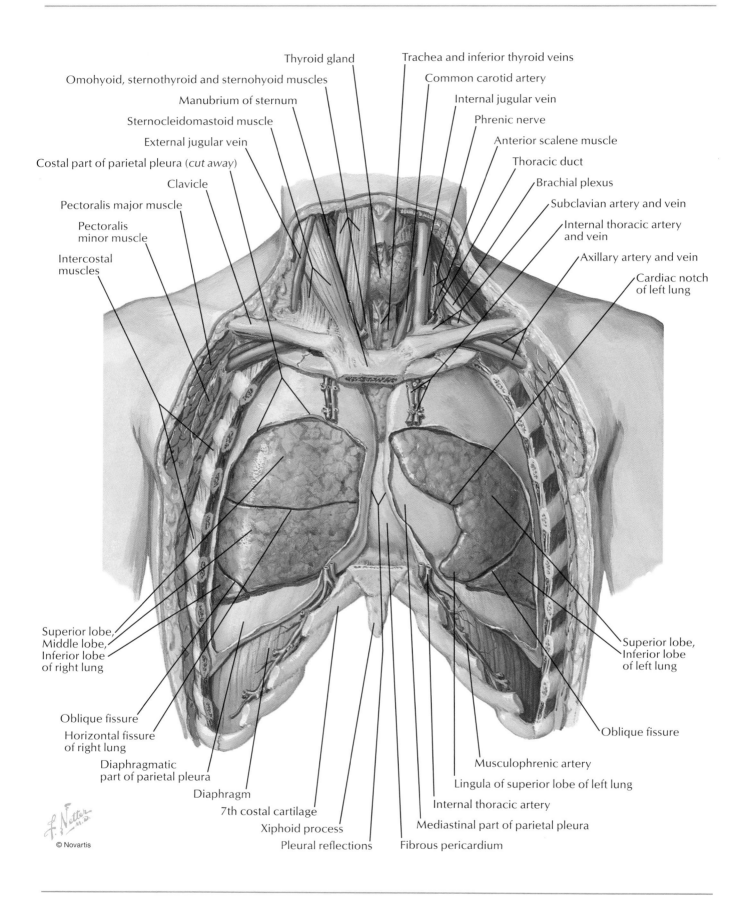

Thyroid gland

Omohyoid, sternothyroid and sternohyoid muscles

Manubrium of sternum

Sternocleidomastoid muscle

External jugular vein

Costal part of parietal pleura (*cut away*)

Clavicle

Pectoralis major muscle

Pectoralis minor muscle

Intercostal muscles

Trachea and inferior thyroid veins

Common carotid artery

Internal jugular vein

Phrenic nerve

Anterior scalene muscle

Thoracic duct

Brachial plexus

Subclavian artery and vein

Internal thoracic artery and vein

Axillary artery and vein

Cardiac notch of left lung

Superior lobe, Middle lobe, Inferior lobe of right lung

Superior lobe, Inferior lobe of left lung

Oblique fissure

Horizontal fissure of right lung

Diaphragmatic part of parietal pleura

Diaphragm

7th costal cartilage

Xiphoid process

Pleural reflections

Oblique fissure

Musculophrenic artery

Lingula of superior lobe of left lung

Internal thoracic artery

Mediastinal part of parietal pleura

Fibrous pericardium

© Novartis

**PLATE 186**

**THORAX**

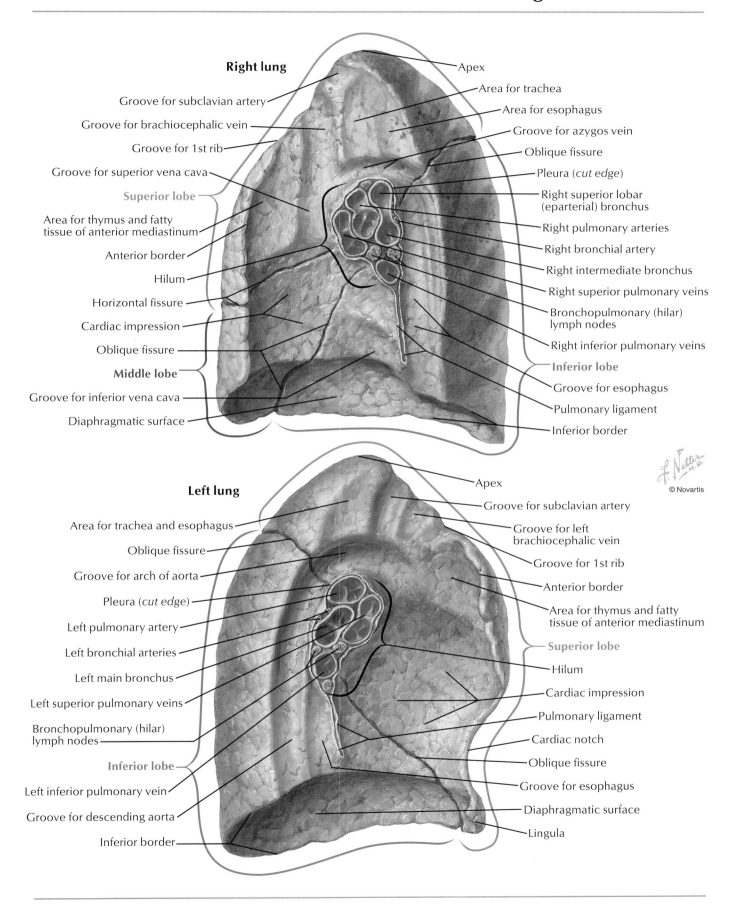

**Right lung**

Groove for subclavian artery
Groove for brachiocephalic vein
Groove for 1st rib
Groove for superior vena cava
Superior lobe
Area for thymus and fatty tissue of anterior mediastinum
Anterior border
Hilum
Horizontal fissure
Cardiac impression
Oblique fissure
**Middle lobe**
Groove for inferior vena cava
Diaphragmatic surface

Apex
Area for trachea
Area for esophagus
Groove for azygos vein
Oblique fissure
Pleura (*cut edge*)
Right superior lobar (eparterial) bronchus
Right pulmonary arteries
Right bronchial artery
Right intermediate bronchus
Right superior pulmonary veins
Bronchopulmonary (hilar) lymph nodes
Right inferior pulmonary veins
Inferior lobe
Groove for esophagus
Pulmonary ligament
Inferior border

**Left lung**

Area for trachea and esophagus
Oblique fissure
Groove for arch of aorta
Pleura (*cut edge*)
Left pulmonary artery
Left bronchial arteries
Left main bronchus
Left superior pulmonary veins
Bronchopulmonary (hilar) lymph nodes
Inferior lobe
Left inferior pulmonary vein
Groove for descending aorta
Inferior border

Apex
Groove for subclavian artery
Groove for left brachiocephalic vein
Groove for 1st rib
Anterior border
Area for thymus and fatty tissue of anterior mediastinum
Superior lobe
Hilum
Cardiac impression
Pulmonary ligament
Cardiac notch
Oblique fissure
Groove for esophagus
Diaphragmatic surface
Lingula

© Novartis

# Bronchopulmonary Segments

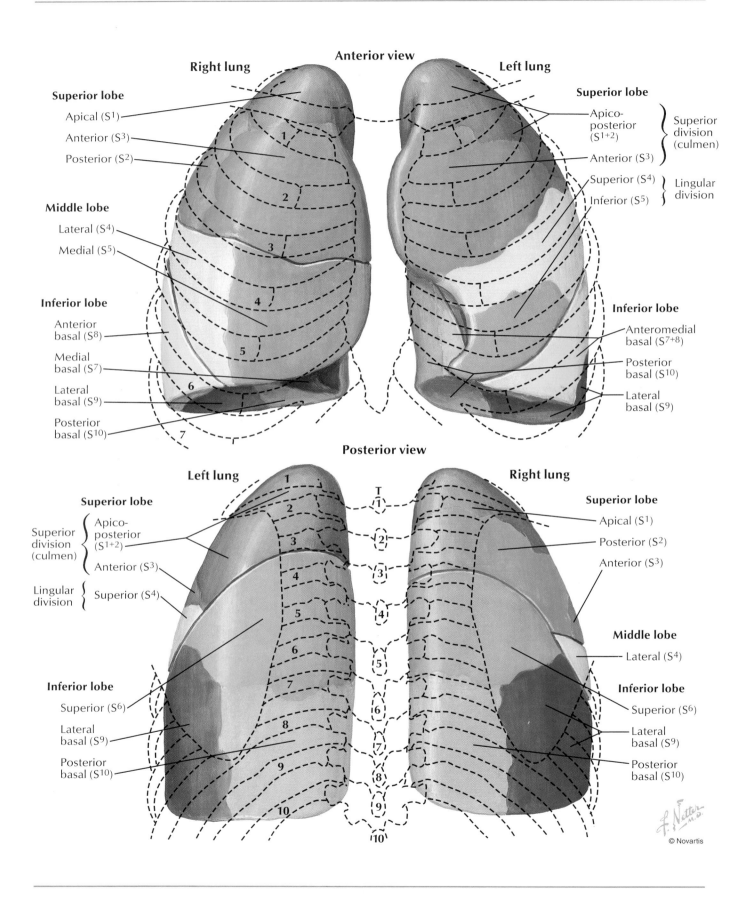

**Anterior view**

**Right lung**

**Left lung**

**Superior lobe**
- Apical (S¹)
- Anterior (S³)
- Posterior (S²)

**Middle lobe**
- Lateral (S⁴)
- Medial (S⁵)

**Inferior lobe**
- Anterior basal (S⁸)
- Medial basal (S⁷)
- Lateral basal (S⁹)
- Posterior basal (S¹⁰)

**Superior lobe**
- Apico-posterior (S¹⁺²) } Superior division (culmen)
- Anterior (S³)
- Superior (S⁴) } Lingular division
- Inferior (S⁵)

**Inferior lobe**
- Anteromedial basal (S⁷⁺⁸)
- Posterior basal (S¹⁰)
- Lateral basal (S⁹)

**Posterior view**

**Left lung**

**Right lung**

**Superior lobe**
- Superior division (culmen) { Apico-posterior (S¹⁺²)
- Anterior (S³)
- Lingular division { Superior (S⁴)

**Inferior lobe**
- Superior (S⁶)
- Lateral basal (S⁹)
- Posterior basal (S¹⁰)

**Superior lobe**
- Apical (S¹)
- Posterior (S²)
- Anterior (S³)

**Middle lobe**
- Lateral (S⁴)

**Inferior lobe**
- Superior (S⁶)
- Lateral basal (S⁹)
- Posterior basal (S¹⁰)

**PLATE 188**

**THORAX**

## Lateral views

### Right lung

**Superior lobe**
- Apical (S$^1$)
- Posterior (S$^2$)
- Anterior (S$^3$)

**Middle lobe**
- Lateral (S$^4$)
- Medial (S$^5$)

**Inferior lobe**
- Superior (S$^6$)
- Anterior basal (S$^8$)
- Lateral basal (S$^9$)

### Left lung

**Superior lobe**
- Apico-posterior (S$^{1+2}$) } Superior division (culmen)
- Anterior (S$^3$) }
- Superior (S$^4$) } Lingular division
- Inferior (S$^5$) }

**Inferior lobe**
- Superior (S$^6$)
- Antero-medial basal (S$^{7+8}$)
- Lateral basal (S$^9$)

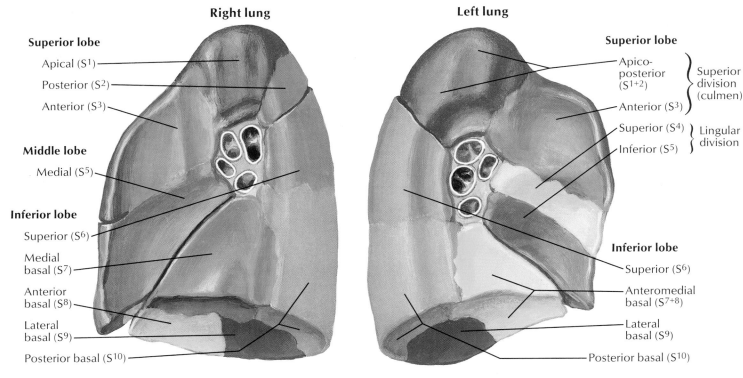

## Medial views

### Right lung

**Superior lobe**
- Apical (S$^1$)
- Posterior (S$^2$)
- Anterior (S$^3$)

**Middle lobe**
- Medial (S$^5$)

**Inferior lobe**
- Superior (S$^6$)
- Medial basal (S$^7$)
- Anterior basal (S$^8$)
- Lateral basal (S$^9$)
- Posterior basal (S$^{10}$)

### Left lung

**Superior lobe**
- Apico-posterior (S$^{1+2}$) } Superior division (culmen)
- Anterior (S$^3$) }
- Superior (S$^4$) } Lingular division
- Inferior (S$^5$) }

**Inferior lobe**
- Superior (S$^6$)
- Anteromedial basal (S$^{7+8}$)
- Lateral basal (S$^9$)
- Posterior basal (S$^{10}$)

**LUNGS**

***PLATE 189***

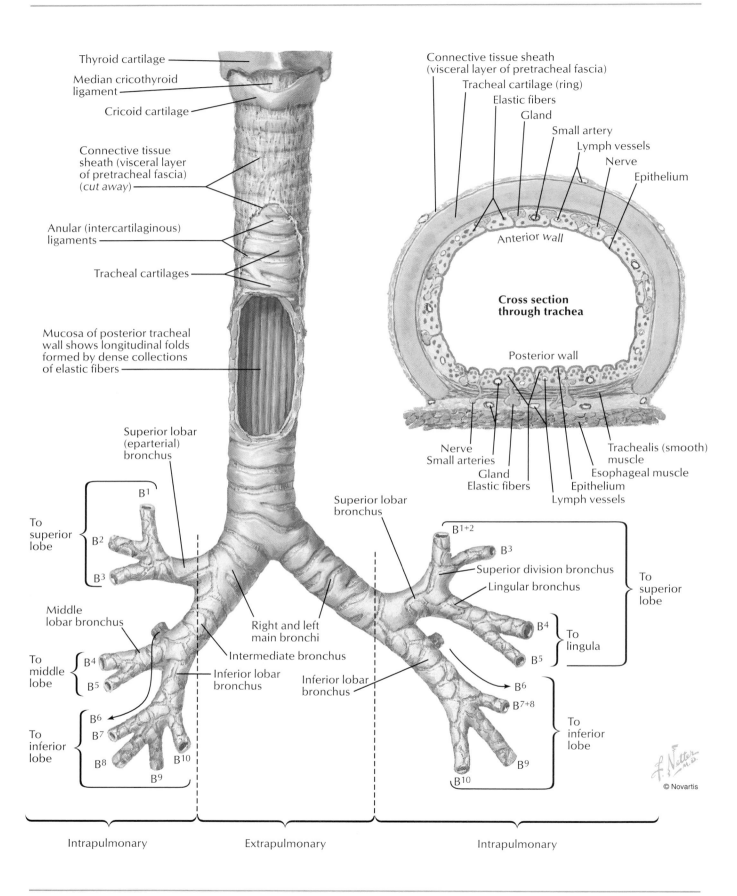

Thyroid cartilage

Median cricothyroid ligament

Cricoid cartilage

Connective tissue sheath (visceral layer of pretracheal fascia) (*cut away*)

Anular (intercartilaginous) ligaments

Tracheal cartilages

Mucosa of posterior tracheal wall shows longitudinal folds formed by dense collections of elastic fibers

Connective tissue sheath (visceral layer of pretracheal fascia)

Tracheal cartilage (ring)

Elastic fibers

Gland

Small artery

Lymph vessels

Nerve

Epithelium

Anterior *wall*

**Cross section through trachea**

Posterior wall

Nerve

Small arteries

Gland

Elastic fibers

Trachealis (smooth) muscle

Esophageal muscle

Epithelium

Lymph vessels

Superior lobar (eparterial) bronchus

B$^1$

To superior lobe

B$^2$

B$^3$

Superior lobar bronchus

B$^{1+2}$

B$^3$

Superior division bronchus

Lingular bronchus

To superior lobe

Middle lobar bronchus

Right and left main bronchi

Intermediate bronchus

B$^4$

To lingula

To middle lobe

B$^4$

B$^5$

Inferior lobar bronchus

Inferior lobar bronchus

B$^5$

B$^6$

B$^{7+8}$

To inferior lobe

To inferior lobe

B$^6$

B$^7$

B$^8$

B$^{10}$

B$^9$

B$^9$

B$^{10}$

Intrapulmonary

Extrapulmonary

Intrapulmonary

© Novartis

**PLATE 190**

**THORAX**

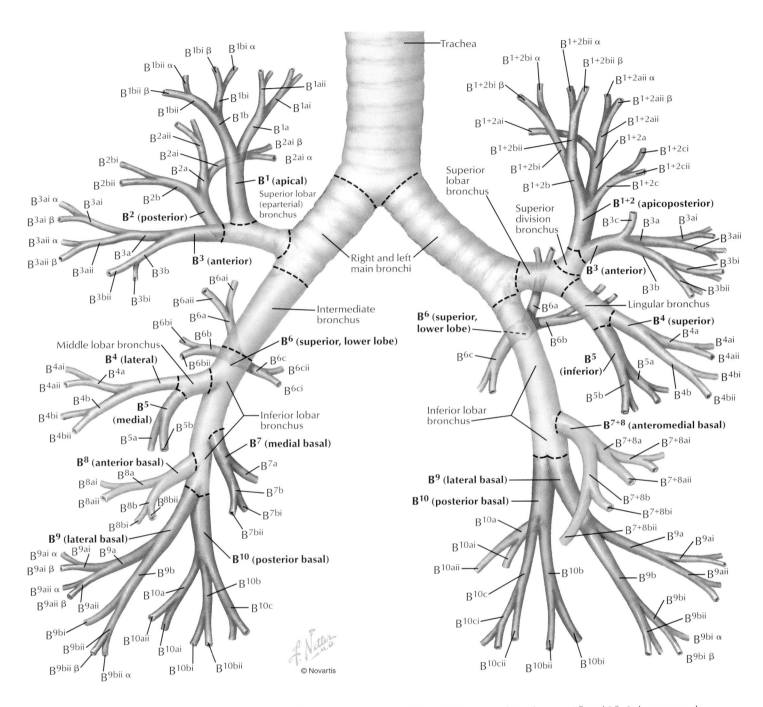

Trachea

B$^{1bi}$ β  B$^{1bi}$ α
B$^{1bii}$ α
B$^{1bii}$ β
B$^{1bii}$
B$^{1bi}$
B$^{1b}$
B$^{1aii}$
B$^{1ai}$
B$^{1a}$
B$^{2aii}$
B$^{2ai}$
B$^{2ai}$ β
B$^{2bi}$
B$^{2a}$
B$^{2ai}$ α
B$^{2bii}$
B$^{2b}$
**B$^1$ (apical)**
Superior lobar
(eparterial)
bronchus
B$^{3ai}$ α  B$^{3ai}$
B$^{3ai}$ β
**B$^2$ (posterior)**
B$^{3aii}$ α
B$^{3aii}$ β
B$^{3a}$
**B$^3$ (anterior)**
B$^{3aii}$  B$^{3b}$
B$^{3bii}$  B$^{3bi}$

B$^{1+2bi}$ α  B$^{1+2bii}$ α
B$^{1+2bi}$ β  B$^{1+2bii}$ β
B$^{1+2aii}$ α
B$^{1+2aii}$ β
B$^{1+2ai}$
B$^{1+2bii}$
B$^{1+2aii}$
B$^{1+2a}$
B$^{1+2bi}$
B$^{1+2b}$
B$^{1+2ci}$
B$^{1+2cii}$
B$^{1+2c}$
Superior
lobar
bronchus
Superior
division
bronchus
**B$^{1+2}$ (apicoposterior)**
B$^{3c}$  B$^{3a}$  B$^{3ai}$
B$^{3aii}$
**B$^3$ (anterior)**  B$^{3bi}$
B$^{3b}$  B$^{3bii}$
Lingular bronchus

Right and left
main bronchi

B$^{6ai}$
B$^{6aii}$
B$^{6a}$
B$^{6bi}$
B$^{6b}$
Middle lobar bronchus
**B$^4$ (lateral)**
B$^{6bii}$
**B$^6$ (superior, lower lobe)**
B$^{6c}$
B$^{6cii}$
B$^{6ci}$
Intermediate
bronchus

**B$^6$ (superior,
lower lobe)**
B$^{6a}$
B$^{6b}$
B$^{6c}$
**B$^4$ (superior)**
**B$^3$ (anterior)**
B$^{4a}$  B$^{4ai}$
B$^{4aii}$
B$^{5a}$  B$^{4bi}$
**B$^5$
(inferior)**
B$^{5b}$  B$^{4b}$  B$^{4bii}$

B$^{4ai}$
B$^{4a}$
B$^{4aii}$
**B$^4$ (lateral)**
B$^{4b}$
B$^{4bi}$
B$^{4bii}$
**B$^5$
(medial)**
B$^{5b}$
B$^{5a}$
Inferior lobar
bronchus
**B$^7$ (medial basal)**
**B$^8$ (anterior basal)**
B$^{8a}$
B$^{8ai}$
B$^{7a}$
B$^{8aii}$
B$^{8b}$  B$^{8bii}$
B$^{8bi}$
B$^{7b}$
B$^{7bi}$
B$^{7bii}$

Inferior lobar
bronchus
**B$^{7+8}$ (anteromedial basal)**
B$^{7+8a}$  B$^{7+8ai}$
**B$^9$ (lateral basal)**
**B$^{10}$ (posterior basal)**
B$^{7+8aii}$
B$^{7+8b}$
B$^{7+8bi}$
B$^{7+8bii}$

**B$^9$ (lateral basal)**
B$^{9ai}$ α  B$^{9ai}$  B$^{9a}$
B$^{9ai}$ β
B$^{9aii}$ α
B$^{9b}$
B$^{9aii}$ β  B$^{9aii}$
B$^{10a}$
**B$^{10}$ (posterior basal)**
B$^{10b}$
B$^{10c}$
B$^{9bi}$
B$^{9bii}$
B$^{10aii}$  B$^{10ai}$
B$^{9bii}$ β
B$^{9bii}$ α  B$^{10bi}$  B$^{10bii}$

B$^{10a}$
B$^{10ai}$
B$^{10aii}$
B$^{10b}$
B$^{10c}$
B$^{10ci}$
B$^{10cii}$  B$^{10bii}$  B$^{10bi}$

B$^{9a}$  B$^{9ai}$
B$^{9aii}$
B$^{9b}$
B$^{9bi}$
B$^{9bii}$
B$^{9bi}$ α
B$^{9bi}$ β

© Novartis

Nomenclature in common usage for bronchopulmonary segments (Plates 188 and 189) is that of Jackson and Huber, and segmental bronchi are named accordingly. Ikeda proposed nomenclature (as demonstrated here) for bronchial subdivisions as far as 6th generation. For simplification on this illustration, only some bronchial subdivisions are labeled as far as 5th or 6th generation. Segmental bronchi (B) are numbered from 1 to 10 in each lung, corresponding to pulmonary segments. In left lung,

B$^1$ and B$^2$ are combined as are B$^7$ and B$^8$. Subsegmental, or 4th order, bronchi are indicated by addition of lower-case letters a, b or c when an additional branch is present. Fifth order bronchi are designated by Roman numerals i (anterior) or ii (posterior) and 6th order bronchi by Greek letters α or β. Several texts use alternate numbers (as proposed by Boyden) for segmental bronchi.

Variations of standard bronchial pattern shown here are common, especially in peripheral airways.

# Intrapulmonary Airways: Schema

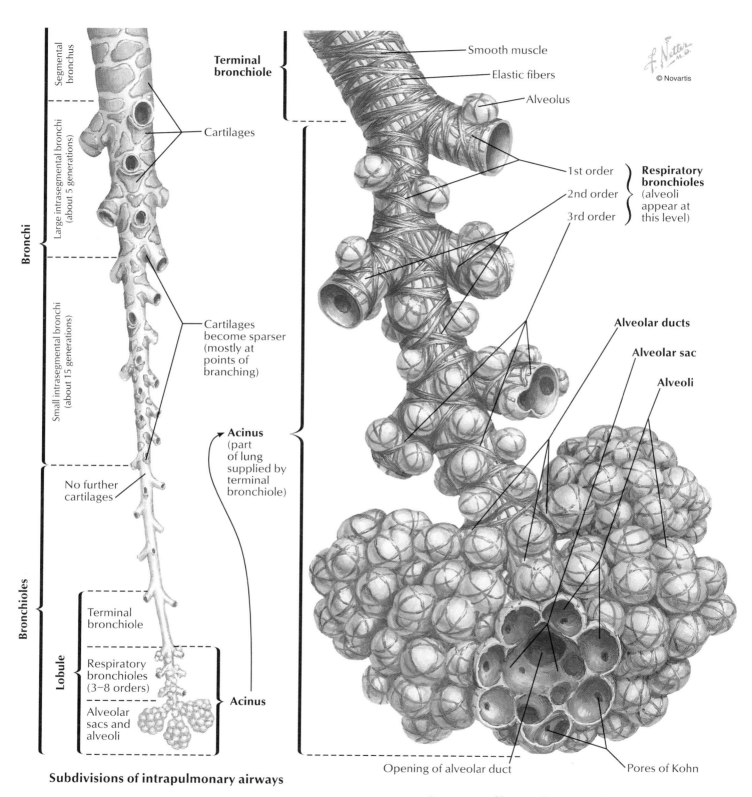

**Bronchi**

Segmental bronchus

Large intrasegmental bronchi (about 5 generations)

Small intrasegmental bronchi (about 15 generations)

**Terminal bronchiole**

Cartilages

Cartilages become sparser (mostly at points of branching)

No further cartilages

**Acinus** (part of lung supplied by terminal bronchiole)

**Bronchioles**

**Lobule**

Terminal bronchiole

Respiratory bronchioles (3–8 orders)

Alveolar sacs and alveoli

**Acinus**

**Subdivisions of intrapulmonary airways**

Smooth muscle

Elastic fibers

Alveolus

1st order

2nd order

3rd order

**Respiratory bronchioles** (alveoli appear at this level)

**Alveolar ducts**

**Alveolar sac**

**Alveoli**

Opening of alveolar duct

Pores of Kohn

**Structure of intrapulmonary airways**

© Novartis

*PLATE 192*

**THORAX**

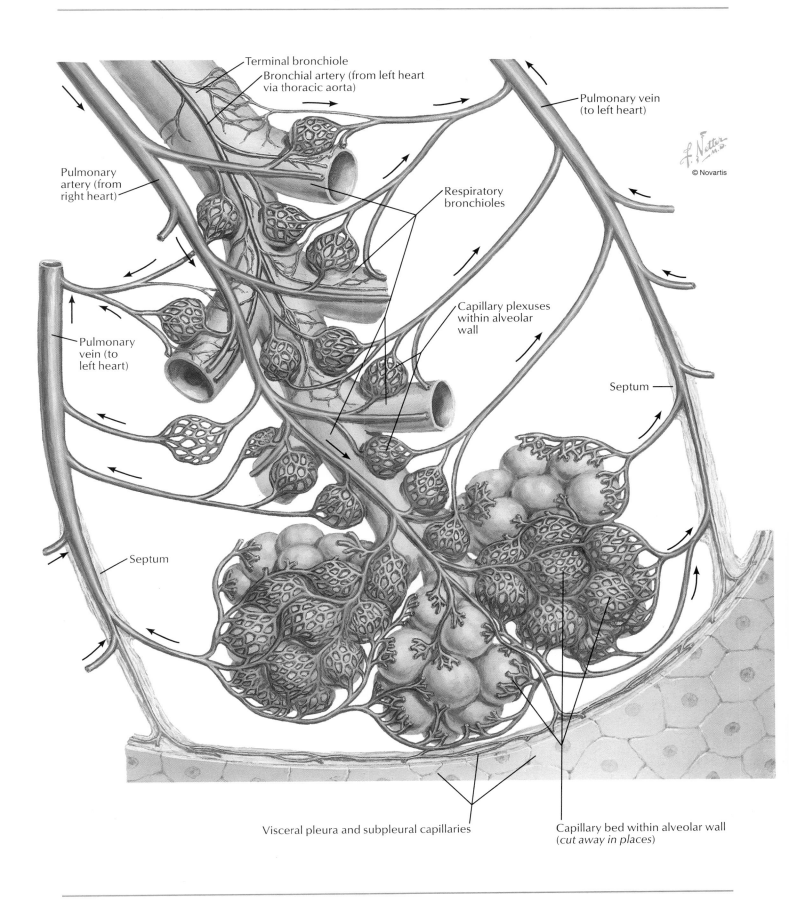

Terminal bronchiole

Bronchial artery (from left heart via thoracic aorta)

Pulmonary vein (to left heart)

Pulmonary artery (from right heart)

Respiratory bronchioles

Pulmonary vein (to left heart)

Capillary plexuses within alveolar wall

Septum

Septum

Visceral pleura and subpleural capillaries

Capillary bed within alveolar wall (*cut away in places*)

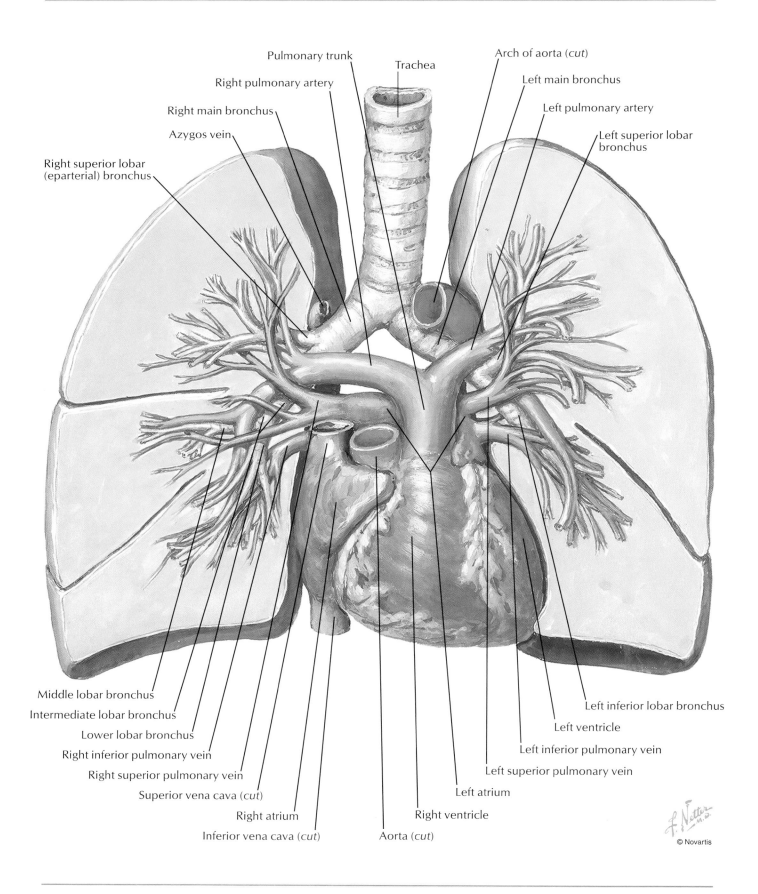

Pulmonary trunk

Trachea

Right pulmonary artery

Arch of aorta (*cut*)

Right main bronchus

Left main bronchus

Azygos vein

Left pulmonary artery

Right superior lobar (eparterial) bronchus

Left superior lobar bronchus

Middle lobar bronchus

Left inferior lobar bronchus

Intermediate lobar bronchus

Left ventricle

Lower lobar bronchus

Left inferior pulmonary vein

Right inferior pulmonary vein

Left superior pulmonary vein

Right superior pulmonary vein

Left atrium

Superior vena cava (*cut*)

Right ventricle

Right atrium

Inferior vena cava (*cut*)

Aorta (*cut*)

*PLATE 194*

**THORAX**

© Novartis

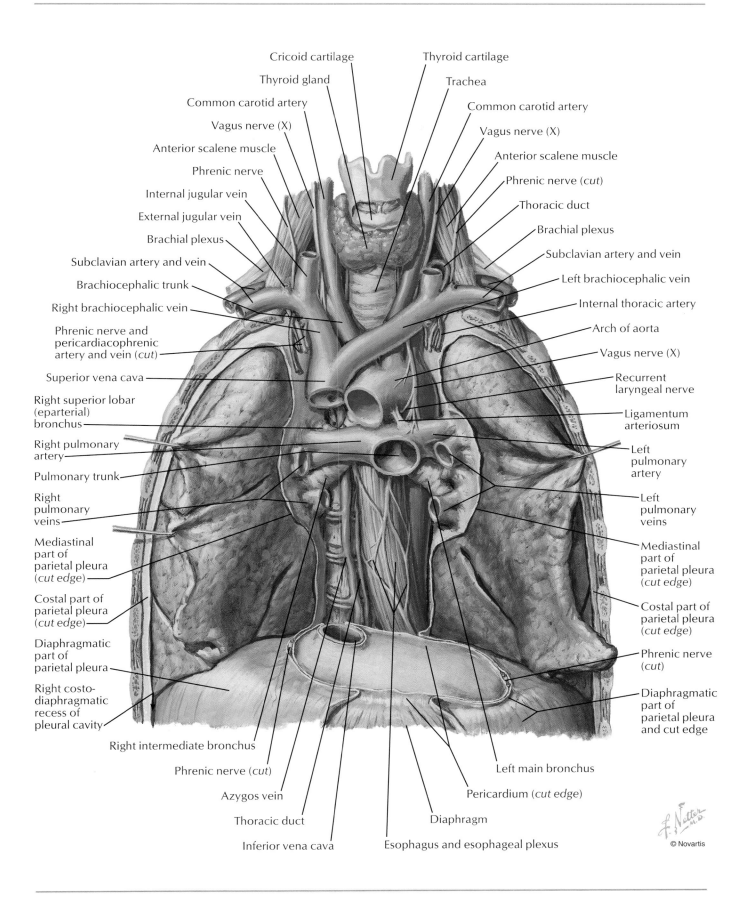

Cricoid cartilage

Thyroid gland

Common carotid artery

Vagus nerve (X)

Anterior scalene muscle

Phrenic nerve

Internal jugular vein

External jugular vein

Brachial plexus

Subclavian artery and vein

Brachiocephalic trunk

Right brachiocephalic vein

Phrenic nerve and pericardiacophrenic artery and vein (*cut*)

Superior vena cava

Right superior lobar (eparterial) bronchus

Right pulmonary artery

Pulmonary trunk

Right pulmonary veins

Mediastinal part of parietal pleura (*cut edge*)

Costal part of parietal pleura (*cut edge*)

Diaphragmatic part of parietal pleura

Right costo-diaphragmatic recess of pleural cavity

Right intermediate bronchus

Phrenic nerve (*cut*)

Azygos vein

Thoracic duct

Inferior vena cava

Thyroid cartilage

Trachea

Common carotid artery

Vagus nerve (X)

Anterior scalene muscle

Phrenic nerve (*cut*)

Thoracic duct

Brachial plexus

Subclavian artery and vein

Left brachiocephalic vein

Internal thoracic artery

Arch of aorta

Vagus nerve (X)

Recurrent laryngeal nerve

Ligamentum arteriosum

Left pulmonary artery

Left pulmonary veins

Mediastinal part of parietal pleura (*cut edge*)

Costal part of parietal pleura (*cut edge*)

Phrenic nerve (*cut*)

Diaphragmatic part of parietal pleura and cut edge

Left main bronchus

Pericardium (*cut edge*)

Diaphragm

Esophagus and esophageal plexus

© Novartis

# *Bronchial Arteries and Veins*

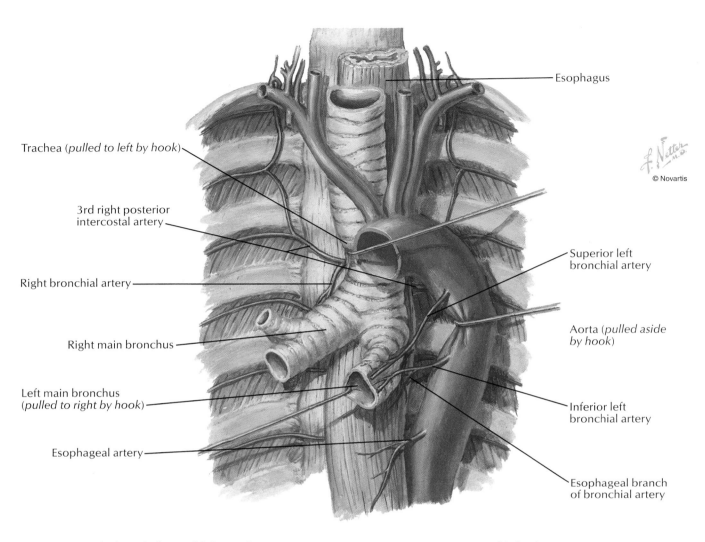

Esophagus

Trachea (*pulled to left by hook*)

3rd right posterior intercostal artery

Right bronchial artery

Right main bronchus

Left main bronchus (*pulled to right by hook*)

Esophageal artery

Superior left bronchial artery

Aorta (*pulled aside by hook*)

Inferior left bronchial artery

Esophageal branch of bronchial artery

F. Netter
© Novartis

**Variations in bronchial arteries**

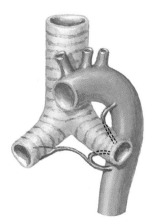

Right and left bronchial arteries originating from aorta by single stem

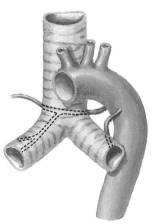

Only single bronchial artery to each bronchus (normally, two to left bronchus)

**Bronchial veins**

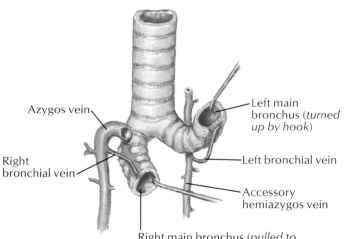

Azygos vein

Right bronchial vein

Left main bronchus (*turned up by hook*)

Left bronchial vein

Accessory hemiazygos vein

Right main bronchus (*pulled to left and rotated by hook*)

**PLATE 196**

**THORAX**

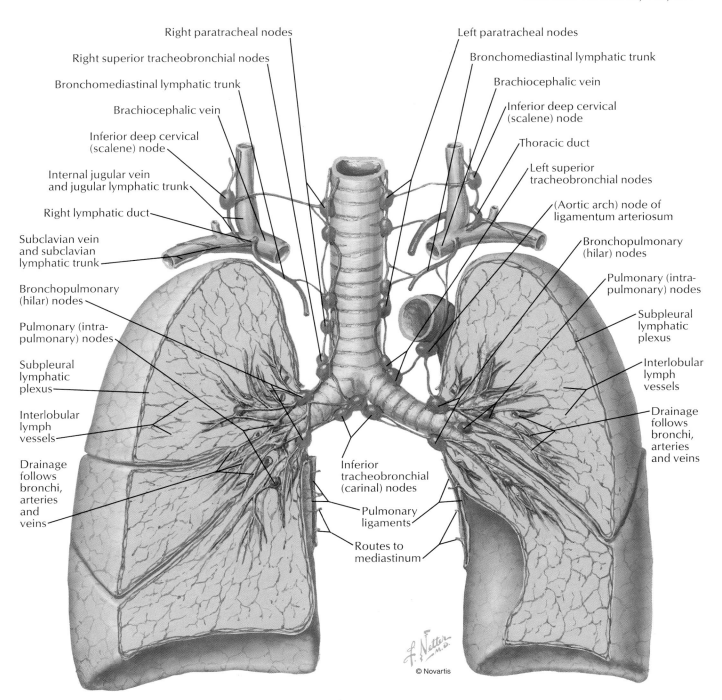

Right paratracheal nodes

Right superior tracheobronchial nodes

Bronchomediastinal lymphatic trunk

Brachiocephalic vein

Inferior deep cervical (scalene) node

Internal jugular vein and jugular lymphatic trunk

Right lymphatic duct

Subclavian vein and subclavian lymphatic trunk

Bronchopulmonary (hilar) nodes

Pulmonary (intra-pulmonary) nodes

Subpleural lymphatic plexus

Interlobular lymph vessels

Drainage follows bronchi, arteries and veins

Left paratracheal nodes

Bronchomediastinal lymphatic trunk

Brachiocephalic vein

Inferior deep cervical (scalene) node

Thoracic duct

Left superior tracheobronchial nodes

(Aortic arch) node of ligamentum arteriosum

Bronchopulmonary (hilar) nodes

Pulmonary (intra-pulmonary) nodes

Subpleural lymphatic plexus

Interlobular lymph vessels

Drainage follows bronchi, arteries and veins

Inferior tracheobronchial (carinal) nodes

Pulmonary ligaments

Routes to mediastinum

**Drainage routes**

**Right lung:** All lobes drain to pulmonary and broncho-pulmonary (hilar) nodes, then to inferior tracheobronchial (carinal) nodes, right superior tracheobronchial nodes and to right paratracheal nodes on way to brachiocephalic vein via bronchomediastinal lymphatic trunk and/or inferior deep cervical (scalene) node.

**Left lung:** Superior lobe drains to pulmonary and broncho-pulmonary (hilar) nodes, inferior tracheobronchial (carinal) nodes, left superior tracheobronchial nodes, left paratracheal nodes and/or (aortic arch) node of ligamentum arteriosum, then to brachiocephalic vein via left bronchomediastinal trunk and thoracic duct. Left inferior lobe drains also to pulmonary and bronchopulmonary (hilar) nodes and to inferior tracheo-bronchial (carinal) nodes, but then mostly to right superior tracheobronchial nodes, where it follows same route as lymph from right lung.

# Autonomic Nerves in Thorax

SEE ALSO PLATES 124, 125, 152, 300

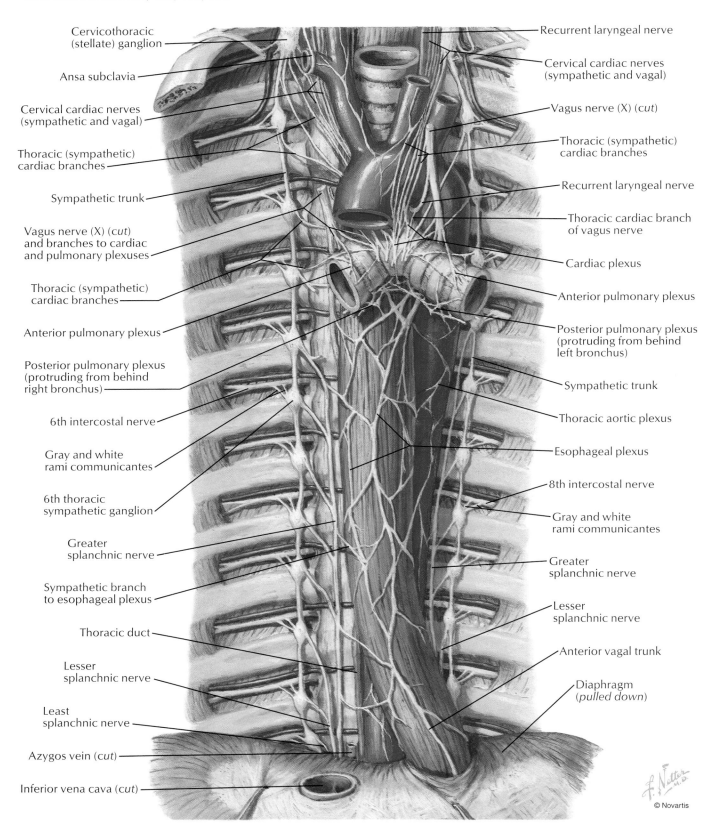

Cervicothoracic (stellate) ganglion

Ansa subclavia

Cervical cardiac nerves (sympathetic and vagal)

Thoracic (sympathetic) cardiac branches

Sympathetic trunk

Vagus nerve (X) (cut) and branches to cardiac and pulmonary plexuses

Thoracic (sympathetic) cardiac branches

Anterior pulmonary plexus

Posterior pulmonary plexus (protruding from behind right bronchus)

6th intercostal nerve

Gray and white rami communicantes

6th thoracic sympathetic ganglion

Greater splanchnic nerve

Sympathetic branch to esophageal plexus

Thoracic duct

Lesser splanchnic nerve

Least splanchnic nerve

Azygos vein (cut)

Inferior vena cava (cut)

Recurrent laryngeal nerve

Cervical cardiac nerves (sympathetic and vagal)

Vagus nerve (X) (cut)

Thoracic (sympathetic) cardiac branches

Recurrent laryngeal nerve

Thoracic cardiac branch of vagus nerve

Cardiac plexus

Anterior pulmonary plexus

Posterior pulmonary plexus (protruding from behind left bronchus)

Sympathetic trunk

Thoracic aortic plexus

Esophageal plexus

8th intercostal nerve

Gray and white rami communicantes

Greater splanchnic nerve

Lesser splanchnic nerve

Anterior vagal trunk

Diaphragm (pulled down)

© Novartis

**PLATE 198**

**THORAX**

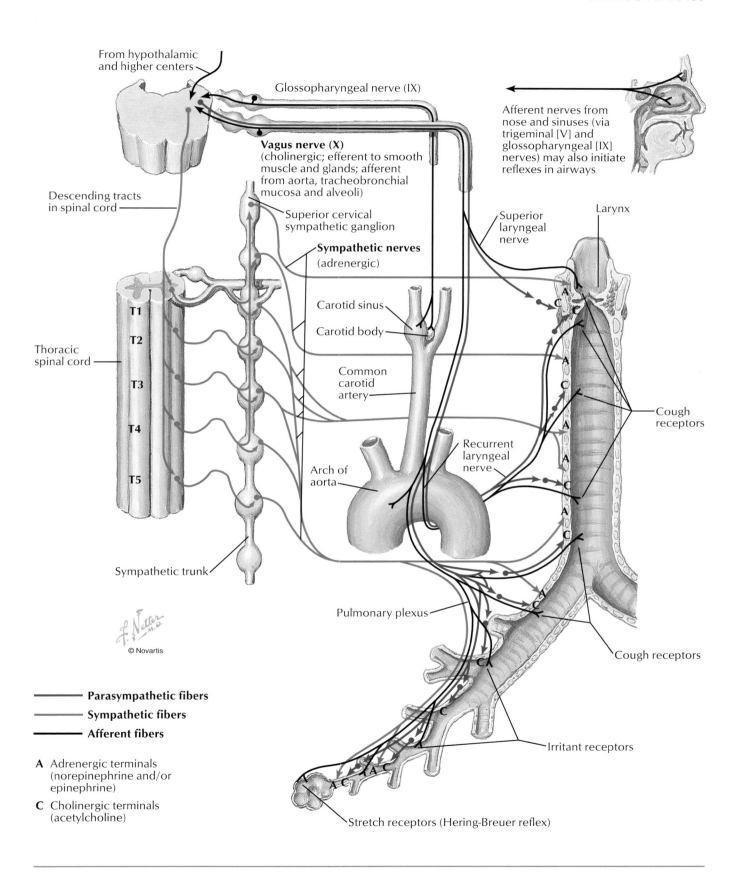

From hypothalamic and higher centers

Glossopharyngeal nerve (IX)

Afferent nerves from nose and sinuses (via trigeminal [V] and glossopharyngeal [IX] nerves) may also initiate reflexes in airways

**Vagus nerve (X)** (cholinergic; efferent to smooth muscle and glands; afferent from aorta, tracheobronchial mucosa and alveoli)

Descending tracts in spinal cord

Superior cervical sympathetic ganglion

Superior laryngeal nerve

Larynx

**Sympathetic nerves** (adrenergic)

T1

T2

Thoracic spinal cord

T3

T4

T5

Carotid sinus

Carotid body

Common carotid artery

Cough receptors

Recurrent laryngeal nerve

Arch of aorta

Sympathetic trunk

Pulmonary plexus

Cough receptors

*f. Netter*
© Novartis

—————— **Parasympathetic fibers**

—————— **Sympathetic fibers**

—————— **Afferent fibers**

Irritant receptors

**A** Adrenergic terminals (norepinephrine and/or epinephrine)

**C** Cholinergic terminals (acetylcholine)

Stretch receptors (Hering-Breuer reflex)

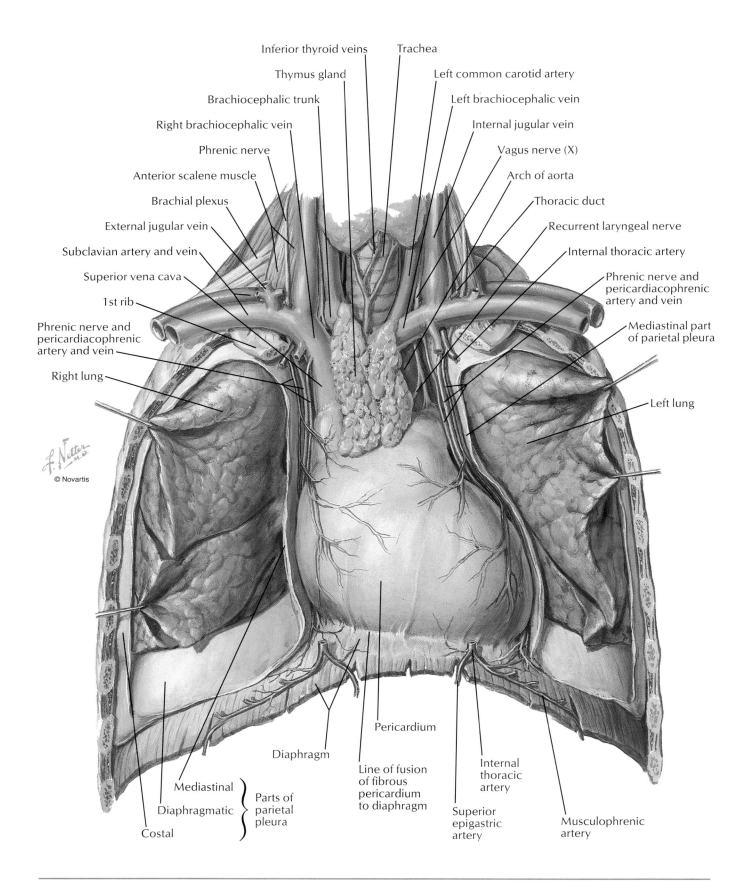

Inferior thyroid veins

Thymus gland

Brachiocephalic trunk

Right brachiocephalic vein

Phrenic nerve

Anterior scalene muscle

Brachial plexus

External jugular vein

Subclavian artery and vein

Superior vena cava

1st rib

Phrenic nerve and pericardiacophrenic artery and vein

Right lung

Trachea

Left common carotid artery

Left brachiocephalic vein

Internal jugular vein

Vagus nerve (X)

Arch of aorta

Thoracic duct

Recurrent laryngeal nerve

Internal thoracic artery

Phrenic nerve and pericardiacophrenic artery and vein

Mediastinal part of parietal pleura

Left lung

Mediastinal
Diaphragmatic
Costal
} Parts of parietal pleura

Diaphragm

Line of fusion of fibrous pericardium to diaphragm

Pericardium

Superior epigastric artery

Internal thoracic artery

Musculophrenic artery

© Novartis

**PLATE 200**

**THORAX**

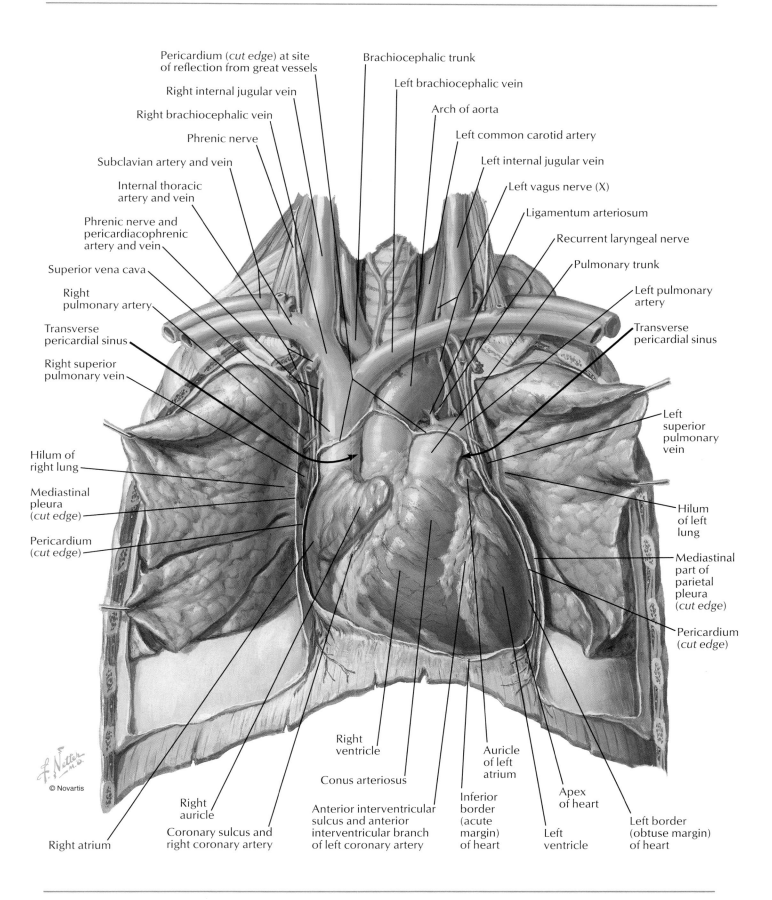

Pericardium (*cut edge*) at site of reflection from great vessels

Right internal jugular vein

Right brachiocephalic vein

Phrenic nerve

Subclavian artery and vein

Internal thoracic artery and vein

Phrenic nerve and pericardiacophrenic artery and vein

Superior vena cava

Right pulmonary artery

Transverse pericardial sinus

Right superior pulmonary vein

Hilum of right lung

Mediastinal pleura (*cut edge*)

Pericardium (*cut edge*)

Brachiocephalic trunk

Left brachiocephalic vein

Arch of aorta

Left common carotid artery

Left internal jugular vein

Left vagus nerve (X)

Ligamentum arteriosum

Recurrent laryngeal nerve

Pulmonary trunk

Left pulmonary artery

Transverse pericardial sinus

Left superior pulmonary vein

Hilum of left lung

Mediastinal part of parietal pleura (*cut edge*)

Pericardium (*cut edge*)

Right ventricle

Conus arteriosus

Right auricle

Coronary sulcus and right coronary artery

Anterior interventricular sulcus and anterior interventricular branch of left coronary artery

Auricle of left atrium

Inferior border (acute margin) of heart

Left ventricle

Apex of heart

Left border (obtuse margin) of heart

Right atrium

f. Netter M.D.

© Novartis

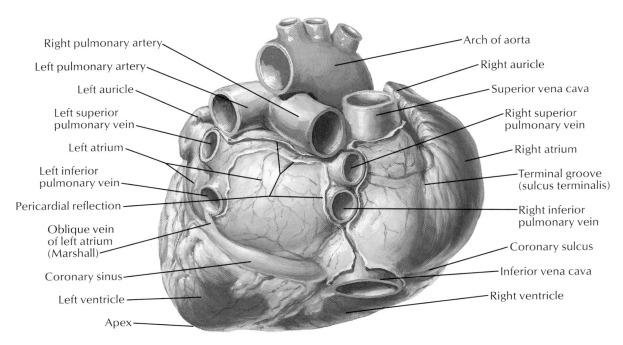

Right pulmonary artery
Left pulmonary artery
Left auricle
Left superior pulmonary vein
Left atrium
Left inferior pulmonary vein
Pericardial reflection
Oblique vein of left atrium (Marshall)
Coronary sinus
Left ventricle
Apex

Arch of aorta
Right auricle
Superior vena cava
Right superior pulmonary vein
Right atrium
Terminal groove (sulcus terminalis)
Right inferior pulmonary vein
Coronary sulcus
Inferior vena cava
Right ventricle

**Base of heart: posterior view**

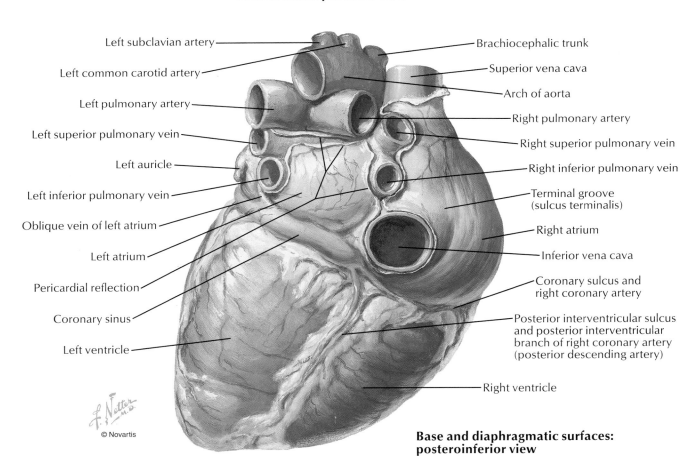

Left subclavian artery
Left common carotid artery
Left pulmonary artery
Left superior pulmonary vein
Left auricle
Left inferior pulmonary vein
Oblique vein of left atrium
Left atrium
Pericardial reflection
Coronary sinus
Left ventricle

Brachiocephalic trunk
Superior vena cava
Arch of aorta
Right pulmonary artery
Right superior pulmonary vein
Right inferior pulmonary vein
Terminal groove (sulcus terminalis)
Right atrium
Inferior vena cava
Coronary sulcus and right coronary artery
Posterior interventricular sulcus and posterior interventricular branch of right coronary artery (posterior descending artery)
Right ventricle

© Novartis

**Base and diaphragmatic surfaces: posteroinferior view**

*PLATE 202*                                                                 **THORAX**

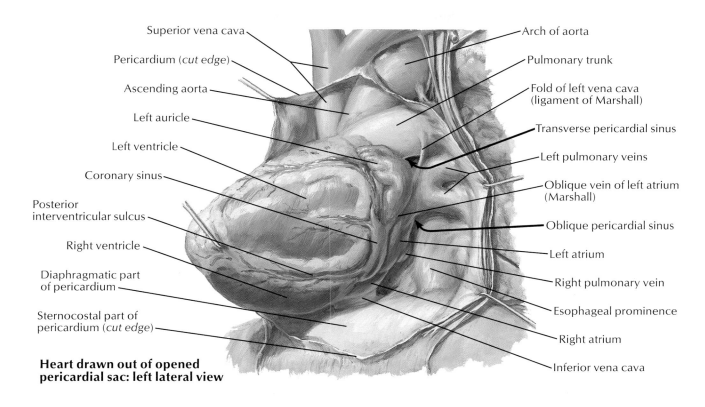

Superior vena cava

Pericardium (*cut edge*)

Ascending aorta

Left auricle

Left ventricle

Coronary sinus

Posterior interventricular sulcus

Right ventricle

Diaphragmatic part of pericardium

Sternocostal part of pericardium (*cut edge*)

Arch of aorta

Pulmonary trunk

Fold of left vena cava (ligament of Marshall)

Transverse pericardial sinus

Left pulmonary veins

Oblique vein of left atrium (Marshall)

Oblique pericardial sinus

Left atrium

Right pulmonary vein

Esophageal prominence

Right atrium

Inferior vena cava

**Heart drawn out of opened pericardial sac: left lateral view**

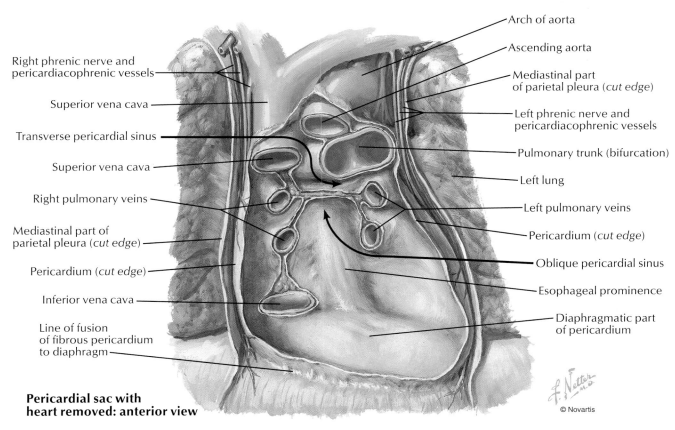

Right phrenic nerve and pericardiacophrenic vessels

Superior vena cava

Transverse pericardial sinus

Superior vena cava

Right pulmonary veins

Mediastinal part of parietal pleura (*cut edge*)

Pericardium (*cut edge*)

Inferior vena cava

Line of fusion of fibrous pericardium to diaphragm

Arch of aorta

Ascending aorta

Mediastinal part of parietal pleura (*cut edge*)

Left phrenic nerve and pericardiacophrenic vessels

Pulmonary trunk (bifurcation)

Left lung

Left pulmonary veins

Pericardium (*cut edge*)

Oblique pericardial sinus

Esophageal prominence

Diaphragmatic part of pericardium

**Pericardial sac with heart removed: anterior view**

© Novartis

**HEART**

**PLATE 203**

# Coronary Arteries and Cardiac Veins

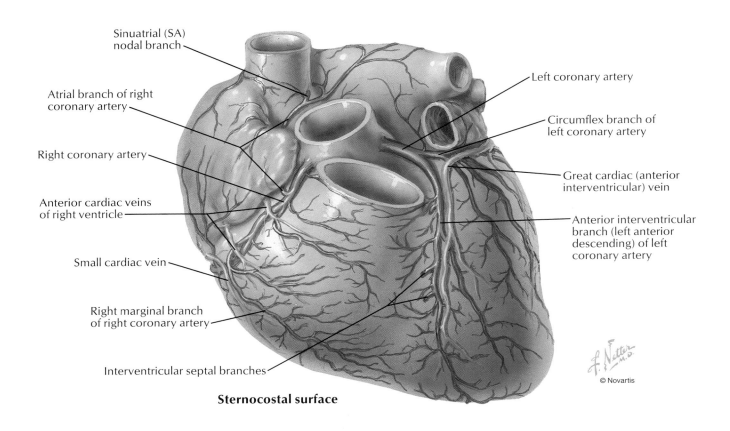

Sinuatrial (SA) nodal branch

Atrial branch of right coronary artery

Right coronary artery

Anterior cardiac veins of right ventricle

Small cardiac vein

Right marginal branch of right coronary artery

Interventricular septal branches

Left coronary artery

Circumflex branch of left coronary artery

Great cardiac (anterior interventricular) vein

Anterior interventricular branch (left anterior descending) of left coronary artery

**Sternocostal surface**

© Novartis

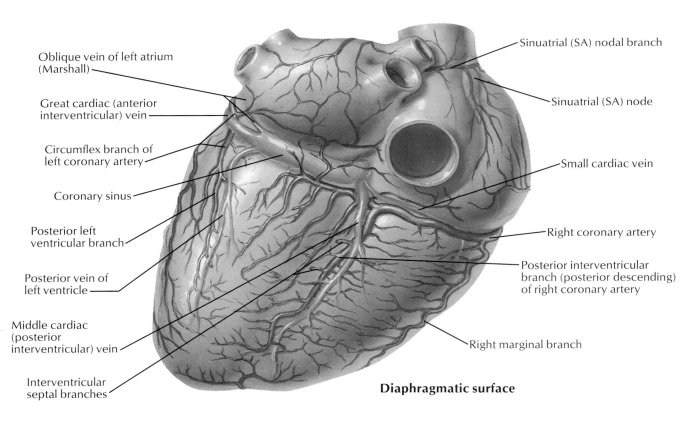

Oblique vein of left atrium (Marshall)

Great cardiac (anterior interventricular) vein

Circumflex branch of left coronary artery

Coronary sinus

Posterior left ventricular branch

Posterior vein of left ventricle

Middle cardiac (posterior interventricular) vein

Interventricular septal branches

Sinuatrial (SA) nodal branch

Sinuatrial (SA) node

Small cardiac vein

Right coronary artery

Posterior interventricular branch (posterior descending) of right coronary artery

Right marginal branch

**Diaphragmatic surface**

*PLATE 204*

**THORAX**

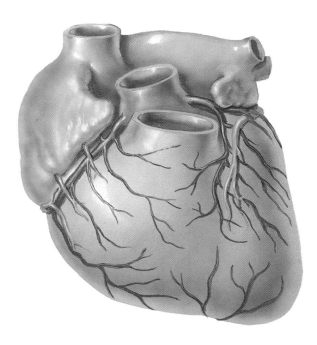

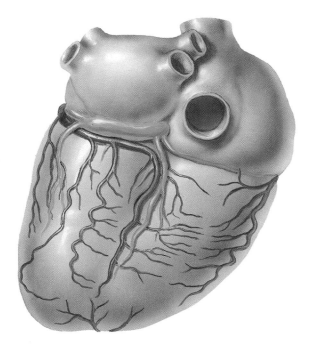

Anterior interventricular (left anterior descending) branch of left coronary artery very short. Apical part of anterior (sternocostal) surface supplied by branches from posterior interventricular (posterior descending) branch of right coronary artery curving around apex

Posterior interventricular (posterior descending) branch derived from circumflex branch of left coronary artery instead of from right coronary artery

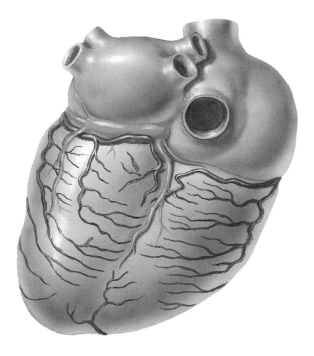

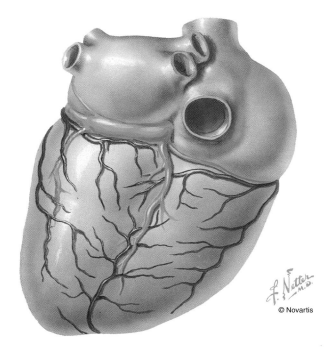

Posterior interventricular (posterior descending) branch absent. Area supplied chiefly by small branches from circumflex branch of left coronary artery and from right coronary artery

Posterior interventricular (posterior descending) branch absent. Area supplied chiefly by elongated anterior interventricular (left anterior descending) branch curving around apex

## Right coronary artery: left anterior oblique view

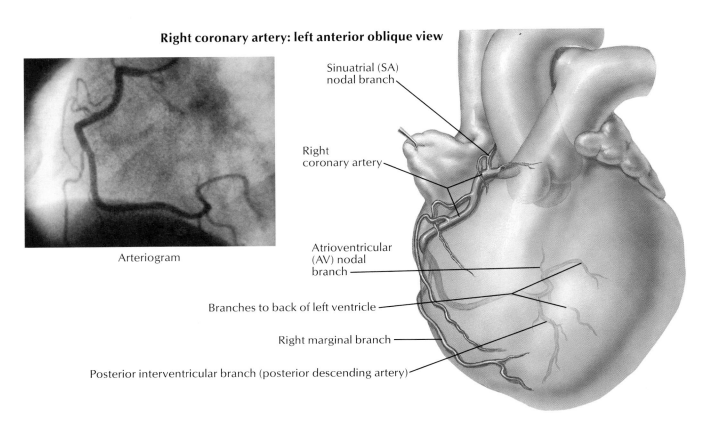

Arteriogram

Sinuatrial (SA) nodal branch

Right coronary artery

Atrioventricular (AV) nodal branch

Branches to back of left ventricle

Right marginal branch

Posterior interventricular branch (posterior descending artery)

## Right coronary artery: right anterior oblique view

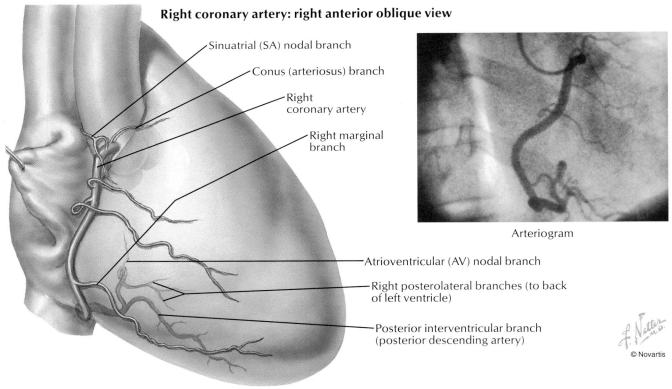

Sinuatrial (SA) nodal branch

Conus (arteriosus) branch

Right coronary artery

Right marginal branch

Arteriogram

Atrioventricular (AV) nodal branch

Right posterolateral branches (to back of left ventricle)

Posterior interventricular branch (posterior descending artery)

© Novartis

**PLATE 206**

**THORAX**

### Left coronary artery: left anterior oblique view

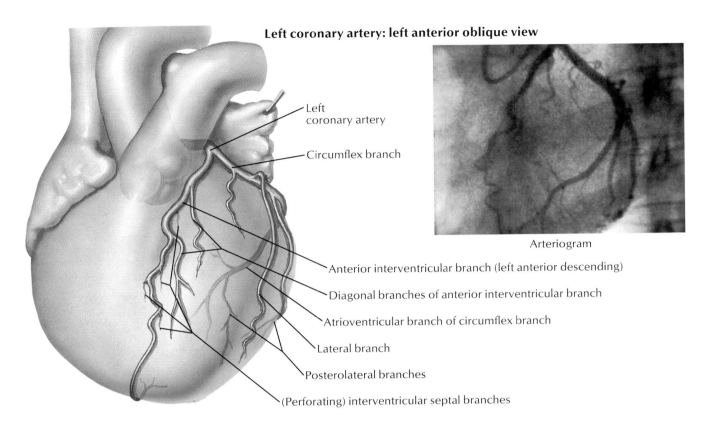

Left coronary artery

Circumflex branch

Arteriogram

Anterior interventricular branch (left anterior descending)

Diagonal branches of anterior interventricular branch

Atrioventricular branch of circumflex branch

Lateral branch

Posterolateral branches

(Perforating) interventricular septal branches

### Left coronary artery: right anterior oblique view

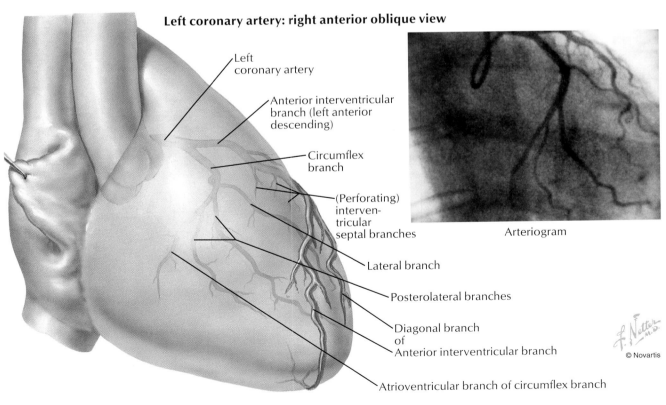

Left coronary artery

Anterior interventricular branch (left anterior descending)

Circumflex branch

(Perforating) interventricular septal branches

Arteriogram

Lateral branch

Posterolateral branches

Diagonal branch of Anterior interventricular branch

Atrioventricular branch of circumflex branch

© Novartis

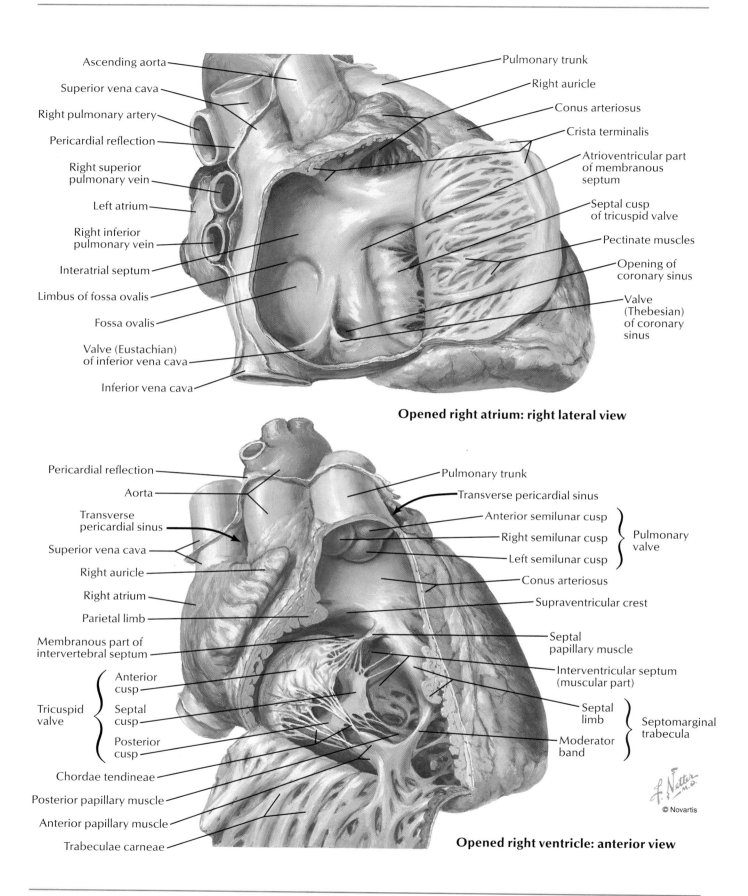

Ascending aorta

Superior vena cava

Right pulmonary artery

Pericardial reflection

Right superior pulmonary vein

Left atrium

Right inferior pulmonary vein

Interatrial septum

Limbus of fossa ovalis

Fossa ovalis

Valve (Eustachian) of inferior vena cava

Inferior vena cava

Pulmonary trunk

Right auricle

Conus arteriosus

Crista terminalis

Atrioventricular part of membranous septum

Septal cusp of tricuspid valve

Pectinate muscles

Opening of coronary sinus

Valve (Thebesian) of coronary sinus

**Opened right atrium: right lateral view**

Pericardial reflection

Aorta

Transverse pericardial sinus

Superior vena cava

Right auricle

Right atrium

Parietal limb

Membranous part of intervertebral septum

Anterior cusp

Tricuspid valve { Septal cusp

Posterior cusp

Chordae tendineae

Posterior papillary muscle

Anterior papillary muscle

Trabeculae carneae

Pulmonary trunk

Transverse pericardial sinus

Anterior semilunar cusp

Right semilunar cusp } Pulmonary valve

Left semilunar cusp

Conus arteriosus

Supraventricular crest

Septal papillary muscle

Interventricular septum (muscular part)

Septal limb } Septomarginal trabecula

Moderator band

© Novartis

**Opened right ventricle: anterior view**

**PLATE 208**

**THORAX**

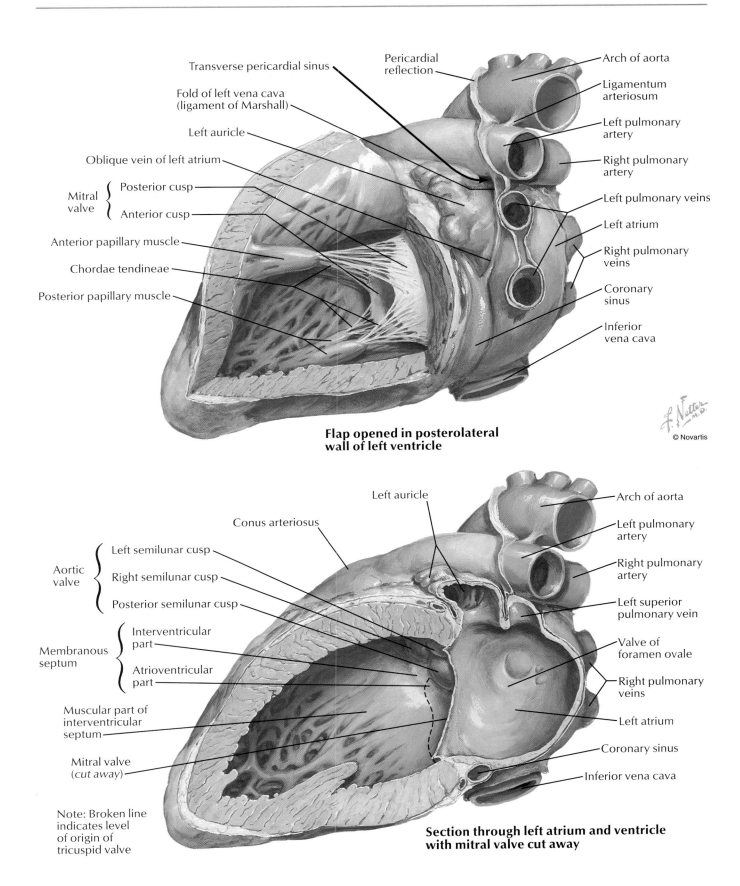

Transverse pericardial sinus

Pericardial reflection

Arch of aorta

Ligamentum arteriosum

Fold of left vena cava (ligament of Marshall)

Left pulmonary artery

Left auricle

Right pulmonary artery

Oblique vein of left atrium

Left pulmonary veins

Mitral { Posterior cusp
valve { Anterior cusp

Left atrium

Right pulmonary veins

Anterior papillary muscle

Chordae tendineae

Coronary sinus

Posterior papillary muscle

Inferior vena cava

**Flap opened in posterolateral wall of left ventricle**

Left auricle

Arch of aorta

Conus arteriosus

Left pulmonary artery

Aortic { Left semilunar cusp
valve { Right semilunar cusp
{ Posterior semilunar cusp

Right pulmonary artery

Left superior pulmonary vein

Membranous { Interventricular part
septum { Atrioventricular part

Valve of foramen ovale

Right pulmonary veins

Muscular part of interventricular septum

Left atrium

Mitral valve (*cut away*)

Coronary sinus

Inferior vena cava

Note: Broken line indicates level of origin of tricuspid valve

**Section through left atrium and ventricle with mitral valve cut away**

© Novartis

# *Valves and Fibrous Skeleton of Heart*

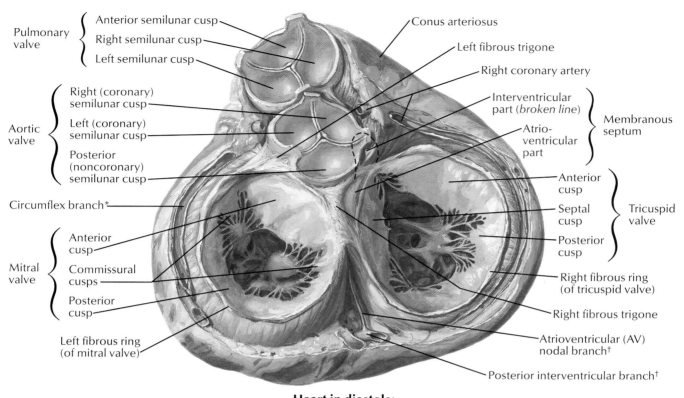

Pulmonary valve
- Anterior semilunar cusp
- Right semilunar cusp
- Left semilunar cusp

Aortic valve
- Right (coronary) semilunar cusp
- Left (coronary) semilunar cusp
- Posterior (noncoronary) semilunar cusp

Circumflex branch*

Mitral valve
- Anterior cusp
- Commissural cusps
- Posterior cusp

Left fibrous ring (of mitral valve)

Conus arteriosus

Left fibrous trigone

Right coronary artery

Membranous septum
- Interventricular part (*broken line*)
- Atrio-ventricular part

Tricuspid valve
- Anterior cusp
- Septal cusp
- Posterior cusp

Right fibrous ring (of tricuspid valve)

Right fibrous trigone

Atrioventricular (AV) nodal branch†

Posterior interventricular branch†

**Heart in diastole:**
**viewed from base with atria removed**

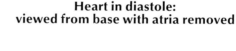
© Novartis

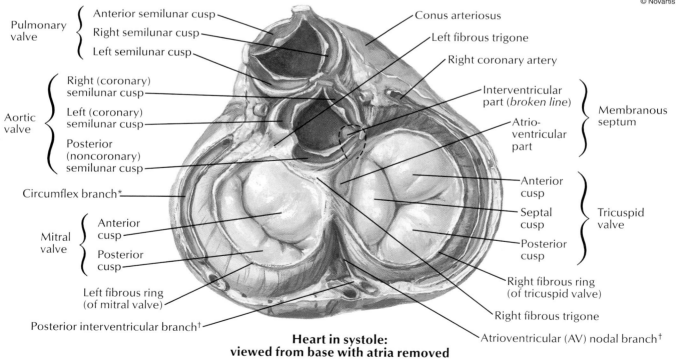

Pulmonary valve
- Anterior semilunar cusp
- Right semilunar cusp
- Left semilunar cusp

Aortic valve
- Right (coronary) semilunar cusp
- Left (coronary) semilunar cusp
- Posterior (noncoronary) semilunar cusp

Circumflex branch*

Mitral valve
- Anterior cusp
- Posterior cusp

Left fibrous ring (of mitral valve)

Posterior interventricular branch†

Conus arteriosus

Left fibrous trigone

Right coronary artery

Membranous septum
- Interventricular part (*broken line*)
- Atrio-ventricular part

Tricuspid valve
- Anterior cusp
- Septal cusp
- Posterior cusp

Right fibrous ring (of tricuspid valve)

Right fibrous trigone

Atrioventricular (AV) nodal branch†

**Heart in systole:**
**viewed from base with atria removed**

*Of left coronary artery
†Of right coronary artery

*PLATE 210*

**THORAX**

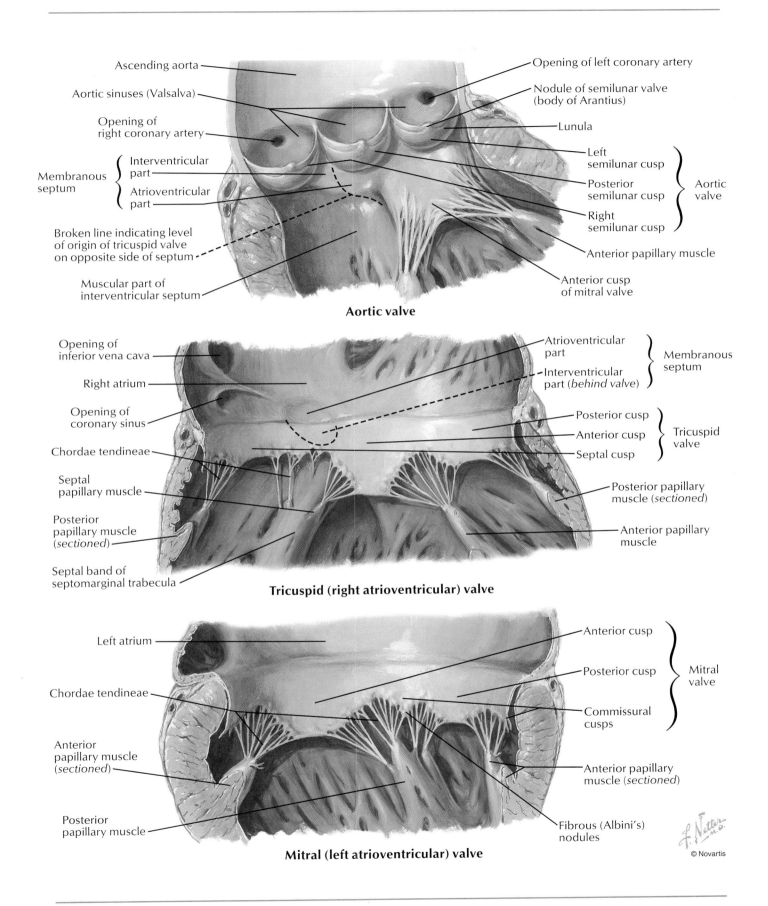

Ascending aorta

Aortic sinuses (Valsalva)

Opening of right coronary artery

Membranous septum { Interventricular part — Atrioventricular part

Broken line indicating level of origin of tricuspid valve on opposite side of septum

Muscular part of interventricular septum

Opening of left coronary artery

Nodule of semilunar valve (body of Arantius)

Lunula

Left semilunar cusp

Posterior semilunar cusp } Aortic valve

Right semilunar cusp

Anterior papillary muscle

Anterior cusp of mitral valve

**Aortic valve**

Opening of inferior vena cava

Right atrium

Opening of coronary sinus

Chordae tendineae

Septal papillary muscle

Posterior papillary muscle (sectioned)

Septal band of septomarginal trabecula

Atrioventricular part

Interventricular part (behind valve) } Membranous septum

Posterior cusp

Anterior cusp } Tricuspid valve

Septal cusp

Posterior papillary muscle (sectioned)

Anterior papillary muscle

**Tricuspid (right atrioventricular) valve**

Left atrium

Chordae tendineae

Anterior papillary muscle (sectioned)

Posterior papillary muscle

Anterior cusp

Posterior cusp } Mitral valve

Commissural cusps

Anterior papillary muscle (sectioned)

Fibrous (Albini's) nodules

**Mitral (left atrioventricular) valve**

© Novartis

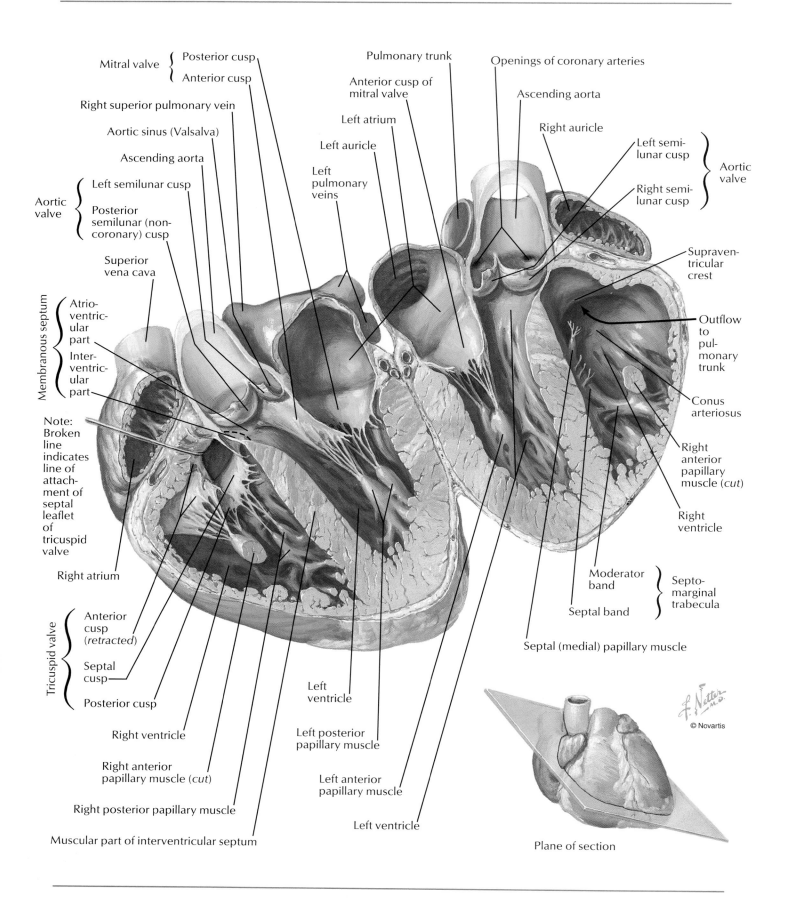

Mitral valve { Posterior cusp
Anterior cusp

Right superior pulmonary vein

Aortic sinus (Valsalva)

Ascending aorta

Aortic valve { Left semilunar cusp
Posterior semilunar (non-coronary) cusp

Superior vena cava

Membranous septum { Atrio-ventricular part
Inter-ventricular part

Note: Broken line indicates line of attachment of septal leaflet of tricuspid valve

Right atrium

Tricuspid valve { Anterior cusp (retracted)
Septal cusp
Posterior cusp

Right ventricle

Right anterior papillary muscle (cut)

Right posterior papillary muscle

Muscular part of interventricular septum

Pulmonary trunk

Anterior cusp of mitral valve

Left atrium

Left auricle

Left pulmonary veins

Openings of coronary arteries

Ascending aorta

Right auricle

Aortic valve { Left semi-lunar cusp
Right semi-lunar cusp

Supraventricular crest

Outflow to pulmonary trunk

Conus arteriosus

Right anterior papillary muscle (cut)

Right ventricle

Moderator band
Septal band } Septo-marginal trabecula

Septal (medial) papillary muscle

Left ventricle

Left posterior papillary muscle

Left anterior papillary muscle

Left ventricle

Plane of section

**PLATE 212**

**THORAX**

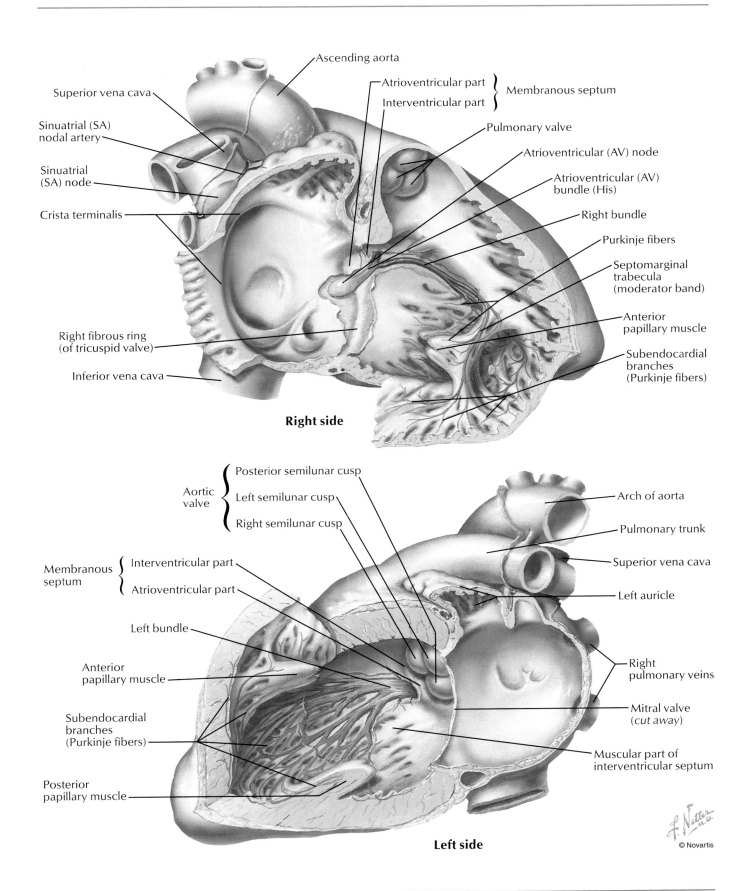

Ascending aorta

Atrioventricular part
Interventricular part } Membranous septum

Superior vena cava

Sinuatrial (SA) nodal artery

Pulmonary valve

Atrioventricular (AV) node

Sinuatrial (SA) node

Atrioventricular (AV) bundle (His)

Crista terminalis

Right bundle

Purkinje fibers

Septomarginal trabecula (moderator band)

Right fibrous ring (of tricuspid valve)

Anterior papillary muscle

Inferior vena cava

Subendocardial branches (Purkinje fibers)

**Right side**

Posterior semilunar cusp

Aortic valve {
Left semilunar cusp

Right semilunar cusp

Arch of aorta

Pulmonary trunk

Superior vena cava

Membranous septum {
Interventricular part

Atrioventricular part

Left auricle

Left bundle

Anterior papillary muscle

Right pulmonary veins

Subendocardial branches (Purkinje fibers)

Mitral valve (*cut away*)

Muscular part of interventricular septum

Posterior papillary muscle

**Left side**

© Novartis

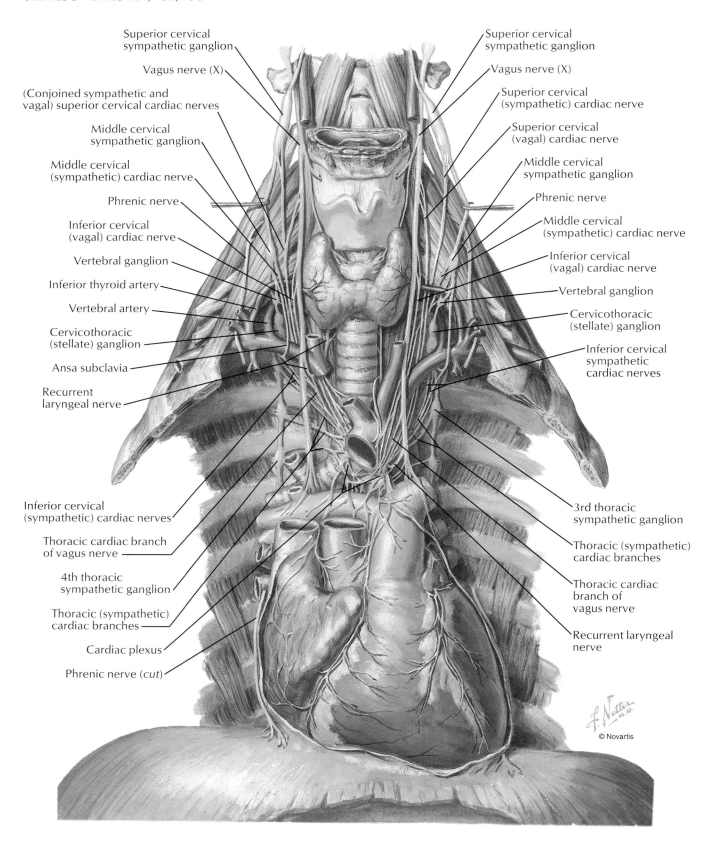

Superior cervical sympathetic ganglion

Vagus nerve (X)

(Conjoined sympathetic and vagal) superior cervical cardiac nerves

Middle cervical sympathetic ganglion

Middle cervical (sympathetic) cardiac nerve

Phrenic nerve

Inferior cervical (vagal) cardiac nerve

Vertebral ganglion

Inferior thyroid artery

Vertebral artery

Cervicothoracic (stellate) ganglion

Ansa subclavia

Recurrent laryngeal nerve

Inferior cervical (sympathetic) cardiac nerves

Thoracic cardiac branch of vagus nerve

4th thoracic sympathetic ganglion

Thoracic (sympathetic) cardiac branches

Cardiac plexus

Phrenic nerve (*cut*)

Superior cervical sympathetic ganglion

Vagus nerve (X)

Superior cervical (sympathetic) cardiac nerve

Superior cervical (vagal) cardiac nerve

Middle cervical sympathetic ganglion

Phrenic nerve

Middle cervical (sympathetic) cardiac nerve

Inferior cervical (vagal) cardiac nerve

Vertebral ganglion

Cervicothoracic (stellate) ganglion

Inferior cervical sympathetic cardiac nerves

3rd thoracic sympathetic ganglion

Thoracic (sympathetic) cardiac branches

Thoracic cardiac branch of vagus nerve

Recurrent laryngeal nerve

© Novartis

**PLATE 214**

**THORAX**

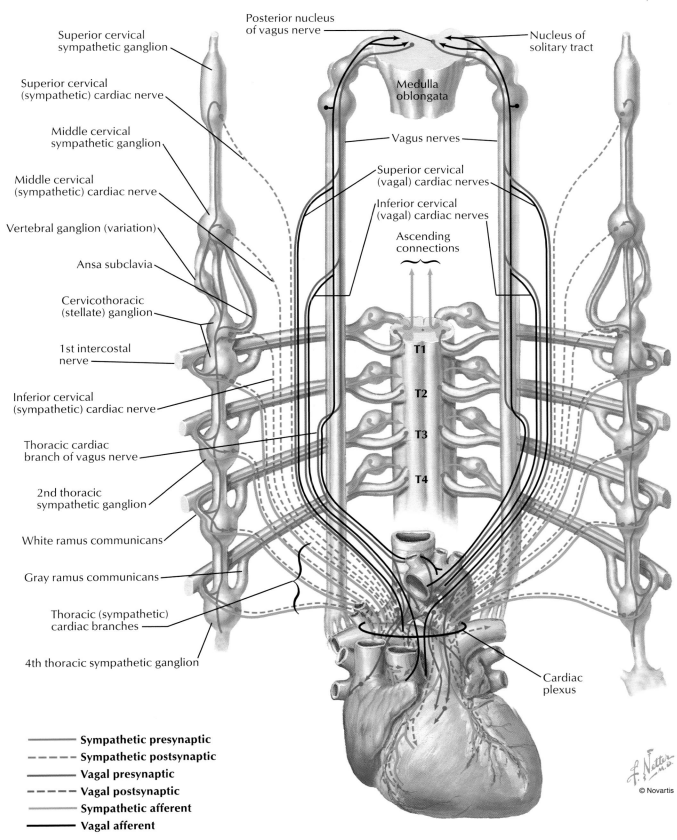

Posterior nucleus of vagus nerve

Nucleus of solitary tract

Medulla oblongata

Vagus nerves

Superior cervical (vagal) cardiac nerves

Inferior cervical (vagal) cardiac nerves

Ascending connections

Superior cervical sympathetic ganglion

Superior cervical (sympathetic) cardiac nerve

Middle cervical sympathetic ganglion

Middle cervical (sympathetic) cardiac nerve

Vertebral ganglion (variation)

Ansa subclavia

Cervicothoracic (stellate) ganglion

1st intercostal nerve

Inferior cervical (sympathetic) cardiac nerve

Thoracic cardiac branch of vagus nerve

2nd thoracic sympathetic ganglion

White ramus communicans

Gray ramus communicans

Thoracic (sympathetic) cardiac branches

4th thoracic sympathetic ganglion

T1

T2

T3

T4

Cardiac plexus

- Sympathetic presynaptic
- Sympathetic postsynaptic
- Vagal presynaptic
- Vagal postsynaptic
- Sympathetic afferent
- Vagal afferent

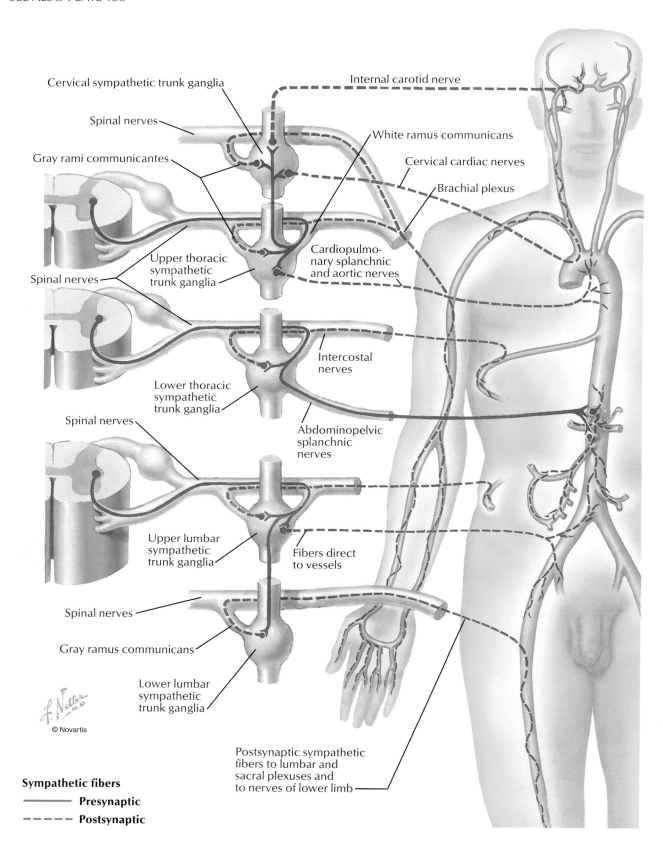

Cervical sympathetic trunk ganglia

Internal carotid nerve

Spinal nerves

White ramus communicans

Gray rami communicantes

Cervical cardiac nerves

Brachial plexus

Upper thoracic sympathetic trunk ganglia

Spinal nerves

Cardiopulmonary splanchnic and aortic nerves

Intercostal nerves

Lower thoracic sympathetic trunk ganglia

Spinal nerves

Abdominopelvic splanchnic nerves

Upper lumbar sympathetic trunk ganglia

Fibers direct to vessels

Spinal nerves

Gray ramus communicans

Lower lumbar sympathetic trunk ganglia

Postsynaptic sympathetic fibers to lumbar and sacral plexuses and to nerves of lower limb

**Sympathetic fibers**

——— **Presynaptic**

– – – – **Postsynaptic**

© Novartis

**PLATE 216**

**THORAX**

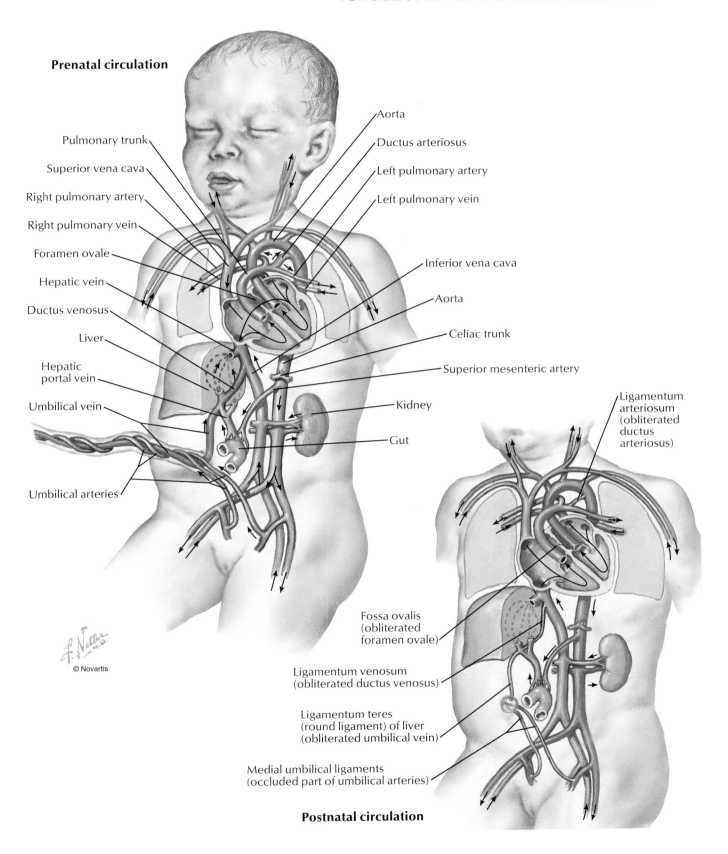

**Prenatal circulation**

Pulmonary trunk

Superior vena cava

Right pulmonary artery

Right pulmonary vein

Foramen ovale

Hepatic vein

Ductus venosus

Liver

Hepatic portal vein

Umbilical vein

Umbilical arteries

Aorta

Ductus arteriosus

Left pulmonary artery

Left pulmonary vein

Inferior vena cava

Aorta

Celiac trunk

Superior mesenteric artery

Kidney

Gut

Ligamentum arteriosum (obliterated ductus arteriosus)

Fossa ovalis (obliterated foramen ovale)

Ligamentum venosum (obliterated ductus venosus)

Ligamentum teres (round ligament) of liver (obliterated umbilical vein)

Medial umbilical ligaments (occluded part of umbilical arteries)

**Postnatal circulation**

© Novartis

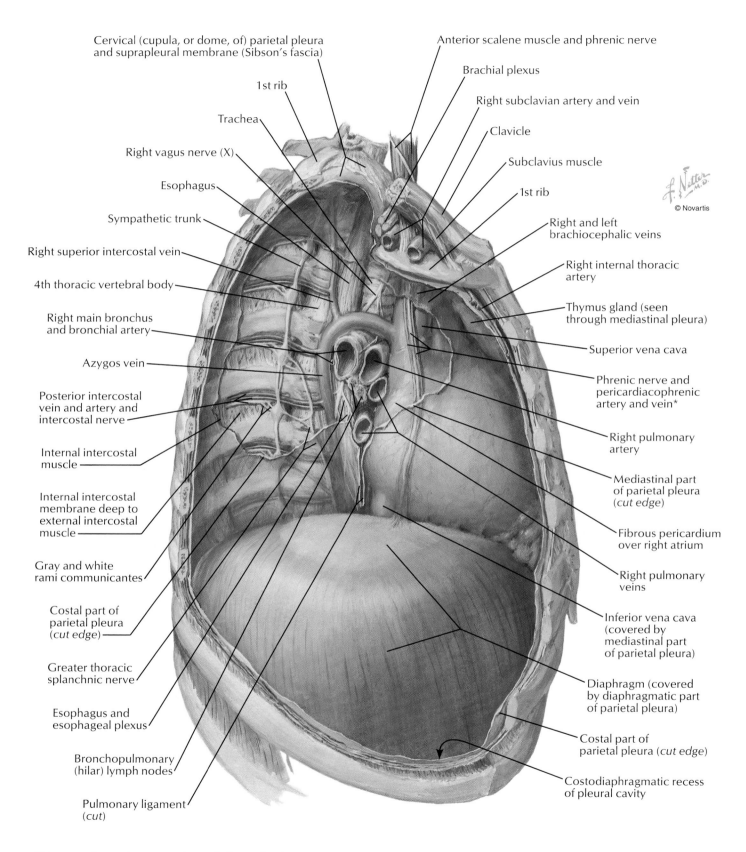

Cervical (cupula, or dome, of) parietal pleura and suprapleural membrane (Sibson's fascia)

1st rib

Trachea

Right vagus nerve (X)

Esophagus

Sympathetic trunk

Right superior intercostal vein

4th thoracic vertebral body

Right main bronchus and bronchial artery

Azygos vein

Posterior intercostal vein and artery and intercostal nerve

Internal intercostal muscle

Internal intercostal membrane deep to external intercostal muscle

Gray and white rami communicantes

Costal part of parietal pleura (*cut edge*)

Greater thoracic splanchnic nerve

Esophagus and esophageal plexus

Bronchopulmonary (hilar) lymph nodes

Pulmonary ligament (*cut*)

Anterior scalene muscle and phrenic nerve

Brachial plexus

Right subclavian artery and vein

Clavicle

Subclavius muscle

1st rib

Right and left brachiocephalic veins

Right internal thoracic artery

Thymus gland (seen through mediastinal pleura)

Superior vena cava

Phrenic nerve and pericardiacophrenic artery and vein*

Right pulmonary artery

Mediastinal part of parietal pleura (*cut edge*)

Fibrous pericardium over right atrium

Right pulmonary veins

Inferior vena cava (covered by mediastinal part of parietal pleura)

Diaphragm (covered by diaphragmatic part of parietal pleura)

Costal part of parietal pleura (*cut edge*)

Costodiaphragmatic recess of pleural cavity

*Nerve and vessels commonly run independently

**PLATE 218**

**THORAX**

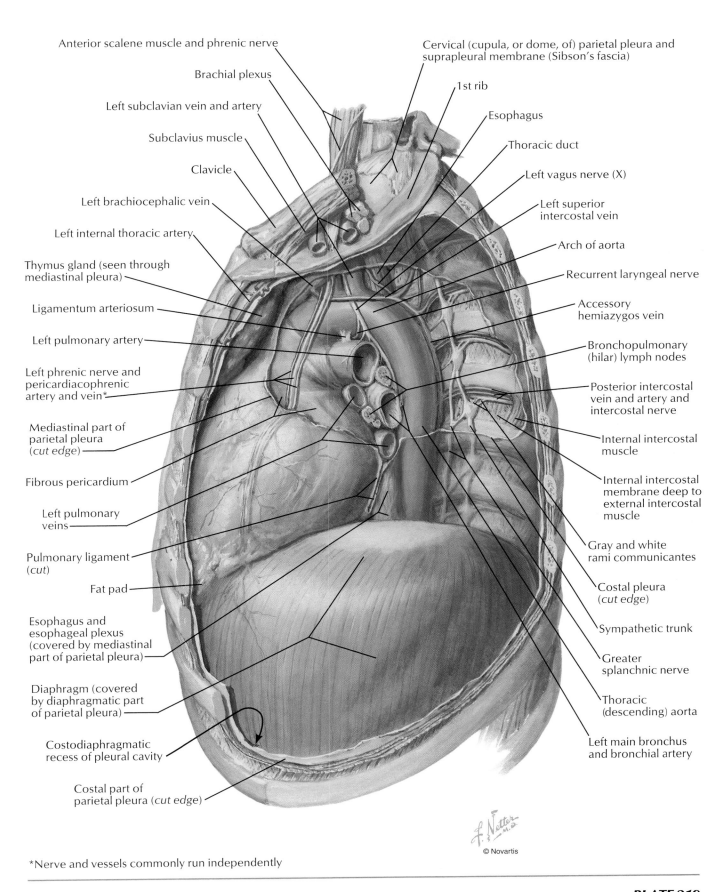

Anterior scalene muscle and phrenic nerve

Brachial plexus

Left subclavian vein and artery

Subclavius muscle

Clavicle

Left brachiocephalic vein

Left internal thoracic artery

Thymus gland (seen through mediastinal pleura)

Ligamentum arteriosum

Left pulmonary artery

Left phrenic nerve and pericardiacophrenic artery and vein*

Mediastinal part of parietal pleura (*cut edge*)

Fibrous pericardium

Left pulmonary veins

Pulmonary ligament (*cut*)

Fat pad

Esophagus and esophageal plexus (covered by mediastinal part of parietal pleura)

Diaphragm (covered by diaphragmatic part of parietal pleura)

Costodiaphragmatic recess of pleural cavity

Costal part of parietal pleura (*cut edge*)

Cervical (cupula, or dome, of) parietal pleura and suprapleural membrane (Sibson's fascia)

1st rib

Esophagus

Thoracic duct

Left vagus nerve (X)

Left superior intercostal vein

Arch of aorta

Recurrent laryngeal nerve

Accessory hemiazygos vein

Bronchopulmonary (hilar) lymph nodes

Posterior intercostal vein and artery and intercostal nerve

Internal intercostal muscle

Internal intercostal membrane deep to external intercostal muscle

Gray and white rami communicantes

Costal pleura (*cut edge*)

Sympathetic trunk

Greater splanchnic nerve

Thoracic (descending) aorta

Left main bronchus and bronchial artery

*Nerve and vessels commonly run independently

© Novartis

# Esophagus In Situ

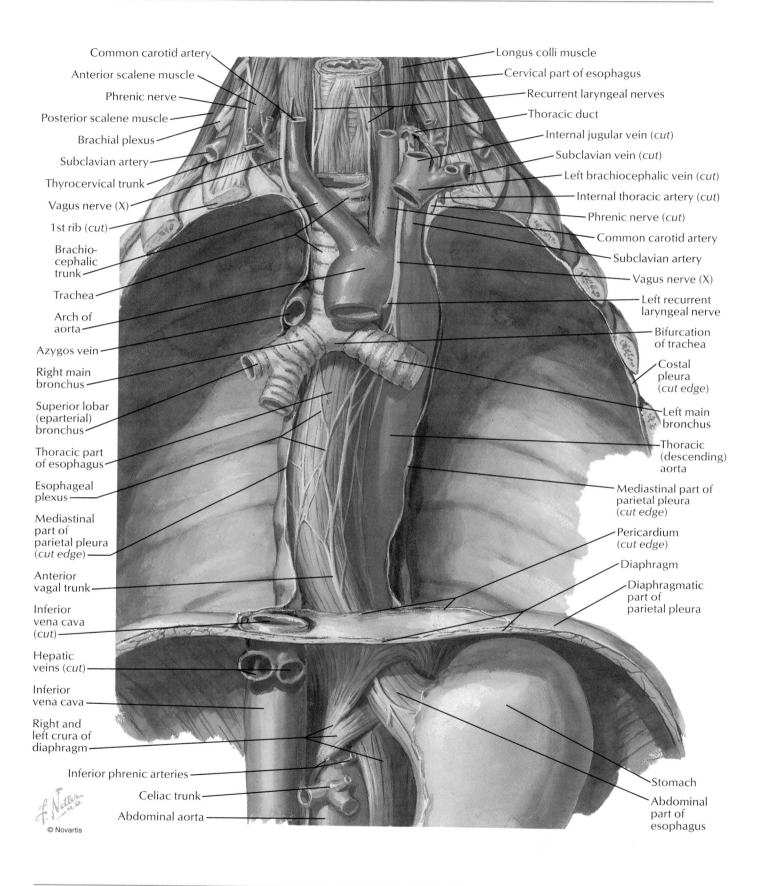

Common carotid artery

Anterior scalene muscle

Phrenic nerve

Posterior scalene muscle

Brachial plexus

Subclavian artery

Thyrocervical trunk

Vagus nerve (X)

1st rib (cut)

Brachio-cephalic trunk

Trachea

Arch of aorta

Azygos vein

Right main bronchus

Superior lobar (eparterial) bronchus

Thoracic part of esophagus

Esophageal plexus

Mediastinal part of parietal pleura (cut edge)

Anterior vagal trunk

Inferior vena cava (cut)

Hepatic veins (cut)

Inferior vena cava

Right and left crura of diaphragm

Inferior phrenic arteries

Celiac trunk

Abdominal aorta

Longus colli muscle

Cervical part of esophagus

Recurrent laryngeal nerves

Thoracic duct

Internal jugular vein (cut)

Subclavian vein (cut)

Left brachiocephalic vein (cut)

Internal thoracic artery (cut)

Phrenic nerve (cut)

Common carotid artery

Subclavian artery

Vagus nerve (X)

Left recurrent laryngeal nerve

Bifurcation of trachea

Costal pleura (cut edge)

Left main bronchus

Thoracic (descending) aorta

Mediastinal part of parietal pleura (cut edge)

Pericardium (cut edge)

Diaphragm

Diaphragmatic part of parietal pleura

Stomach

Abdominal part of esophagus

**PLATE 220**

**THORAX**

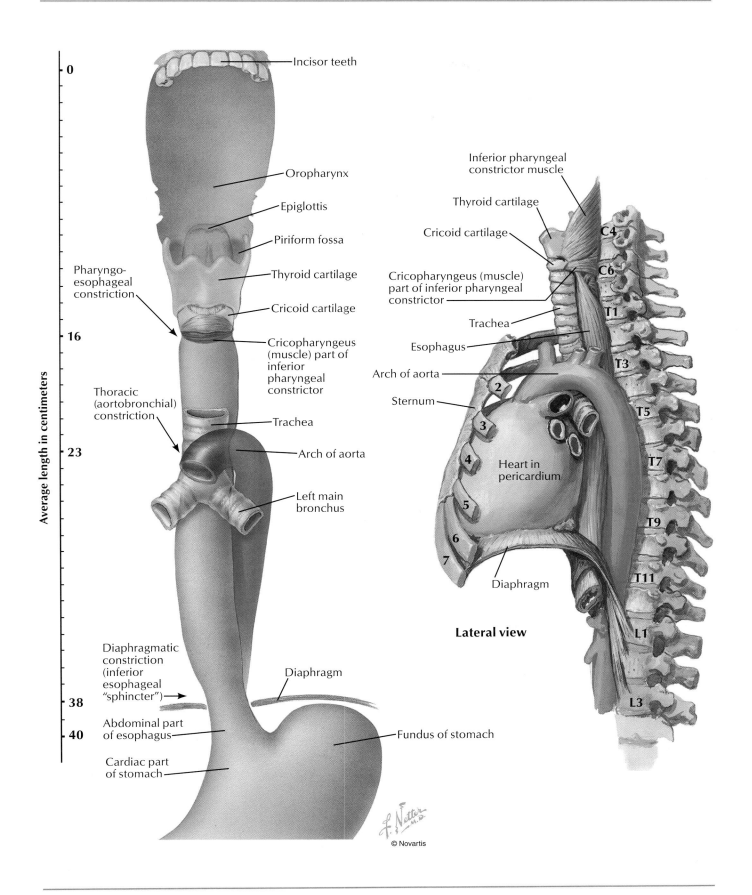

Incisor teeth

Oropharynx

Epiglottis

Piriform fossa

Thyroid cartilage

Cricoid cartilage

Pharyngo-esophageal constriction

Cricopharyngeus (muscle) part of inferior pharyngeal constrictor

Thoracic (aortobronchial) constriction

Trachea

Arch of aorta

Left main bronchus

Diaphragmatic constriction (inferior esophageal "sphincter")

Diaphragm

Abdominal part of esophagus

Fundus of stomach

Cardiac part of stomach

Average length in centimeters

0

16

23

38

40

Inferior pharyngeal constrictor muscle

Thyroid cartilage

Cricoid cartilage

Cricopharyngeus (muscle) part of inferior pharyngeal constrictor

Trachea

Esophagus

Arch of aorta

Sternum

Heart in pericardium

Diaphragm

**Lateral view**

C4

C6

T1

T3

T5

T7

T9

T11

L1

L3

2

3

4

5

6

7

*f. Netter*
M.D.

© Novartis

# Musculature of Esophagus

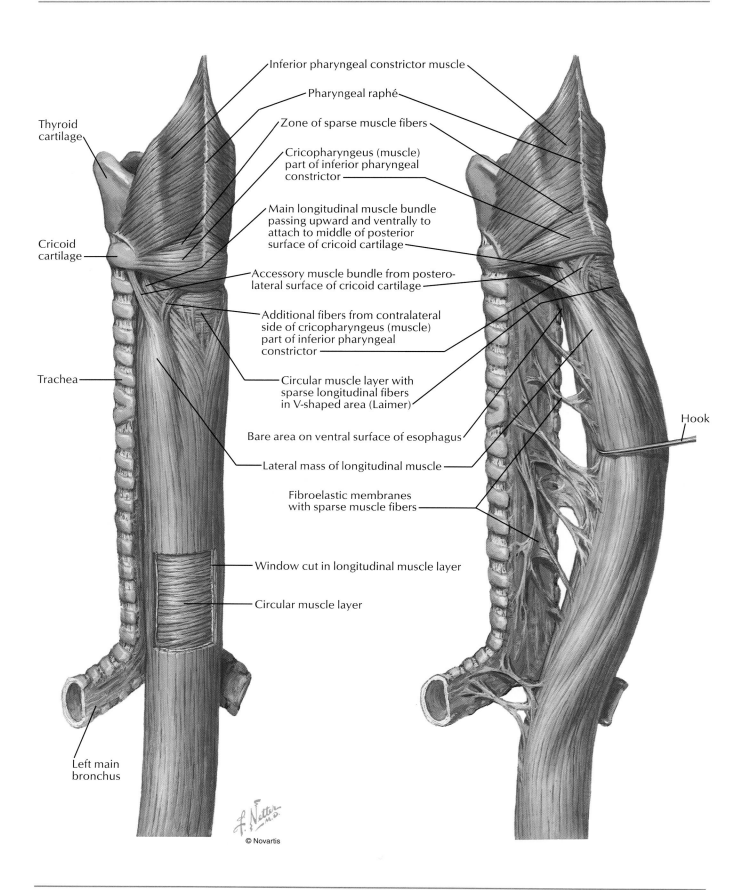

Inferior pharyngeal constrictor muscle

Pharyngeal raphé

Zone of sparse muscle fibers

Thyroid cartilage

Cricopharyngeus (muscle) part of inferior pharyngeal constrictor

Main longitudinal muscle bundle passing upward and ventrally to attach to middle of posterior surface of cricoid cartilage

Cricoid cartilage

Accessory muscle bundle from posterolateral surface of cricoid cartilage

Additional fibers from contralateral side of cricopharyngeus (muscle) part of inferior pharyngeal constrictor

Trachea

Circular muscle layer with sparse longitudinal fibers in V-shaped area (Laimer)

Bare area on ventral surface of esophagus

Lateral mass of longitudinal muscle

Fibroelastic membranes with sparse muscle fibers

Hook

Window cut in longitudinal muscle layer

Circular muscle layer

Left main bronchus

© Novartis

PLATE 222

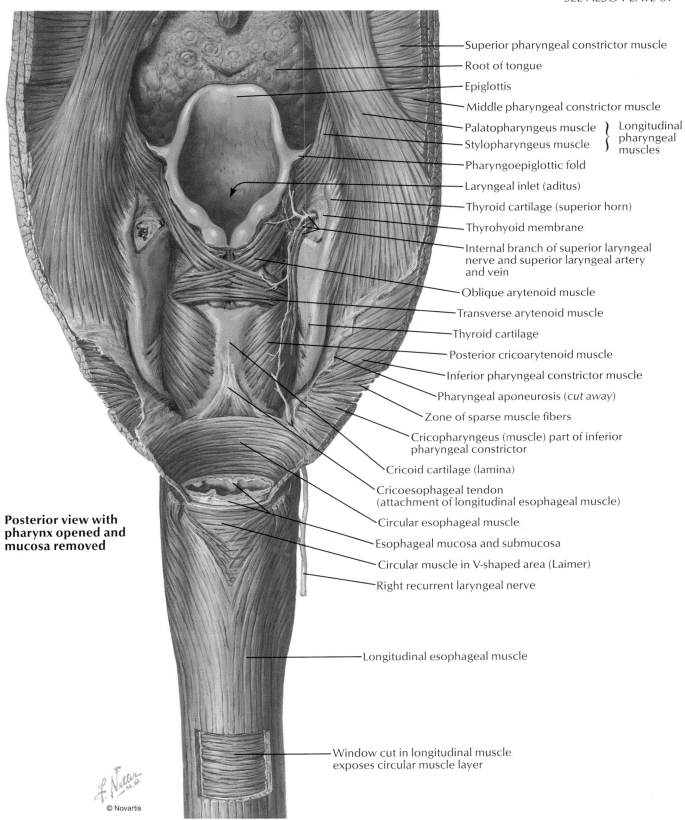

Superior pharyngeal constrictor muscle

Root of tongue

Epiglottis

Middle pharyngeal constrictor muscle

Palatopharyngeus muscle ⎫ Longitudinal
Stylopharyngeus muscle ⎬ pharyngeal
                        ⎭ muscles

Pharyngoepiglottic fold

Laryngeal inlet (aditus)

Thyroid cartilage (superior horn)

Thyrohyoid membrane

Internal branch of superior laryngeal nerve and superior laryngeal artery and vein

Oblique arytenoid muscle

Transverse arytenoid muscle

Thyroid cartilage

Posterior cricoarytenoid muscle

Inferior pharyngeal constrictor muscle

Pharyngeal aponeurosis (*cut away*)

Zone of sparse muscle fibers

Cricopharyngeus (muscle) part of inferior pharyngeal constrictor

Cricoid cartilage (lamina)

Cricoesophageal tendon (attachment of longitudinal esophageal muscle)

Circular esophageal muscle

Esophageal mucosa and submucosa

Circular muscle in V-shaped area (Laimer)

Right recurrent laryngeal nerve

Longitudinal esophageal muscle

Window cut in longitudinal muscle exposes circular muscle layer

**Posterior view with pharynx opened and mucosa removed**

© Novartis

# Esophagogastric Junction

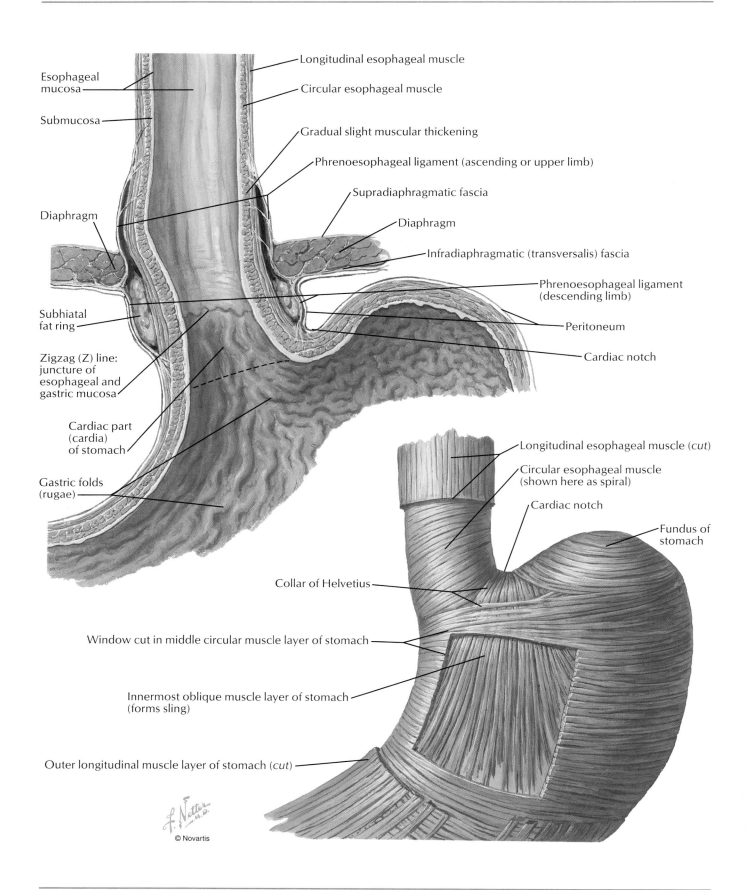

Esophageal mucosa

Submucosa

Diaphragm

Subhiatal fat ring

Zigzag (Z) line: juncture of esophageal and gastric mucosa

Cardiac part (cardia) of stomach

Gastric folds (rugae)

Longitudinal esophageal muscle

Circular esophageal muscle

Gradual slight muscular thickening

Phrenoesophageal ligament (ascending or upper limb)

Supradiaphragmatic fascia

Diaphragm

Infradiaphragmatic (transversalis) fascia

Phrenoesophageal ligament (descending limb)

Peritoneum

Cardiac notch

Longitudinal esophageal muscle (cut)

Circular esophageal muscle (shown here as spiral)

Cardiac notch

Fundus of stomach

Collar of Helvetius

Window cut in middle circular muscle layer of stomach

Innermost oblique muscle layer of stomach (forms sling)

Outer longitudinal muscle layer of stomach (cut)

f. Netter
M.D.

© Novartis

**PLATE 224**

**THORAX**

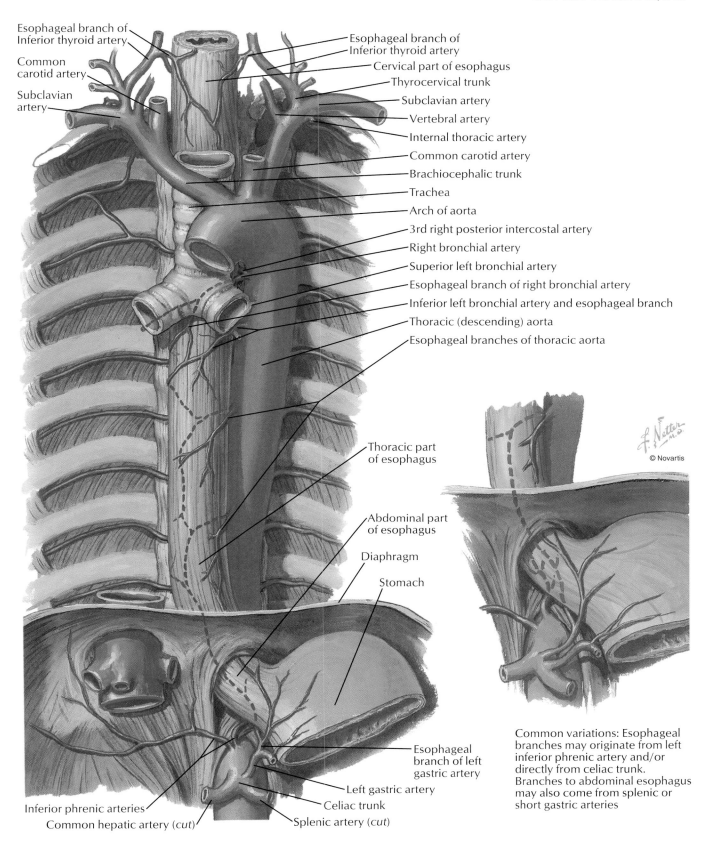

Esophageal branch of Inferior thyroid artery

Common carotid artery

Subclavian artery

Esophageal branch of Inferior thyroid artery

Cervical part of esophagus

Thyrocervical trunk

Subclavian artery

Vertebral artery

Internal thoracic artery

Common carotid artery

Brachiocephalic trunk

Trachea

Arch of aorta

3rd right posterior intercostal artery

Right bronchial artery

Superior left bronchial artery

Esophageal branch of right bronchial artery

Inferior left bronchial artery and esophageal branch

Thoracic (descending) aorta

Esophageal branches of thoracic aorta

Thoracic part of esophagus

Abdominal part of esophagus

Diaphragm

Stomach

Esophageal branch of left gastric artery

Left gastric artery

Celiac trunk

Splenic artery (cut)

Inferior phrenic arteries

Common hepatic artery (cut)

Common variations: Esophageal branches may originate from left inferior phrenic artery and/or directly from celiac trunk. Branches to abdominal esophagus may also come from splenic or short gastric arteries

© Novartis

*SEE ALSO PLATE 297*

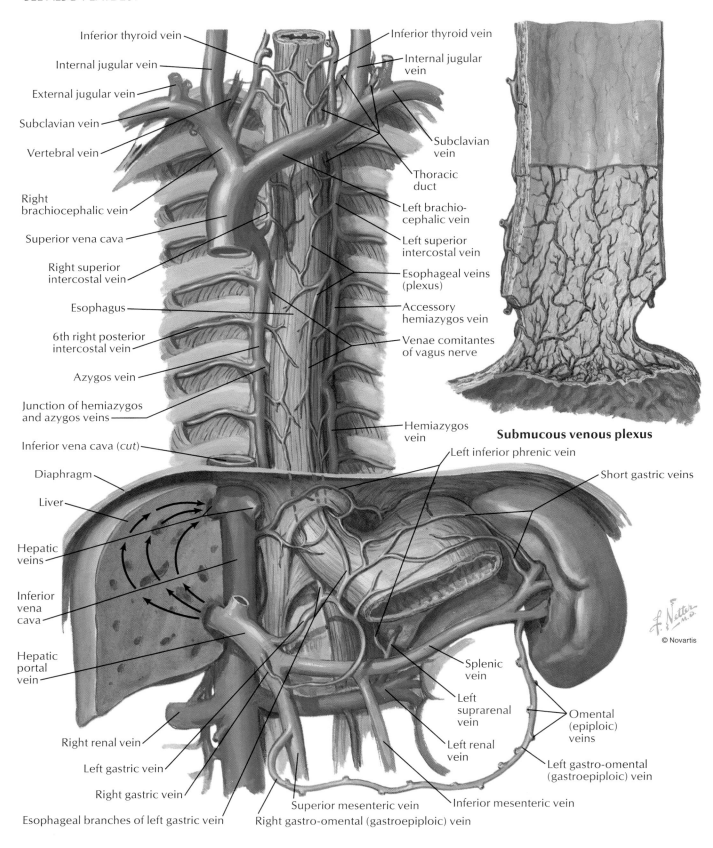

Inferior thyroid vein

Internal jugular vein

External jugular vein

Subclavian vein

Vertebral vein

Right brachiocephalic vein

Superior vena cava

Right superior intercostal vein

Esophagus

6th right posterior intercostal vein

Azygos vein

Junction of hemiazygos and azygos veins

Inferior vena cava (*cut*)

Diaphragm

Liver

Hepatic veins

Inferior vena cava

Hepatic portal vein

Right renal vein

Left gastric vein

Right gastric vein

Esophageal branches of left gastric vein

Inferior thyroid vein

Internal jugular vein

Subclavian vein

Thoracic duct

Left brachio-cephalic vein

Left superior intercostal vein

Esophageal veins (plexus)

Accessory hemiazygos vein

Venae comitantes of vagus nerve

Hemiazygos vein

**Submucous venous plexus**

Left inferior phrenic vein

Short gastric veins

Splenic vein

Left suprarenal vein

Left renal vein

Omental (epiploic) veins

Left gastro-omental (gastroepiploic) vein

Inferior mesenteric vein

Superior mesenteric vein

Right gastro-omental (gastroepiploic) vein

© Novartis

**PLATE 226**                                                                                         **THORAX**

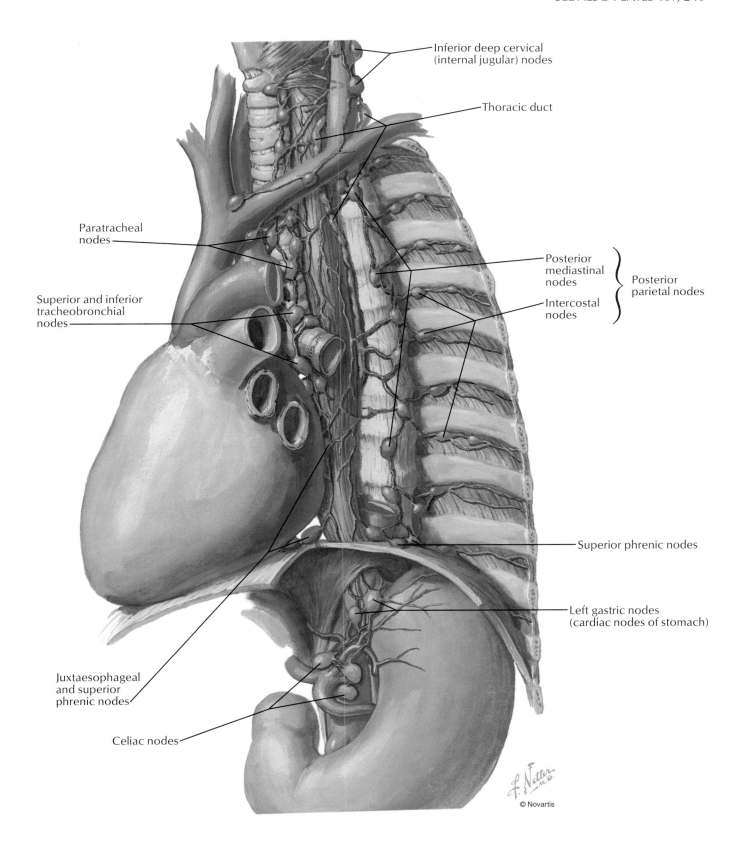

Inferior deep cervical (internal jugular) nodes

Thoracic duct

Paratracheal nodes

Posterior mediastinal nodes

Posterior parietal nodes

Intercostal nodes

Superior and inferior tracheobronchial nodes

Superior phrenic nodes

Left gastric nodes (cardiac nodes of stomach)

Juxtaesophageal and superior phrenic nodes

Celiac nodes

SEE ALSO PLATES 152, 198

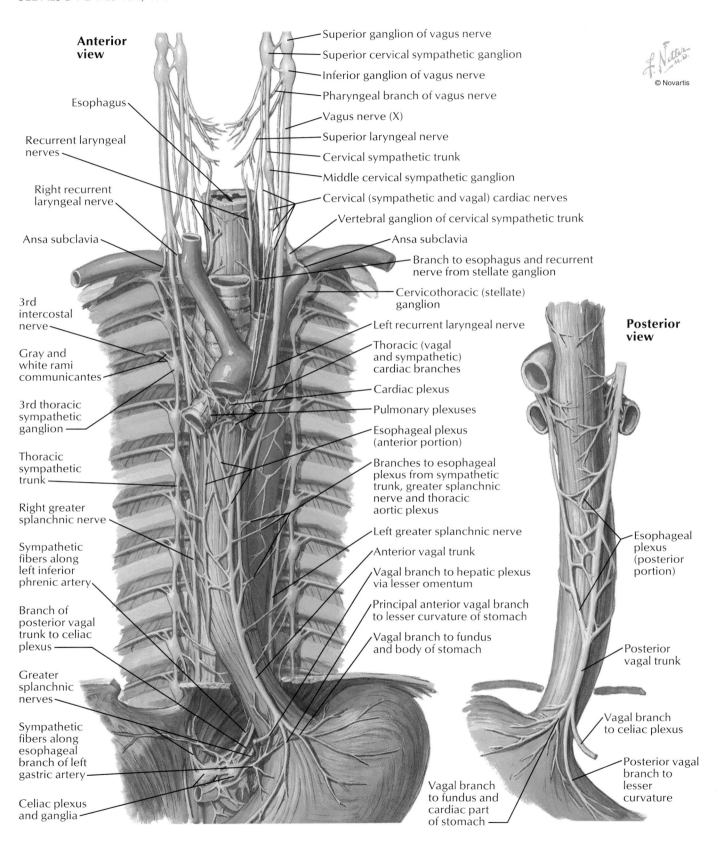

**Anterior view**

Superior ganglion of vagus nerve

Superior cervical sympathetic ganglion

Inferior ganglion of vagus nerve

Pharyngeal branch of vagus nerve

Vagus nerve (X)

Superior laryngeal nerve

Cervical sympathetic trunk

Middle cervical sympathetic ganglion

Cervical (sympathetic and vagal) cardiac nerves

Vertebral ganglion of cervical sympathetic trunk

Ansa subclavia

Branch to esophagus and recurrent nerve from stellate ganglion

Cervicothoracic (stellate) ganglion

Left recurrent laryngeal nerve

Thoracic (vagal and sympathetic) cardiac branches

Cardiac plexus

Pulmonary plexuses

Esophageal plexus (anterior portion)

Branches to esophageal plexus from sympathetic trunk, greater splanchnic nerve and thoracic aortic plexus

Left greater splanchnic nerve

Anterior vagal trunk

Vagal branch to hepatic plexus via lesser omentum

Principal anterior vagal branch to lesser curvature of stomach

Vagal branch to fundus and body of stomach

Esophagus

Recurrent laryngeal nerves

Right recurrent laryngeal nerve

Ansa subclavia

3rd intercostal nerve

Gray and white rami communicantes

3rd thoracic sympathetic ganglion

Thoracic sympathetic trunk

Right greater splanchnic nerve

Sympathetic fibers along left inferior phrenic artery

Branch of posterior vagal trunk to celiac plexus

Greater splanchnic nerves

Sympathetic fibers along esophageal branch of left gastric artery

Celiac plexus and ganglia

**Posterior view**

Esophageal plexus (posterior portion)

Posterior vagal trunk

Vagal branch to celiac plexus

Posterior vagal branch to lesser curvature

Vagal branch to fundus and cardiac part of stomach

**PLATE 228**                                                                 **THORAX**

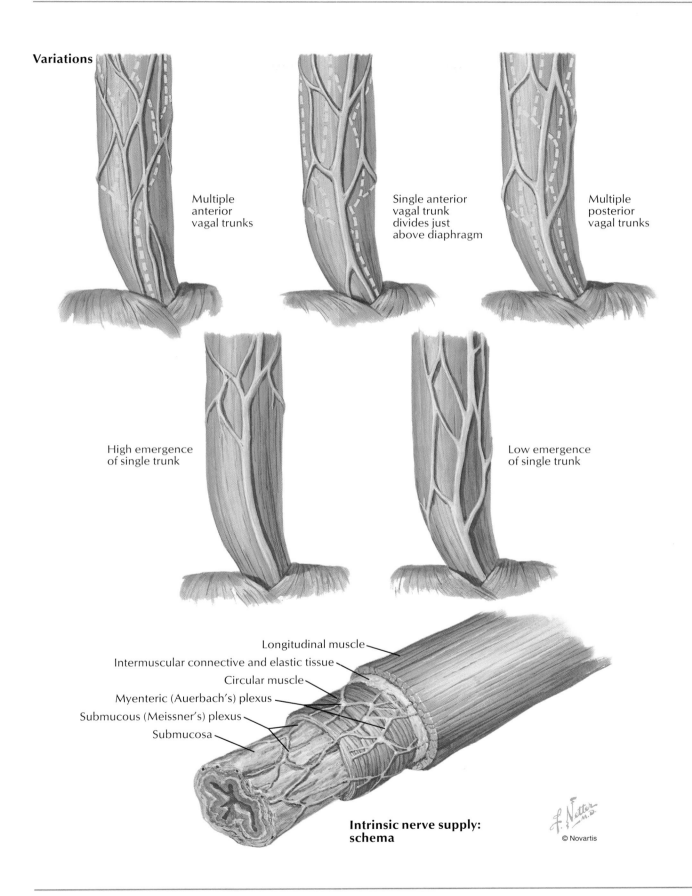

**Variations**

Multiple anterior vagal trunks

Single anterior vagal trunk divides just above diaphragm

Multiple posterior vagal trunks

High emergence of single trunk

Low emergence of single trunk

Longitudinal muscle

Intermuscular connective and elastic tissue

Circular muscle

Myenteric (Auerbach's) plexus

Submucous (Meissner's) plexus

Submucosa

**Intrinsic nerve supply: schema**

© Novartis

# *Mediastinum: Cross Section (Superior View)*

SEE ALSO PLATE 516

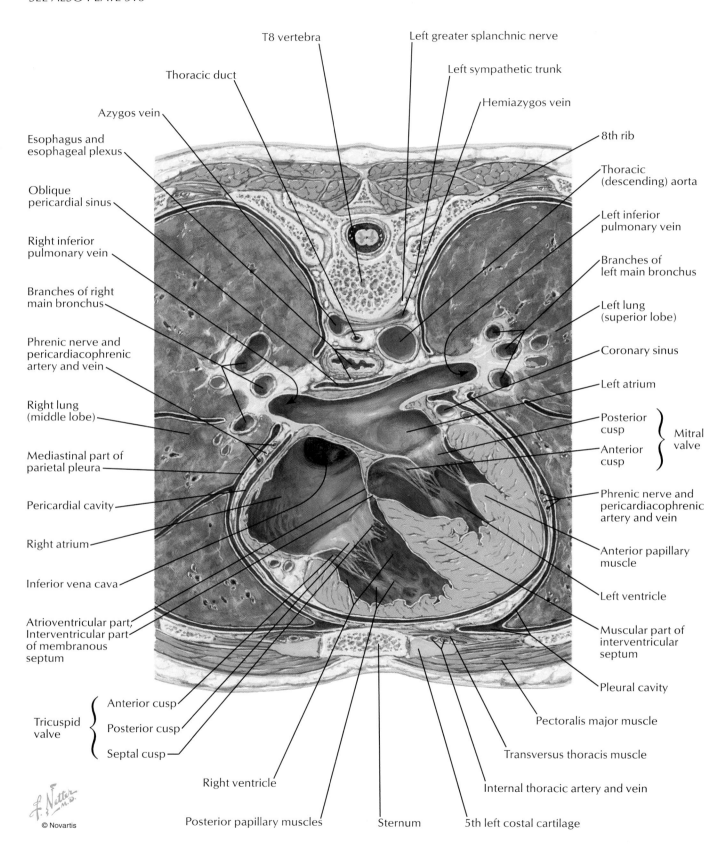

T8 vertebra

Thoracic duct

Azygos vein

Esophagus and esophageal plexus

Oblique pericardial sinus

Right inferior pulmonary vein

Branches of right main bronchus

Phrenic nerve and pericardiacophrenic artery and vein

Right lung (middle lobe)

Mediastinal part of parietal pleura

Pericardial cavity

Right atrium

Inferior vena cava

Atrioventricular part; Interventricular part of membranous septum

Tricuspid valve
{
Anterior cusp
Posterior cusp
Septal cusp
}

Right ventricle

Posterior papillary muscles

Left greater splanchnic nerve

Left sympathetic trunk

Hemiazygos vein

8th rib

Thoracic (descending) aorta

Left inferior pulmonary vein

Branches of left main bronchus

Left lung (superior lobe)

Coronary sinus

Left atrium

Posterior cusp
Anterior cusp
} Mitral valve

Phrenic nerve and pericardiacophrenic artery and vein

Anterior papillary muscle

Left ventricle

Muscular part of interventricular septum

Pleural cavity

Pectoralis major muscle

Transversus thoracis muscle

Internal thoracic artery and vein

Sternum

5th left costal cartilage

**PLATE 230**

**THORAX**

# Section IV
# ABDOMEN

**BODY WALL**
*Plates 231 – 250*

231. Bony Framework of Abdomen
232. Anterior Abdominal Wall:
    Superficial Dissection
233. Anterior Abdominal Wall:
    Intermediate Dissection
234. Anterior Abdominal Wall:
    Deep Dissection
235. Rectus Sheath: Cross Sections
236. Anterior Abdominal Wall:
    Internal View
237. Posterolateral Abdominal Wall
238. Arteries of Anterior Abdominal Wall
239. Veins of Anterior Abdominal Wall
240. Nerves of Anterior Abdominal Wall
241. Thoracoabdominal Nerves
242. Inguinal and Femoral Regions
243. Inguinal Region: Dissections

244. Femoral Sheath and Inguinal Canal
245. Inguinal Canal and Spermatic Cord
246. Posterior Abdominal Wall:
    Internal View
247. Arteries of Posterior Abdominal Wall
248. Veins of Posterior Abdominal Wall
249. Lymph Vessels and Nodes of
    Posterior Abdominal Wall
250. Nerves of Posterior Abdominal Wall

**PERITONEAL CAVITY**
*Plates 251 – 257*

251. Regions and Planes of Abdomen
252. Greater Omentum and
    Abdominal Viscera
253. Mesenteric Relations of Intestines
254. Mesenteric Relations of Intestines
    (*continued*)
255. Omental Bursa: Stomach Reflected

256. Omental Bursa: Cross Section
257. Peritoneum of Posterior
     Abdominal Wall

**VISCERA (GUT)**
*Plates 258 – 268*
258. Stomach In Situ
259. Mucosa of Stomach
260. Musculature of Stomach
261. Duodenum In Situ
262. Mucosa and Musculature
     of Duodenum
263. Mucosa and Musculature
     of Small Intestine
264. Ileocecal Region
265. Ileocecal Region (*continued*)
266. (Vermiform) Appendix
267. Mucosa and Musculature
     of Large Intestine
268. Sigmoid Colon: Variations in Position

**VISCERA (ACCESSORY ORGANS)**
*Plates 269 – 281*
269. Topography of Liver
270. Surfaces and Bed of Liver
271. Liver In Situ and Variations in Form
272. Liver Segments and Lobes: Vessel
     and Duct Distribution
273. Intrahepatic Vascular and Duct
     Systems
274. Liver Structure: Schema
275. Intrahepatic Biliary System: Schema
276. Gallbladder and Extrahepatic
     Bile Ducts
277. Variations in Cystic and
     Hepatic Ducts

278. Junction of (Common) Bile Duct
     and Duodenum
279. Pancreas In Situ
280. Variations in Pancreatic Ducts
281. Spleen

**VISCERAL VASCULATURE**
*Plates 282 – 299*
282. Arteries of Stomach, Liver and Spleen
283. Arteries of Stomach, Duodenum,
     Pancreas and Spleen
284. Arteries of Liver, Pancreas,
     Duodenum and Spleen
285. Arteries of Duodenum and Head
     of Pancreas
286. Arteries of Small Intestine
287. Arteries of Large Intestine
288. Arterial Variations and Collateral
     Supply of Liver and Gallbladder
289. Variations in Colic Arteries
290. Veins of Stomach, Duodenum,
     Pancreas and Spleen
291. Veins of Small Intestine
292. Veins of Large Intestine
293. Hepatic Portal Vein Tributaries:
     Portocaval Anastomoses
294. Variations and Anomalies of
     Hepatic Portal Vein
295. Lymph Vessels and Nodes of Stomach
296. Lymph Vessels and Nodes
     of Small Intestine
297. Lymph Vessels and Nodes
     of Large Intestine
298. Lymph Vessels and Nodes of Liver
299. Lymph Vessels and Nodes
     of Pancreas

**INNERVATION**
*Plates 300 – 310*

300. Autonomic Nerves and Ganglia of Abdomen
301. Nerves of Stomach and Duodenum
302. Nerves of Stomach and Duodenum (*continued*)
303. Innervation of Stomach and Duodenum: Schema
304. Nerves of Small Intestine
305. Nerves of Large Intestine
306. Innervation of Small and Large Intestines: Schema
307. Autonomic Reflex Pathways: Schema
308. Intrinsic Autonomic Plexuses of Intestine: Schema
309. Innervation of Liver and Biliary Tract: Schema
310. Innervation of Pancreas: Schema

**KIDNEYS AND SUPRARENAL GLANDS**
*Plates 311 – 329*

311. Kidneys In Situ: Anterior Views
312. Kidneys In Situ: Posterior Views
313. Gross Structure of Kidney
314. Renal Artery and Vein In Situ
315. Intrarenal Arteries and Renal Segments

316. Variations in Renal Artery and Vein
317. Nephron and Collecting Tubule: Schema
318. Blood Vessels in Parenchyma of Kidney: Schema
319. Ureters
320. Arteries of Ureters and Urinary Bladder
321. Lymph Vessels and Nodes of Kidneys and Urinary Bladder
312. Nerves of Kidneys, Ureters and Urinary Bladder
323. Innervation of Kidneys and Upper Ureters: Schema
324. Renal Fascia
325. Arteries and Veins of Suprarenal Glands In Situ
326. Nerves of Suprarenal Glands: Dissection and Schema
327. Schematic Cross Section of Abdomen at T12 (Superior View)
328. Schematic Cross Section of Abdomen at L2, 3 (Superior View)
329. Abdominal Wall and Viscera: Median (Sagittal) Section

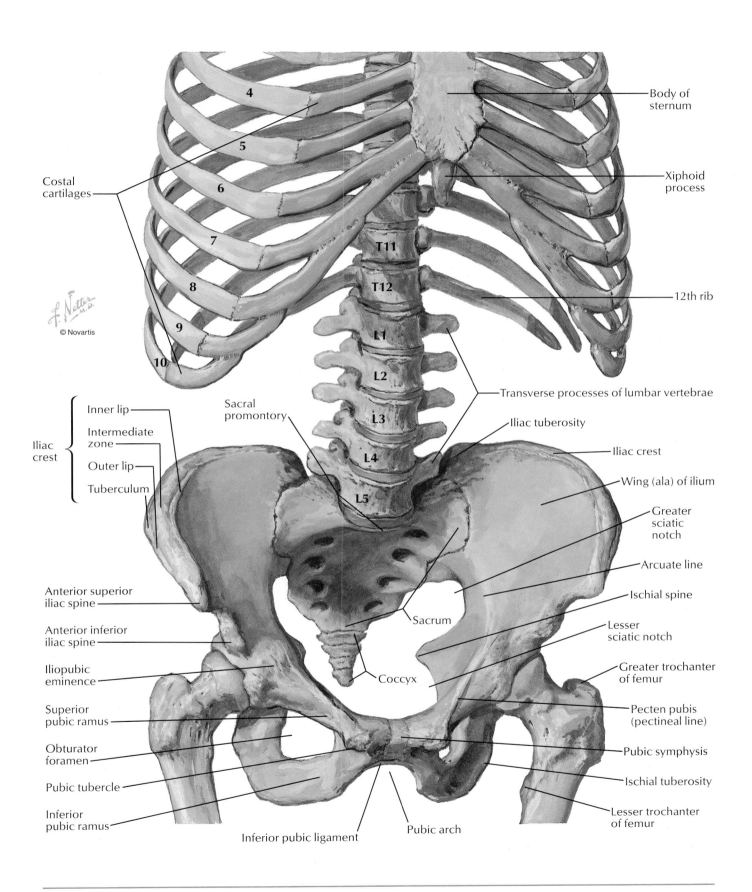

4

5

6

7

8

9

10

Costal
cartilages

f. Netter
M.D.

© Novartis

Body of
sternum

Xiphoid
process

T11

T12

12th rib

L1

L2

L3

L4

L5

Transverse processes of lumbar vertebrae

Sacral
promontory

Iliac tuberosity

Iliac crest

Wing (ala) of ilium

Greater
sciatic
notch

Arcuate line

Ischial spine

Lesser
sciatic
notch

Greater trochanter
of femur

Pecten pubis
(pectineal line)

Pubic symphysis

Ischial tuberosity

Lesser trochanter
of femur

Iliac
crest

Inner lip

Intermediate
zone

Outer lip

Tuberculum

Anterior superior
iliac spine

Anterior inferior
iliac spine

Iliopubic
eminence

Superior
pubic ramus

Obturator
foramen

Pubic tubercle

Inferior
pubic ramus

Sacrum

Coccyx

Inferior pubic ligament

Pubic arch

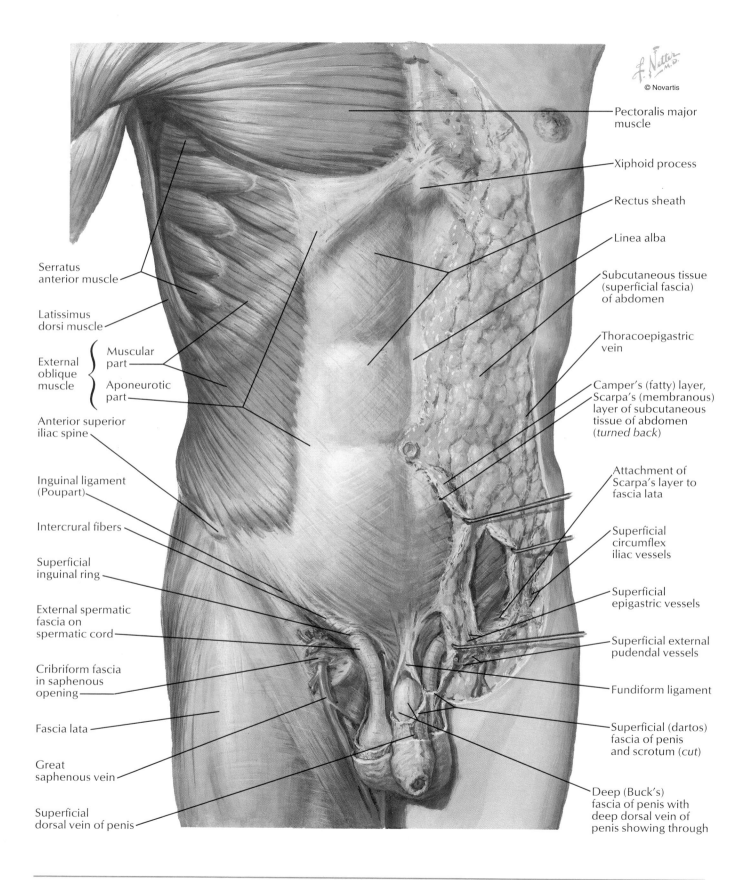

Pectoralis major muscle

Xiphoid process

Rectus sheath

Linea alba

Subcutaneous tissue (superficial fascia) of abdomen

Thoracoepigastric vein

Camper's (fatty) layer, Scarpa's (membranous) layer of subcutaneous tissue of abdomen (*turned back*)

Attachment of Scarpa's layer to fascia lata

Superficial circumflex iliac vessels

Superficial epigastric vessels

Superficial external pudendal vessels

Fundiform ligament

Superficial (dartos) fascia of penis and scrotum (*cut*)

Deep (Buck's) fascia of penis with deep dorsal vein of penis showing through

Serratus anterior muscle

Latissimus dorsi muscle

External oblique muscle
{ Muscular part
  Aponeurotic part

Anterior superior iliac spine

Inguinal ligament (Poupart)

Intercrural fibers

Superficial inguinal ring

External spermatic fascia on spermatic cord

Cribriform fascia in saphenous opening

Fascia lata

Great saphenous vein

Superficial dorsal vein of penis

*PLATE 232*

**ABDOMEN**

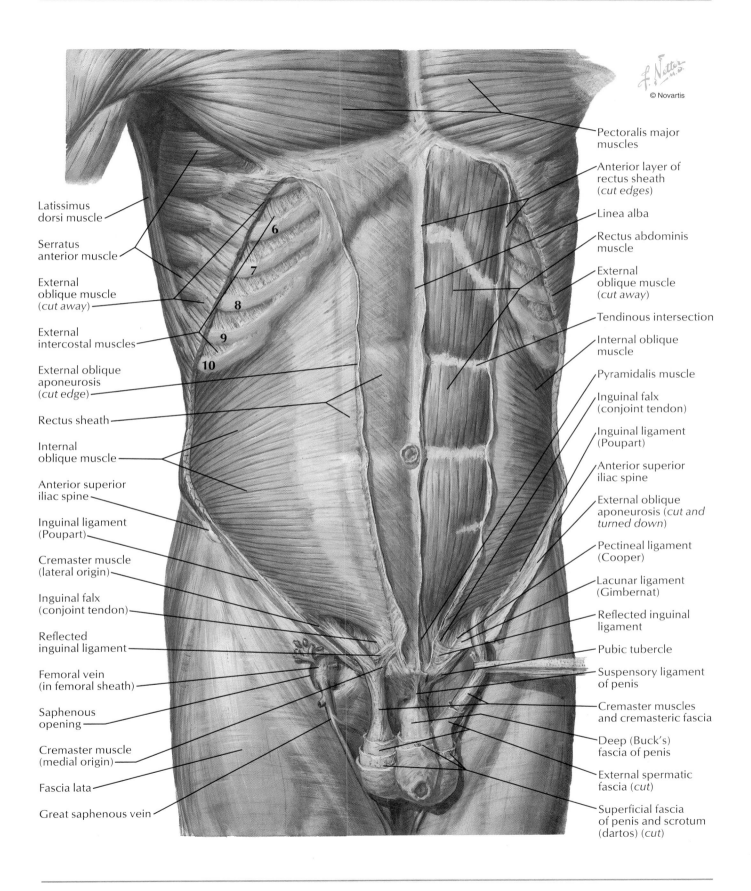

Latissimus
dorsi muscle

Serratus
anterior muscle

External
oblique muscle
(*cut away*)

External
intercostal muscles

External oblique
aponeurosis
(*cut edge*)

Rectus sheath

Internal
oblique muscle

Anterior superior
iliac spine

Inguinal ligament
(Poupart)

Cremaster muscle
(lateral origin)

Inguinal falx
(conjoint tendon)

Reflected
inguinal ligament

Femoral vein
(in femoral sheath)

Saphenous
opening

Cremaster muscle
(medial origin)

Fascia lata

Great saphenous vein

6
7
8
9
10

Pectoralis major
muscles

Anterior layer of
rectus sheath
(*cut edges*)

Linea alba

Rectus abdominis
muscle

External
oblique muscle
(*cut away*)

Tendinous intersection

Internal oblique
muscle

Pyramidalis muscle

Inguinal falx
(conjoint tendon)

Inguinal ligament
(Poupart)

Anterior superior
iliac spine

External oblique
aponeurosis (*cut and
turned down*)

Pectineal ligament
(Cooper)

Lacunar ligament
(Gimbernat)

Reflected inguinal
ligament

Pubic tubercle

Suspensory ligament
of penis

Cremaster muscles
and cremasteric fascia

Deep (Buck's)
fascia of penis

External spermatic
fascia (*cut*)

Superficial fascia
of penis and scrotum
(dartos) (*cut*)

*f. Netter*
© Novartis

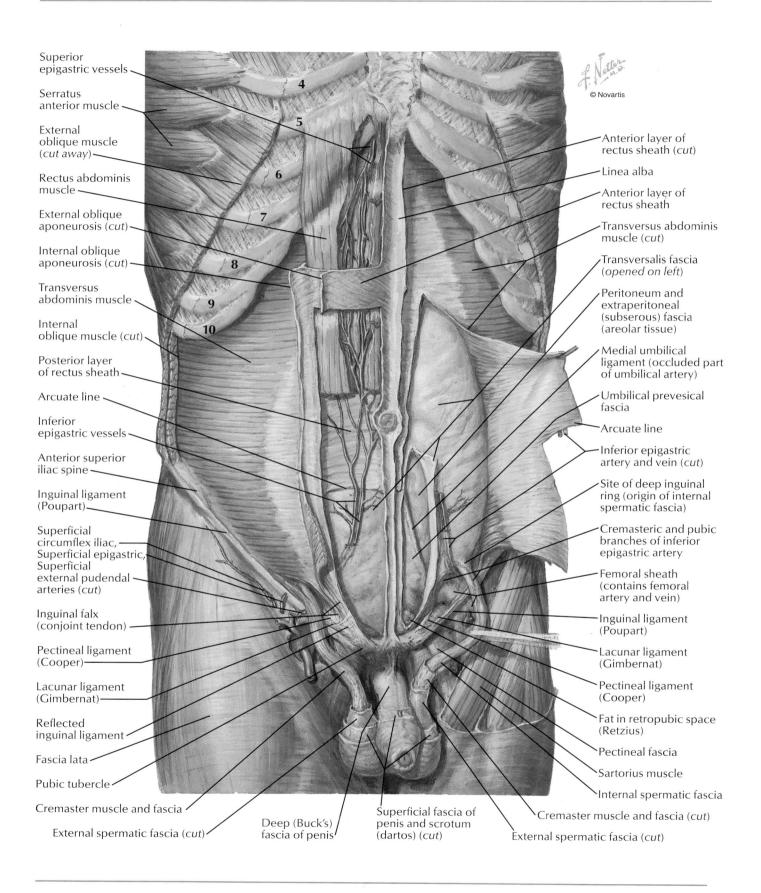

Superior epigastric vessels

Serratus anterior muscle

External oblique muscle (*cut away*)

Rectus abdominis muscle

External oblique aponeurosis (*cut*)

Internal oblique aponeurosis (*cut*)

Transversus abdominis muscle

Internal oblique muscle (*cut*)

Posterior layer of rectus sheath

Arcuate line

Inferior epigastric vessels

Anterior superior iliac spine

Inguinal ligament (Poupart)

Superficial circumflex iliac, Superficial epigastric, Superficial external pudendal arteries (*cut*)

Inguinal falx (conjoint tendon)

Pectineal ligament (Cooper)

Lacunar ligament (Gimbernat)

Reflected inguinal ligament

Fascia lata

Pubic tubercle

Cremaster muscle and fascia

External spermatic fascia (*cut*)

Deep (Buck's) fascia of penis

Superficial fascia of penis and scrotum (dartos) (*cut*)

Anterior layer of rectus sheath (*cut*)

Linea alba

Anterior layer of rectus sheath

Transversus abdominis muscle (*cut*)

Transversalis fascia (*opened on left*)

Peritoneum and extraperitoneal (subserous) fascia (areolar tissue)

Medial umbilical ligament (occluded part of umbilical artery)

Umbilical prevesical fascia

Arcuate line

Inferior epigastric artery and vein (*cut*)

Site of deep inguinal ring (origin of internal spermatic fascia)

Cremasteric and pubic branches of inferior epigastric artery

Femoral sheath (contains femoral artery and vein)

Inguinal ligament (Poupart)

Lacunar ligament (Gimbernat)

Pectineal ligament (Cooper)

Fat in retropubic space (Retzius)

Pectineal fascia

Sartorius muscle

Internal spermatic fascia

Cremaster muscle and fascia (*cut*)

External spermatic fascia (*cut*)

**PLATE 234**

**ABDOMEN**

## Section above arcuate line

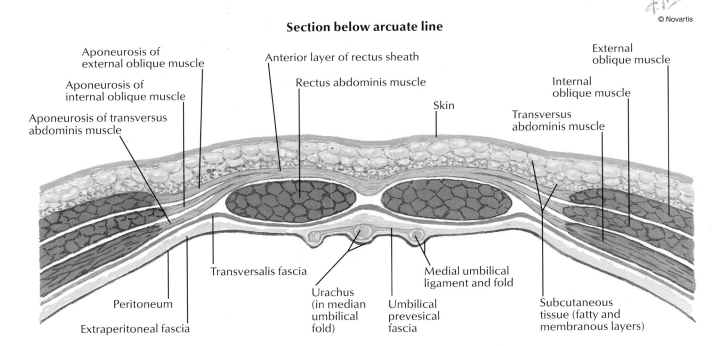

Aponeurosis of external oblique muscle

Aponeurosis of internal oblique muscle

Aponeurosis of transversus abdominis muscle

Anterior layer of rectus sheath

Rectus abdominis muscle

Linea alba

Skin

External oblique muscle

Internal oblique muscle

Transversus abdominis muscle

Peritoneum

Extraperitoneal fascia

Transversalis fascia

Posterior layer of rectus sheath

Falciform ligament

Subcutaneous tissue (fatty layer)

Aponeurosis of internal oblique muscle splits to form anterior and posterior layers of rectus sheath. Aponeurosis of external oblique muscle joins anterior layer of sheath; aponeurosis of transversus abdominis muscle joins posterior layer. Anterior and posterior layers of rectus sheath unite medially to form linea alba

## Section below arcuate line

Aponeurosis of external oblique muscle

Aponeurosis of internal oblique muscle

Aponeurosis of transversus abdominis muscle

Anterior layer of rectus sheath

Rectus abdominis muscle

Skin

External oblique muscle

Internal oblique muscle

Transversus abdominis muscle

Transversalis fascia

Medial umbilical ligament and fold

Peritoneum

Extraperitoneal fascia

Urachus (in median umbilical fold)

Umbilical prevesical fascia

Subcutaneous tissue (fatty and membranous layers)

Aponeurosis of internal oblique muscle does not split at this level but passes completely anterior to rectus abdominis muscle and is fused there with both aponeurosis of external oblique muscle and that of transversus abdominis muscle. Thus, posterior wall of rectus sheath is absent below arcuate line and rectus abdominis muscle lies on transversalis fascia

© Novartis

FOR UMBILICAL VESSELS SEE PLATE 217

Diaphragm

Diaphragmatic fascia

Falciform ligament

Peritoneum (*cut edges*)

Transversalis fascia and its cut edge

Arcuate line

Rectus abdominis muscle

Inferior epigastric vessels

Inguinal triangle (Hesselbach)

Transversalis fascia (*cut*)

Interfoveolar ligament

Deep circumflex iliac vessels

Deep inguinal ring

Cremasteric and pubic branches of inferior epigastric artery

External iliac vessels

Spermatic cord

Femoral ring

Femoral sheath

Lacunar ligament (Gimbernat)

Pectineal ligament (Cooper)

Inguinal falx (conjoint tendon)

Umbilical artery (occluded part distal to this point)

Obturator nerve and vessels

Obturator canal

Ureter (*cut*)

Anterior recess of ischioanal fossa

Superior vesical artery

Ductus (vas) deferens

Parietal pleura

Round ligament (ligamentum teres) of liver and paraumbilical veins

Umbilicus

Peritoneum

Transversalis fascia

External and Internal oblique muscles

Transversus abdominis muscle

Left medial umbilical ligament (obliterated left umbilical artery)

Right medial umbilical fold

Median umbilical ligament (obliterated urachus) and paraumbilical veins in median umbilical fold

Umbilical pre-vesical fascia

Lateral umbilical fold (contains inferior epigastric vessels)

Femoral nerve

Iliopsoas fascia

Iliopsoas muscle

External iliac vessels

Supravesical fossa

Transverse vesical fold

Obturator internus muscle

Tendinous arch of Levator ani muscle

Bulbourethral gland (Cowper) embedded in deep transverse perineal muscle

Seminal vesicle

Prostate and sphincter urethrae muscle

Urinary bladder

Perineal membrane

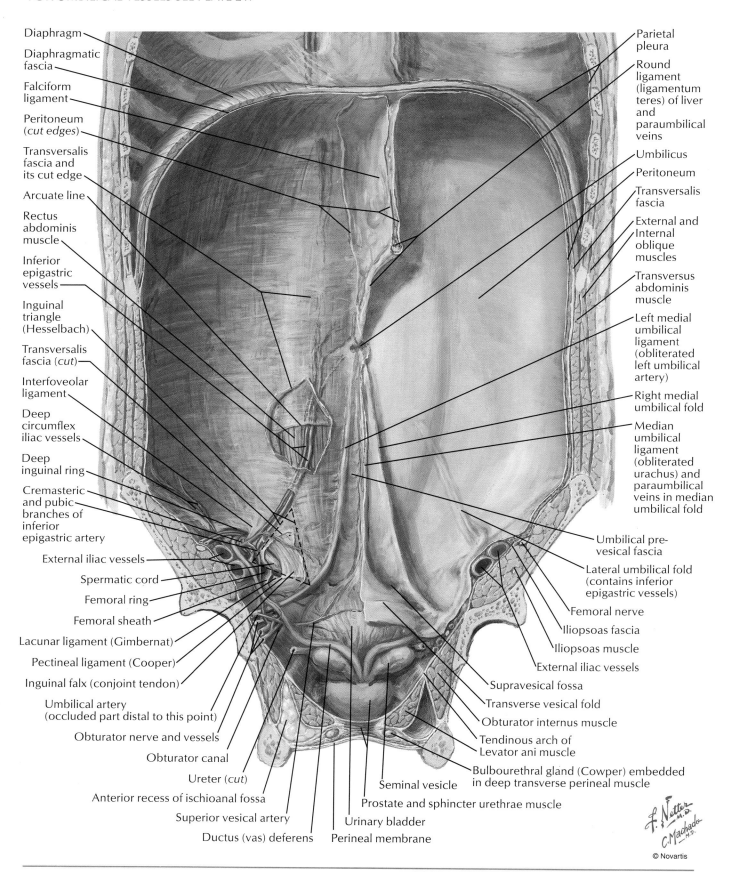

*F. Netter M.D.*
*C. Machado M.D.*

© Novartis

**PLATE 236**

**ABDOMEN**

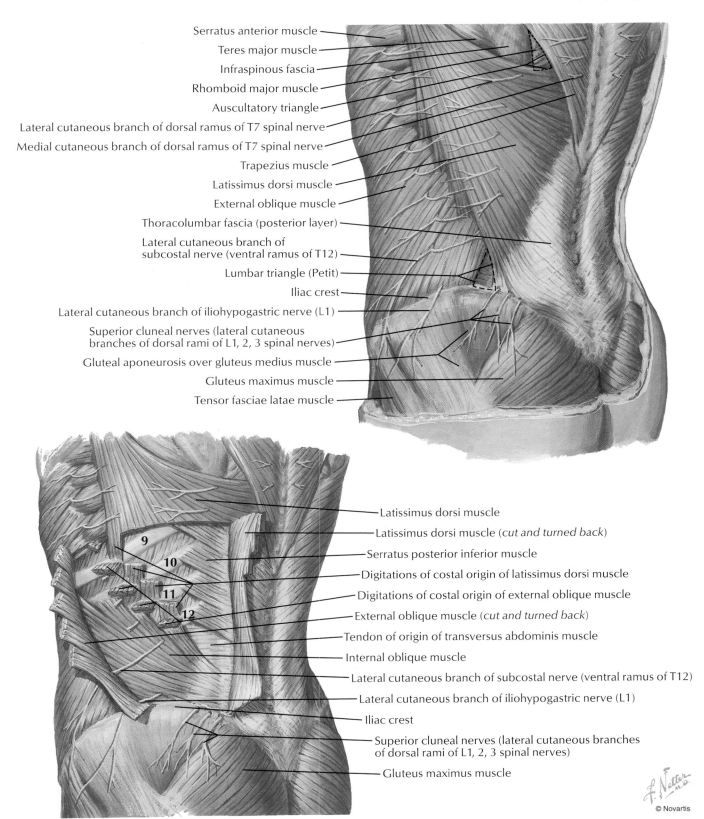

Serratus anterior muscle

Teres major muscle

Infraspinous fascia

Rhomboid major muscle

Auscultatory triangle

Lateral cutaneous branch of dorsal ramus of T7 spinal nerve

Medial cutaneous branch of dorsal ramus of T7 spinal nerve

Trapezius muscle

Latissimus dorsi muscle

External oblique muscle

Thoracolumbar fascia (posterior layer)

Lateral cutaneous branch of subcostal nerve (ventral ramus of T12)

Lumbar triangle (Petit)

Iliac crest

Lateral cutaneous branch of iliohypogastric nerve (L1)

Superior cluneal nerves (lateral cutaneous branches of dorsal rami of L1, 2, 3 spinal nerves)

Gluteal aponeurosis over gluteus medius muscle

Gluteus maximus muscle

Tensor fasciae latae muscle

Latissimus dorsi muscle

Latissimus dorsi muscle (*cut and turned back*)

Serratus posterior inferior muscle

Digitations of costal origin of latissimus dorsi muscle

Digitations of costal origin of external oblique muscle

External oblique muscle (*cut and turned back*)

Tendon of origin of transversus abdominis muscle

Internal oblique muscle

Lateral cutaneous branch of subcostal nerve (ventral ramus of T12)

Lateral cutaneous branch of iliohypogastric nerve (L1)

Iliac crest

Superior cluneal nerves (lateral cutaneous branches of dorsal rami of L1, 2, 3 spinal nerves)

Gluteus maximus muscle

9

10

11

12

© Novartis

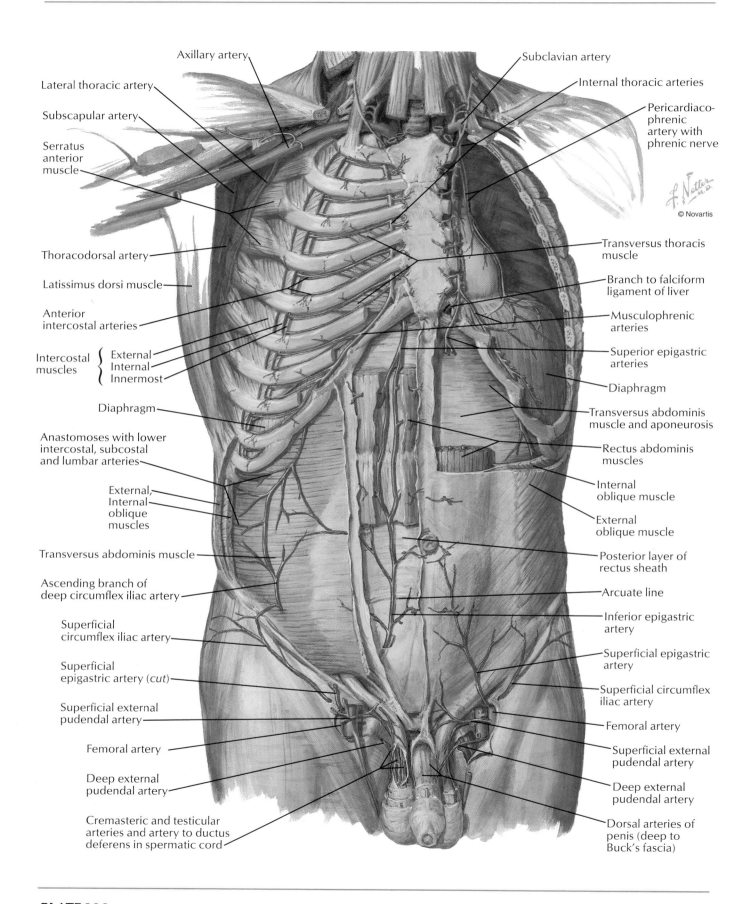

Axillary artery

Subclavian artery

Lateral thoracic artery

Internal thoracic arteries

Subscapular artery

Pericardiaco-phrenic artery with phrenic nerve

Serratus anterior muscle

Thoracodorsal artery

Transversus thoracis muscle

Latissimus dorsi muscle

Branch to falciform ligament of liver

Anterior intercostal arteries

Musculophrenic arteries

Intercostal muscles { External Internal Innermost

Superior epigastric arteries

Diaphragm

Diaphragm

Transversus abdominis muscle and aponeurosis

Anastomoses with lower intercostal, subcostal and lumbar arteries

Rectus abdominis muscles

External, Internal oblique muscles

Internal oblique muscle

External oblique muscle

Transversus abdominis muscle

Posterior layer of rectus sheath

Ascending branch of deep circumflex iliac artery

Arcuate line

Superficial circumflex iliac artery

Inferior epigastric artery

Superficial epigastric artery (cut)

Superficial epigastric artery

Superficial external pudendal artery

Superficial circumflex iliac artery

Femoral artery

Femoral artery

Superficial external pudendal artery

Deep external pudendal artery

Deep external pudendal artery

Cremasteric and testicular arteries and artery to ductus deferens in spermatic cord

Dorsal arteries of penis (deep to Buck's fascia)

**PLATE 238**

**ABDOMEN**

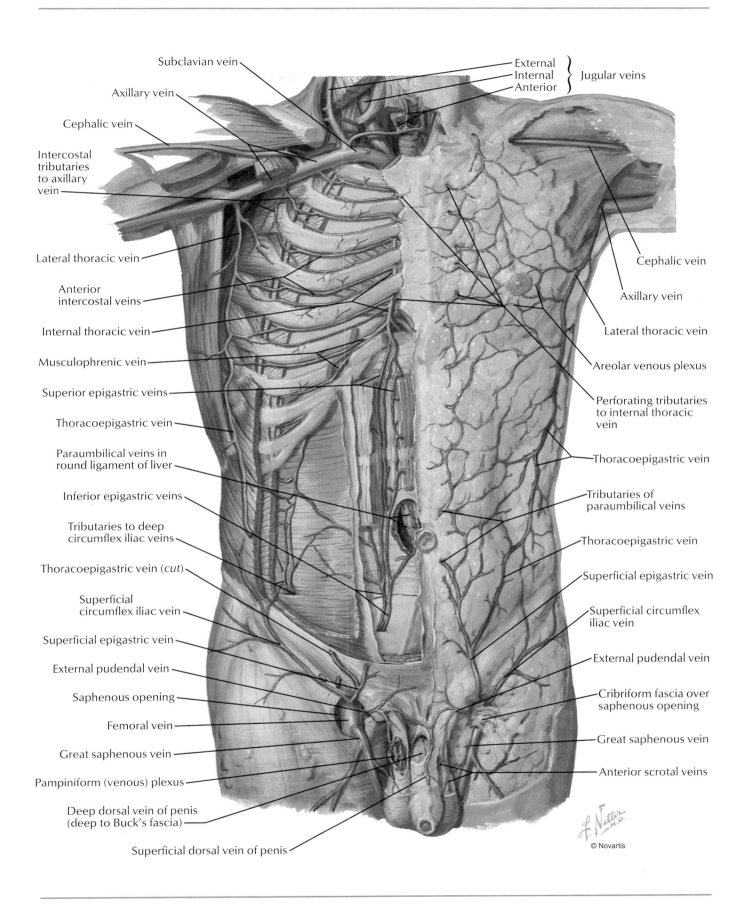

Subclavian vein

Axillary vein

Cephalic vein

Intercostal tributaries to axillary vein

Lateral thoracic vein

Anterior intercostal veins

Internal thoracic vein

Musculophrenic vein

Superior epigastric veins

Thoracoepigastric vein

Paraumbilical veins in round ligament of liver

Inferior epigastric veins

Tributaries to deep circumflex iliac veins

Thoracoepigastric vein (cut)

Superficial circumflex iliac vein

Superficial epigastric vein

External pudendal vein

Saphenous opening

Femoral vein

Great saphenous vein

Pampiniform (venous) plexus

Deep dorsal vein of penis (deep to Buck's fascia)

Superficial dorsal vein of penis

External
Internal      } Jugular veins
Anterior

Cephalic vein

Axillary vein

Lateral thoracic vein

Areolar venous plexus

Perforating tributaries to internal thoracic vein

Thoracoepigastric vein

Tributaries of paraumbilical veins

Thoracoepigastric vein

Superficial epigastric vein

Superficial circumflex iliac vein

External pudendal vein

Cribriform fascia over saphenous opening

Great saphenous vein

Anterior scrotal veins

© Novartis

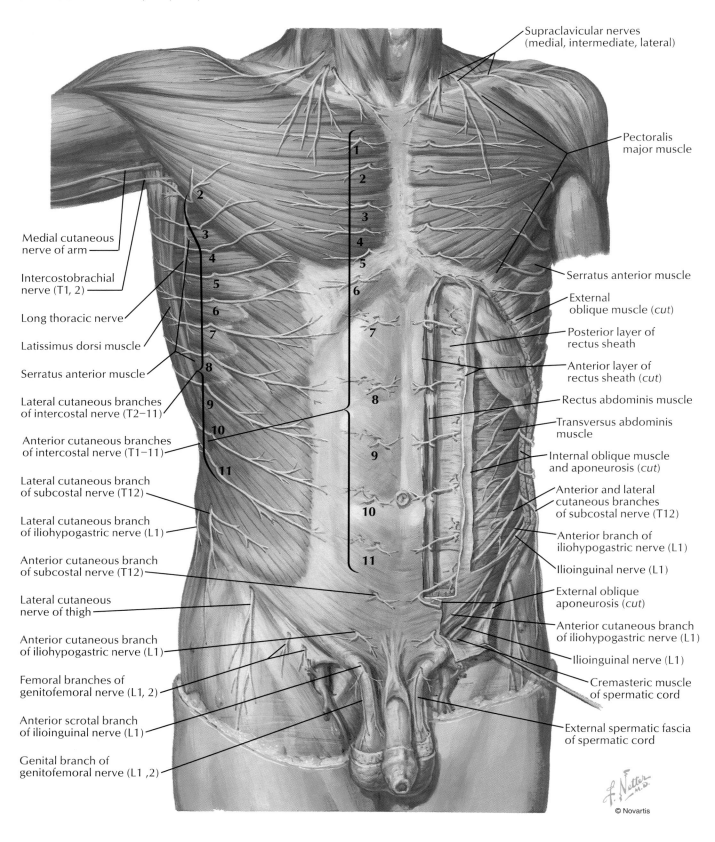

Supraclavicular nerves
(medial, intermediate, lateral)

Pectoralis
major muscle

Medial cutaneous
nerve of arm

Intercostobrachial
nerve (T1, 2)

Long thoracic nerve

Latissimus dorsi muscle

Serratus anterior muscle

Lateral cutaneous branches
of intercostal nerve (T2−11)

Anterior cutaneous branches
of intercostal nerve (T1−11)

Lateral cutaneous branch
of subcostal nerve (T12)

Lateral cutaneous branch
of iliohypogastric nerve (L1)

Anterior cutaneous branch
of subcostal nerve (T12)

Lateral cutaneous
nerve of thigh

Anterior cutaneous branch
of iliohypogastric nerve (L1)

Femoral branches of
genitofemoral nerve (L1, 2)

Anterior scrotal branch
of ilioinguinal nerve (L1)

Genital branch of
genitofemoral nerve (L1 ,2)

Serratus anterior muscle

External
oblique muscle (*cut*)

Posterior layer of
rectus sheath

Anterior layer of
rectus sheath (*cut*)

Rectus abdominis muscle

Transversus abdominis
muscle

Internal oblique muscle
and aponeurosis (*cut*)

Anterior and lateral
cutaneous branches
of subcostal nerve (T12)

Anterior branch of
iliohypogastric nerve (L1)

Ilioinguinal nerve (L1)

External oblique
aponeurosis (*cut*)

Anterior cutaneous branch
of iliohypogastric nerve (L1)

Ilioinguinal nerve (L1)

Cremasteric muscle
of spermatic cord

External spermatic fascia
of spermatic cord

**PLATE 240**

**ABDOMEN**

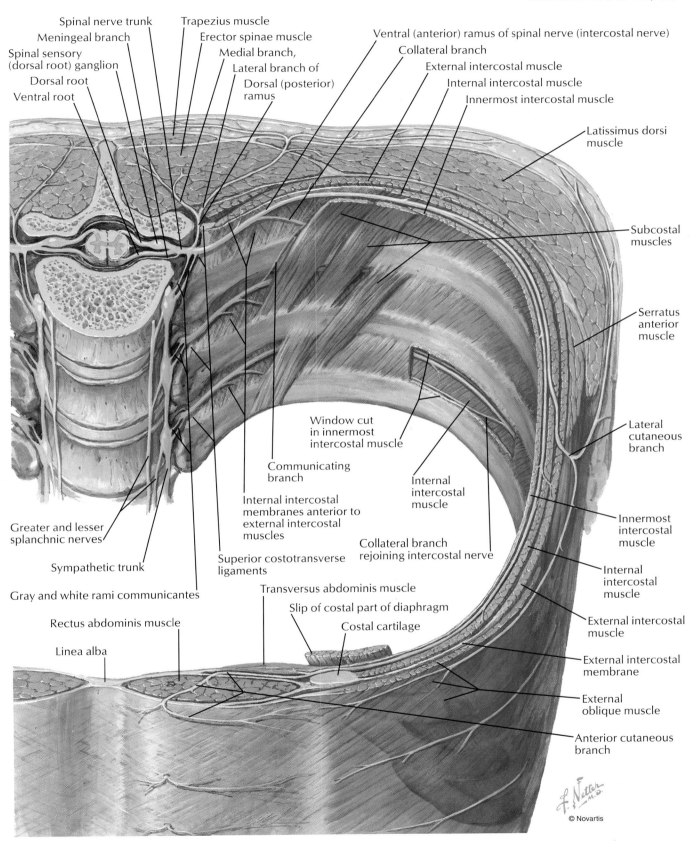

Spinal nerve trunk

Meningeal branch

Spinal sensory (dorsal root) ganglion

Dorsal root

Ventral root

Trapezius muscle

Erector spinae muscle

Medial branch,

Lateral branch of

Dorsal (posterior) ramus

Ventral (anterior) ramus of spinal nerve (intercostal nerve)

Collateral branch

External intercostal muscle

Internal intercostal muscle

Innermost intercostal muscle

Latissimus dorsi muscle

Subcostal muscles

Serratus anterior muscle

Lateral cutaneous branch

Innermost intercostal muscle

Internal intercostal muscle

External intercostal muscle

External intercostal membrane

External oblique muscle

Anterior cutaneous branch

Window cut in innermost intercostal muscle

Communicating branch

Internal intercostal membranes anterior to external intercostal muscles

Superior costotransverse ligaments

Greater and lesser splanchnic nerves

Sympathetic trunk

Gray and white rami communicantes

Rectus abdominis muscle

Linea alba

Internal intercostal muscle

Collateral branch rejoining intercostal nerve

Transversus abdominis muscle

Slip of costal part of diaphragm

Costal cartilage

© Novartis

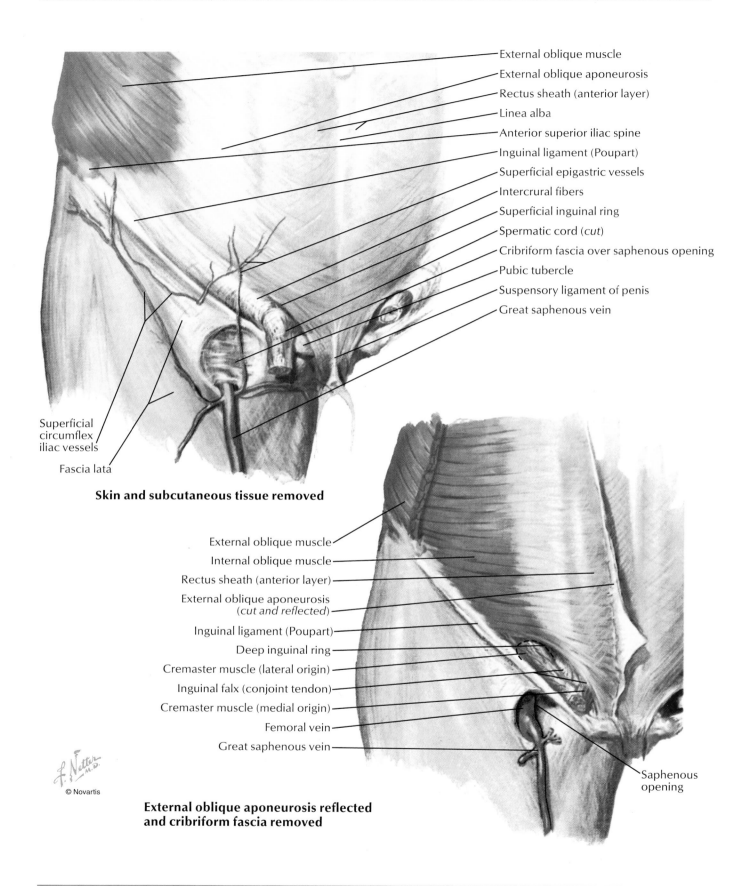

Skin and subcutaneous tissue removed

- External oblique muscle
- External oblique aponeurosis
- Rectus sheath (anterior layer)
- Linea alba
- Anterior superior iliac spine
- Inguinal ligament (Poupart)
- Superficial epigastric vessels
- Intercrural fibers
- Superficial inguinal ring
- Spermatic cord (*cut*)
- Cribriform fascia over saphenous opening
- Pubic tubercle
- Suspensory ligament of penis
- Great saphenous vein

Superficial circumflex iliac vessels

Fascia lata

External oblique aponeurosis reflected and cribriform fascia removed

- External oblique muscle
- Internal oblique muscle
- Rectus sheath (anterior layer)
- External oblique aponeurosis (*cut and reflected*)
- Inguinal ligament (Poupart)
- Deep inguinal ring
- Cremaster muscle (lateral origin)
- Inguinal falx (conjoint tendon)
- Cremaster muscle (medial origin)
- Femoral vein
- Great saphenous vein
- Saphenous opening

© Novartis

**PLATE 242**

**ABDOMEN**

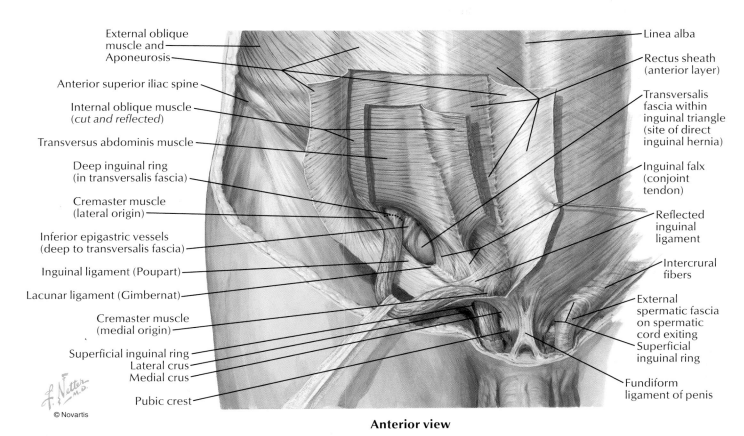

External oblique muscle and Aponeurosis

Anterior superior iliac spine

Internal oblique muscle (*cut and reflected*)

Transversus abdominis muscle

Deep inguinal ring (in transversalis fascia)

Cremaster muscle (lateral origin)

Inferior epigastric vessels (deep to transversalis fascia)

Inguinal ligament (Poupart)

Lacunar ligament (Gimbernat)

Cremaster muscle (medial origin)

Superficial inguinal ring

Lateral crus

Medial crus

Pubic crest

Linea alba

Rectus sheath (anterior layer)

Transversalis fascia within inguinal triangle (site of direct inguinal hernia)

Inguinal falx (conjoint tendon)

Reflected inguinal ligament

Intercrural fibers

External spermatic fascia on spermatic cord exiting

Superficial inguinal ring

Fundiform ligament of penis

© Novartis

**Anterior view**

**Posterior (internal) view**

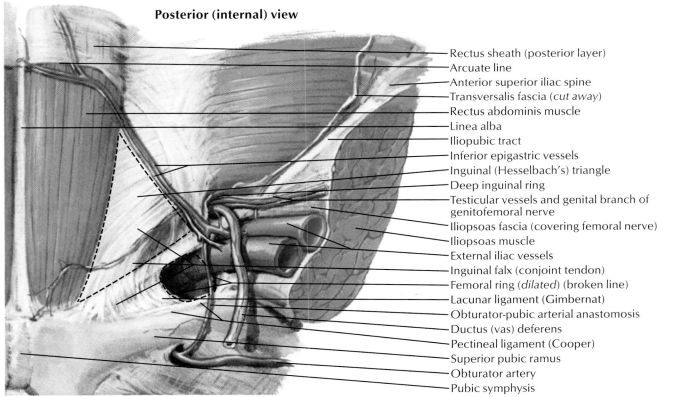

Rectus sheath (posterior layer)

Arcuate line

Anterior superior iliac spine

Transversalis fascia (*cut away*)

Rectus abdominis muscle

Linea alba

Iliopubic tract

Inferior epigastric vessels

Inguinal (Hesselbach's) triangle

Deep inguinal ring

Testicular vessels and genital branch of genitofemoral nerve

Iliopsoas fascia (covering femoral nerve)

Iliopsoas muscle

External iliac vessels

Inguinal falx (conjoint tendon)

Femoral ring (*dilated*) (broken line)

Lacunar ligament (Gimbernat)

Obturator-pubic arterial anastomosis

Ductus (vas) deferens

Pectineal ligament (Cooper)

Superior pubic ramus

Obturator artery

Pubic symphysis

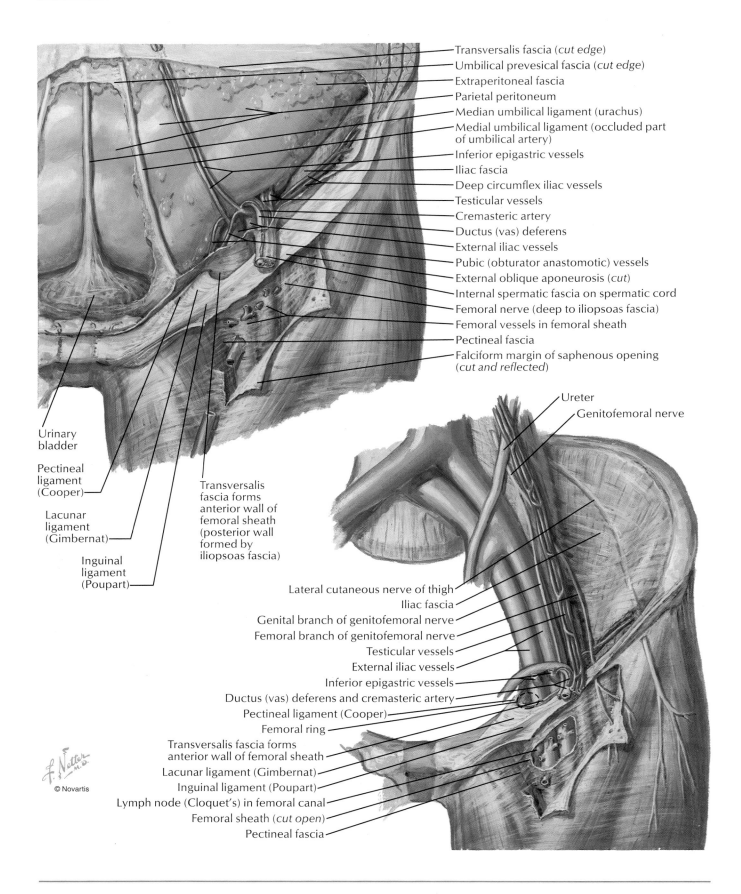

Transversalis fascia (*cut edge*)

Umbilical prevesical fascia (*cut edge*)

Extraperitoneal fascia

Parietal peritoneum

Median umbilical ligament (urachus)

Medial umbilical ligament (occluded part of umbilical artery)

Inferior epigastric vessels

Iliac fascia

Deep circumflex iliac vessels

Testicular vessels

Cremasteric artery

Ductus (vas) deferens

External iliac vessels

Pubic (obturator anastomotic) vessels

External oblique aponeurosis (*cut*)

Internal spermatic fascia on spermatic cord

Femoral nerve (deep to iliopsoas fascia)

Femoral vessels in femoral sheath

Pectineal fascia

Falciform margin of saphenous opening (*cut and reflected*)

Ureter

Genitofemoral nerve

Urinary bladder

Pectineal ligament (Cooper)

Lacunar ligament (Gimbernat)

Inguinal ligament (Poupart)

Transversalis fascia forms anterior wall of femoral sheath (posterior wall formed by iliopsoas fascia)

Lateral cutaneous nerve of thigh

Iliac fascia

Genital branch of genitofemoral nerve

Femoral branch of genitofemoral nerve

Testicular vessels

External iliac vessels

Inferior epigastric vessels

Ductus (vas) deferens and cremasteric artery

Pectineal ligament (Cooper)

Femoral ring

Transversalis fascia forms anterior wall of femoral sheath

Lacunar ligament (Gimbernat)

Inguinal ligament (Poupart)

Lymph node (Cloquet's) in femoral canal

Femoral sheath (*cut open*)

Pectineal fascia

© Novartis

**PLATE 244**

**ABDOMEN**

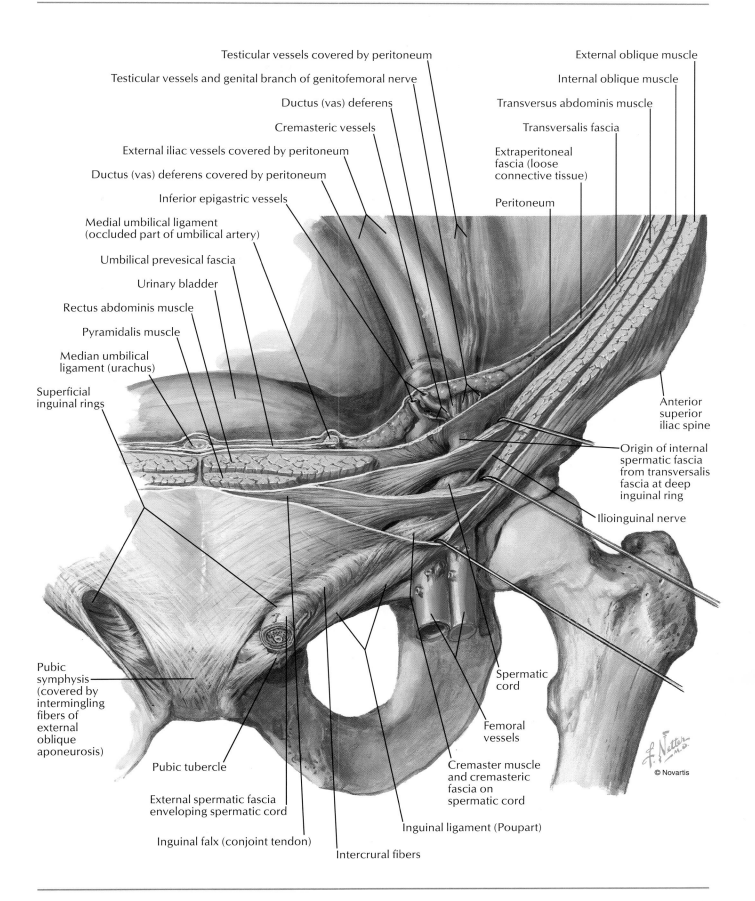

Testicular vessels covered by peritoneum

Testicular vessels and genital branch of genitofemoral nerve

Ductus (vas) deferens

Cremasteric vessels

External iliac vessels covered by peritoneum

Ductus (vas) deferens covered by peritoneum

Inferior epigastric vessels

Medial umbilical ligament (occluded part of umbilical artery)

Umbilical prevesical fascia

Urinary bladder

Rectus abdominis muscle

Pyramidalis muscle

Median umbilical ligament (urachus)

Superficial inguinal rings

Pubic symphysis (covered by intermingling fibers of external oblique aponeurosis)

Pubic tubercle

External spermatic fascia enveloping spermatic cord

Inguinal falx (conjoint tendon)

Intercrural fibers

External oblique muscle

Internal oblique muscle

Transversus abdominis muscle

Transversalis fascia

Extraperitoneal fascia (loose connective tissue)

Peritoneum

Anterior superior iliac spine

Origin of internal spermatic fascia from transversalis fascia at deep inguinal ring

Ilioinguinal nerve

Spermatic cord

Femoral vessels

Cremaster muscle and cremasteric fascia on spermatic cord

Inguinal ligament (Poupart)

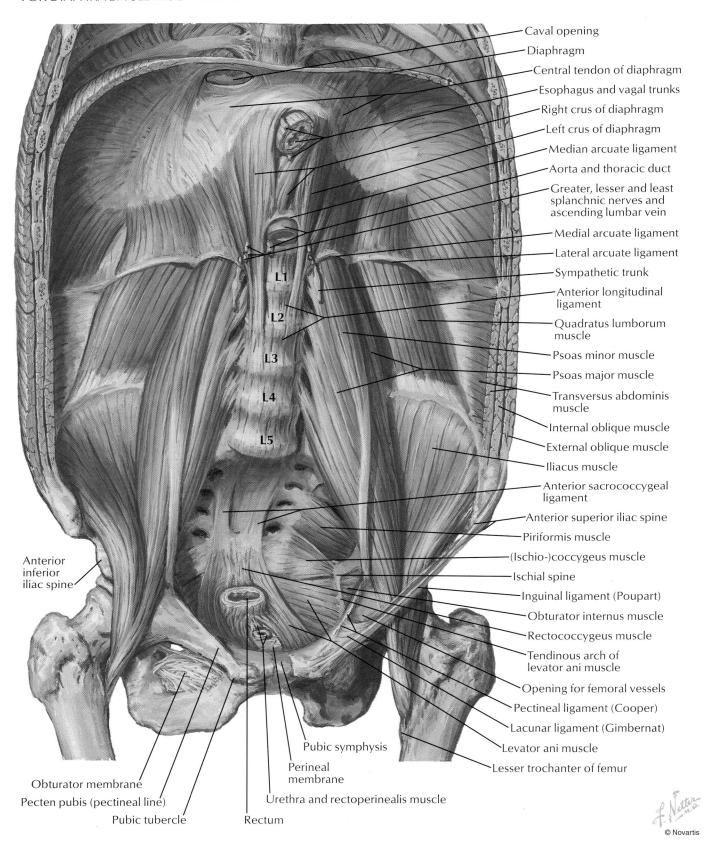

Caval opening
Diaphragm
Central tendon of diaphragm
Esophagus and vagal trunks
Right crus of diaphragm
Left crus of diaphragm
Median arcuate ligament
Aorta and thoracic duct
Greater, lesser and least splanchnic nerves and ascending lumbar vein
Medial arcuate ligament
Lateral arcuate ligament
Sympathetic trunk
Anterior longitudinal ligament
Quadratus lumborum muscle
Psoas minor muscle
Psoas major muscle
Transversus abdominis muscle
Internal oblique muscle
External oblique muscle
Iliacus muscle
Anterior sacrococcygeal ligament
Anterior superior iliac spine
Piriformis muscle
(Ischio-)coccygeus muscle
Ischial spine
Inguinal ligament (Poupart)
Obturator internus muscle
Rectococcygeus muscle
Tendinous arch of levator ani muscle
Opening for femoral vessels
Pectineal ligament (Cooper)
Lacunar ligament (Gimbernat)
Levator ani muscle
Lesser trochanter of femur

L1
L2
L3
L4
L5

Anterior inferior iliac spine

Obturator membrane
Pecten pubis (pectineal line)
Pubic tubercle
Rectum
Pubic symphysis
Perineal membrane
Urethra and rectoperinealis muscle

© Novartis

**PLATE 246**

**ABDOMEN**

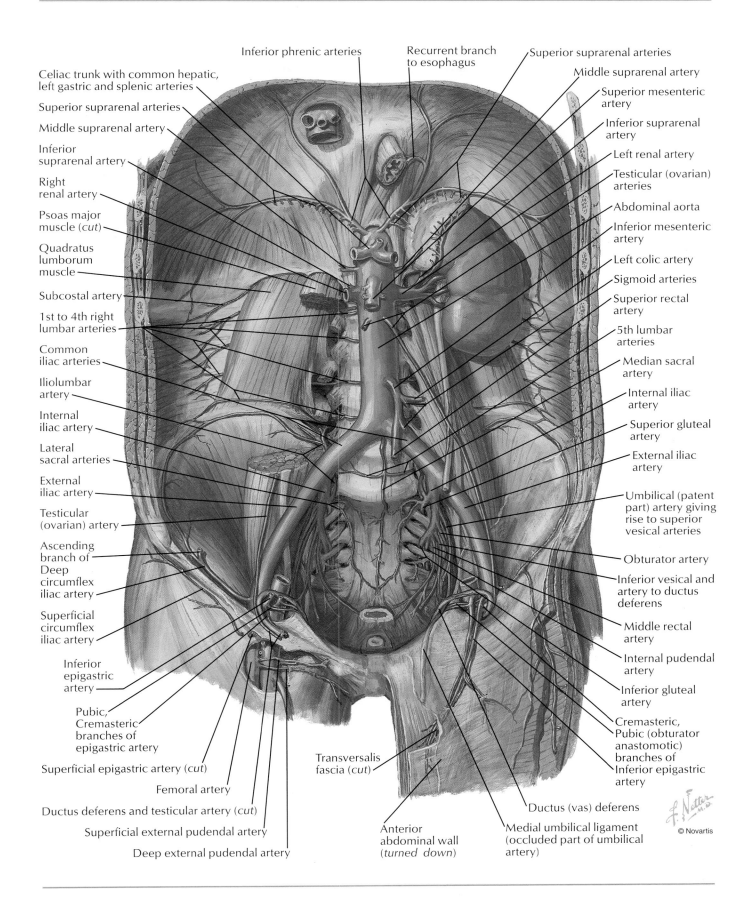

Inferior phrenic arteries

Recurrent branch to esophagus

Superior suprarenal arteries

Middle suprarenal artery

Celiac trunk with common hepatic, left gastric and splenic arteries

Superior suprarenal arteries

Middle suprarenal artery

Inferior suprarenal artery

Right renal artery

Psoas major muscle (cut)

Quadratus lumborum muscle

Subcostal artery

1st to 4th right lumbar arteries

Common iliac arteries

Iliolumbar artery

Internal iliac artery

Lateral sacral arteries

External iliac artery

Testicular (ovarian) artery

Ascending branch of Deep circumflex iliac artery

Superficial circumflex iliac artery

Inferior epigastric artery

Pubic, Cremasteric branches of epigastric artery

Superficial epigastric artery (cut)

Femoral artery

Ductus deferens and testicular artery (cut)

Superficial external pudendal artery

Deep external pudendal artery

Superior mesenteric artery

Inferior suprarenal artery

Left renal artery

Testicular (ovarian) arteries

Abdominal aorta

Inferior mesenteric artery

Left colic artery

Sigmoid arteries

Superior rectal artery

5th lumbar arteries

Median sacral artery

Internal iliac artery

Superior gluteal artery

External iliac artery

Umbilical (patent part) artery giving rise to superior vesical arteries

Obturator artery

Inferior vesical and artery to ductus deferens

Middle rectal artery

Internal pudendal artery

Inferior gluteal artery

Cremasteric, Pubic (obturator anastomotic) branches of Inferior epigastric artery

Ductus (vas) deferens

Medial umbilical ligament (occluded part of umbilical artery)

Transversalis fascia (cut)

Anterior abdominal wall (turned down)

© Novartis

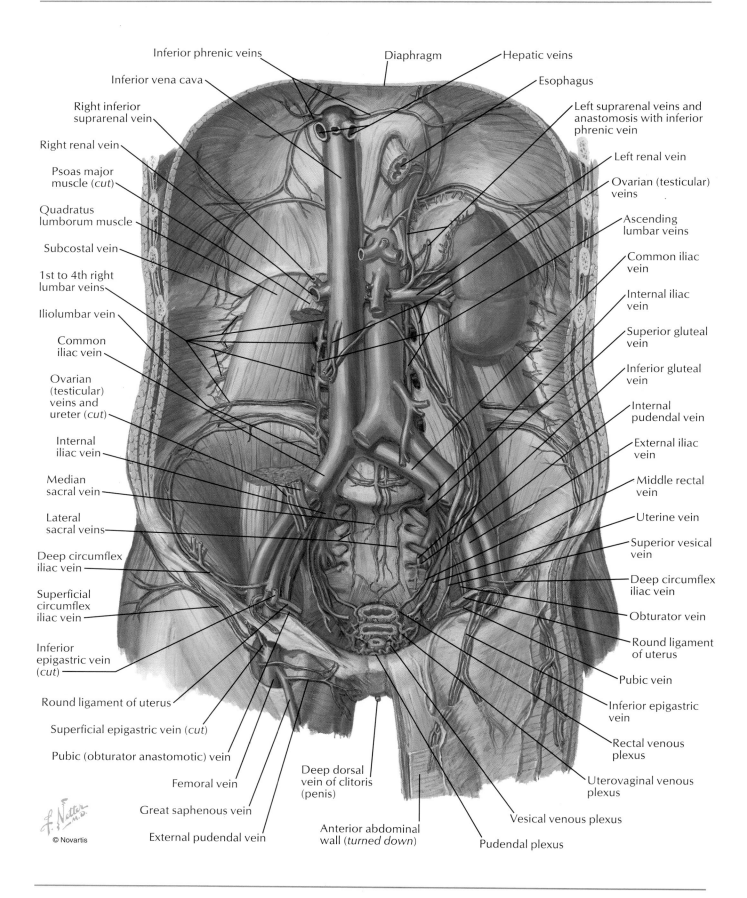

Inferior phrenic veins

Diaphragm

Hepatic veins

Inferior vena cava

Esophagus

Right inferior suprarenal vein

Left suprarenal veins and anastomosis with inferior phrenic vein

Right renal vein

Left renal vein

Psoas major muscle (cut)

Ovarian (testicular) veins

Quadratus lumborum muscle

Ascending lumbar veins

Subcostal vein

Common iliac vein

1st to 4th right lumbar veins

Internal iliac vein

Iliolumbar vein

Superior gluteal vein

Common iliac vein

Inferior gluteal vein

Ovarian (testicular) veins and ureter (cut)

Internal pudendal vein

Internal iliac vein

External iliac vein

Median sacral vein

Middle rectal vein

Lateral sacral veins

Uterine vein

Deep circumflex iliac vein

Superior vesical vein

Superficial circumflex iliac vein

Deep circumflex iliac vein

Inferior epigastric vein (cut)

Obturator vein

Round ligament of uterus

Round ligament of uterus

Pubic vein

Superficial epigastric vein (cut)

Inferior epigastric vein

Pubic (obturator anastomotic) vein

Rectal venous plexus

Femoral vein

Uterovaginal venous plexus

Deep dorsal vein of clitoris (penis)

Great saphenous vein

Vesical venous plexus

External pudendal vein

Anterior abdominal wall (turned down)

Pudendal plexus

© Novartis

**PLATE 248**

**ABDOMEN**

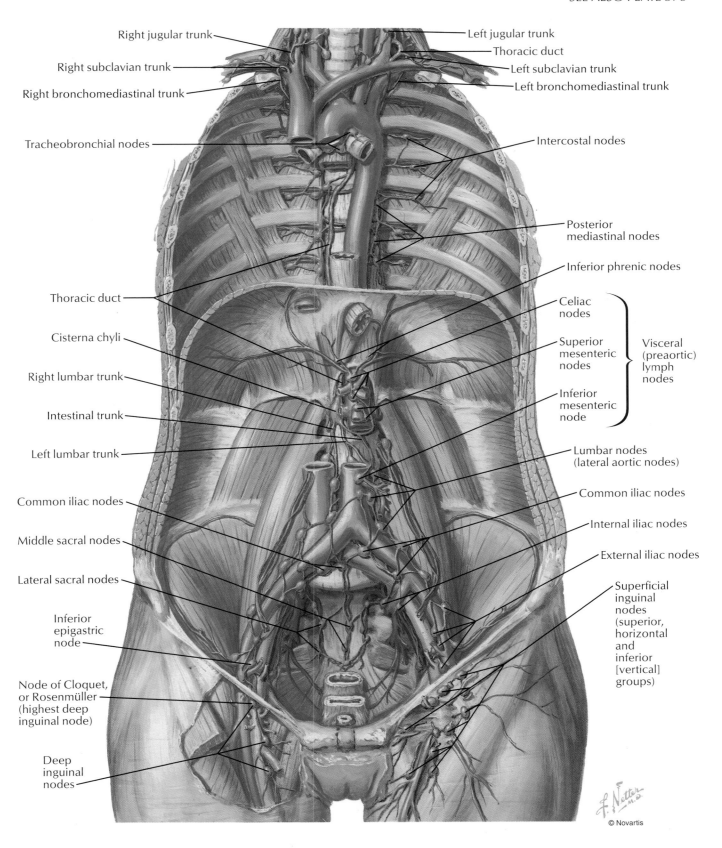

Right jugular trunk

Right subclavian trunk

Right bronchomediastinal trunk

Tracheobronchial nodes

Thoracic duct

Cisterna chyli

Right lumbar trunk

Intestinal trunk

Left lumbar trunk

Common iliac nodes

Middle sacral nodes

Lateral sacral nodes

Inferior epigastric node

Node of Cloquet, or Rosenmüller (highest deep inguinal node)

Deep inguinal nodes

Left jugular trunk

Thoracic duct

Left subclavian trunk

Left bronchomediastinal trunk

Intercostal nodes

Posterior mediastinal nodes

Inferior phrenic nodes

Celiac nodes

Superior mesenteric nodes

Inferior mesenteric node

Visceral (preaortic) lymph nodes

Lumbar nodes (lateral aortic nodes)

Common iliac nodes

Internal iliac nodes

External iliac nodes

Superficial inguinal nodes (superior, horizontal and inferior [vertical] groups)

© Novartis

# Nerves of Posterior Abdominal Wall

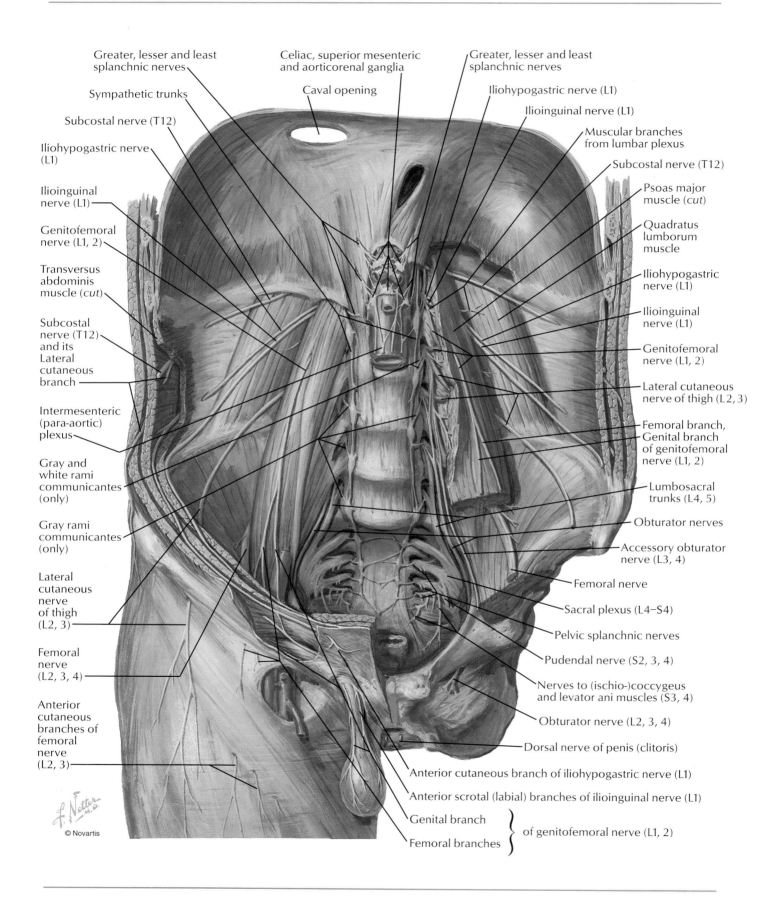

Greater, lesser and least splanchnic nerves

Sympathetic trunks

Subcostal nerve (T12)

Iliohypogastric nerve (L1)

Ilioinguinal nerve (L1)

Genitofemoral nerve (L1, 2)

Transversus abdominis muscle (cut)

Subcostal nerve (T12) and its Lateral cutaneous branch

Intermesenteric (para-aortic) plexus

Gray and white rami communicantes (only)

Gray rami communicantes (only)

Lateral cutaneous nerve of thigh (L2, 3)

Femoral nerve (L2, 3, 4)

Anterior cutaneous branches of femoral nerve (L2, 3)

Celiac, superior mesenteric and aorticorenal ganglia

Caval opening

Greater, lesser and least splanchnic nerves

Iliohypogastric nerve (L1)

Ilioinguinal nerve (L1)

Muscular branches from lumbar plexus

Subcostal nerve (T12)

Psoas major muscle (cut)

Quadratus lumborum muscle

Iliohypogastric nerve (L1)

Ilioinguinal nerve (L1)

Genitofemoral nerve (L1, 2)

Lateral cutaneous nerve of thigh (L2, 3)

Femoral branch, Genital branch of genitofemoral nerve (L1, 2)

Lumbosacral trunks (L4, 5)

Obturator nerves

Accessory obturator nerve (L3, 4)

Femoral nerve

Sacral plexus (L4–S4)

Pelvic splanchnic nerves

Pudendal nerve (S2, 3, 4)

Nerves to (ischio-)coccygeus and levator ani muscles (S3, 4)

Obturator nerve (L2, 3, 4)

Dorsal nerve of penis (clitoris)

Anterior cutaneous branch of iliohypogastric nerve (L1)

Anterior scrotal (labial) branches of ilioinguinal nerve (L1)

Genital branch  } of genitofemoral nerve (L1, 2)
Femoral branches  }

f. Netter
© Novartis

**PLATE 250**

**ABDOMEN**

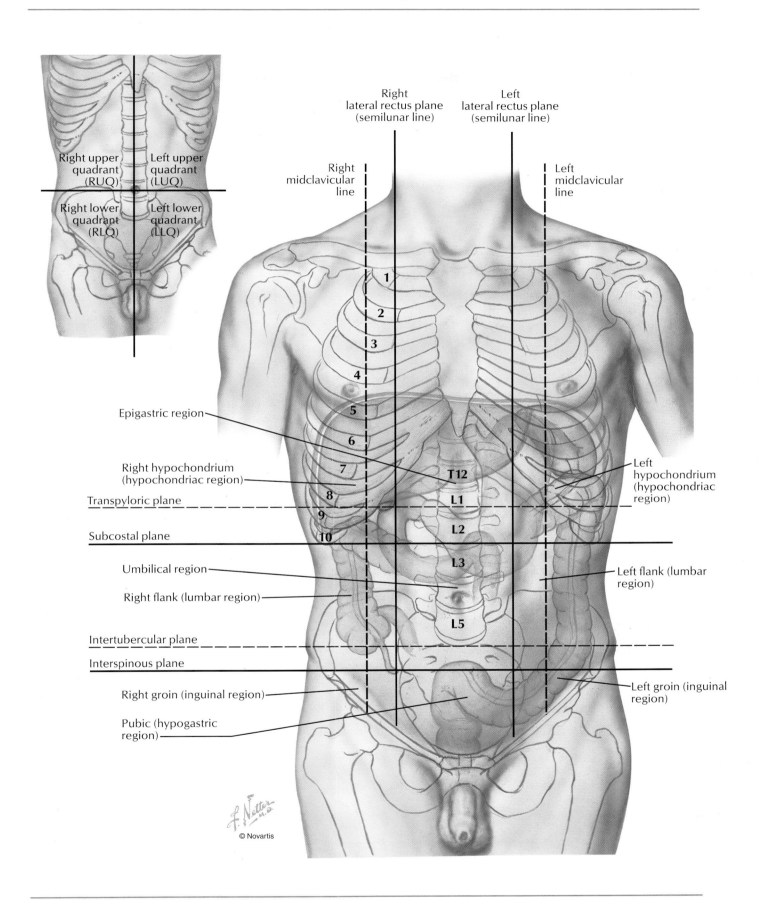

Right upper quadrant (RUQ)

Left upper quadrant (LUQ)

Right lower quadrant (RLQ)

Left lower quadrant (LLQ)

Right lateral rectus plane (semilunar line)

Left lateral rectus plane (semilunar line)

Right midclavicular line

Left midclavicular line

Epigastric region

Right hypochondrium (hypochondriac region)

Transpyloric plane

Subcostal plane

Umbilical region

Right flank (lumbar region)

Intertubercular plane

Interspinous plane

Right groin (inguinal region)

Pubic (hypogastric region)

Left hypochondrium (hypochondriac region)

Left flank (lumbar region)

Left groin (inguinal region)

T12

L1

L2

L3

L5

© Novartis

# Greater Omentum and Abdominal Viscera

SEE ALSO PLATES 258, 328, 329

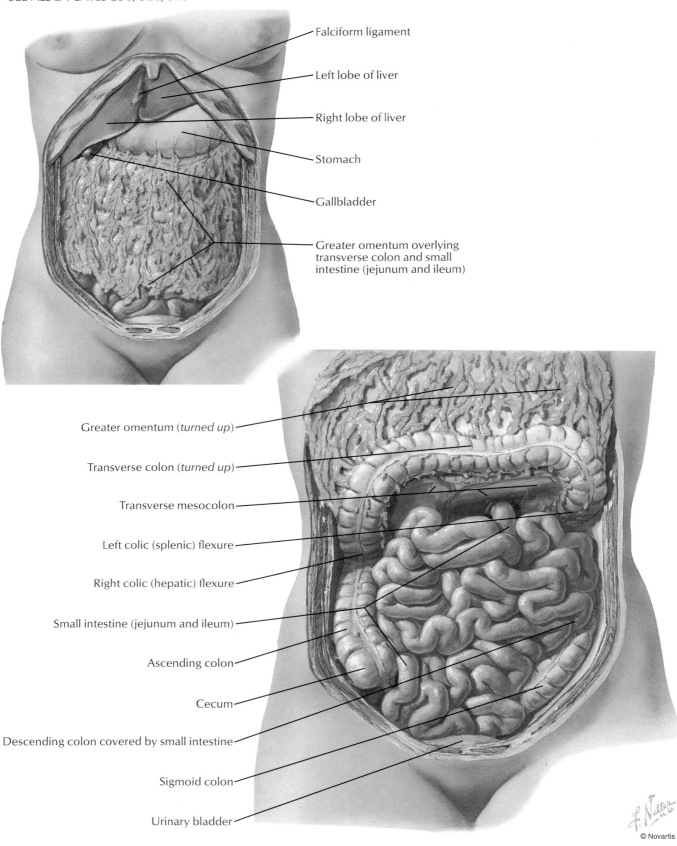

Falciform ligament

Left lobe of liver

Right lobe of liver

Stomach

Gallbladder

Greater omentum overlying transverse colon and small intestine (jejunum and ileum)

Greater omentum (*turned up*)

Transverse colon (*turned up*)

Transverse mesocolon

Left colic (splenic) flexure

Right colic (hepatic) flexure

Small intestine (jejunum and ileum)

Ascending colon

Cecum

Descending colon covered by small intestine

Sigmoid colon

Urinary bladder

© Novartis

**PLATE 252**                                                                **ABDOMEN**

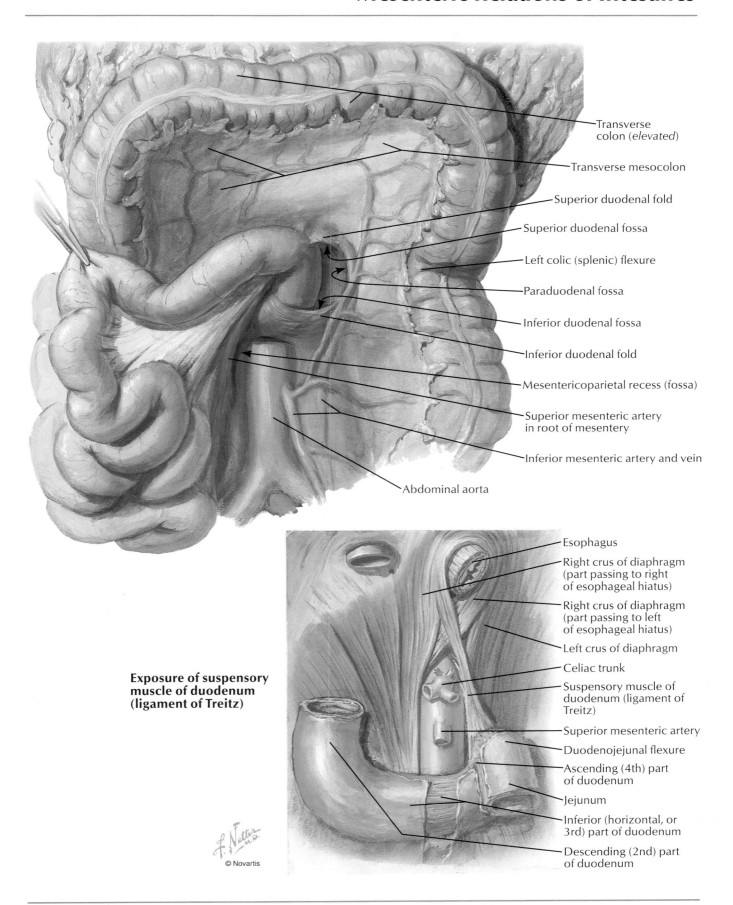

Transverse colon (*elevated*)

Transverse mesocolon

Superior duodenal fold

Superior duodenal fossa

Left colic (splenic) flexure

Paraduodenal fossa

Inferior duodenal fossa

Inferior duodenal fold

Mesentericoparietal recess (fossa)

Superior mesenteric artery in root of mesentery

Inferior mesenteric artery and vein

Abdominal aorta

Esophagus

Right crus of diaphragm (part passing to right of esophageal hiatus)

Right crus of diaphragm (part passing to left of esophageal hiatus)

Left crus of diaphragm

Celiac trunk

Suspensory muscle of duodenum (ligament of Treitz)

Superior mesenteric artery

Duodenojejunal flexure

Ascending (4th) part of duodenum

Jejunum

Inferior (horizontal, or 3rd) part of duodenum

Descending (2nd) part of duodenum

**Exposure of suspensory muscle of duodenum (ligament of Treitz)**

© Novartis

# Mesenteric Relations of Intestines (continued)

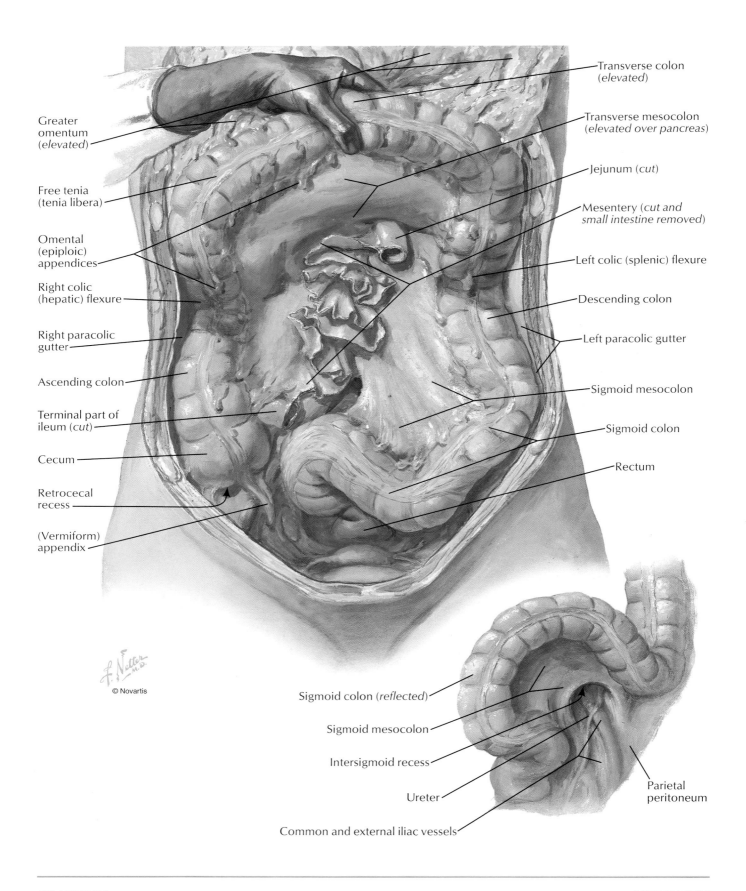

Transverse colon (*elevated*)

Transverse mesocolon (*elevated over pancreas*)

Jejunum (*cut*)

Mesentery (*cut and small intestine removed*)

Left colic (splenic) flexure

Descending colon

Left paracolic gutter

Sigmoid mesocolon

Sigmoid colon

Rectum

Greater omentum (*elevated*)

Free tenia (tenia libera)

Omental (epiploic) appendices

Right colic (hepatic) flexure

Right paracolic gutter

Ascending colon

Terminal part of ileum (*cut*)

Cecum

Retrocecal recess

(Vermiform) appendix

Sigmoid colon (*reflected*)

Sigmoid mesocolon

Intersigmoid recess

Ureter

Common and external iliac vessels

Parietal peritoneum

© Novartis

**PLATE 254**

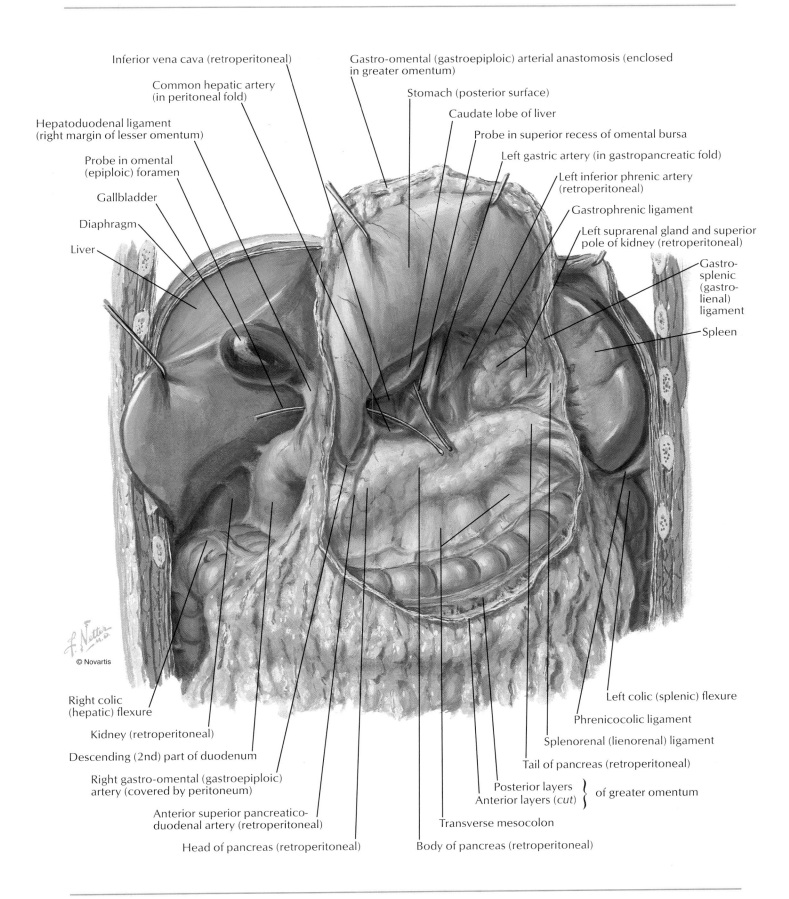

Inferior vena cava (retroperitoneal)

Common hepatic artery (in peritoneal fold)

Hepatoduodenal ligament (right margin of lesser omentum)

Probe in omental (epiploic) foramen

Gallbladder

Diaphragm

Liver

Gastro-omental (gastroepiploic) arterial anastomosis (enclosed in greater omentum)

Stomach (posterior surface)

Caudate lobe of liver

Probe in superior recess of omental bursa

Left gastric artery (in gastropancreatic fold)

Left inferior phrenic artery (retroperitoneal)

Gastrophrenic ligament

Left suprarenal gland and superior pole of kidney (retroperitoneal)

Gastro-splenic (gastro-lienal) ligament

Spleen

Right colic (hepatic) flexure

Kidney (retroperitoneal)

Descending (2nd) part of duodenum

Right gastro-omental (gastroepiploic) artery (covered by peritoneum)

Anterior superior pancreatico-duodenal artery (retroperitoneal)

Head of pancreas (retroperitoneal)

Left colic (splenic) flexure

Phrenicocolic ligament

Splenorenal (lienorenal) ligament

Tail of pancreas (retroperitoneal)

Posterior layers
Anterior layers (cut) } of greater omentum

Transverse mesocolon

Body of pancreas (retroperitoneal)

© Novartis

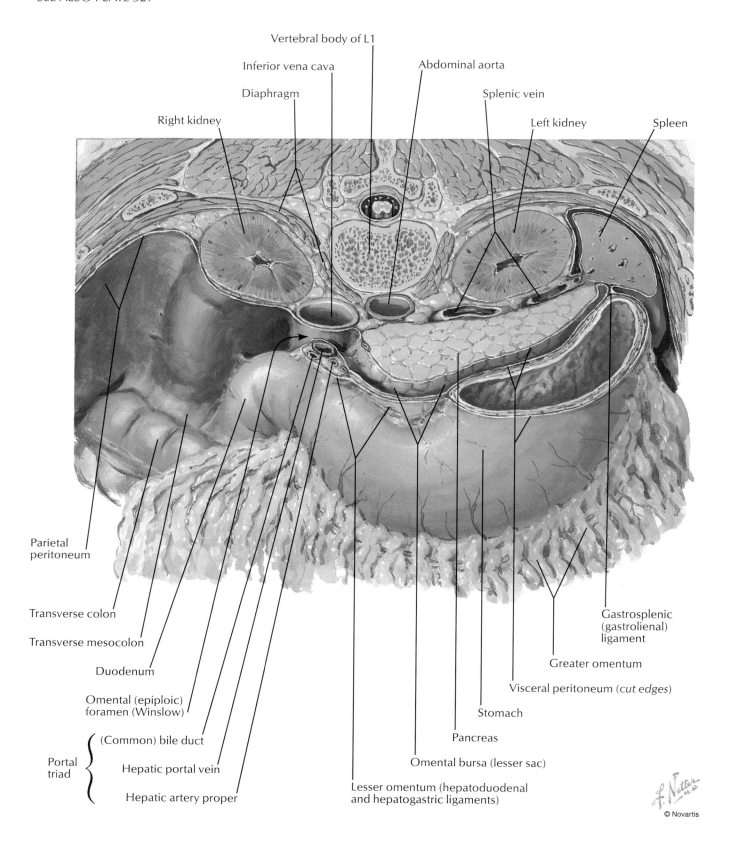

Vertebral body of L1

Inferior vena cava

Diaphragm

Abdominal aorta

Splenic vein

Right kidney

Left kidney

Spleen

Parietal peritoneum

Transverse colon

Transverse mesocolon

Duodenum

Omental (epiploic) foramen (Winslow)

(Common) bile duct

Portal triad

Hepatic portal vein

Hepatic artery proper

Lesser omentum (hepatoduodenal and hepatogastric ligaments)

Omental bursa (lesser sac)

Pancreas

Stomach

Visceral peritoneum (*cut edges*)

Greater omentum

Gastrosplenic (gastrolienal) ligament

© Novartis

**PLATE 256**

**ABDOMEN**

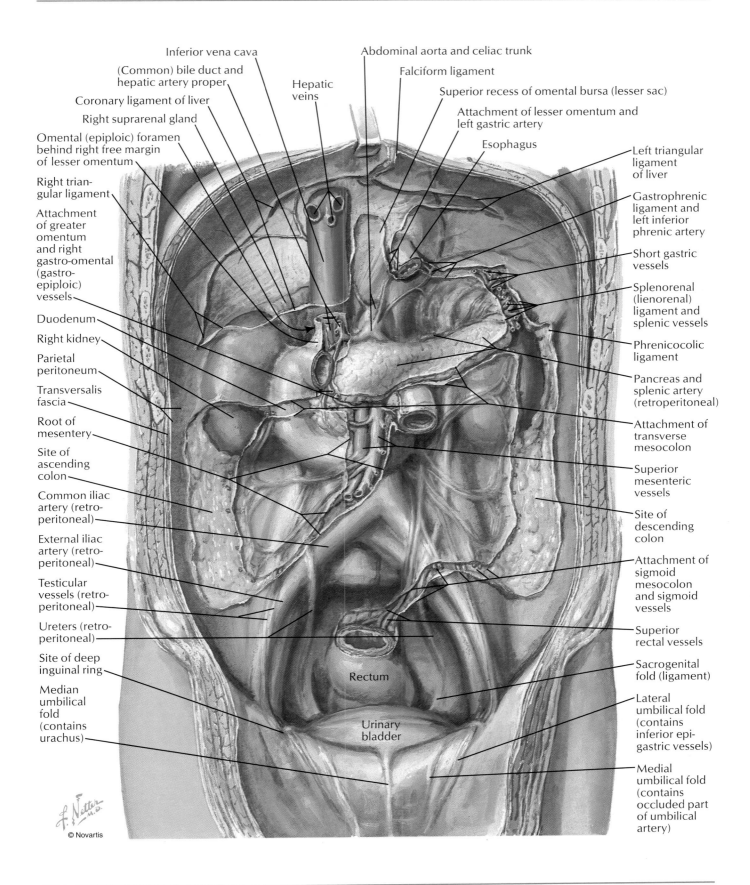

Inferior vena cava

(Common) bile duct and hepatic artery proper

Coronary ligament of liver

Right suprarenal gland

Omental (epiploic) foramen behind right free margin of lesser omentum

Right trian-gular ligament

Attachment of greater omentum and right gastro-omental (gastro-epiploic) vessels

Duodenum

Right kidney

Parietal peritoneum

Transversalis fascia

Root of mesentery

Site of ascending colon

Common iliac artery (retro-peritoneal)

External iliac artery (retro-peritoneal)

Testicular vessels (retro-peritoneal)

Ureters (retro-peritoneal)

Site of deep inguinal ring

Median umbilical fold (contains urachus)

Hepatic veins

Abdominal aorta and celiac trunk

Falciform ligament

Superior recess of omental bursa (lesser sac)

Attachment of lesser omentum and left gastric artery

Esophagus

Left triangular ligament of liver

Gastrophrenic ligament and left inferior phrenic artery

Short gastric vessels

Splenorenal (lienorenal) ligament and splenic vessels

Phrenicocolic ligament

Pancreas and splenic artery (retroperitoneal)

Attachment of transverse mesocolon

Superior mesenteric vessels

Site of descending colon

Attachment of sigmoid mesocolon and sigmoid vessels

Superior rectal vessels

Sacrogenital fold (ligament)

Lateral umbilical fold (contains inferior epi-gastric vessels)

Medial umbilical fold (contains occluded part of umbilical artery)

Rectum

Urinary bladder

© Novartis

**PERITONEAL CAVITY**

**PLATE 257**

# Stomach In Situ

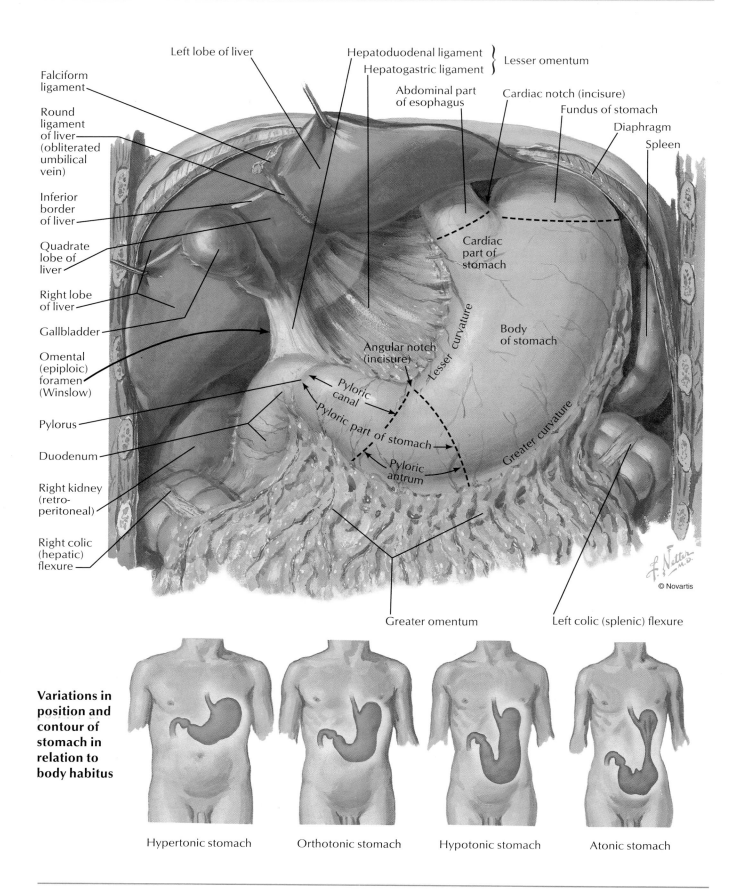

Falciform ligament

Round ligament of liver (obliterated umbilical vein)

Inferior border of liver

Quadrate lobe of liver

Right lobe of liver

Gallbladder

Omental (epiploic) foramen (Winslow)

Pylorus

Duodenum

Right kidney (retroperitoneal)

Right colic (hepatic) flexure

Left lobe of liver

Hepatoduodenal ligament
Hepatogastric ligament } Lesser omentum

Abdominal part of esophagus

Cardiac notch (incisure)

Fundus of stomach

Diaphragm

Spleen

Cardiac part of stomach

Lesser curvature

Body of stomach

Angular notch (incisure)

Pyloric canal

Pyloric part of stomach

Pyloric antrum

Greater curvature

Greater omentum

Left colic (splenic) flexure

**Variations in position and contour of stomach in relation to body habitus**

Hypertonic stomach

Orthotonic stomach

Hypotonic stomach

Atonic stomach

*PLATE 258*

**ABDOMEN**

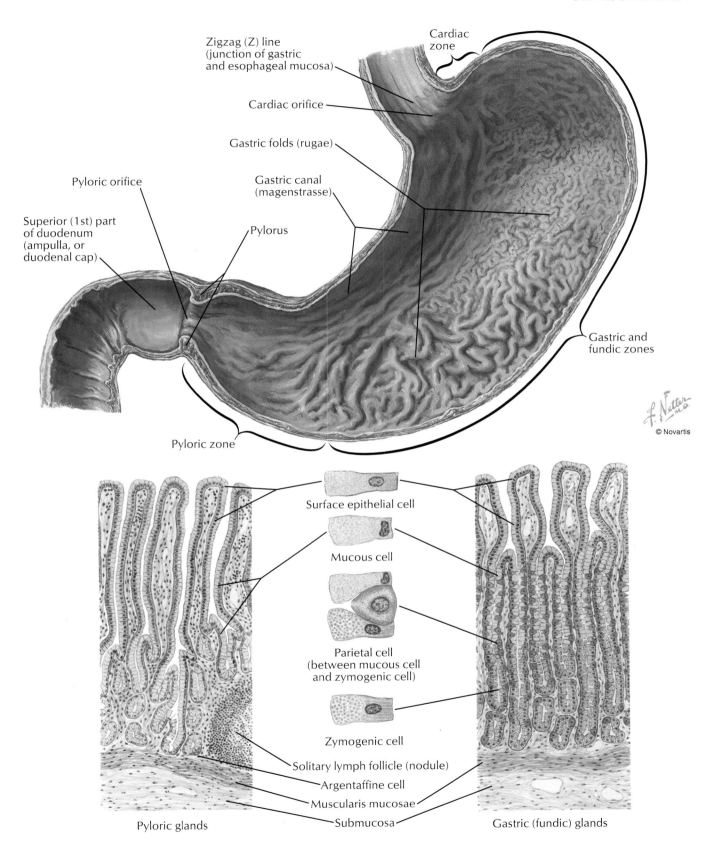

Zigzag (Z) line
(junction of gastric
and esophageal mucosa)

Cardiac
zone

Cardiac orifice

Gastric folds (rugae)

Pyloric orifice

Gastric canal
(magenstrasse)

Superior (1st) part
of duodenum
(ampulla, or
duodenal cap)

Pylorus

Gastric and
fundic zones

Pyloric zone

© Novartis

Surface epithelial cell

Mucous cell

Parietal cell
(between mucous cell
and zymogenic cell)

Zymogenic cell

Solitary lymph follicle (nodule)

Argentaffine cell

Muscularis mucosae

Pyloric glands

Submucosa

Gastric (fundic) glands

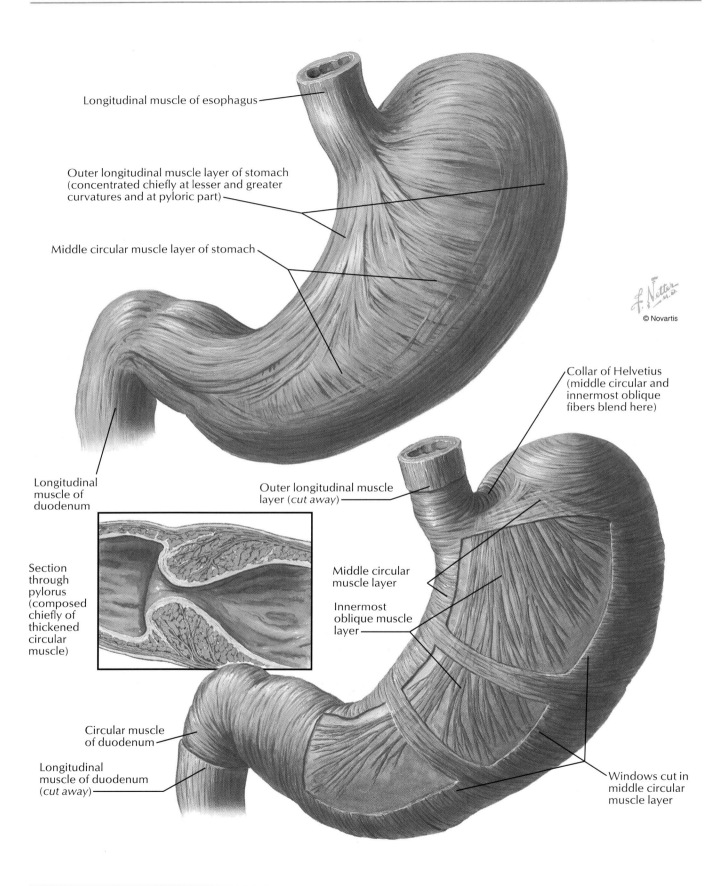

Longitudinal muscle of esophagus

Outer longitudinal muscle layer of stomach (concentrated chiefly at lesser and greater curvatures and at pyloric part)

Middle circular muscle layer of stomach

Longitudinal muscle of duodenum

Section through pylorus (composed chiefly of thickened circular muscle)

Circular muscle of duodenum

Longitudinal muscle of duodenum (*cut away*)

Collar of Helvetius (middle circular and innermost oblique fibers blend here)

Outer longitudinal muscle layer (*cut away*)

Middle circular muscle layer

Innermost oblique muscle layer

Windows cut in middle circular muscle layer

© Novartis

*PLATE 260*     **ABDOMEN**

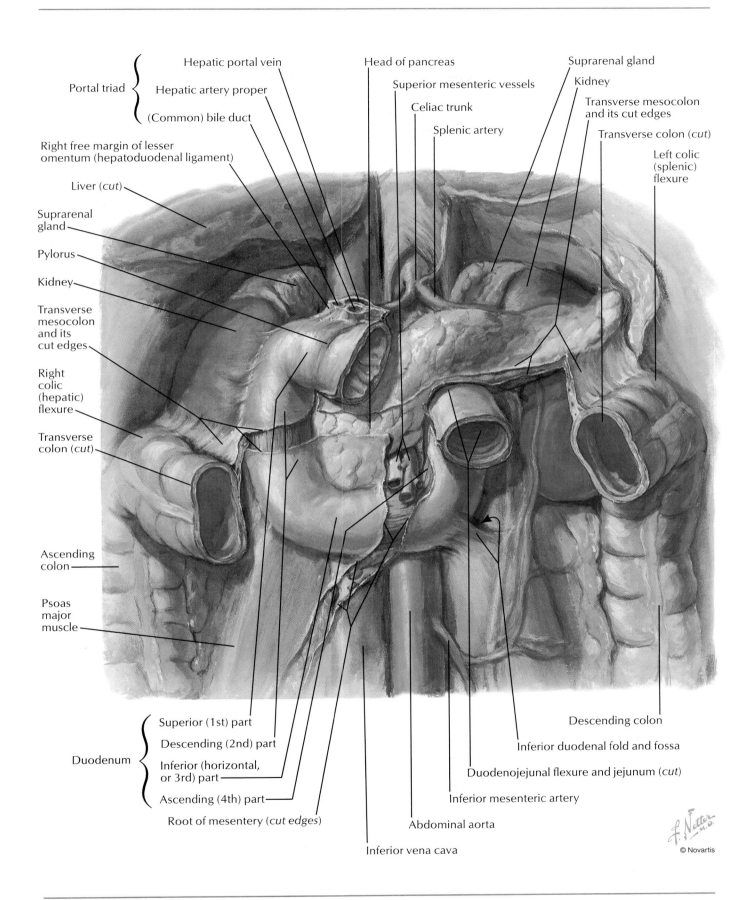

Portal triad
{
Hepatic portal vein

Hepatic artery proper

(Common) bile duct
}

Head of pancreas

Superior mesenteric vessels

Celiac trunk

Splenic artery

Suprarenal gland

Kidney

Transverse mesocolon and its cut edges

Transverse colon (*cut*)

Left colic (splenic) flexure

Right free margin of lesser omentum (hepatoduodenal ligament)

Liver (*cut*)

Suprarenal gland

Pylorus

Kidney

Transverse mesocolon and its cut edges

Right colic (hepatic) flexure

Transverse colon (*cut*)

Ascending colon

Psoas major muscle

Descending colon

Inferior duodenal fold and fossa

Duodenojejunal flexure and jejunum (*cut*)

Inferior mesenteric artery

Abdominal aorta

Inferior vena cava

Duodenum
{
Superior (1st) part

Descending (2nd) part

Inferior (horizontal, or 3rd) part

Ascending (4th) part
}

Root of mesentery (*cut edges*)

F. Netter M.D.

© Novartis

# Mucosa and Musculature of Duodenum

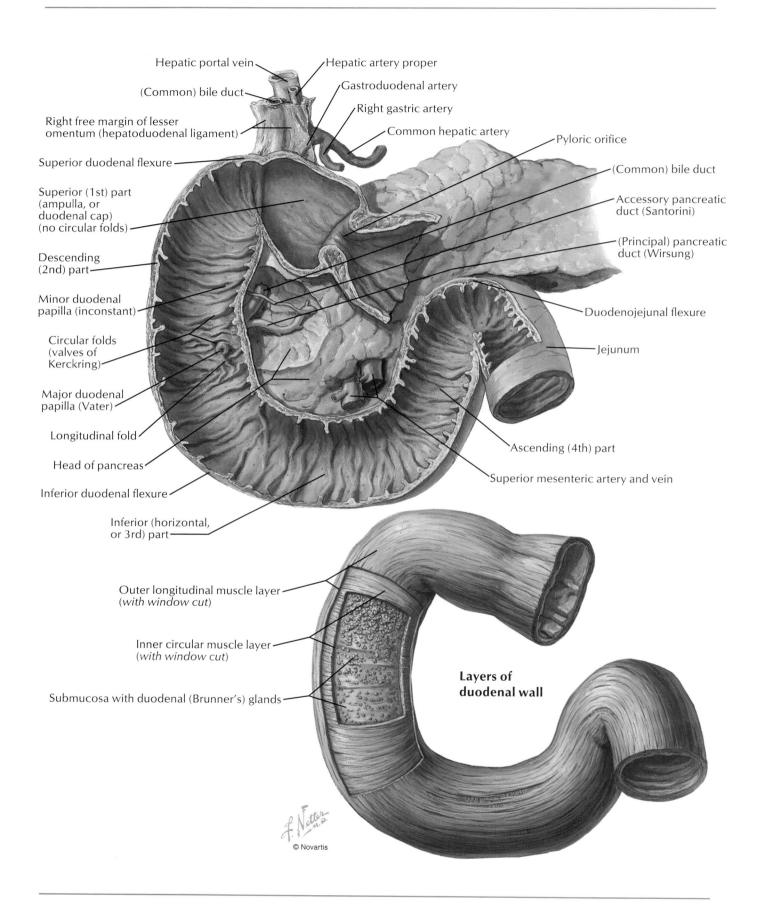

Hepatic portal vein

Hepatic artery proper

(Common) bile duct

Gastroduodenal artery

Right gastric artery

Right free margin of lesser omentum (hepatoduodenal ligament)

Common hepatic artery

Pyloric orifice

Superior duodenal flexure

(Common) bile duct

Superior (1st) part (ampulla, or duodenal cap) (no circular folds)

Accessory pancreatic duct (Santorini)

(Principal) pancreatic duct (Wirsung)

Descending (2nd) part

Minor duodenal papilla (inconstant)

Duodenojejunal flexure

Circular folds (valves of Kerckring)

Jejunum

Major duodenal papilla (Vater)

Longitudinal fold

Head of pancreas

Ascending (4th) part

Inferior duodenal flexure

Superior mesenteric artery and vein

Inferior (horizontal, or 3rd) part

Outer longitudinal muscle layer (*with window cut*)

Inner circular muscle layer (*with window cut*)

**Layers of duodenal wall**

Submucosa with duodenal (Brunner's) glands

© Novartis

*PLATE 262*

**ABDOMEN**

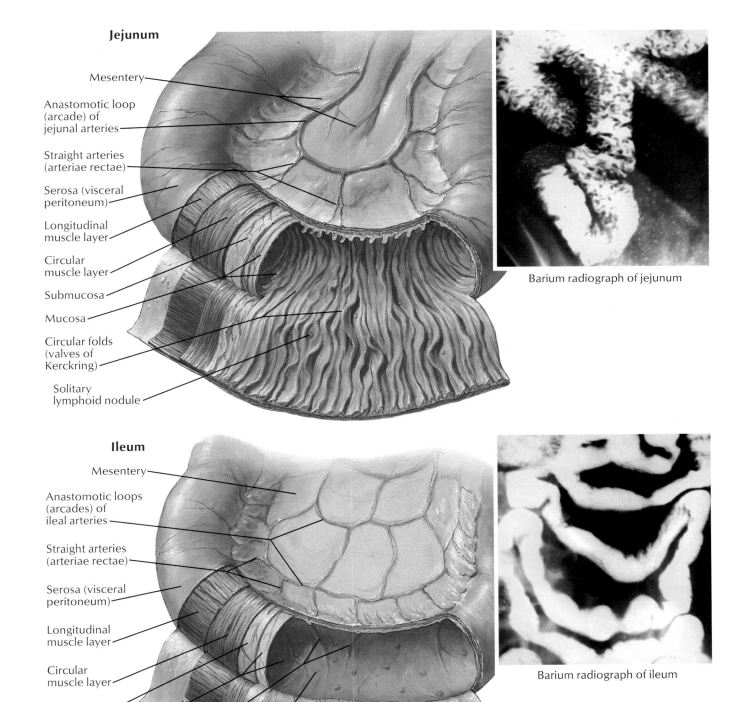

**Jejunum**

Mesentery

Anastomotic loop (arcade) of jejunal arteries

Straight arteries (arteriae rectae)

Serosa (visceral peritoneum)

Longitudinal muscle layer

Circular muscle layer

Submucosa

Mucosa

Circular folds (valves of Kerckring)

Solitary lymphoid nodule

Barium radiograph of jejunum

**Ileum**

Mesentery

Anastomotic loops (arcades) of ileal arteries

Straight arteries (arteriae rectae)

Serosa (visceral peritoneum)

Longitudinal muscle layer

Circular muscle layer

Submucosa

Mucosa

Circular folds

Solitary lymphoid nodules

Aggregate lymphoid nodules (Peyer's patches)

Barium radiograph of ileum

© Novartis

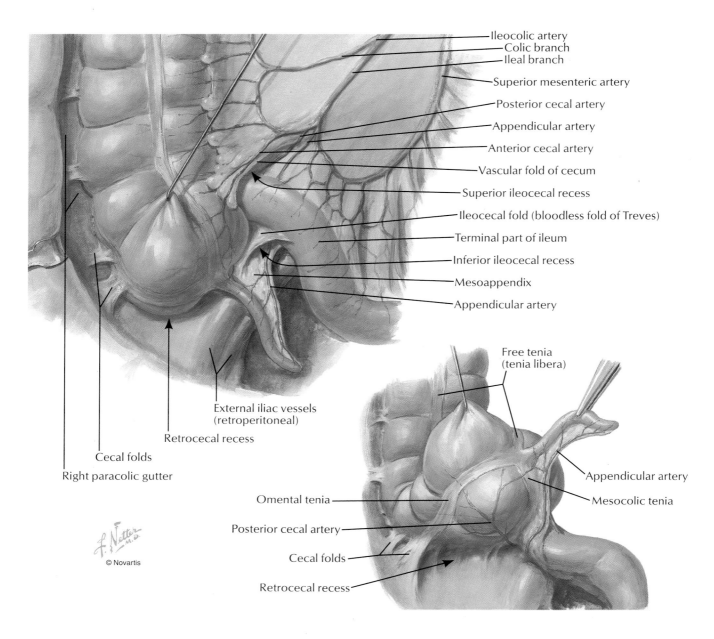

Ileocolic artery
Colic branch
Ileal branch
Superior mesenteric artery
Posterior cecal artery
Appendicular artery
Anterior cecal artery
Vascular fold of cecum
Superior ileocecal recess
Ileocecal fold (bloodless fold of Treves)
Terminal part of ileum
Inferior ileocecal recess
Mesoappendix
Appendicular artery

External iliac vessels (retroperitoneal)

Retrocecal recess

Cecal folds

Right paracolic gutter

Free tenia (tenia libera)

Appendicular artery

Mesocolic tenia

Omental tenia

Posterior cecal artery

Cecal folds

Retrocecal recess

**Some variations in posterior peritoneal attachment of cecum**

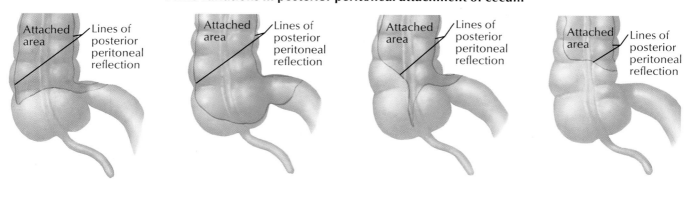

Attached area — Lines of posterior peritoneal reflection

Attached area — Lines of posterior peritoneal reflection

Attached area — Lines of posterior peritoneal reflection

Attached area — Lines of posterior peritoneal reflection

*PLATE 264*

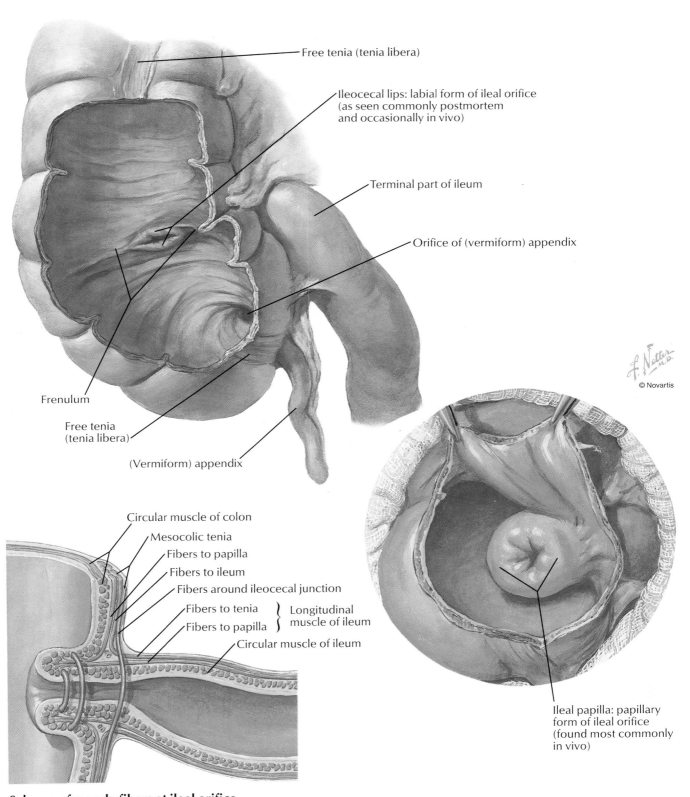

Free tenia (tenia libera)

Ileocecal lips: labial form of ileal orifice
(as seen commonly postmortem
and occasionally in vivo)

Terminal part of ileum

Orifice of (vermiform) appendix

Frenulum

Free tenia
(tenia libera)

(Vermiform) appendix

Ileal papilla: papillary
form of ileal orifice
(found most commonly
in vivo)

Circular muscle of colon
Mesocolic tenia
Fibers to papilla
Fibers to ileum
Fibers around ileocecal junction
Fibers to tenia } Longitudinal
Fibers to papilla } muscle of ileum
Circular muscle of ileum

**Schema of muscle fibers at ileal orifice**

© Novartis

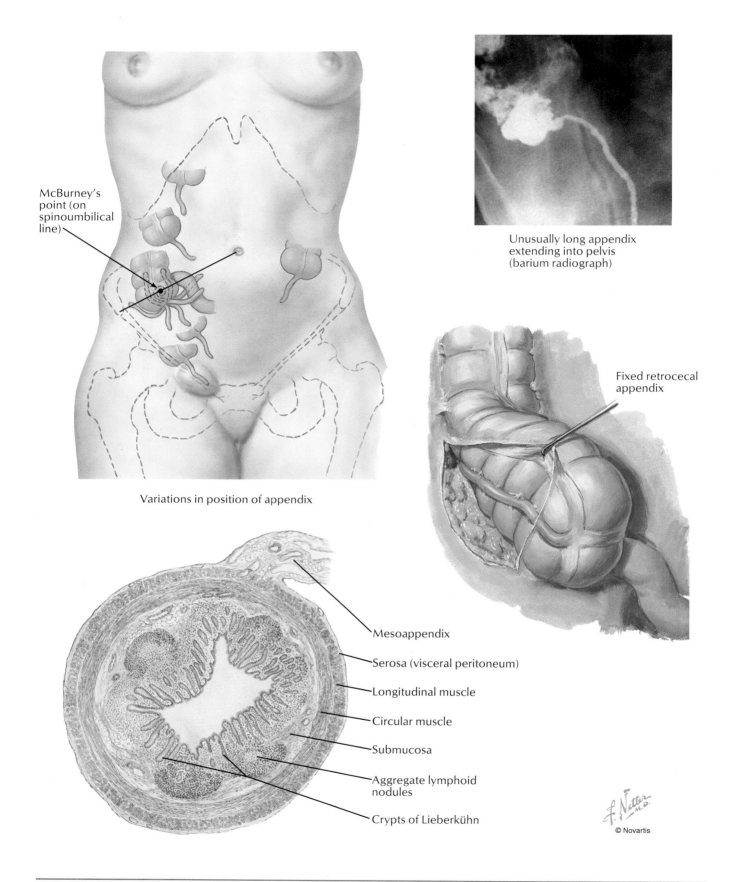

McBurney's point (on spinoumbilical line)

Variations in position of appendix

Unusually long appendix extending into pelvis (barium radiograph)

Fixed retrocecal appendix

Mesoappendix

Serosa (visceral peritoneum)

Longitudinal muscle

Circular muscle

Submucosa

Aggregate lymphoid nodules

Crypts of Lieberkühn

© Novartis

*PLATE 266*

**ABDOMEN**

*FOR RECTUM AND ANAL CANAL SEE PLATES 363–368*

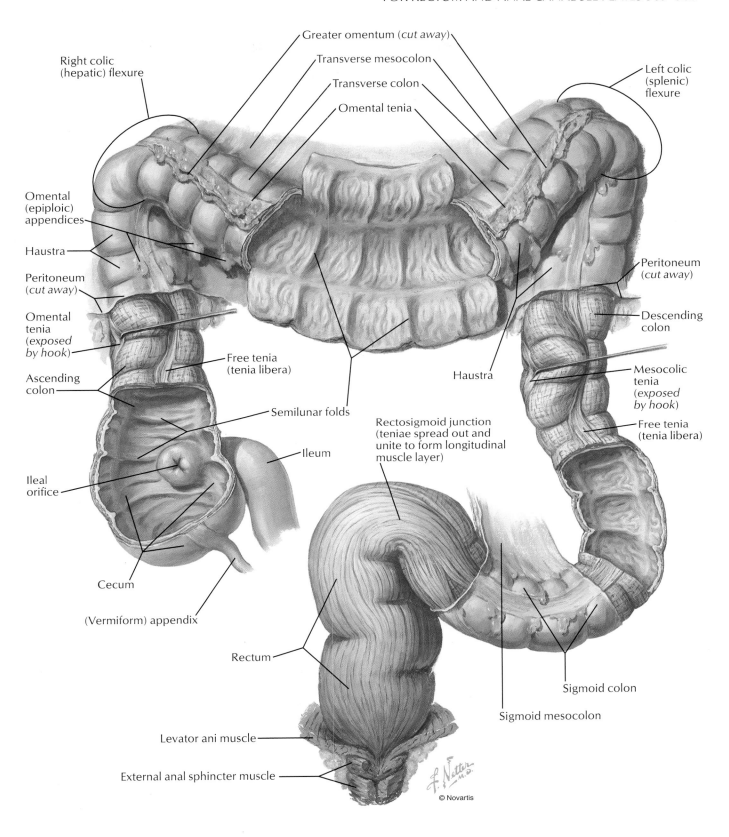

Right colic (hepatic) flexure

Greater omentum (*cut away*)

Transverse mesocolon

Transverse colon

Omental tenia

Left colic (splenic) flexure

Omental (epiploic) appendices

Haustra

Peritoneum (*cut away*)

Omental tenia (*exposed by hook*)

Ascending colon

Ileal orifice

Free tenia (tenia libera)

Semilunar folds

Ileum

Cecum

(Vermiform) appendix

Rectum

Peritoneum (*cut away*)

Descending colon

Haustra

Mesocolic tenia (*exposed by hook*)

Free tenia (tenia libera)

Rectosigmoid junction (teniae spread out and unite to form longitudinal muscle layer)

Sigmoid colon

Sigmoid mesocolon

Levator ani muscle

External anal sphincter muscle

*F. Netter*
© Novartis

# Sigmoid Colon: Variations in Position

FOR RECTUM SEE PLATES 337, 338, 363, 364, 365, 366

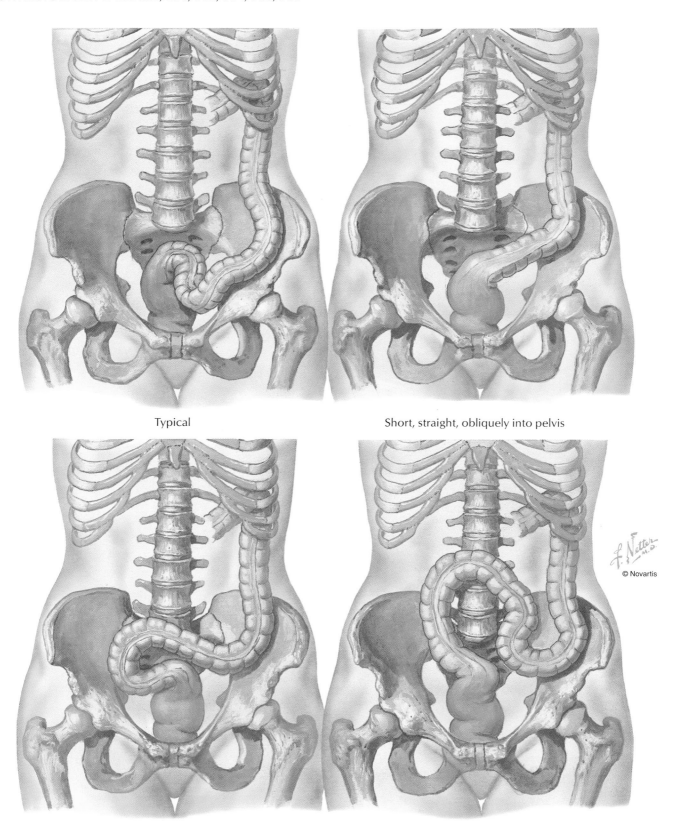

Typical

Short, straight, obliquely into pelvis

Looping to right side

Ascending high into abdomen

**PLATE 268**

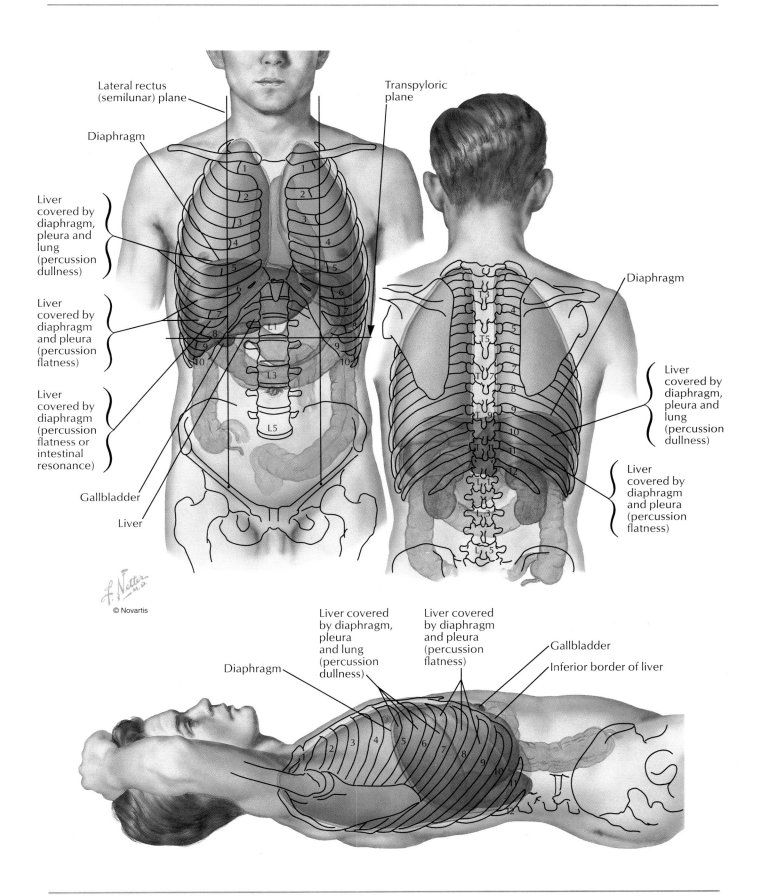

Lateral rectus (semilunar) plane

Transpyloric plane

Diaphragm

Liver covered by diaphragm, pleura and lung (percussion dullness)

Liver covered by diaphragm and pleura (percussion flatness)

Liver covered by diaphragm (percussion flatness or intestinal resonance)

Gallbladder

Liver

Diaphragm

Liver covered by diaphragm, pleura and lung (percussion dullness)

Liver covered by diaphragm and pleura (percussion flatness)

© Novartis

Liver covered by diaphragm, pleura and lung (percussion dullness)

Liver covered by diaphragm and pleura (percussion flatness)

Diaphragm

Gallbladder

Inferior border of liver

**VISCERA (ACCESSORY ORGANS)**

**PLATE 269**

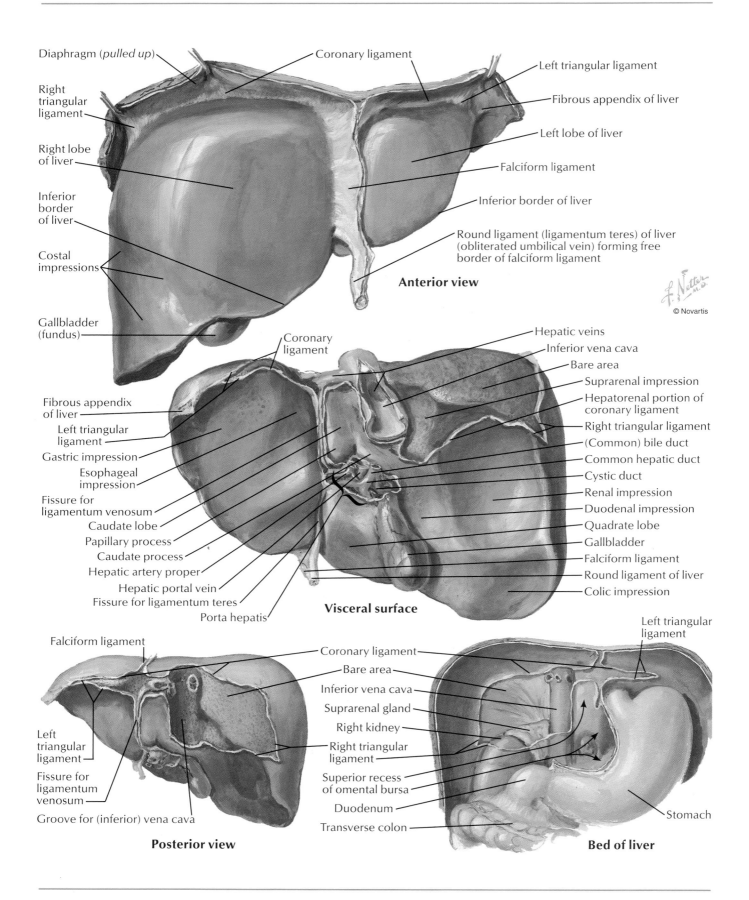

Diaphragm (*pulled up*)

Coronary ligament

Left triangular ligament

Right triangular ligament

Fibrous appendix of liver

Right lobe of liver

Left lobe of liver

Inferior border of liver

Falciform ligament

Inferior border of liver

Costal impressions

Round ligament (ligamentum teres) of liver (obliterated umbilical vein) forming free border of falciform ligament

Gallbladder (fundus)

**Anterior view**

© Novartis

Coronary ligament

Hepatic veins

Inferior vena cava

Bare area

Suprarenal impression

Fibrous appendix of liver

Hepatorenal portion of coronary ligament

Left triangular ligament

Right triangular ligament

Gastric impression

(Common) bile duct

Esophageal impression

Common hepatic duct

Fissure for ligamentum venosum

Cystic duct

Caudate lobe

Renal impression

Papillary process

Duodenal impression

Caudate process

Quadrate lobe

Hepatic artery proper

Gallbladder

Hepatic portal vein

Falciform ligament

Fissure for ligamentum teres

Round ligament of liver

Porta hepatis

Colic impression

**Visceral surface**

Falciform ligament

Coronary ligament

Left triangular ligament

Bare area

Inferior vena cava

Suprarenal gland

Right kidney

Left triangular ligament

Right triangular ligament

Fissure for ligamentum venosum

Superior recess of omental bursa

Groove for (inferior) vena cava

Duodenum

Transverse colon

Stomach

**Posterior view**

**Bed of liver**

**PLATE 270**

**ABDOMEN**

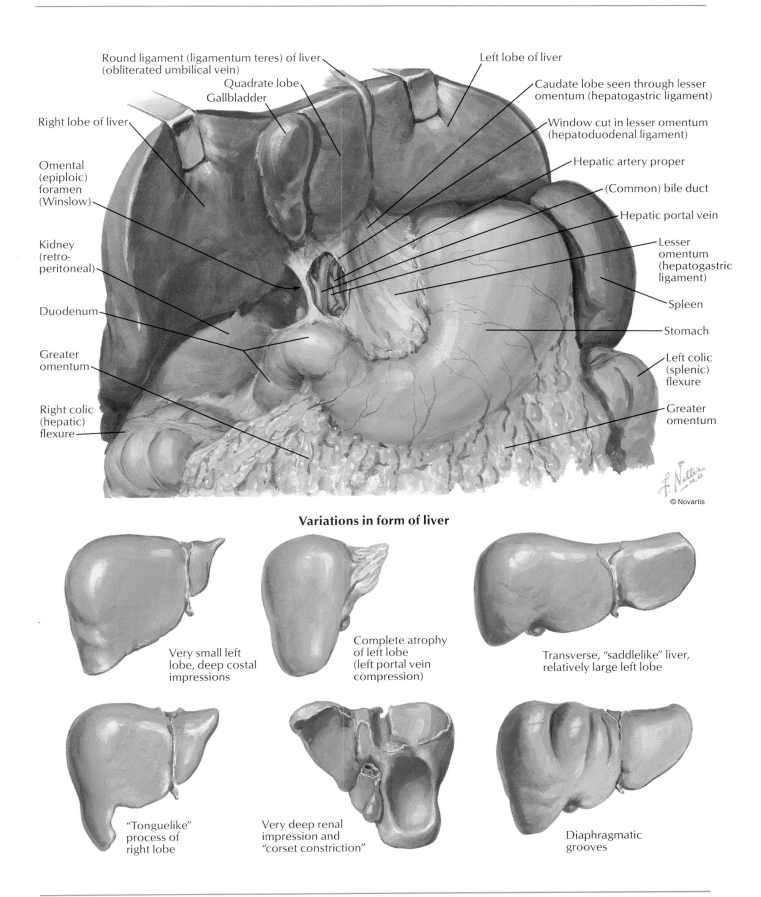

Round ligament (ligamentum teres) of liver (obliterated umbilical vein)

Quadrate lobe

Gallbladder

Right lobe of liver

Omental (epiploic) foramen (Winslow)

Kidney (retroperitoneal)

Duodenum

Greater omentum

Right colic (hepatic) flexure

Left lobe of liver

Caudate lobe seen through lesser omentum (hepatogastric ligament)

Window cut in lesser omentum (hepatoduodenal ligament)

Hepatic artery proper

(Common) bile duct

Hepatic portal vein

Lesser omentum (hepatogastric ligament)

Spleen

Stomach

Left colic (splenic) flexure

Greater omentum

© Novartis

**Variations in form of liver**

Very small left lobe, deep costal impressions

Complete atrophy of left lobe (left portal vein compression)

Transverse, "saddlelike" liver, relatively large left lobe

"Tonguelike" process of right lobe

Very deep renal impression and "corset constriction"

Diaphragmatic grooves

# Liver Segments and Lobes: Vessel and Duct Distribution

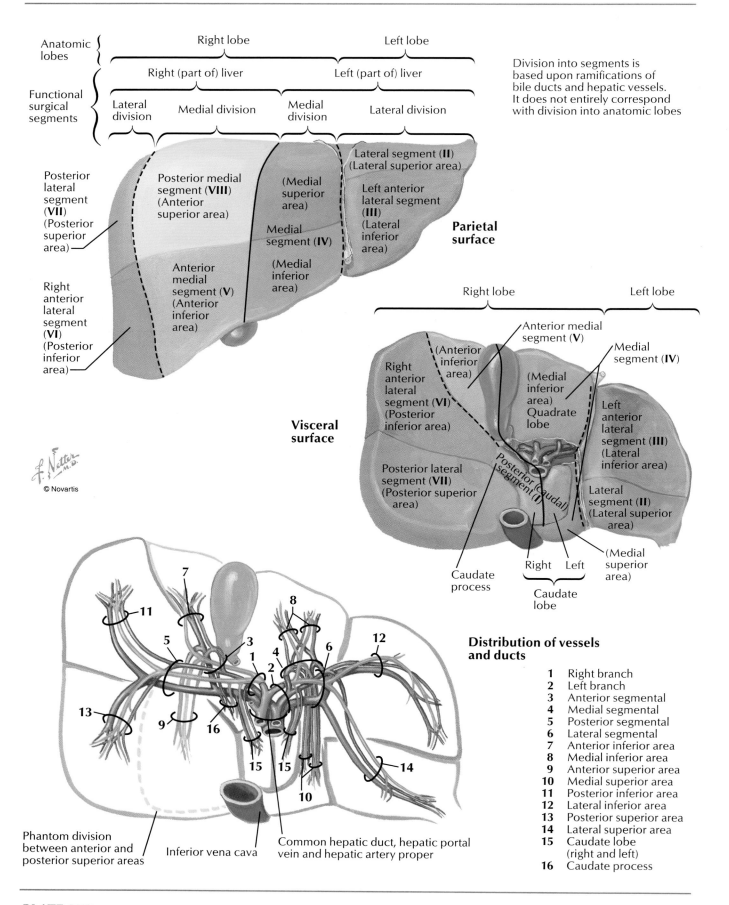

Anatomic lobes

Right lobe

Left lobe

Functional surgical segments

Right (part of) liver

Left (part of) liver

Lateral division

Medial division

Medial division

Lateral division

Division into segments is based upon ramifications of bile ducts and hepatic vessels. It does not entirely correspond with division into anatomic lobes

Posterior lateral segment (**VII**) (Posterior superior area)

Right anterior lateral segment (**VI**) (Posterior inferior area)

Posterior medial segment (**VIII**) (Anterior superior area)

Anterior medial segment (**V**) (Anterior inferior area)

(Medial superior area)

Medial segment (**IV**)

(Medial inferior area)

Lateral segment (**II**) (Lateral superior area)

Left anterior lateral segment (**III**) (Lateral inferior area)

**Parietal surface**

**Visceral surface**

Right lobe

Left lobe

Anterior medial segment (**V**)

Medial segment (**IV**)

Right anterior lateral segment (**VI**) (Posterior inferior area)

(Anterior inferior area)

(Medial inferior area) Quadrate lobe

Left anterior lateral segment (**III**) (Lateral inferior area)

Posterior lateral segment (**VII**) (Posterior superior area)

Posterior (Caudal) segment (**I**)

Lateral segment (**II**) (Lateral superior area)

Right    Left

Caudate lobe

(Medial superior area)

Caudate process

Phantom division between anterior and posterior superior areas

Inferior vena cava

Common hepatic duct, hepatic portal vein and hepatic artery proper

**Distribution of vessels and ducts**

**1** Right branch
**2** Left branch
**3** Anterior segmental
**4** Medial segmental
**5** Posterior segmental
**6** Lateral segmental
**7** Anterior inferior area
**8** Medial inferior area
**9** Anterior superior area
**10** Medial superior area
**11** Posterior inferior area
**12** Lateral inferior area
**13** Posterior superior area
**14** Lateral superior area
**15** Caudate lobe (right and left)
**16** Caudate process

**PLATE 272**

**ABDOMEN**

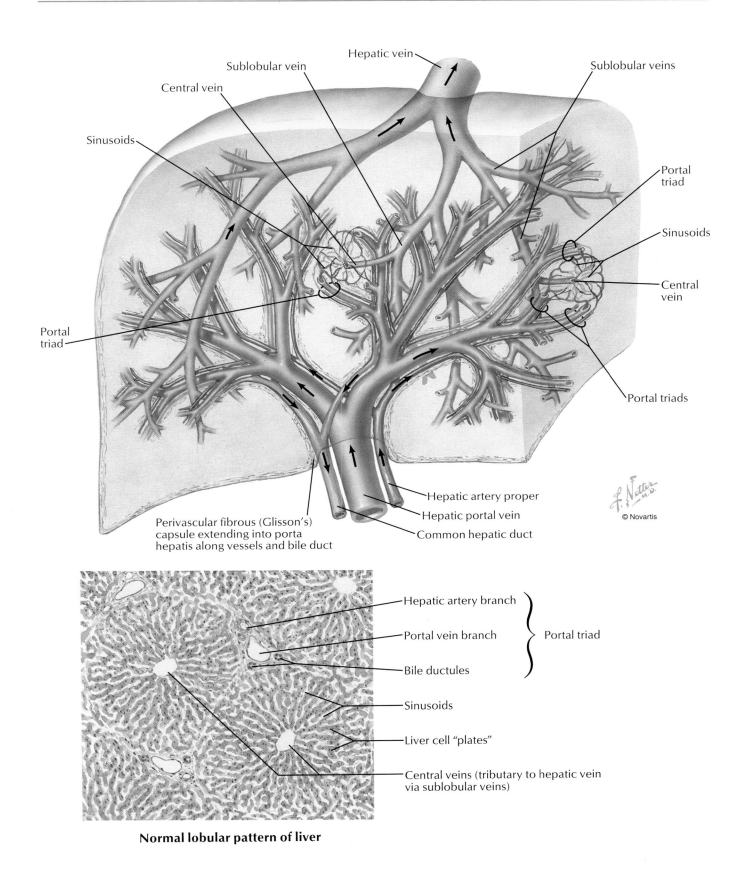

Hepatic vein

Sublobular vein

Central vein

Sinusoids

Sublobular veins

Portal triad

Sinusoids

Central vein

Portal triad

Portal triads

Perivascular fibrous (Glisson's) capsule extending into porta hepatis along vessels and bile duct

Hepatic artery proper

Hepatic portal vein

Common hepatic duct

Hepatic artery branch

Portal vein branch

Bile ductules

Portal triad

Sinusoids

Liver cell "plates"

Central veins (tributary to hepatic vein via sublobular veins)

© Novartis

**Normal lobular pattern of liver**

# Liver Structure: Schema

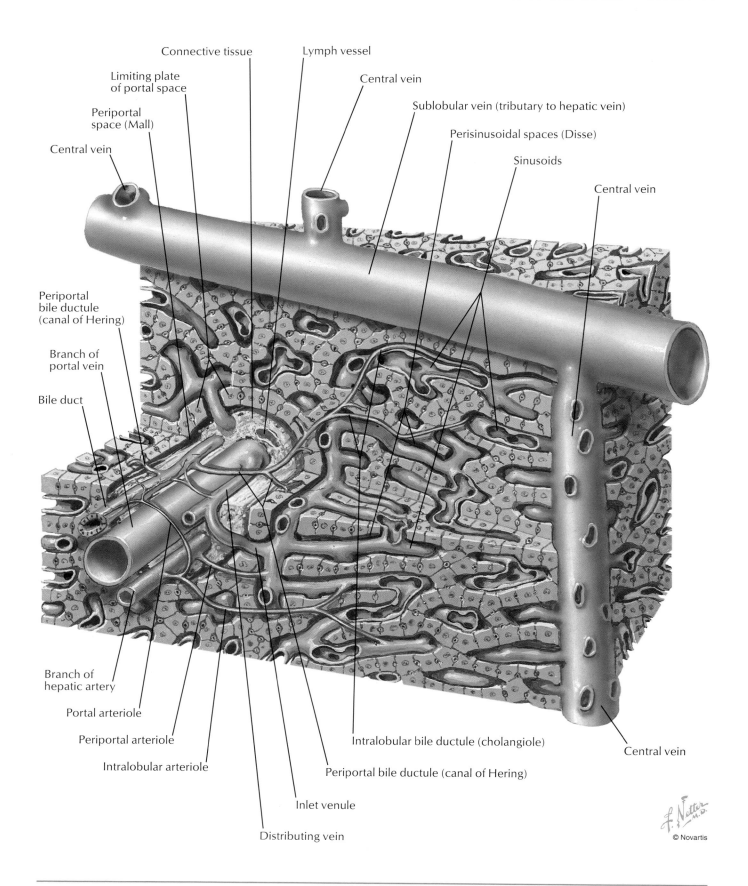

Connective tissue

Limiting plate
of portal space

Lymph vessel

Central vein

Periportal
space (Mall)

Sublobular vein (tributary to hepatic vein)

Central vein

Perisinusoidal spaces (Disse)

Sinusoids

Central vein

Periportal
bile ductule
(canal of Hering)

Branch of
portal vein

Bile duct

Branch of
hepatic artery

Portal arteriole

Periportal arteriole

Intralobular arteriole

Intralobular bile ductule (cholangiole)

Central vein

Periportal bile ductule (canal of Hering)

Inlet venule

Distributing vein

**PLATE 274**

**ABDOMEN**

© Novartis

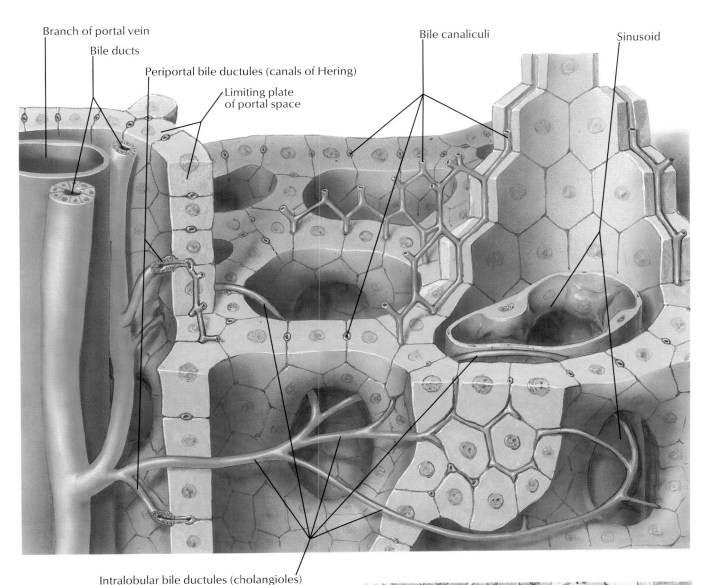

Branch of portal vein

Bile ducts

Periportal bile ductules (canals of Hering)

Limiting plate of portal space

Bile canaliculi

Sinusoid

Intralobular bile ductules (cholangioles)

Note: In above illustration, bile canaliculi appear as structures with walls of their own. However, as shown in histologic section at right, boundaries of canaliculi are actually a specialization of surface membranes of adjoining liver parenchymal cells

© Novartis

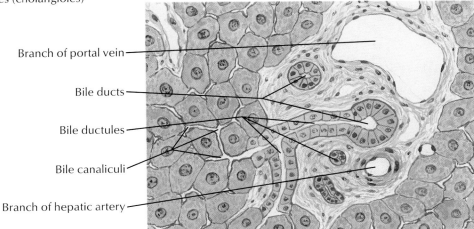

Branch of portal vein

Bile ducts

Bile ductules

Bile canaliculi

Branch of hepatic artery

**Low-power section of liver**

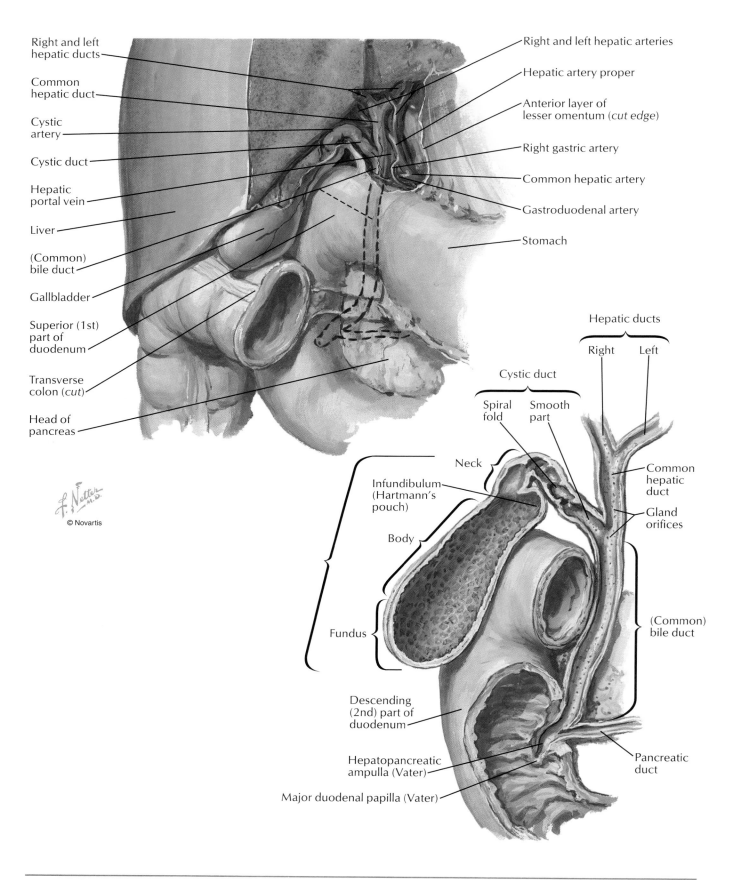

Right and left
hepatic ducts

Common
hepatic duct

Cystic
artery

Cystic duct

Hepatic
portal vein

Liver

(Common)
bile duct

Gallbladder

Superior (1st)
part of
duodenum

Transverse
colon (*cut*)

Head of
pancreas

© Novartis

Right and left hepatic arteries

Hepatic artery proper

Anterior layer of
lesser omentum (*cut edge*)

Right gastric artery

Common hepatic artery

Gastroduodenal artery

Stomach

Hepatic ducts

Right        Left

Cystic duct

Spiral     Smooth
fold        part

Neck

Infundibulum
(Hartmann's
pouch)

Body

Fundus

Descending
(2nd) part of
duodenum

Hepatopancreatic
ampulla (Vater)

Major duodenal papilla (Vater)

Common
hepatic
duct

Gland
orifices

(Common)
bile duct

Pancreatic
duct

*PLATE 276*

**ABDOMEN**

## Variations in cystic duct

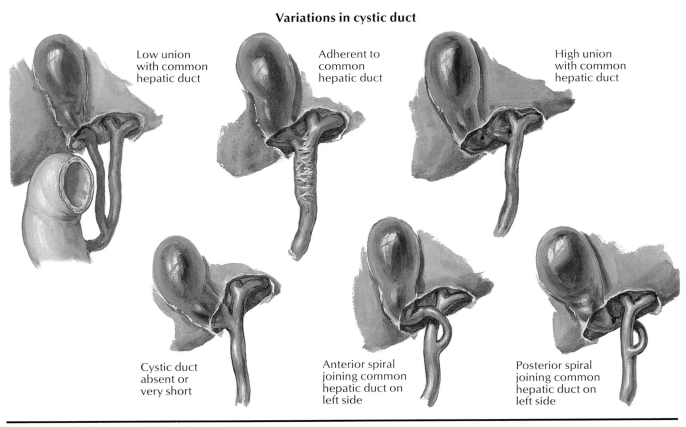

Low union with common hepatic duct

Adherent to common hepatic duct

High union with common hepatic duct

Cystic duct absent or very short

Anterior spiral joining common hepatic duct on left side

Posterior spiral joining common hepatic duct on left side

## Accessory (aberrant) hepatic ducts

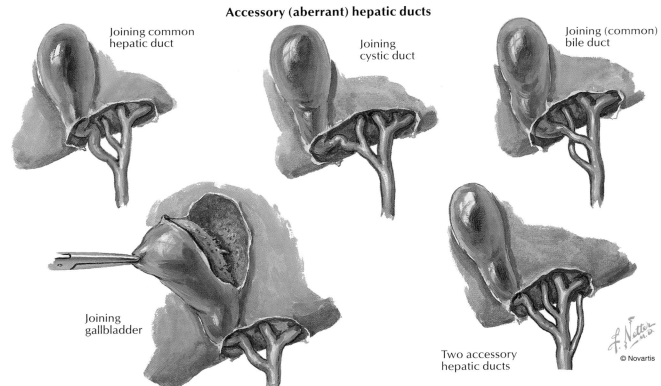

Joining common hepatic duct

Joining cystic duct

Joining (common) bile duct

Joining gallbladder

Two accessory hepatic ducts

© Novartis

# Junction of (Common) Bile Duct and Duodenum

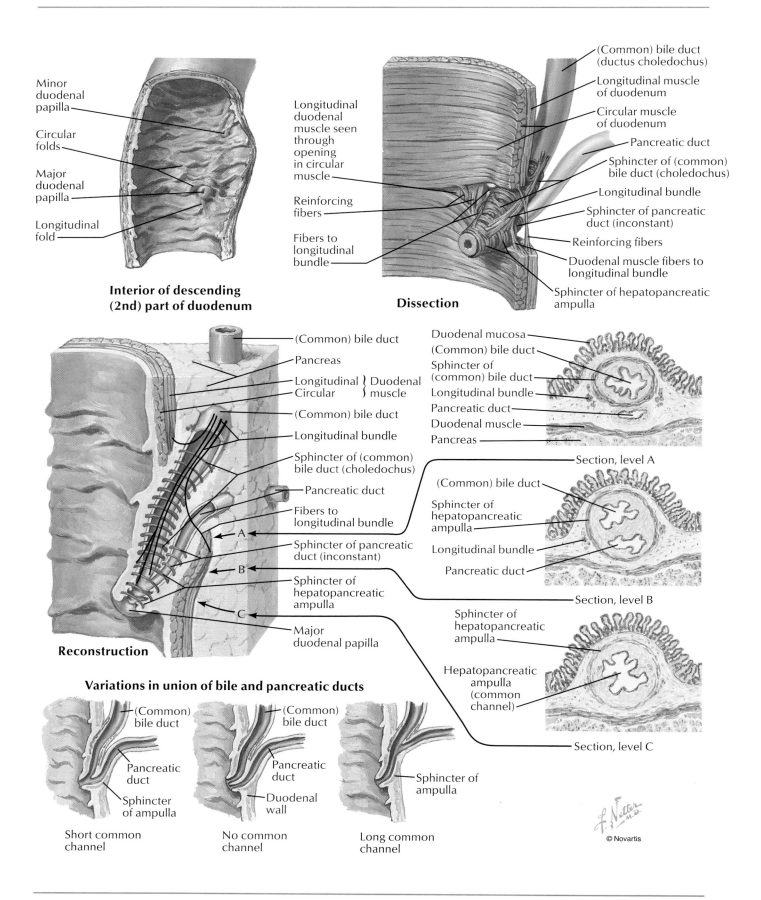

**Interior of descending (2nd) part of duodenum**

Minor duodenal papilla

Circular folds

Major duodenal papilla

Longitudinal fold

**Dissection**

Longitudinal duodenal muscle seen through opening in circular muscle

Reinforcing fibers

Fibers to longitudinal bundle

(Common) bile duct (ductus choledochus)

Longitudinal muscle of duodenum

Circular muscle of duodenum

Pancreatic duct

Sphincter of (common) bile duct (choledochus)

Longitudinal bundle

Sphincter of pancreatic duct (inconstant)

Reinforcing fibers

Duodenal muscle fibers to longitudinal bundle

Sphincter of hepatopancreatic ampulla

**Reconstruction**

(Common) bile duct

Pancreas

Longitudinal  } Duodenal
Circular      } muscle

(Common) bile duct

Longitudinal bundle

Sphincter of (common) bile duct (choledochus)

Pancreatic duct

Fibers to longitudinal bundle

Sphincter of pancreatic duct (inconstant)

Sphincter of hepatopancreatic ampulla

Major duodenal papilla

Duodenal mucosa

(Common) bile duct

Sphincter of (common) bile duct

Longitudinal bundle

Pancreatic duct

Duodenal muscle

Pancreas

**Section, level A**

(Common) bile duct

Sphincter of hepatopancreatic ampulla

Longitudinal bundle

Pancreatic duct

**Section, level B**

Sphincter of hepatopancreatic ampulla

Hepatopancreatic ampulla (common channel)

**Section, level C**

## Variations in union of bile and pancreatic ducts

(Common) bile duct

Pancreatic duct

Sphincter of ampulla

**Short common channel**

(Common) bile duct

Pancreatic duct

Duodenal wall

**No common channel**

Sphincter of ampulla

**Long common channel**

© Novartis

**PLATE 278**

**ABDOMEN**

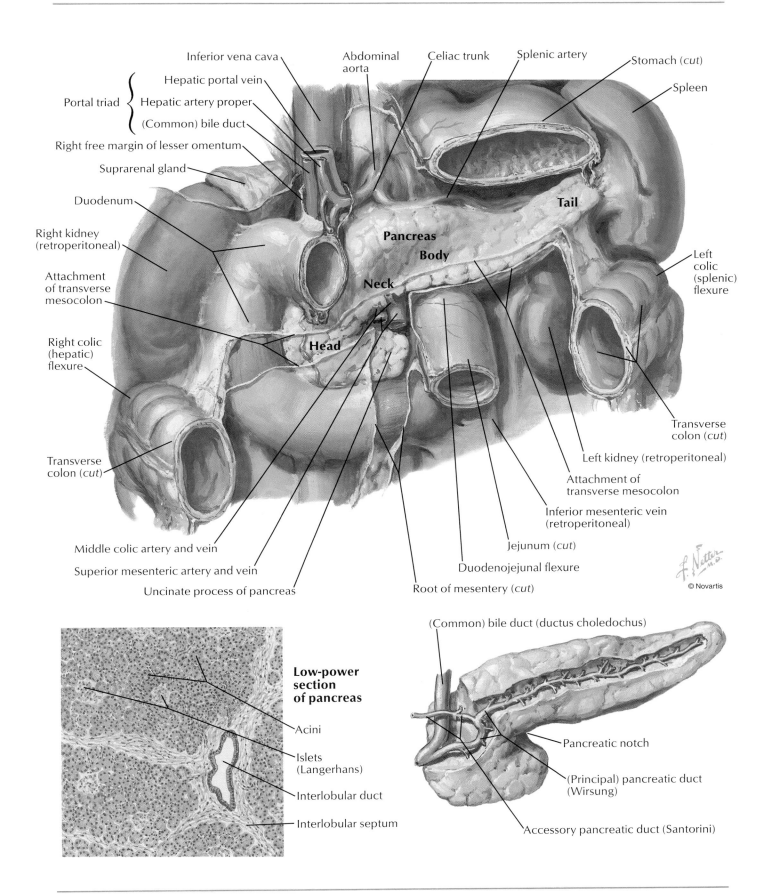

Inferior vena cava

Abdominal aorta

Celiac trunk

Splenic artery

Stomach (*cut*)

Spleen

Portal triad {
Hepatic portal vein
Hepatic artery proper
(Common) bile duct
}

Right free margin of lesser omentum

Suprarenal gland

Duodenum

Right kidney (retroperitoneal)

Attachment of transverse mesocolon

Right colic (hepatic) flexure

Transverse colon (*cut*)

Middle colic artery and vein

Superior mesenteric artery and vein

Uncinate process of pancreas

**Pancreas Body**

**Tail**

**Neck**

**Head**

Left colic (splenic) flexure

Transverse colon (*cut*)

Left kidney (retroperitoneal)

Attachment of transverse mesocolon

Inferior mesenteric vein (retroperitoneal)

Jejunum (*cut*)

Duodenojejunal flexure

Root of mesentery (*cut*)

**Low-power section of pancreas**

Acini

Islets (Langerhans)

Interlobular duct

Interlobular septum

(Common) bile duct (ductus choledochus)

Pancreatic notch

(Principal) pancreatic duct (Wirsung)

Accessory pancreatic duct (Santorini)

*F. Netter M.D.*
© Novartis

**VISCERA (ACCESSORY ORGANS)**

*PLATE 279*

# Variations in Pancreatic Ducts

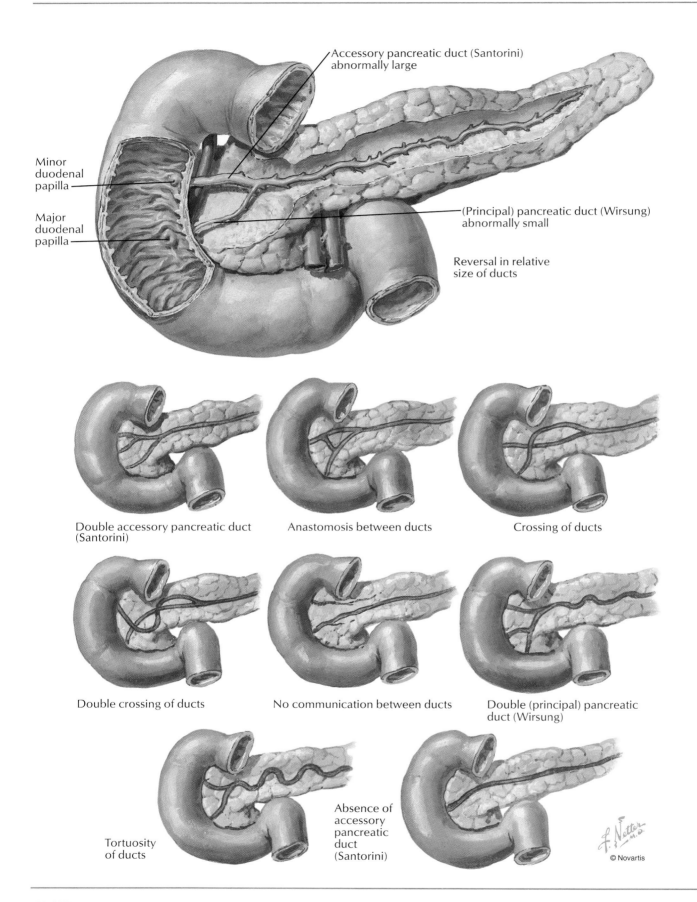

Accessory pancreatic duct (Santorini) abnormally large

Minor duodenal papilla

Major duodenal papilla

(Principal) pancreatic duct (Wirsung) abnormally small

Reversal in relative size of ducts

Double accessory pancreatic duct (Santorini)

Anastomosis between ducts

Crossing of ducts

Double crossing of ducts

No communication between ducts

Double (principal) pancreatic duct (Wirsung)

Tortuosity of ducts

Absence of accessory pancreatic duct (Santorini)

© Novartis

**PLATE 280**    **ABDOMEN**

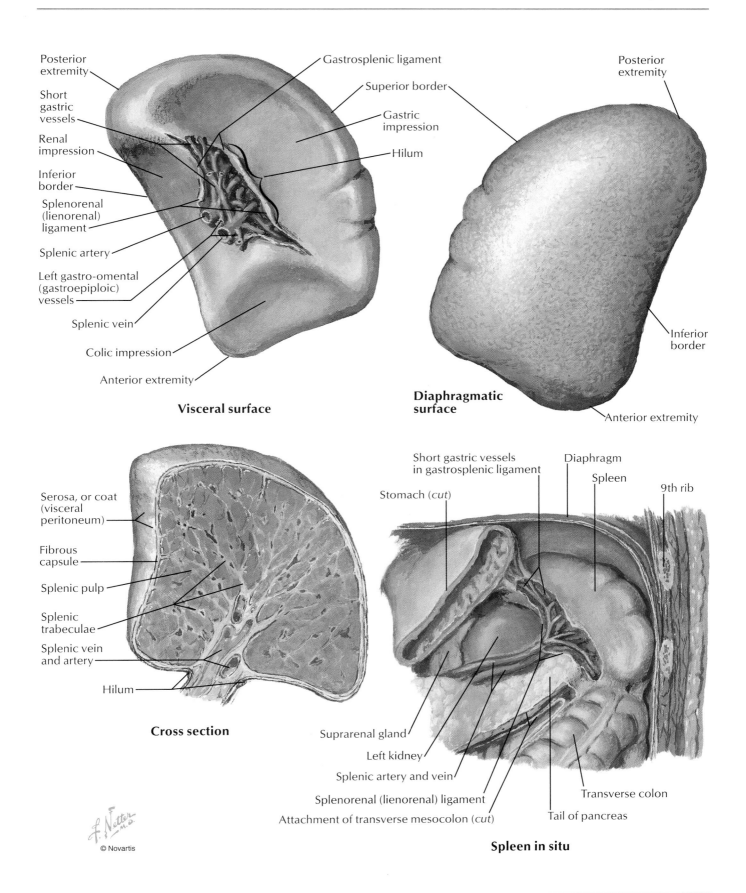

Posterior extremity

Short gastric vessels

Renal impression

Inferior border

Splenorenal (lienorenal) ligament

Splenic artery

Left gastro-omental (gastroepiploic) vessels

Splenic vein

Colic impression

Anterior extremity

Gastrosplenic ligament

Superior border

Gastric impression

Hilum

**Visceral surface**

Posterior extremity

Inferior border

Anterior extremity

**Diaphragmatic surface**

Serosa, or coat (visceral peritoneum)

Fibrous capsule

Splenic pulp

Splenic trabeculae

Splenic vein and artery

Hilum

**Cross section**

Short gastric vessels in gastrosplenic ligament

Stomach (*cut*)

Diaphragm

Spleen

9th rib

Suprarenal gland

Left kidney

Splenic artery and vein

Splenorenal (lienorenal) ligament

Attachment of transverse mesocolon (*cut*)

Transverse colon

Tail of pancreas

**Spleen in situ**

© Novartis

# Arteries of Stomach, Liver and Spleen

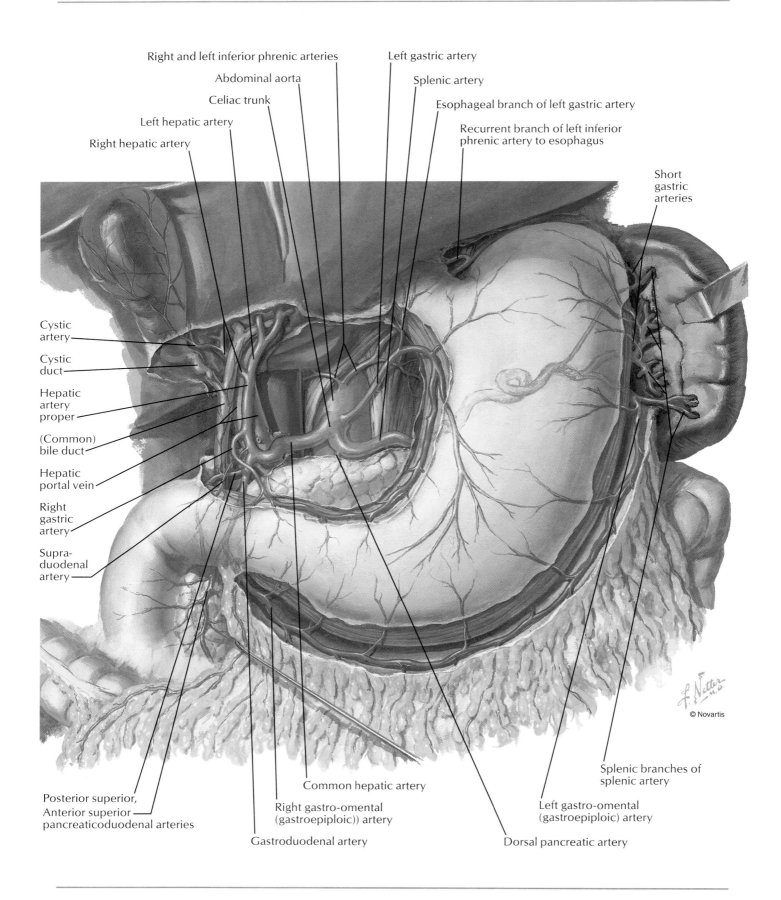

Right and left inferior phrenic arteries

Abdominal aorta

Celiac trunk

Left hepatic artery

Right hepatic artery

Left gastric artery

Splenic artery

Esophageal branch of left gastric artery

Recurrent branch of left inferior phrenic artery to esophagus

Short gastric arteries

Cystic artery

Cystic duct

Hepatic artery proper

(Common) bile duct

Hepatic portal vein

Right gastric artery

Supra-duodenal artery

Posterior superior, Anterior superior pancreaticoduodenal arteries

Common hepatic artery

Right gastro-omental (gastroepiploic)) artery

Gastroduodenal artery

Dorsal pancreatic artery

Left gastro-omental (gastroepiploic) artery

Splenic branches of splenic artery

F. Netter M.D.

© Novartis

**PLATE 282**

**ABDOMEN**

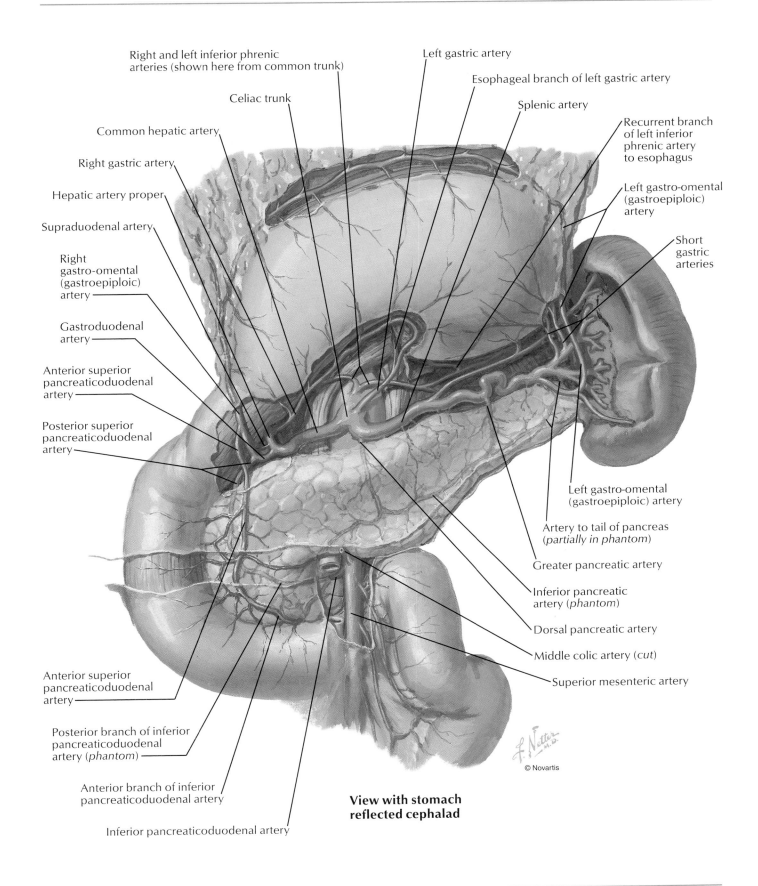

Right and left inferior phrenic arteries (shown here from common trunk)

Left gastric artery

Esophageal branch of left gastric artery

Celiac trunk

Splenic artery

Common hepatic artery

Recurrent branch of left inferior phrenic artery to esophagus

Right gastric artery

Hepatic artery proper

Left gastro-omental (gastroepiploic) artery

Supraduodenal artery

Short gastric arteries

Right gastro-omental (gastroepiploic) artery

Gastroduodenal artery

Anterior superior pancreaticoduodenal artery

Posterior superior pancreaticoduodenal artery

Left gastro-omental (gastroepiploic) artery

Artery to tail of pancreas (partially in phantom)

Greater pancreatic artery

Inferior pancreatic artery (phantom)

Dorsal pancreatic artery

Middle colic artery (cut)

Superior mesenteric artery

Anterior superior pancreaticoduodenal artery

Posterior branch of inferior pancreaticoduodenal artery (phantom)

Anterior branch of inferior pancreaticoduodenal artery

Inferior pancreaticoduodenal artery

**View with stomach reflected cephalad**

© Novartis

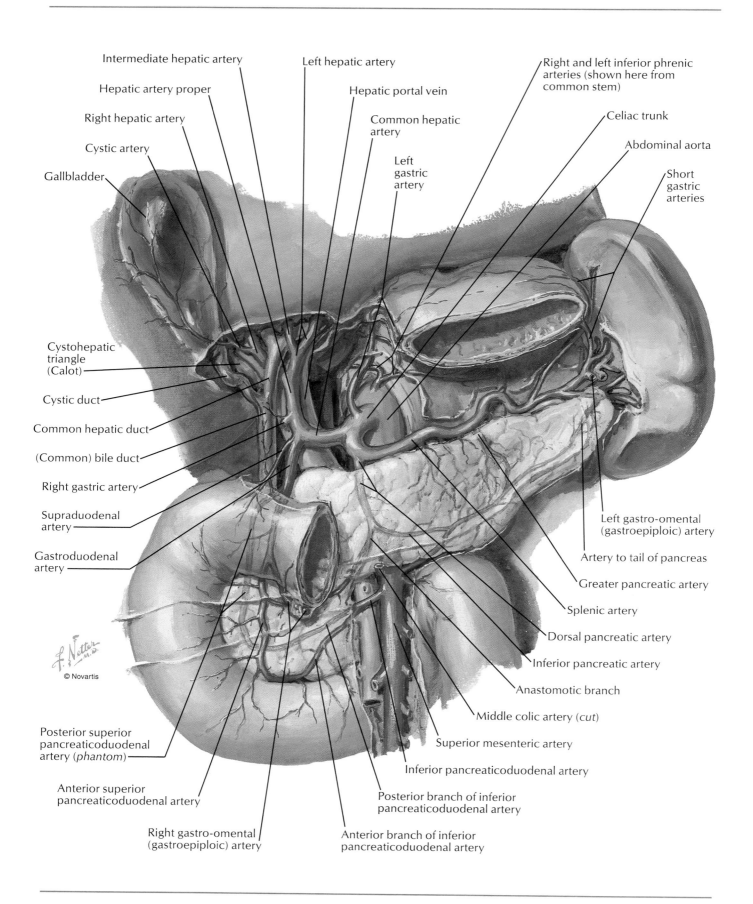

Intermediate hepatic artery

Hepatic artery proper

Right hepatic artery

Cystic artery

Gallbladder

Left hepatic artery

Hepatic portal vein

Common hepatic artery

Left gastric artery

Right and left inferior phrenic arteries (shown here from common stem)

Celiac trunk

Abdominal aorta

Short gastric arteries

Cystohepatic triangle (Calot)

Cystic duct

Common hepatic duct

(Common) bile duct

Right gastric artery

Supraduodenal artery

Gastroduodenal artery

Posterior superior pancreaticoduodenal artery (*phantom*)

Anterior superior pancreaticoduodenal artery

Right gastro-omental (gastroepiploic) artery

Anterior branch of inferior pancreaticoduodenal artery

Posterior branch of inferior pancreaticoduodenal artery

Inferior pancreaticoduodenal artery

Superior mesenteric artery

Middle colic artery (*cut*)

Anastomotic branch

Inferior pancreatic artery

Dorsal pancreatic artery

Splenic artery

Greater pancreatic artery

Artery to tail of pancreas

Left gastro-omental (gastroepiploic) artery

**PLATE 284**

**ABDOMEN**

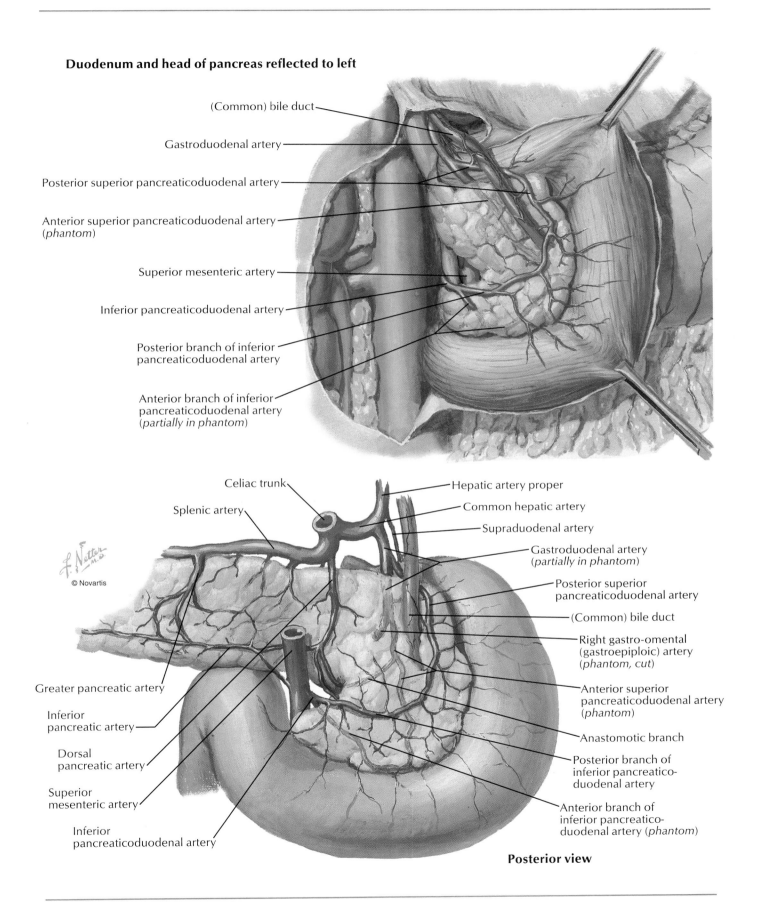

**Duodenum and head of pancreas reflected to left**

(Common) bile duct

Gastroduodenal artery

Posterior superior pancreaticoduodenal artery

Anterior superior pancreaticoduodenal artery
(*phantom*)

Superior mesenteric artery

Inferior pancreaticoduodenal artery

Posterior branch of inferior
pancreaticoduodenal artery

Anterior branch of inferior
pancreaticoduodenal artery
(*partially in phantom*)

Celiac trunk

Splenic artery

© Novartis

Greater pancreatic artery

Inferior
pancreatic artery

Dorsal
pancreatic artery

Superior
mesenteric artery

Inferior
pancreaticoduodenal artery

Hepatic artery proper

Common hepatic artery

Supraduodenal artery

Gastroduodenal artery
(*partially in phantom*)

Posterior superior
pancreaticoduodenal artery

(Common) bile duct

Right gastro-omental
(gastroepiploic) artery
(*phantom, cut*)

Anterior superior
pancreaticoduodenal artery
(*phantom*)

Anastomotic branch

Posterior branch of
inferior pancreatico-
duodenal artery

Anterior branch of
inferior pancreatico-
duodenal artery (*phantom*)

**Posterior view**

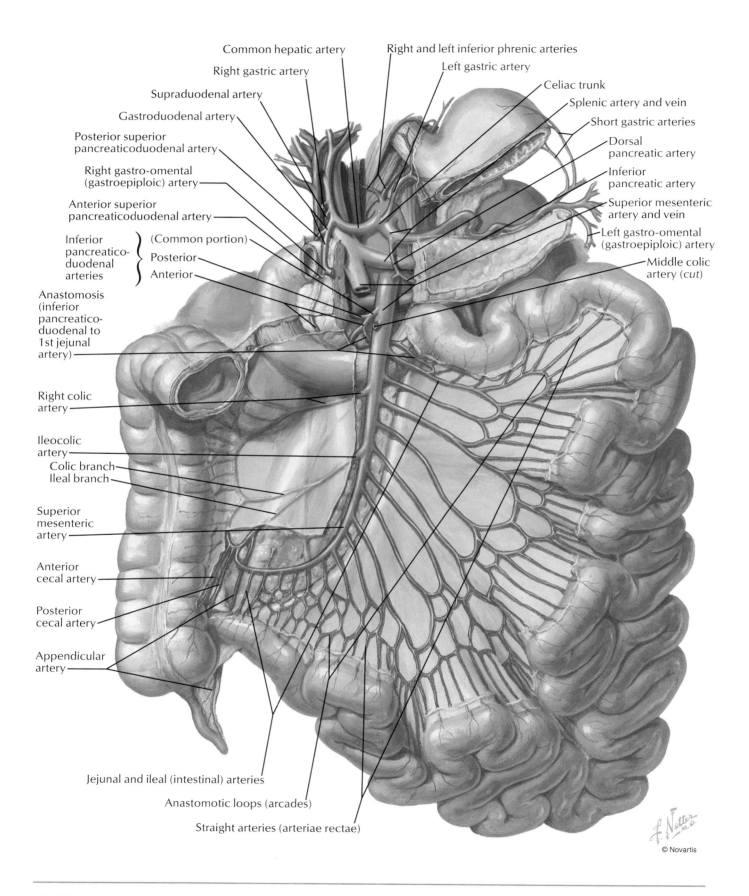

Common hepatic artery

Right gastric artery

Supraduodenal artery

Gastroduodenal artery

Posterior superior pancreaticoduodenal artery

Right gastro-omental (gastroepiploic) artery

Anterior superior pancreaticoduodenal artery

Inferior pancreatico-duodenal arteries { (Common portion) / Posterior / Anterior

Anastomosis (inferior pancreatico-duodenal to 1st jejunal artery)

Right colic artery

Ileocolic artery

Colic branch

Ileal branch

Superior mesenteric artery

Anterior cecal artery

Posterior cecal artery

Appendicular artery

Jejunal and ileal (intestinal) arteries

Anastomotic loops (arcades)

Straight arteries (arteriae rectae)

Right and left inferior phrenic arteries

Left gastric artery

Celiac trunk

Splenic artery and vein

Short gastric arteries

Dorsal pancreatic artery

Inferior pancreatic artery

Superior mesenteric artery and vein

Left gastro-omental (gastroepiploic) artery

Middle colic artery (*cut*)

© Novartis

**PLATE 286**

**ABDOMEN**

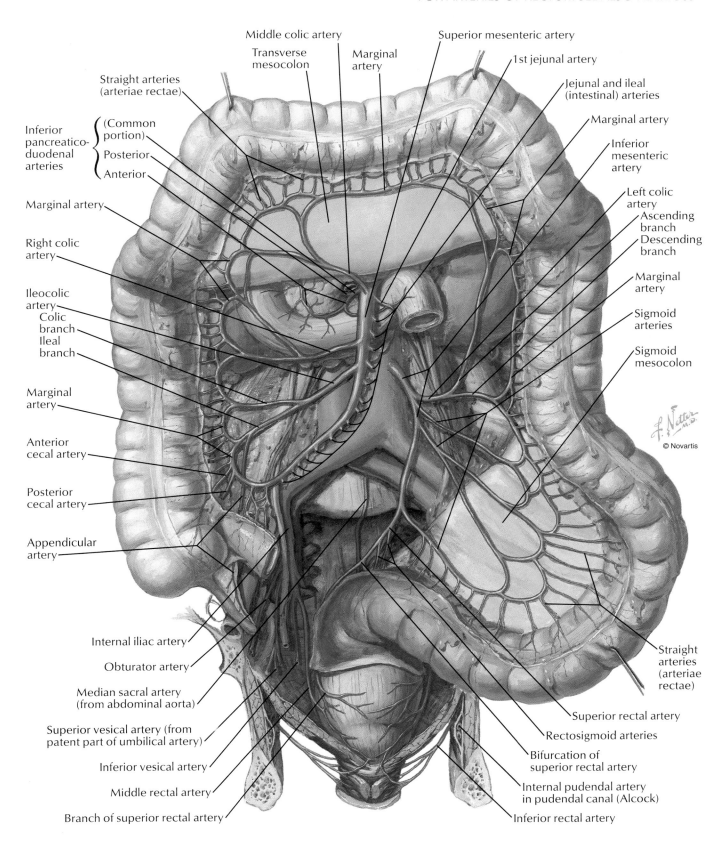

Middle colic artery

Superior mesenteric artery

Transverse mesocolon

Marginal artery

1st jejunal artery

Jejunal and ileal (intestinal) arteries

Straight arteries (arteriae rectae)

Marginal artery

Inferior pancreaticoduodenal arteries

(Common portion)

Posterior

Anterior

Inferior mesenteric artery

Left colic artery

Ascending branch

Descending branch

Marginal artery

Right colic artery

Marginal artery

Sigmoid arteries

Ileocolic artery

Colic branch

Ileal branch

Sigmoid mesocolon

Marginal artery

Anterior cecal artery

Posterior cecal artery

Appendicular artery

Internal iliac artery

Obturator artery

Straight arteries (arteriae rectae)

Median sacral artery (from abdominal aorta)

Superior vesical artery (from patent part of umbilical artery)

Superior rectal artery

Rectosigmoid arteries

Inferior vesical artery

Middle rectal artery

Bifurcation of superior rectal artery

Internal pudendal artery in pudendal canal (Alcock)

Branch of superior rectal artery

Inferior rectal artery

© Novartis

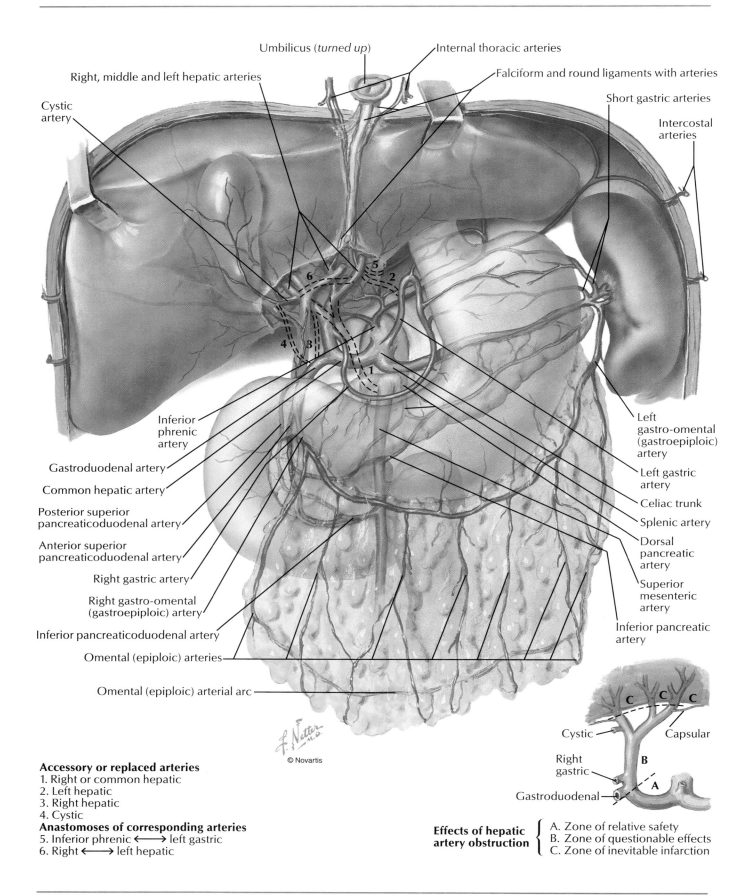

Umbilicus (*turned up*)

Internal thoracic arteries

Right, middle and left hepatic arteries

Falciform and round ligaments with arteries

Short gastric arteries

Cystic artery

Intercostal arteries

Inferior phrenic artery

Gastroduodenal artery

Common hepatic artery

Posterior superior pancreaticoduodenal artery

Anterior superior pancreaticoduodenal artery

Right gastric artery

Right gastro-omental (gastroepiploic) artery

Inferior pancreaticoduodenal artery

Omental (epiploic) arteries

Omental (epiploic) arterial arc

Left gastro-omental (gastroepiploic) artery

Left gastric artery

Celiac trunk

Splenic artery

Dorsal pancreatic artery

Superior mesenteric artery

Inferior pancreatic artery

*f. Netter*
© Novartis

**Accessory or replaced arteries**
1. Right or common hepatic
2. Left hepatic
3. Right hepatic
4. Cystic
**Anastomoses of corresponding arteries**
5. Inferior phrenic ⟷ left gastric
6. Right ⟷ left hepatic

Cystic

Capsular

Right gastric

B

Gastroduodenal

A

C  C  C

**Effects of hepatic artery obstruction**
A. Zone of relative safety
B. Zone of questionable effects
C. Zone of inevitable infarction

**PLATE 288**

**ABDOMEN**

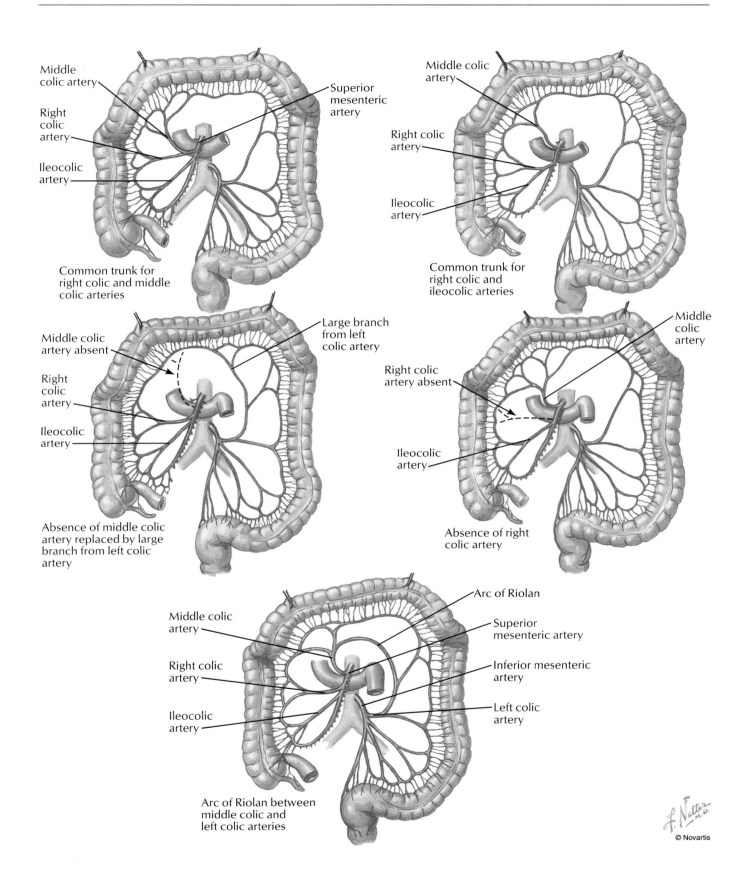

Middle colic artery

Right colic artery

Ileocolic artery

Superior mesenteric artery

Common trunk for right colic and middle colic arteries

Middle colic artery

Right colic artery

Ileocolic artery

Common trunk for right colic and ileocolic arteries

Middle colic artery absent

Right colic artery

Ileocolic artery

Large branch from left colic artery

Absence of middle colic artery replaced by large branch from left colic artery

Right colic artery absent

Ileocolic artery

Middle colic artery

Absence of right colic artery

Middle colic artery

Right colic artery

Ileocolic artery

Arc of Riolan

Superior mesenteric artery

Inferior mesenteric artery

Left colic artery

Arc of Riolan between middle colic and left colic arteries

# Veins of Stomach, Duodenum, Pancreas and Spleen

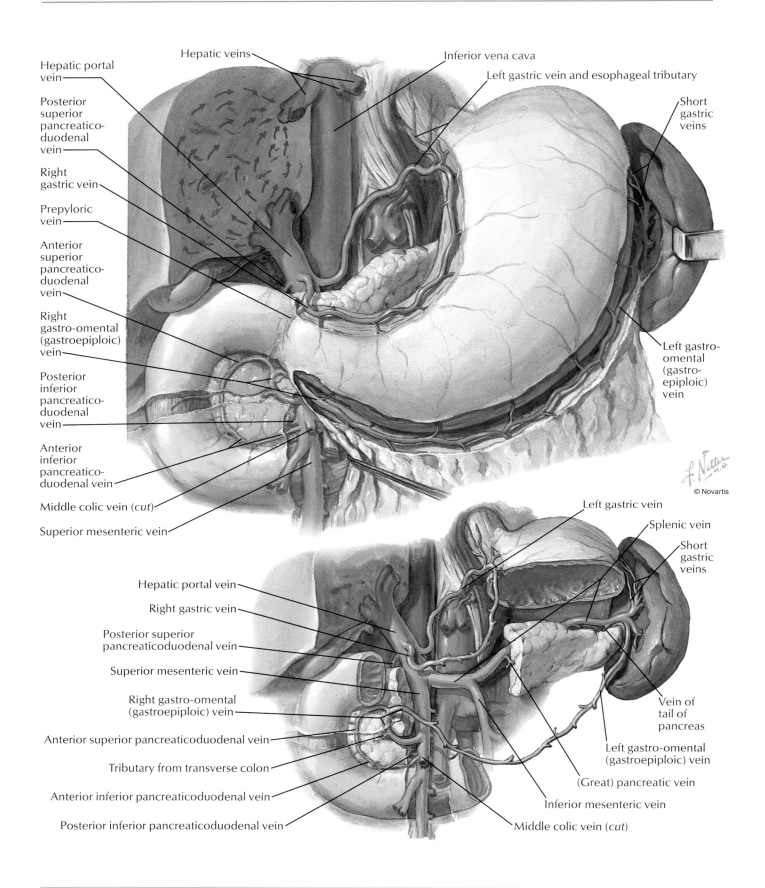

Hepatic veins

Inferior vena cava

Left gastric vein and esophageal tributary

Short gastric veins

Hepatic portal vein

Posterior superior pancreaticoduodenal vein

Right gastric vein

Prepyloric vein

Anterior superior pancreaticoduodenal vein

Right gastro-omental (gastroepiploic) vein

Posterior inferior pancreaticoduodenal vein

Anterior inferior pancreaticoduodenal vein

Middle colic vein (cut)

Superior mesenteric vein

Left gastro-omental (gastro-epiploic) vein

Left gastric vein

Splenic vein

Short gastric veins

Hepatic portal vein

Right gastric vein

Posterior superior pancreaticoduodenal vein

Superior mesenteric vein

Right gastro-omental (gastroepiploic) vein

Anterior superior pancreaticoduodenal vein

Tributary from transverse colon

Anterior inferior pancreaticoduodenal vein

Posterior inferior pancreaticoduodenal vein

Vein of tail of pancreas

Left gastro-omental (gastroepiploic) vein

(Great) pancreatic vein

Inferior mesenteric vein

Middle colic vein (cut)

© Novartis

PLATE 290

ABDOMEN

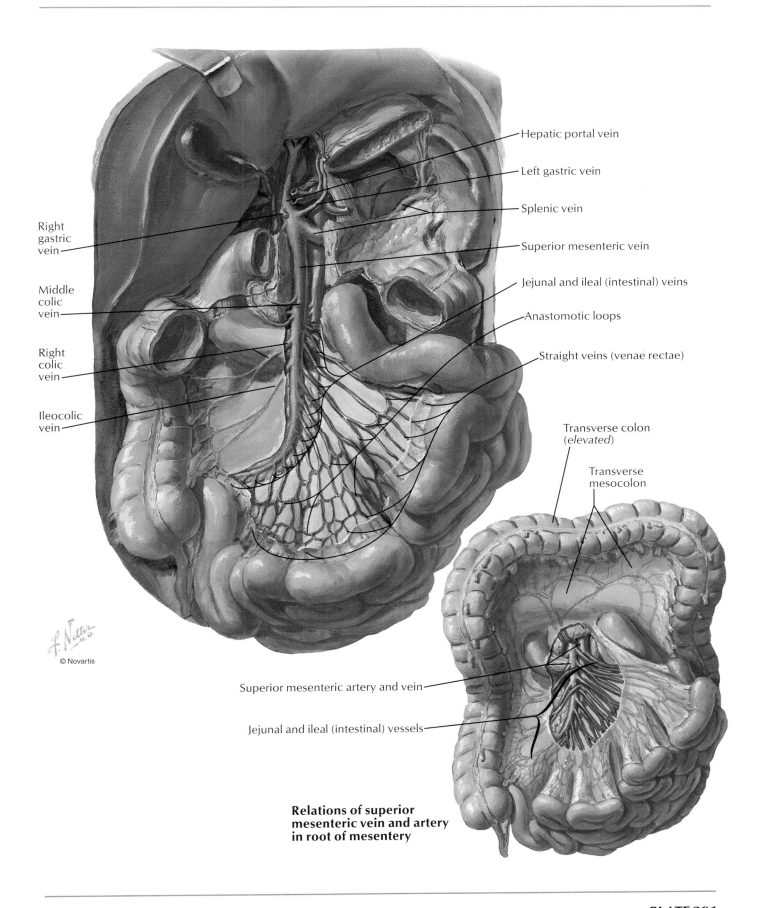

Hepatic portal vein

Left gastric vein

Splenic vein

Superior mesenteric vein

Jejunal and ileal (intestinal) veins

Anastomotic loops

Straight veins (venae rectae)

Transverse colon (*elevated*)

Transverse mesocolon

Right gastric vein

Middle colic vein

Right colic vein

Ileocolic vein

Superior mesenteric artery and vein

Jejunal and ileal (intestinal) vessels

**Relations of superior mesenteric vein and artery in root of mesentery**

*FOR VEINS OF RECTUM SEE ALSO PLATE 370*

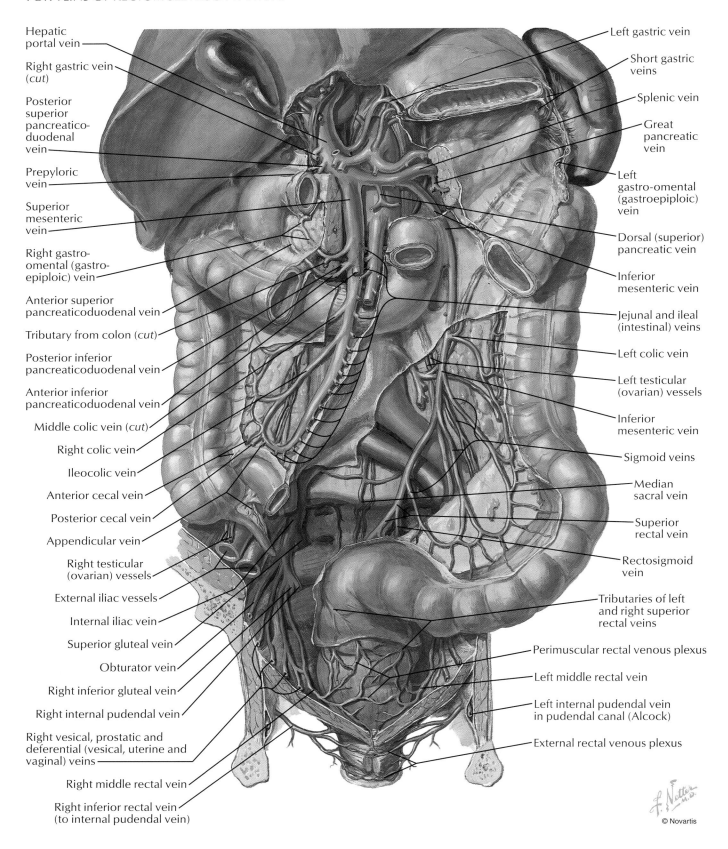

Hepatic portal vein

Right gastric vein (*cut*)

Posterior superior pancreatico-duodenal vein

Prepyloric vein

Superior mesenteric vein

Right gastro-omental (gastro-epiploic) vein

Anterior superior pancreaticoduodenal vein

Tributary from colon (*cut*)

Posterior inferior pancreaticoduodenal vein

Anterior inferior pancreaticoduodenal vein

Middle colic vein (*cut*)

Right colic vein

Ileocolic vein

Anterior cecal vein

Posterior cecal vein

Appendicular vein

Right testicular (ovarian) vessels

External iliac vessels

Internal iliac vein

Superior gluteal vein

Obturator vein

Right inferior gluteal vein

Right internal pudendal vein

Right vesical, prostatic and deferential (vesical, uterine and vaginal) veins

Right middle rectal vein

Right inferior rectal vein (to internal pudendal vein)

Left gastric vein

Short gastric veins

Splenic vein

Great pancreatic vein

Left gastro-omental (gastroepiploic) vein

Dorsal (superior) pancreatic vein

Inferior mesenteric vein

Jejunal and ileal (intestinal) veins

Left colic vein

Left testicular (ovarian) vessels

Inferior mesenteric vein

Sigmoid veins

Median sacral vein

Superior rectal vein

Rectosigmoid vein

Tributaries of left and right superior rectal veins

Perimuscular rectal venous plexus

Left middle rectal vein

Left internal pudendal vein in pudendal canal (Alcock)

External rectal venous plexus

*f. Netter M.D.*

© Novartis

**PLATE 292**

**ABDOMEN**

# Hepatic Portal Vein Tributaries: Portocaval Anastomoses

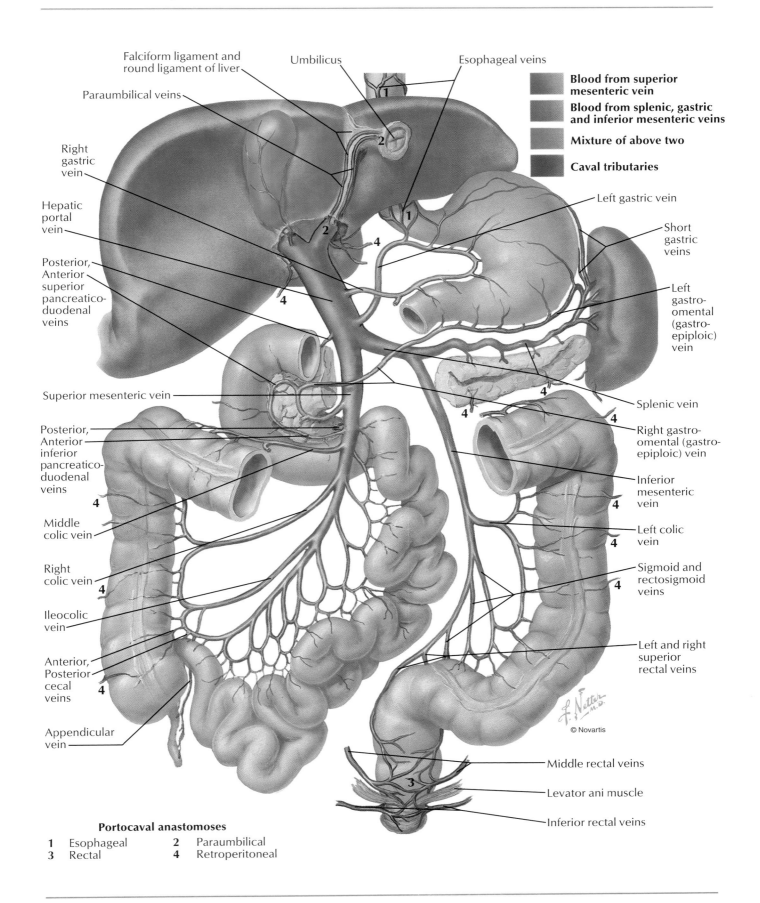

Falciform ligament and round ligament of liver

Umbilicus

Esophageal veins

Paraumbilical veins

**Blood from superior mesenteric vein**

**Blood from splenic, gastric and inferior mesenteric veins**

**Mixture of above two**

**Caval tributaries**

Right gastric vein

Left gastric vein

Short gastric veins

Hepatic portal vein

Posterior, Anterior superior pancreaticoduodenal veins

Left gastro-omental (gastro-epiploic) vein

Splenic vein

Superior mesenteric vein

Posterior, Anterior inferior pancreaticoduodenal veins

Right gastro-omental (gastro-epiploic) vein

Inferior mesenteric vein

Middle colic vein

Left colic vein

Right colic vein

Sigmoid and rectosigmoid veins

Ileocolic vein

Left and right superior rectal veins

Anterior, Posterior cecal veins

Appendicular vein

Middle rectal veins

Levator ani muscle

Inferior rectal veins

*f. Netter* M.D.

© Novartis

**Portocaval anastomoses**

| | | | |
|---|---|---|---|
| **1** | Esophageal | **2** | Paraumbilical |
| **3** | Rectal | **4** | Retroperitoneal |

**VISCERAL VASCULATURE**

*PLATE 293*

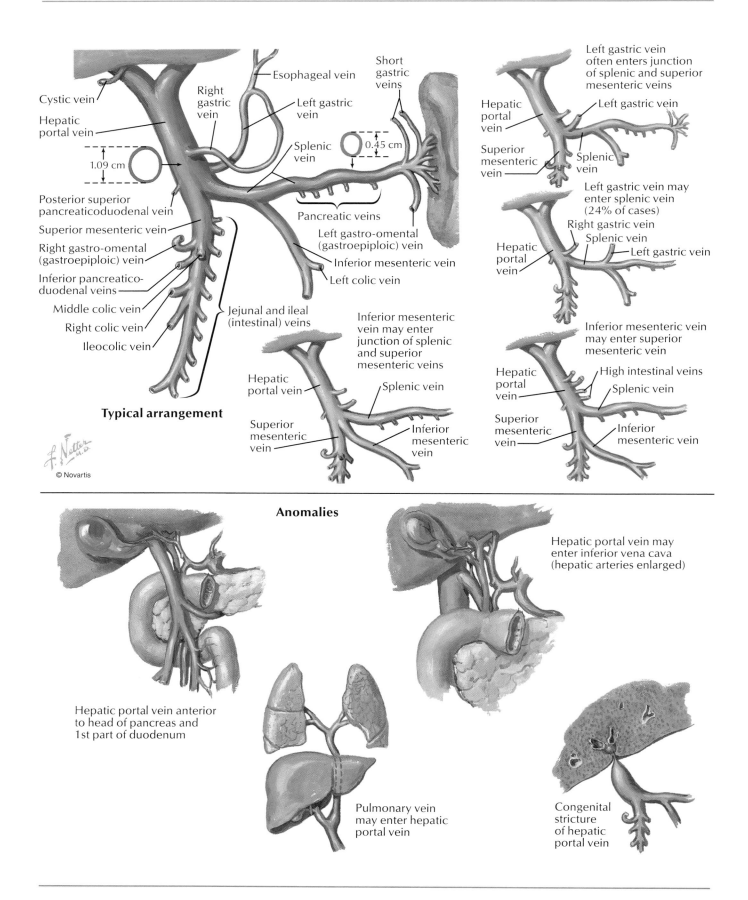

Cystic vein

Hepatic portal vein

1.09 cm

Posterior superior pancreaticoduodenal vein

Superior mesenteric vein

Right gastro-omental (gastroepiploic) vein

Inferior pancreatico-duodenal veins

Middle colic vein

Right colic vein

Ileocolic vein

Right gastric vein

Esophageal vein

Left gastric vein

Splenic vein

Short gastric veins

0.45 cm

Pancreatic veins

Left gastro-omental (gastroepiploic) vein

Inferior mesenteric vein

Left colic vein

Jejunal and ileal (intestinal) veins

**Typical arrangement**

© Novartis

Left gastric vein often enters junction of splenic and superior mesenteric veins

Hepatic portal vein

Left gastric vein

Superior mesenteric vein

Splenic vein

Left gastric vein may enter splenic vein (24% of cases)

Right gastric vein

Splenic vein

Hepatic portal vein

Left gastric vein

Inferior mesenteric vein may enter junction of splenic and superior mesenteric veins

Hepatic portal vein

Splenic vein

Superior mesenteric vein

Inferior mesenteric vein

Inferior mesenteric vein may enter superior mesenteric vein

Hepatic portal vein

High intestinal veins

Splenic vein

Superior mesenteric vein

Inferior mesenteric vein

**Anomalies**

Hepatic portal vein anterior to head of pancreas and 1st part of duodenum

Pulmonary vein may enter hepatic portal vein

Hepatic portal vein may enter inferior vena cava (hepatic arteries enlarged)

Congenital stricture of hepatic portal vein

*PLATE 294*

**ABDOMEN**

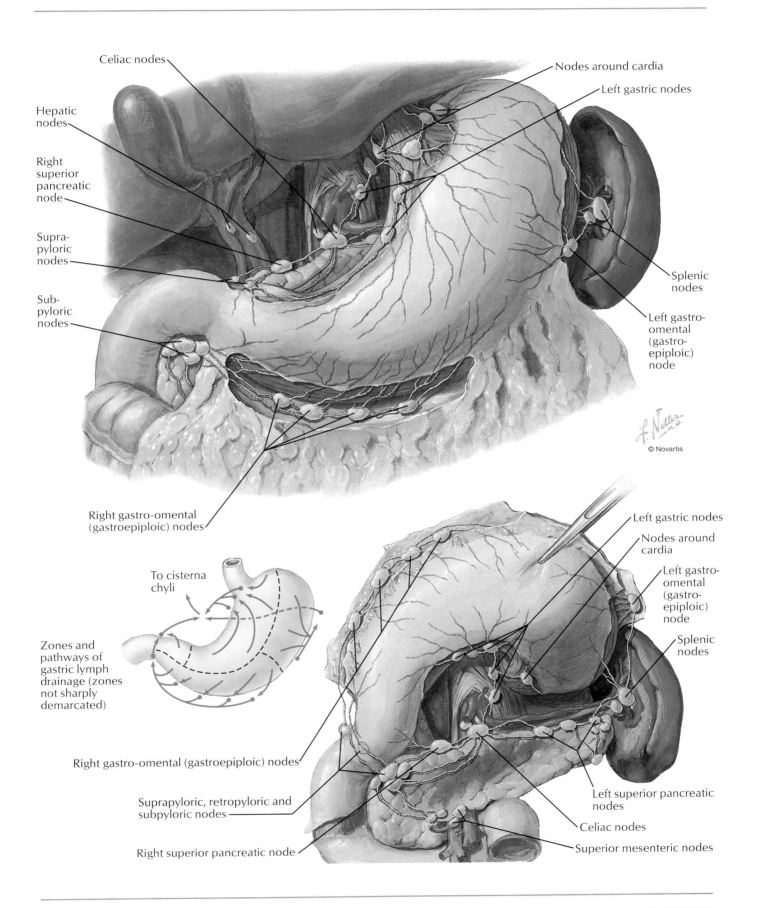

Celiac nodes

Nodes around cardia

Left gastric nodes

Hepatic nodes

Right superior pancreatic node

Supra-pyloric nodes

Sub-pyloric nodes

Splenic nodes

Left gastro-omental (gastro-epiploic) node

Right gastro-omental (gastroepiploic) nodes

To cisterna chyli

Zones and pathways of gastric lymph drainage (zones not sharply demarcated)

Left gastric nodes

Nodes around cardia

Left gastro-omental (gastro-epiploic) node

Splenic nodes

Right gastro-omental (gastroepiploic) nodes

Suprapyloric, retropyloric and subpyloric nodes

Right superior pancreatic node

Left superior pancreatic nodes

Celiac nodes

Superior mesenteric nodes

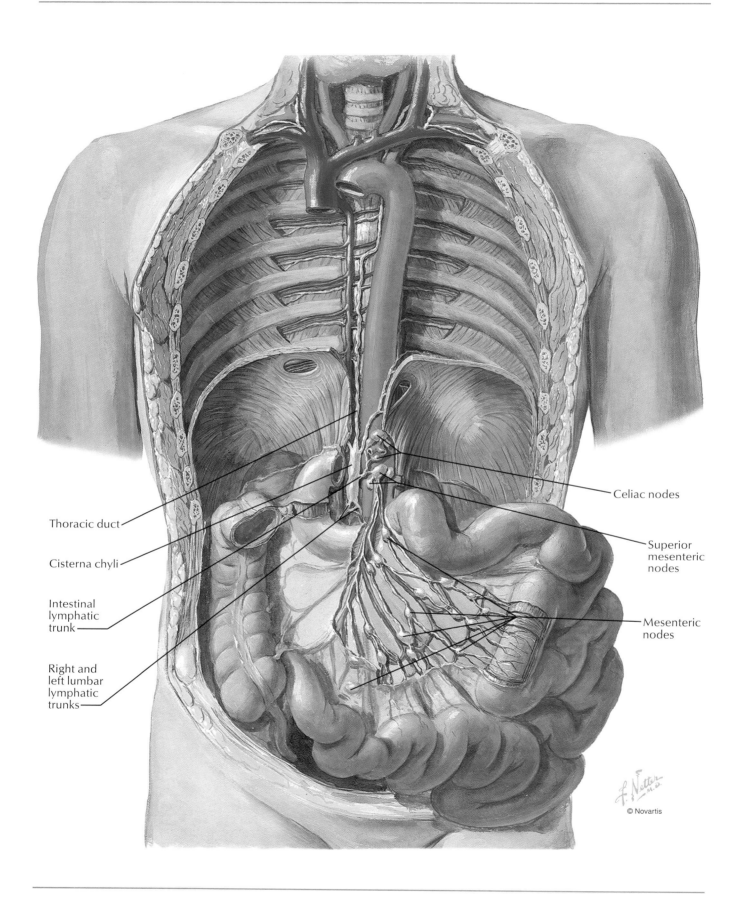

Celiac nodes

Superior
mesenteric
nodes

Mesenteric
nodes

Thoracic duct

Cisterna chyli

Intestinal
lymphatic
trunk

Right and
left lumbar
lymphatic
trunks

© Novartis

**PLATE 296**

**ABDOMEN**

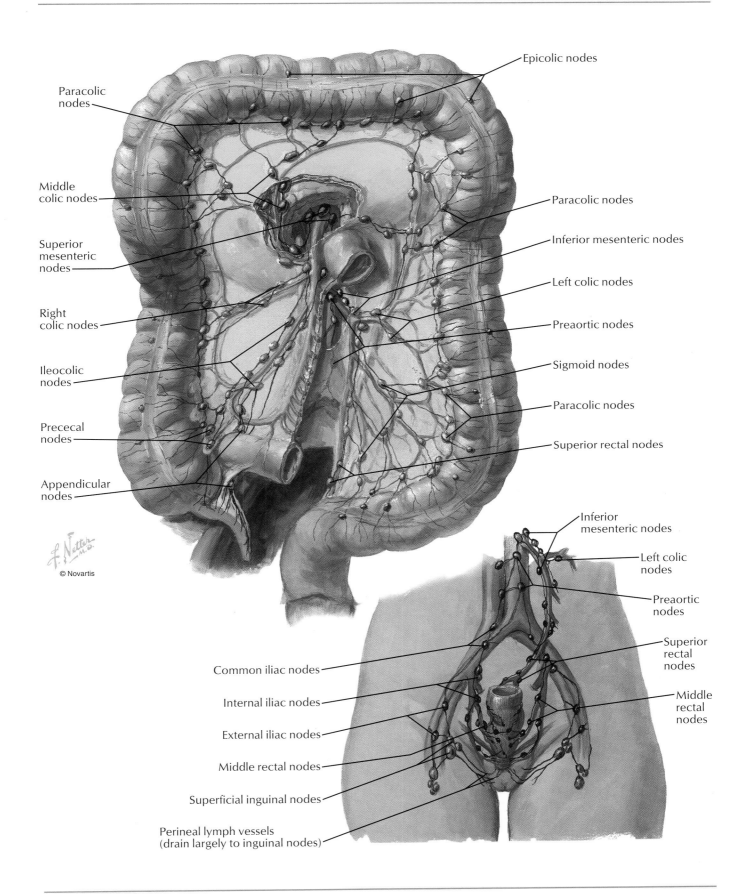

Epicolic nodes

Paracolic nodes

Middle colic nodes

Superior mesenteric nodes

Right colic nodes

Ileocolic nodes

Prececal nodes

Appendicular nodes

Paracolic nodes

Inferior mesenteric nodes

Left colic nodes

Preaortic nodes

Sigmoid nodes

Paracolic nodes

Superior rectal nodes

Inferior mesenteric nodes

Left colic nodes

Preaortic nodes

Superior rectal nodes

Middle rectal nodes

Common iliac nodes

Internal iliac nodes

External iliac nodes

Middle rectal nodes

Superficial inguinal nodes

Perineal lymph vessels (drain largely to inguinal nodes)

© Novartis

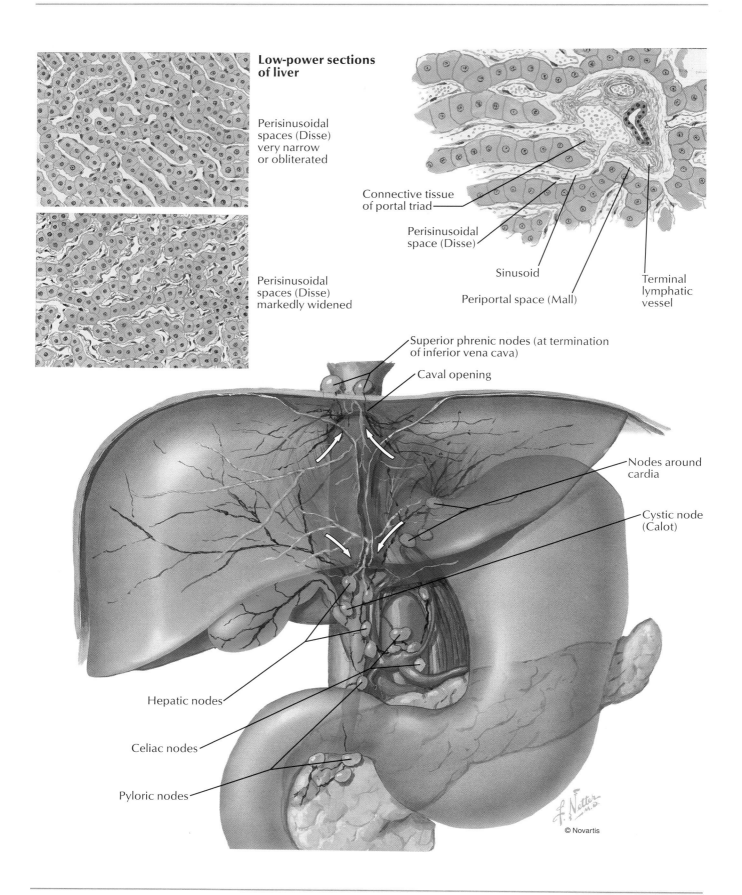

**Low-power sections of liver**

Perisinusoidal spaces (Disse) very narrow or obliterated

Perisinusoidal spaces (Disse) markedly widened

Connective tissue of portal triad

Perisinusoidal space (Disse)

Sinusoid

Periportal space (Mall)

Terminal lymphatic vessel

Superior phrenic nodes (at termination of inferior vena cava)

Caval opening

Nodes around cardia

Cystic node (Calot)

Hepatic nodes

Celiac nodes

Pyloric nodes

© Novartis

**PLATE 298**

**ABDOMEN**

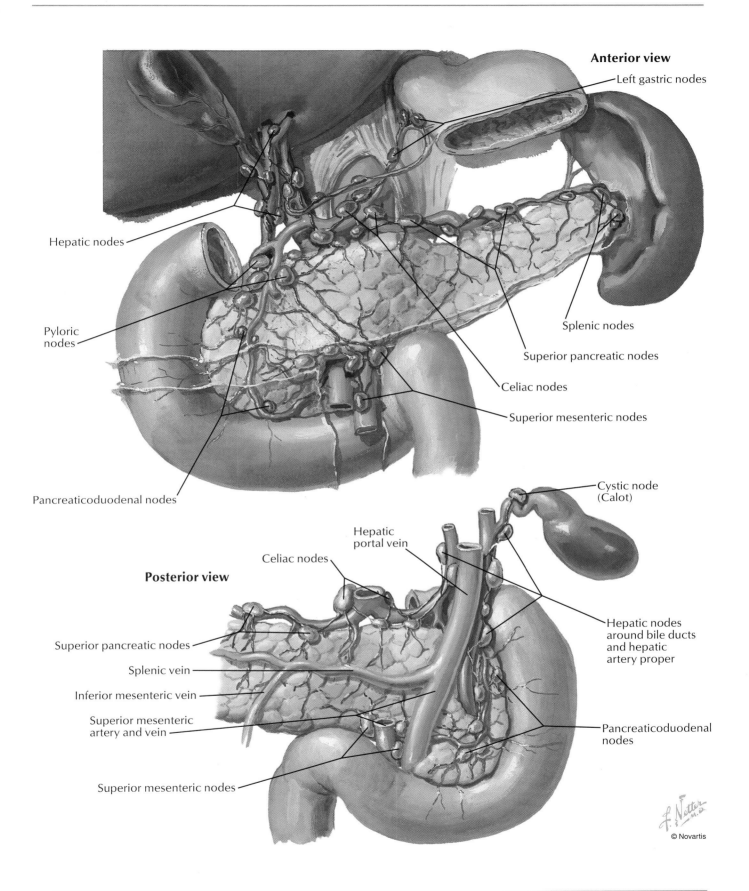

**Anterior view**

Left gastric nodes

Hepatic nodes

Pyloric nodes

Splenic nodes

Superior pancreatic nodes

Celiac nodes

Superior mesenteric nodes

Pancreaticoduodenal nodes

Cystic node (Calot)

Hepatic portal vein

Celiac nodes

**Posterior view**

Hepatic nodes around bile ducts and hepatic artery proper

Superior pancreatic nodes

Splenic vein

Inferior mesenteric vein

Superior mesenteric artery and vein

Pancreaticoduodenal nodes

Superior mesenteric nodes

© Novartis

SEE ALSO PLATE 152

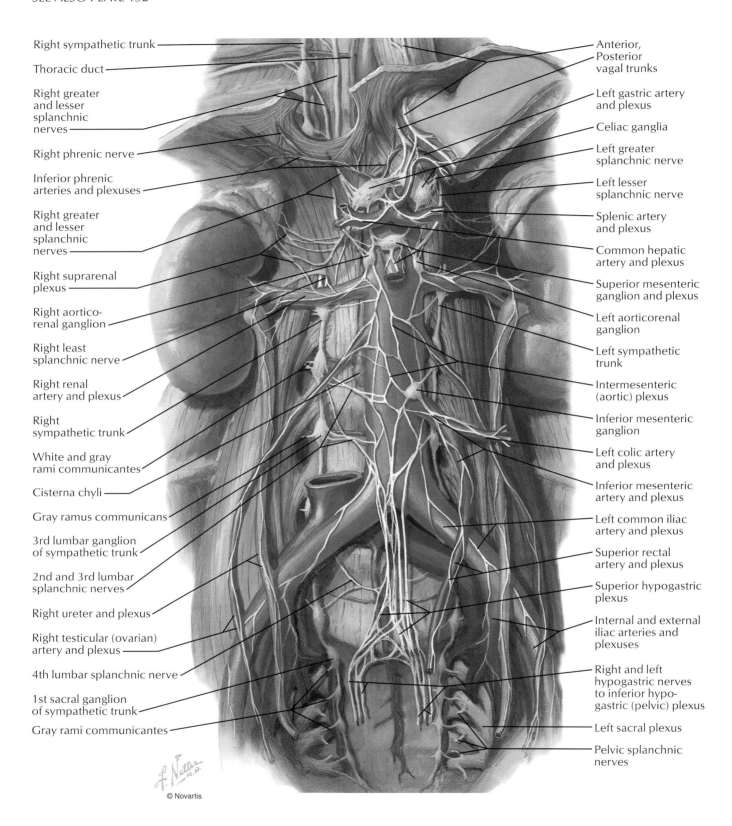

Right sympathetic trunk

Thoracic duct

Right greater and lesser splanchnic nerves

Right phrenic nerve

Inferior phrenic arteries and plexuses

Right greater and lesser splanchnic nerves

Right suprarenal plexus

Right aortico-renal ganglion

Right least splanchnic nerve

Right renal artery and plexus

Right sympathetic trunk

White and gray rami communicantes

Cisterna chyli

Gray ramus communicans

3rd lumbar ganglion of sympathetic trunk

2nd and 3rd lumbar splanchnic nerves

Right ureter and plexus

Right testicular (ovarian) artery and plexus

4th lumbar splanchnic nerve

1st sacral ganglion of sympathetic trunk

Gray rami communicantes

Anterior, Posterior vagal trunks

Left gastric artery and plexus

Celiac ganglia

Left greater splanchnic nerve

Left lesser splanchnic nerve

Splenic artery and plexus

Common hepatic artery and plexus

Superior mesenteric ganglion and plexus

Left aorticorenal ganglion

Left sympathetic trunk

Intermesenteric (aortic) plexus

Inferior mesenteric ganglion

Left colic artery and plexus

Inferior mesenteric artery and plexus

Left common iliac artery and plexus

Superior rectal artery and plexus

Superior hypogastric plexus

Internal and external iliac arteries and plexuses

Right and left hypogastric nerves to inferior hypo-gastric (pelvic) plexus

Left sacral plexus

Pelvic splanchnic nerves

**PLATE 300**

**ABDOMEN**

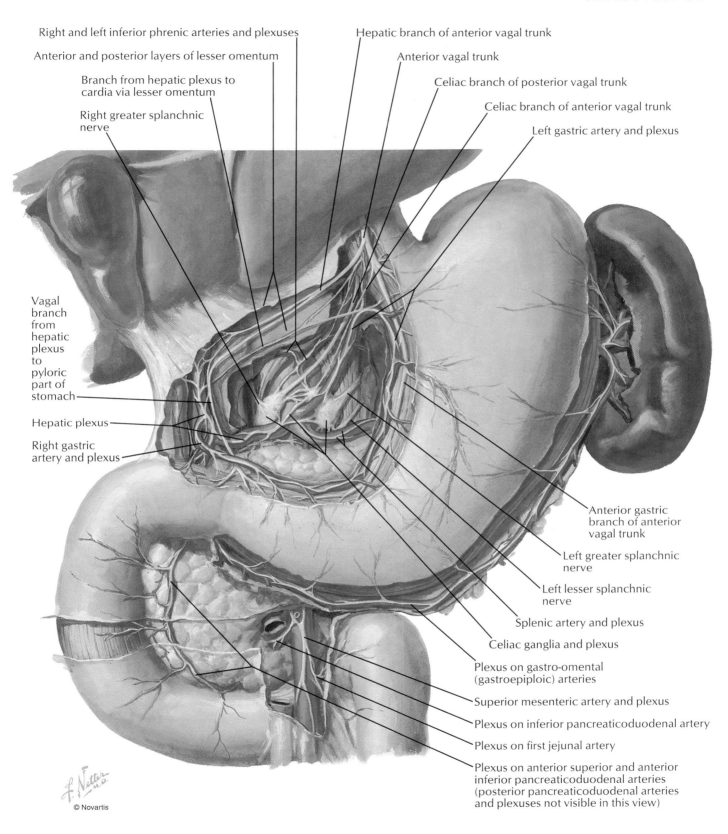

Right and left inferior phrenic arteries and plexuses

Anterior and posterior layers of lesser omentum

Branch from hepatic plexus to cardia via lesser omentum

Right greater splanchnic nerve

Hepatic branch of anterior vagal trunk

Anterior vagal trunk

Celiac branch of posterior vagal trunk

Celiac branch of anterior vagal trunk

Left gastric artery and plexus

Vagal branch from hepatic plexus to pyloric part of stomach

Hepatic plexus

Right gastric artery and plexus

Anterior gastric branch of anterior vagal trunk

Left greater splanchnic nerve

Left lesser splanchnic nerve

Splenic artery and plexus

Celiac ganglia and plexus

Plexus on gastro-omental (gastroepiploic) arteries

Superior mesenteric artery and plexus

Plexus on inferior pancreaticoduodenal artery

Plexus on first jejunal artery

Plexus on anterior superior and anterior inferior pancreaticoduodenal arteries (posterior pancreaticoduodenal arteries and plexuses not visible in this view)

*f. Netter*
M.D.

© Novartis

# Nerves of Stomach and Duodenum (continued)

SEE ALSO PLATE 152

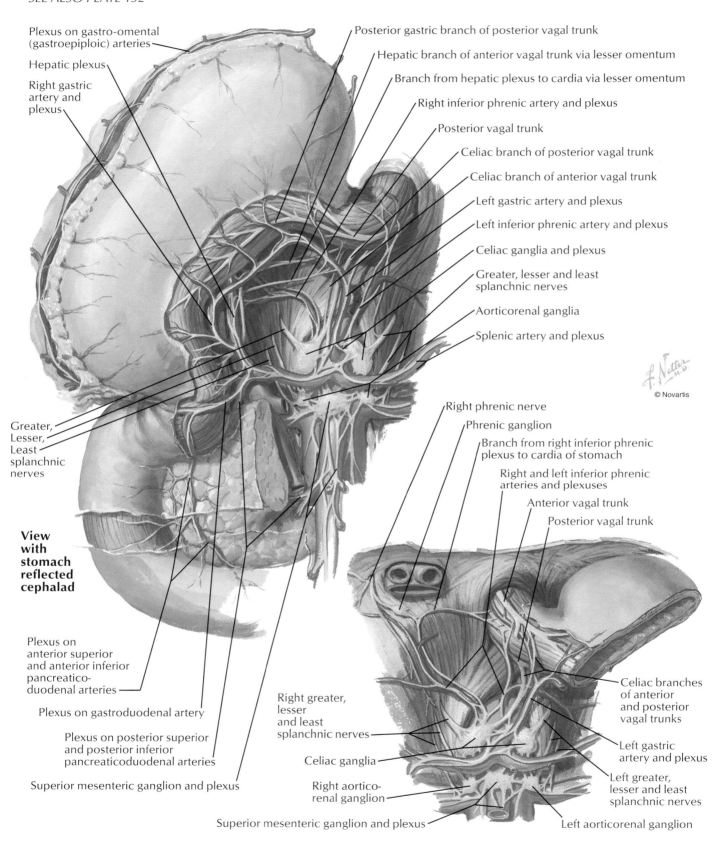

Plexus on gastro-omental (gastroepiploic) arteries

Hepatic plexus

Right gastric artery and plexus

Posterior gastric branch of posterior vagal trunk

Hepatic branch of anterior vagal trunk via lesser omentum

Branch from hepatic plexus to cardia via lesser omentum

Right inferior phrenic artery and plexus

Posterior vagal trunk

Celiac branch of posterior vagal trunk

Celiac branch of anterior vagal trunk

Left gastric artery and plexus

Left inferior phrenic artery and plexus

Celiac ganglia and plexus

Greater, lesser and least splanchnic nerves

Aorticorenal ganglia

Splenic artery and plexus

Greater, Lesser, Least splanchnic nerves

**View with stomach reflected cephalad**

Right phrenic nerve

Phrenic ganglion

Branch from right inferior phrenic plexus to cardia of stomach

Right and left inferior phrenic arteries and plexuses

Anterior vagal trunk

Posterior vagal trunk

Plexus on anterior superior and anterior inferior pancreatico- duodenal arteries

Plexus on gastroduodenal artery

Plexus on posterior superior and posterior inferior pancreaticoduodenal arteries

Superior mesenteric ganglion and plexus

Right greater, lesser and least splanchnic nerves

Celiac ganglia

Right aortico- renal ganglion

Superior mesenteric ganglion and plexus

Celiac branches of anterior and posterior vagal trunks

Left gastric artery and plexus

Left greater, lesser and least splanchnic nerves

Left aorticorenal ganglion

© Novartis

**PLATE 302**　　　　　　　　　　　　　　　　　　　**ABDOMEN**

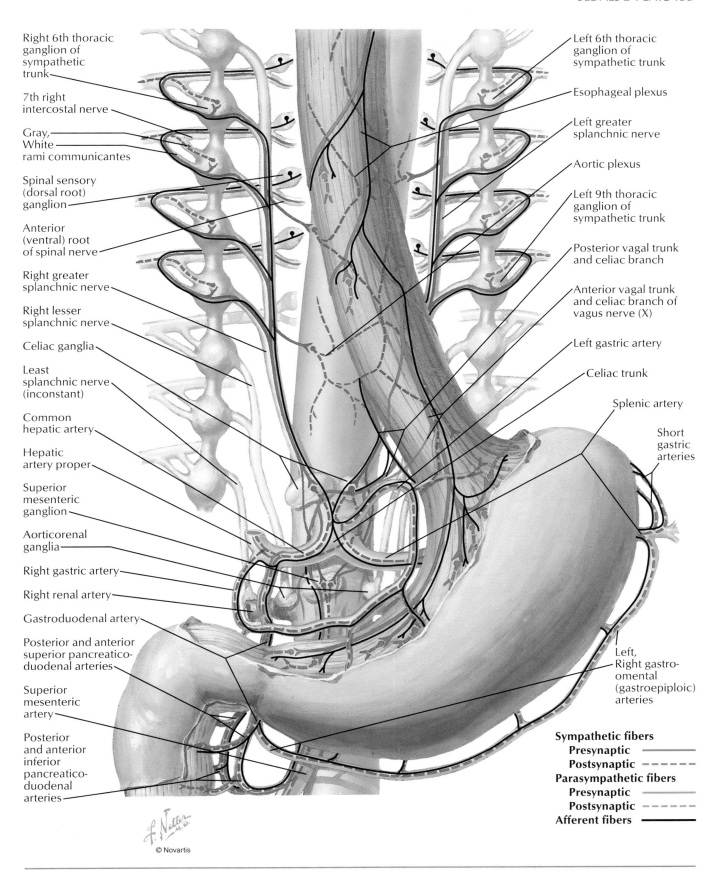

Right 6th thoracic ganglion of sympathetic trunk

7th right intercostal nerve

Gray, White rami communicantes

Spinal sensory (dorsal root) ganglion

Anterior (ventral) root of spinal nerve

Right greater splanchnic nerve

Right lesser splanchnic nerve

Celiac ganglia

Least splanchnic nerve (inconstant)

Common hepatic artery

Hepatic artery proper

Superior mesenteric ganglion

Aorticorenal ganglia

Right gastric artery

Right renal artery

Gastroduodenal artery

Posterior and anterior superior pancreaticoduodenal arteries

Superior mesenteric artery

Posterior and anterior inferior pancreaticoduodenal arteries

Left 6th thoracic ganglion of sympathetic trunk

Esophageal plexus

Left greater splanchnic nerve

Aortic plexus

Left 9th thoracic ganglion of sympathetic trunk

Posterior vagal trunk and celiac branch

Anterior vagal trunk and celiac branch of vagus nerve (X)

Left gastric artery

Celiac trunk

Splenic artery

Short gastric arteries

Left, Right gastro-omental (gastroepiploic) arteries

**Sympathetic fibers**
  Presynaptic ———
  Postsynaptic – – –
**Parasympathetic fibers**
  Presynaptic ———
  Postsynaptic – – –
**Afferent fibers** ━━━

*F. Netter M.D.*

© Novartis

SEE ALSO PLATE 152

Recurrent branch of left inferior phrenic artery and plexus to esophagus

Anterior vagal trunk

Posterior vagal trunk

Hepatic branch of anterior vagal trunk (courses in lesser omentum, removed here)

Celiac branches of anterior and posterior vagal trunks

Inferior phrenic arteries and plexuses

Left gastric artery and plexus

Hepatic plexus

Greater splanchnic nerves

Right gastric artery and plexus (*cut*)

Celiac ganglia and plexus

Gastroduodenal artery and plexus

Lesser splanchnic nerves

Least splanchnic nerves

Aorticorenal ganglia

Superior mesenteric ganglion

Intermesenteric (aortic) plexus

Inferior pancreaticoduodenal arteries and plexuses

Superior mesenteric artery and plexus

Middle colic artery and plexus (*cut*)

Right colic artery and plexus

Ileocolic artery and plexus

Superior mesenteric artery and plexus

Peritoneum (*cut edge*)

Mesenteric branches

Mesoappendix (contains appendicular artery and nerve plexus)

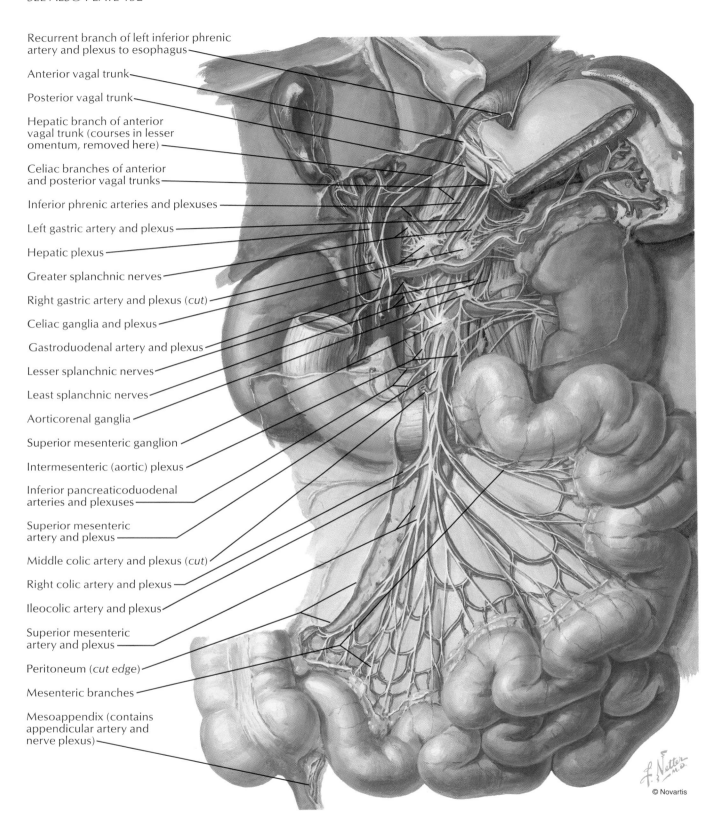

© Novartis

**PLATE 304**

**ABDOMEN**

FOR NERVES OF RECTUM SEE PLATES 152, 381, 382, 383, 384

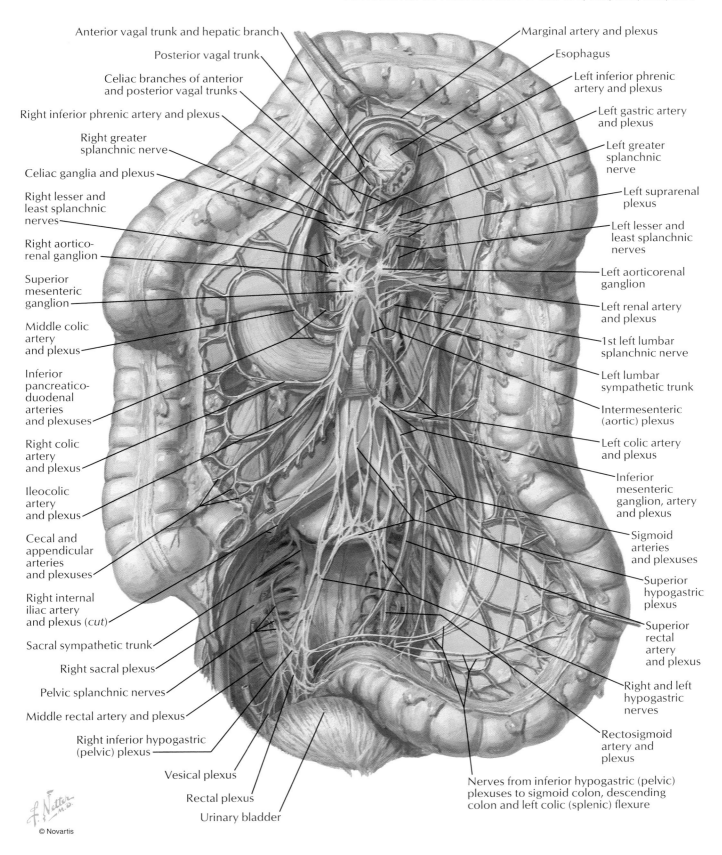

Anterior vagal trunk and hepatic branch

Posterior vagal trunk

Celiac branches of anterior and posterior vagal trunks

Right inferior phrenic artery and plexus

Right greater splanchnic nerve

Celiac ganglia and plexus

Right lesser and least splanchnic nerves

Right aortico-renal ganglion

Superior mesenteric ganglion

Middle colic artery and plexus

Inferior pancreatico-duodenal arteries and plexuses

Right colic artery and plexus

Ileocolic artery and plexus

Cecal and appendicular arteries and plexuses

Right internal iliac artery and plexus (cut)

Sacral sympathetic trunk

Right sacral plexus

Pelvic splanchnic nerves

Middle rectal artery and plexus

Right inferior hypogastric (pelvic) plexus

Vesical plexus

Rectal plexus

Urinary bladder

Marginal artery and plexus

Esophagus

Left inferior phrenic artery and plexus

Left gastric artery and plexus

Left greater splanchnic nerve

Left suprarenal plexus

Left lesser and least splanchnic nerves

Left aorticorenal ganglion

Left renal artery and plexus

1st left lumbar splanchnic nerve

Left lumbar sympathetic trunk

Intermesenteric (aortic) plexus

Left colic artery and plexus

Inferior mesenteric ganglion, artery and plexus

Sigmoid arteries and plexuses

Superior hypogastric plexus

Superior rectal artery and plexus

Right and left hypogastric nerves

Rectosigmoid artery and plexus

Nerves from inferior hypogastric (pelvic) plexuses to sigmoid colon, descending colon and left colic (splenic) flexure

f. Netter M.D.

© Novartis

**INNERVATION**

*PLATE 305*

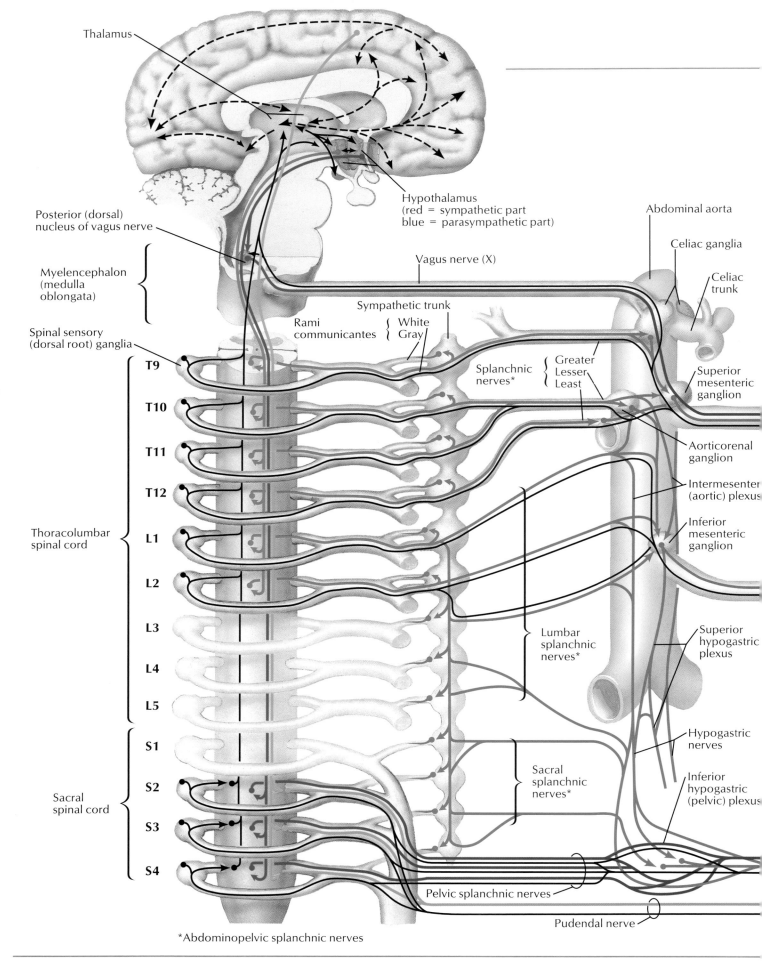

Thalamus

Hypothalamus
(red = sympathetic part
blue = parasympathetic part)

Abdominal aorta

Celiac ganglia

Celiac trunk

Posterior (dorsal)
nucleus of vagus nerve

Myelencephalon
(medulla
oblongata)

Vagus nerve (X)

Sympathetic trunk

Spinal sensory
(dorsal root) ganglia

Rami
communicantes { White
Gray

Splanchnic
nerves* { Greater
Lesser
Least

Superior
mesenteric
ganglion

T9

T10

T11

Aorticorenal
ganglion

T12

Intermesenteric
(aortic) plexus

Thoracolumbar
spinal cord

L1

Inferior
mesenteric
ganglion

L2

L3

Lumbar
splanchnic
nerves*

Superior
hypogastric
plexus

L4

L5

S1

Hypogastric
nerves

Sacral
spinal cord

S2

Sacral
splanchnic
nerves*

Inferior
hypogastric
(pelvic) plexus

S3

S4

Pelvic splanchnic nerves

Pudendal nerve

*Abdominopelvic splanchnic nerves

**PLATE 306**

**ABDOMEN**

**Sympathetic efferents** ——————
**Parasympathetic efferents** ——————
**Somatic efferents** ——————
**Afferents and CNS connections** ——————
**Indefinite paths** – – – – –

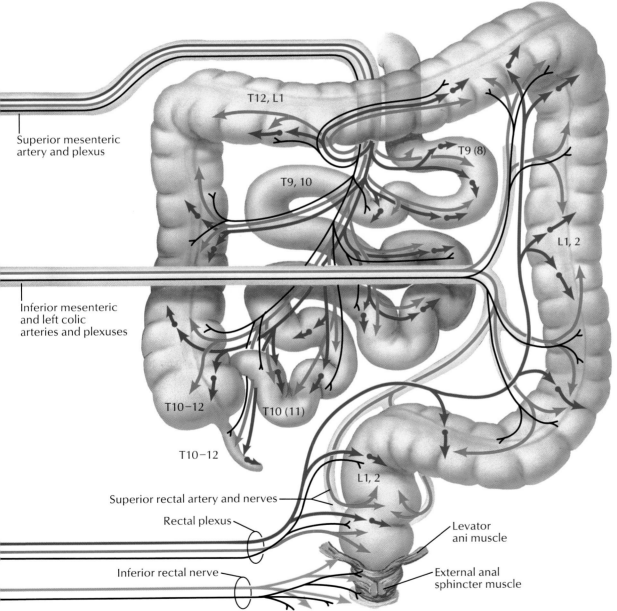

Superior mesenteric
artery and plexus

T12, L1

T9 (8)

T9, 10

L1, 2

Inferior mesenteric
and left colic
arteries and plexuses

T10–12

T10 (11)

T10–12

L1, 2

Superior rectal artery and nerves

Rectal plexus

Levator
ani muscle

Inferior rectal nerve

External anal
sphincter muscle

Chief segmental sources
of sympathetic fibers
innervating different
regions of intestinal
tract are indicated.
Numerous afferent fibers
are carried centripetally
through approximately
the same sympathetic
splanchnic nerves
that transmit
presynaptic fibers

© Novartis

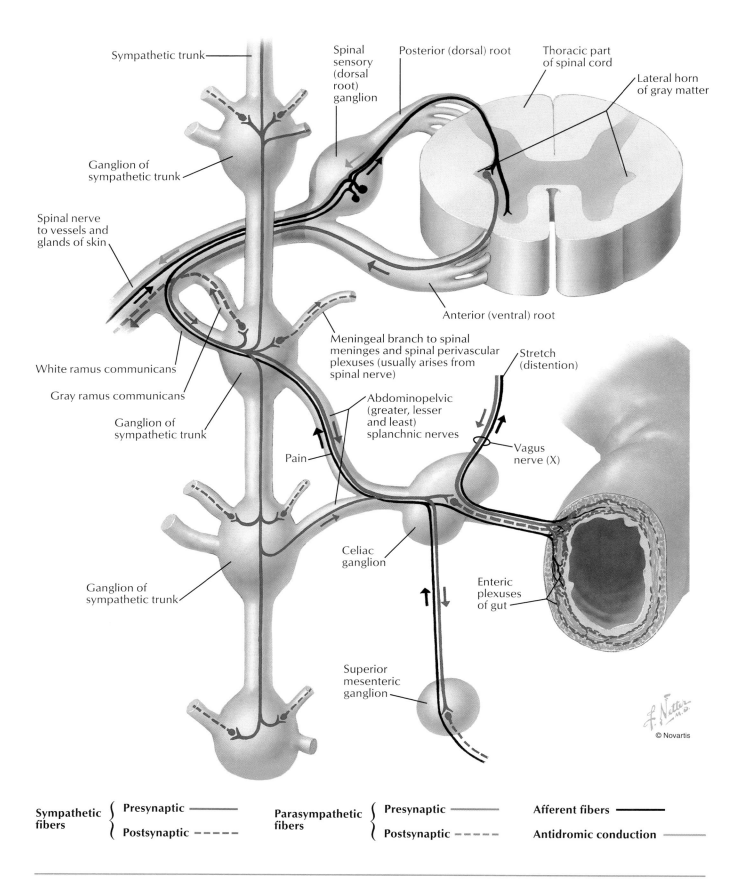

Sympathetic trunk

Ganglion of sympathetic trunk

Spinal nerve to vessels and glands of skin

White ramus communicans

Gray ramus communicans

Ganglion of sympathetic trunk

Ganglion of sympathetic trunk

Spinal sensory (dorsal root) ganglion

Posterior (dorsal) root

Thoracic part of spinal cord

Lateral horn of gray matter

Anterior (ventral) root

Meningeal branch to spinal meninges and spinal perivascular plexuses (usually arises from spinal nerve)

Abdominopelvic (greater, lesser and least) splanchnic nerves

Pain

Stretch (distention)

Vagus nerve (X)

Celiac ganglion

Enteric plexuses of gut

Superior mesenteric ganglion

| Sympathetic fibers | Presynaptic ——— |
| | Postsynaptic − − − |

| Parasympathetic fibers | Presynaptic ——— |
| | Postsynaptic − − − |

Afferent fibers ———

Antidromic conduction ———

© Novartis

**PLATE 307**                                                          **ABDOMEN**

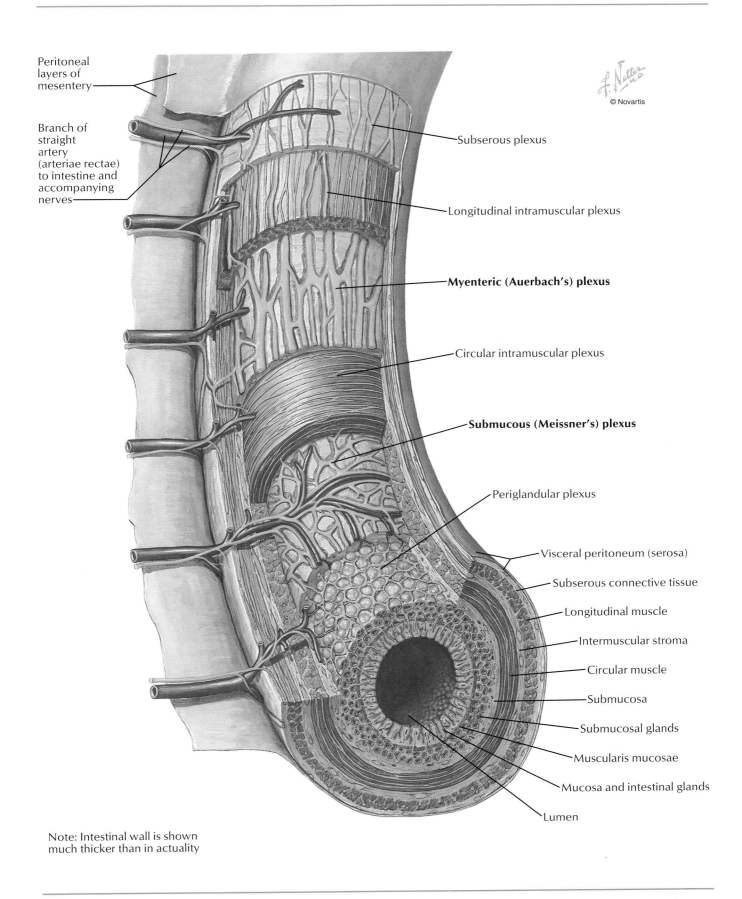

Peritoneal layers of mesentery

Branch of straight artery (arteriae rectae) to intestine and accompanying nerves

Subserous plexus

Longitudinal intramuscular plexus

**Myenteric (Auerbach's) plexus**

Circular intramuscular plexus

**Submucous (Meissner's) plexus**

Periglandular plexus

Visceral peritoneum (serosa)

Subserous connective tissue

Longitudinal muscle

Intermuscular stroma

Circular muscle

Submucosa

Submucosal glands

Muscularis mucosae

Mucosa and intestinal glands

Lumen

Note: Intestinal wall is shown much thicker than in actuality

# Innervation of Liver and Biliary Tract: Schema

*SEE ALSO PLATE 153*

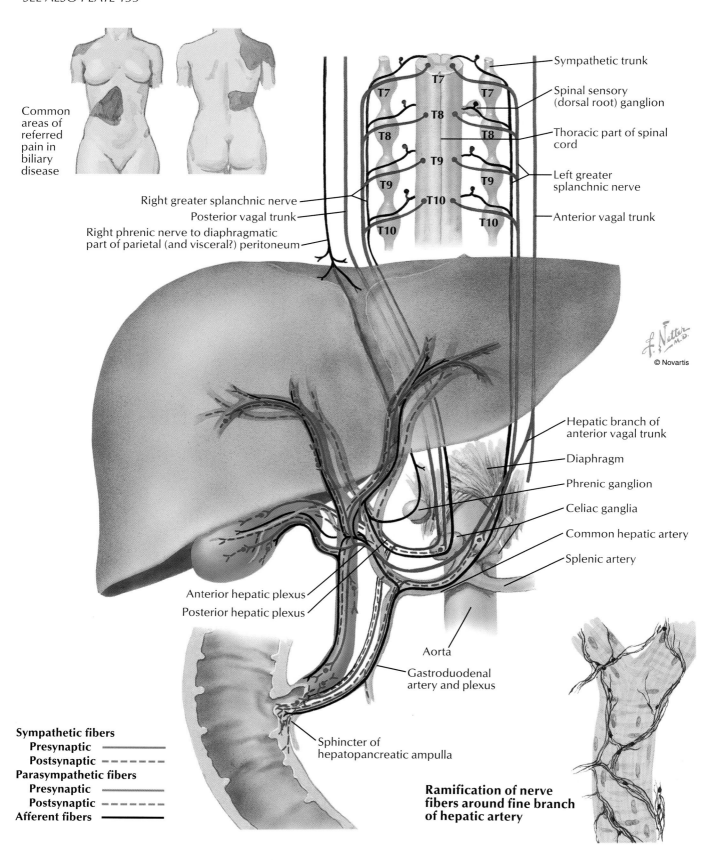

Common areas of referred pain in biliary disease

Sympathetic trunk

Spinal sensory (dorsal root) ganglion

Thoracic part of spinal cord

Left greater splanchnic nerve

Anterior vagal trunk

T7

T8

T9

T10

Right greater splanchnic nerve

Posterior vagal trunk

Right phrenic nerve to diaphragmatic part of parietal (and visceral?) peritoneum

Hepatic branch of anterior vagal trunk

Diaphragm

Phrenic ganglion

Celiac ganglia

Common hepatic artery

Splenic artery

Anterior hepatic plexus

Posterior hepatic plexus

Aorta

Gastroduodenal artery and plexus

Sphincter of hepatopancreatic ampulla

**Sympathetic fibers**
  **Presynaptic** ————
  **Postsynaptic** – – – –
**Parasympathetic fibers**
  **Presynaptic** ————
  **Postsynaptic** – – – –
**Afferent fibers** ————

**Ramification of nerve fibers around fine branch of hepatic artery**

© Novartis

*PLATE 309*                                        **ABDOMEN**

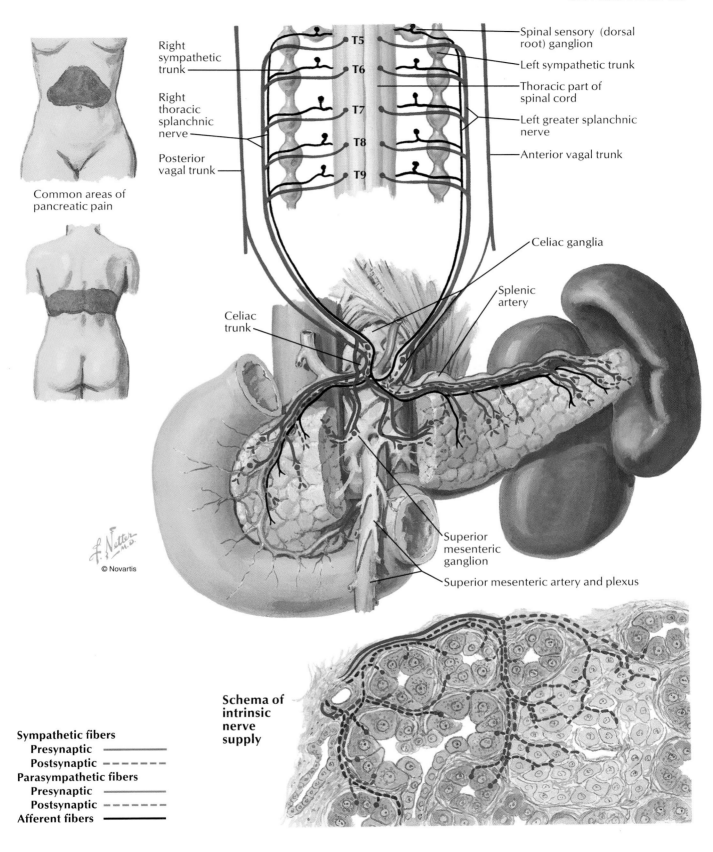

Common areas of pancreatic pain

Right sympathetic trunk

Right thoracic splanchnic nerve

Posterior vagal trunk

Celiac trunk

T5
T6
T7
T8
T9

Spinal sensory (dorsal root) ganglion

Left sympathetic trunk

Thoracic part of spinal cord

Left greater splanchnic nerve

Anterior vagal trunk

Celiac ganglia

Splenic artery

Superior mesenteric ganglion

Superior mesenteric artery and plexus

Schema of intrinsic nerve supply

**Sympathetic fibers**
  Presynaptic
  Postsynaptic
**Parasympathetic fibers**
  Presynaptic
  Postsynaptic
**Afferent fibers**

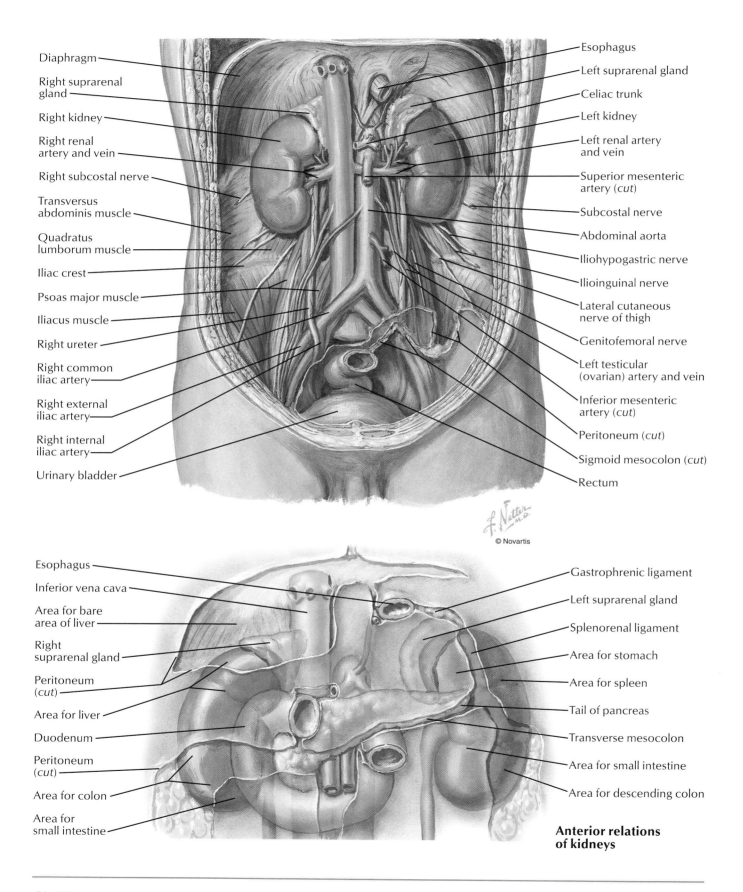

Diaphragm

Right suprarenal gland

Right kidney

Right renal artery and vein

Right subcostal nerve

Transversus abdominis muscle

Quadratus lumborum muscle

Iliac crest

Psoas major muscle

Iliacus muscle

Right ureter

Right common iliac artery

Right external iliac artery

Right internal iliac artery

Urinary bladder

Esophagus

Left suprarenal gland

Celiac trunk

Left kidney

Left renal artery and vein

Superior mesenteric artery (cut)

Subcostal nerve

Abdominal aorta

Iliohypogastric nerve

Ilioinguinal nerve

Lateral cutaneous nerve of thigh

Genitofemoral nerve

Left testicular (ovarian) artery and vein

Inferior mesenteric artery (cut)

Peritoneum (cut)

Sigmoid mesocolon (cut)

Rectum

© Novartis

Esophagus

Inferior vena cava

Area for bare area of liver

Right suprarenal gland

Peritoneum (cut)

Area for liver

Duodenum

Peritoneum (cut)

Area for colon

Area for small intestine

Gastrophrenic ligament

Left suprarenal gland

Splenorenal ligament

Area for stomach

Area for spleen

Tail of pancreas

Transverse mesocolon

Area for small intestine

Area for descending colon

**Anterior relations of kidneys**

**PLATE 311**

**ABDOMEN**

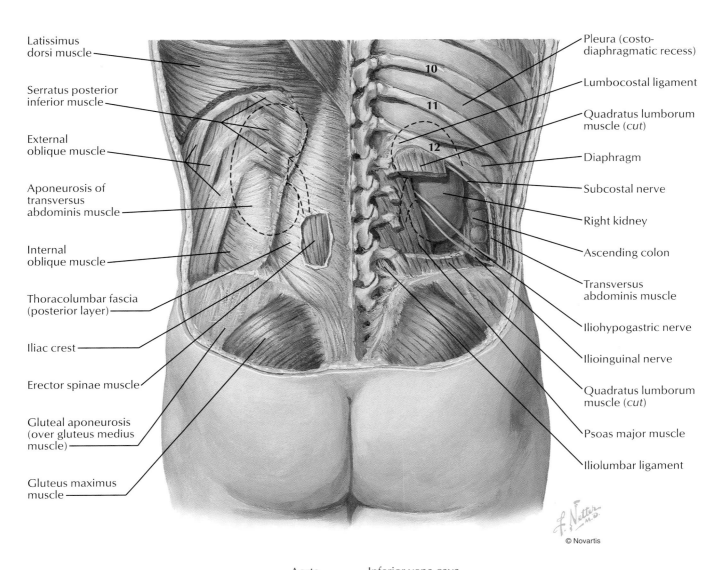

Latissimus dorsi muscle

Serratus posterior inferior muscle

External oblique muscle

Aponeurosis of transversus abdominis muscle

Internal oblique muscle

Thoracolumbar fascia (posterior layer)

Iliac crest

Erector spinae muscle

Gluteal aponeurosis (over gluteus medius muscle)

Gluteus maximus muscle

Pleura (costo-diaphragmatic recess)

Lumbocostal ligament

Quadratus lumborum muscle (*cut*)

Diaphragm

Subcostal nerve

Right kidney

Ascending colon

Transversus abdominis muscle

Iliohypogastric nerve

Ilioinguinal nerve

Quadratus lumborum muscle (*cut*)

Psoas major muscle

Iliolumbar ligament

10

11

12

© Novartis

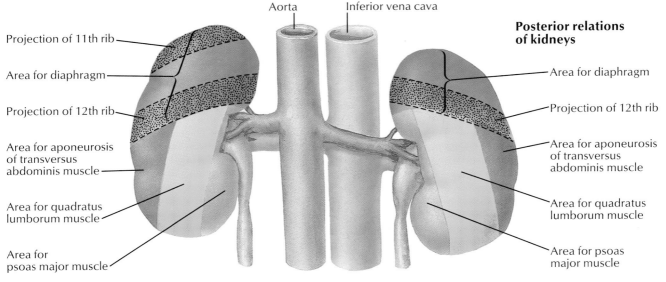

Aorta

Inferior vena cava

**Posterior relations of kidneys**

Projection of 11th rib

Area for diaphragm

Projection of 12th rib

Area for aponeurosis of transversus abdominis muscle

Area for quadratus lumborum muscle

Area for psoas major muscle

Area for diaphragm

Projection of 12th rib

Area for aponeurosis of transversus abdominis muscle

Area for quadratus lumborum muscle

Area for psoas major muscle

# Gross Structure of Kidney

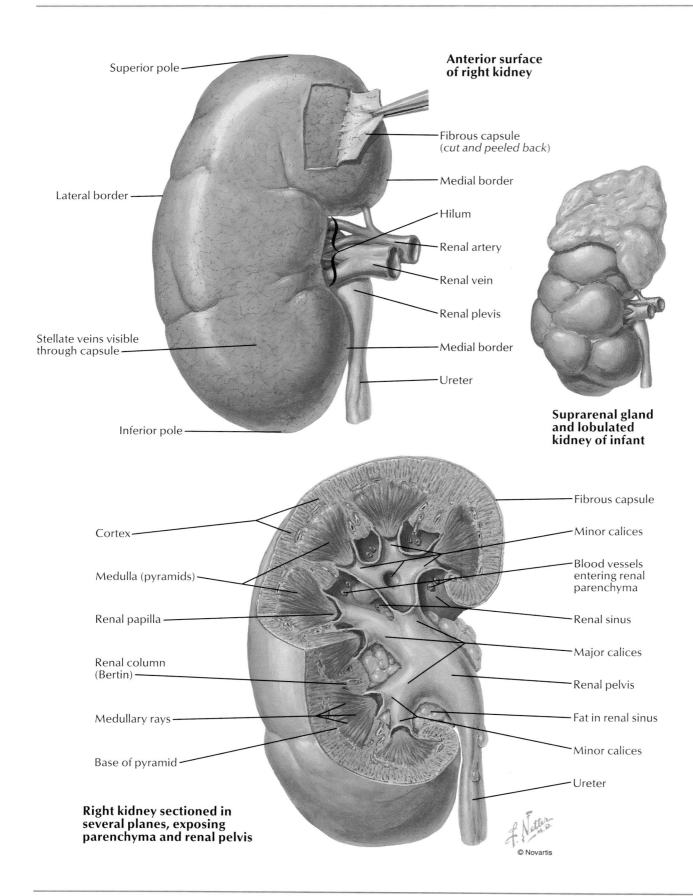

Superior pole

**Anterior surface of right kidney**

Fibrous capsule (*cut and peeled back*)

Medial border

Hilum

Renal artery

Renal vein

Renal plevis

Lateral border

Stellate veins visible through capsule

Medial border

Ureter

Inferior pole

**Suprarenal gland and lobulated kidney of infant**

Cortex

Fibrous capsule

Minor calices

Medulla (pyramids)

Blood vessels entering renal parenchyma

Renal papilla

Renal sinus

Renal column (Bertin)

Major calices

Renal pelvis

Medullary rays

Fat in renal sinus

Base of pyramid

Minor calices

Ureter

**Right kidney sectioned in several planes, exposing parenchyma and renal pelvis**

© Novartis

**PLATE 313**

**ABDOMEN**

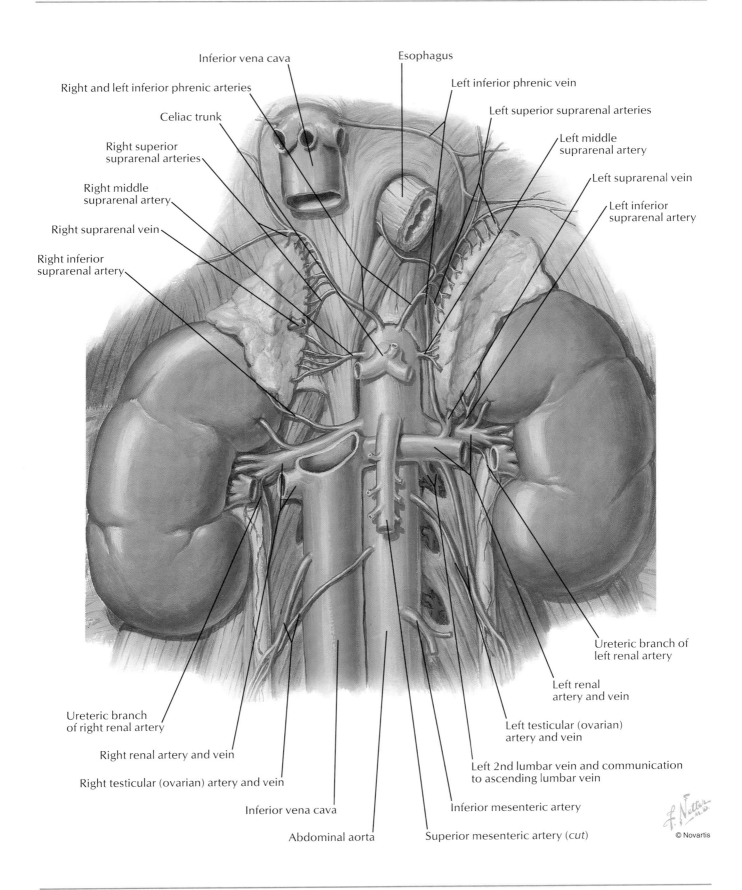

Inferior vena cava

Right and left inferior phrenic arteries

Celiac trunk

Right superior suprarenal arteries

Right middle suprarenal artery

Right suprarenal vein

Right inferior suprarenal artery

Esophagus

Left inferior phrenic vein

Left superior suprarenal arteries

Left middle suprarenal artery

Left suprarenal vein

Left inferior suprarenal artery

Ureteric branch of left renal artery

Left renal artery and vein

Left testicular (ovarian) artery and vein

Left 2nd lumbar vein and communication to ascending lumbar vein

Inferior mesenteric artery

Superior mesenteric artery (cut)

Ureteric branch of right renal artery

Right renal artery and vein

Right testicular (ovarian) artery and vein

Inferior vena cava

Abdominal aorta

© Novartis

# *Intrarenal Arteries and Renal Segments*

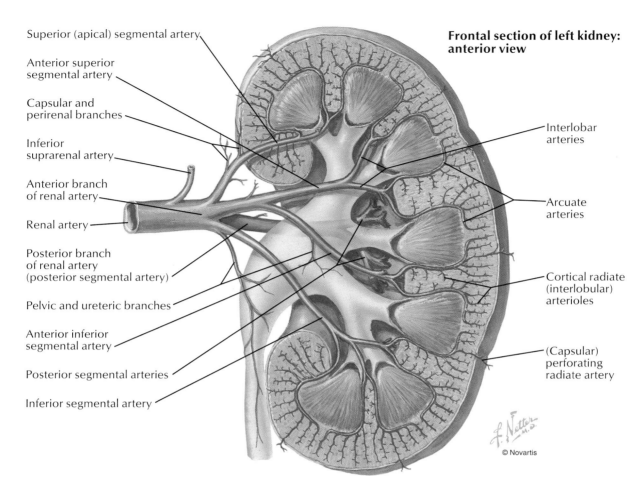

Superior (apical) segmental artery

Anterior superior segmental artery

Capsular and perirenal branches

Inferior suprarenal artery

Anterior branch of renal artery

Renal artery

Posterior branch of renal artery (posterior segmental artery)

Pelvic and ureteric branches

Anterior inferior segmental artery

Posterior segmental arteries

Inferior segmental artery

**Frontal section of left kidney: anterior view**

Interlobar arteries

Arcuate arteries

Cortical radiate (interlobular) arterioles

(Capsular) perforating radiate artery

© Novartis

**Vascular renal segments**

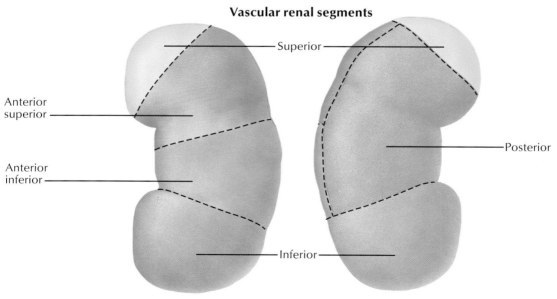

Superior

Anterior superior

Posterior

Anterior inferior

Inferior

Anterior surface of left kidney

Posterior surface of left kidney

*PLATE 315*

**ABDOMEN**

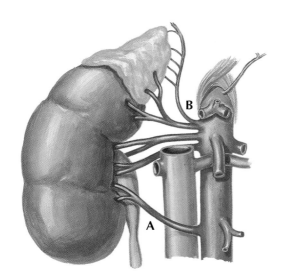

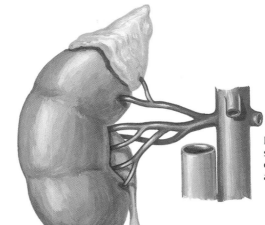

Proximal subdivision of renal artery

**A** Low accessory right renal artery may pass anterior to inferior vena cava instead of posterior to it

**B** Inferior phrenic artery with superior suprarenal arteries may arise from renal artery (middle suprarenal artery absent)

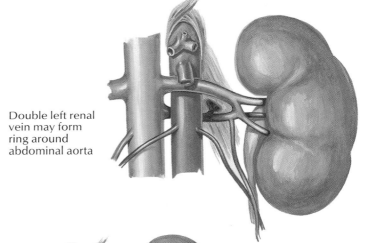

Double left renal vein may form ring around abdominal aorta

Multiple renal veins

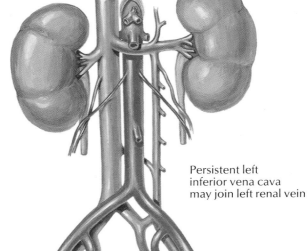

Persistent left inferior vena cava may join left renal vein

© Novartis

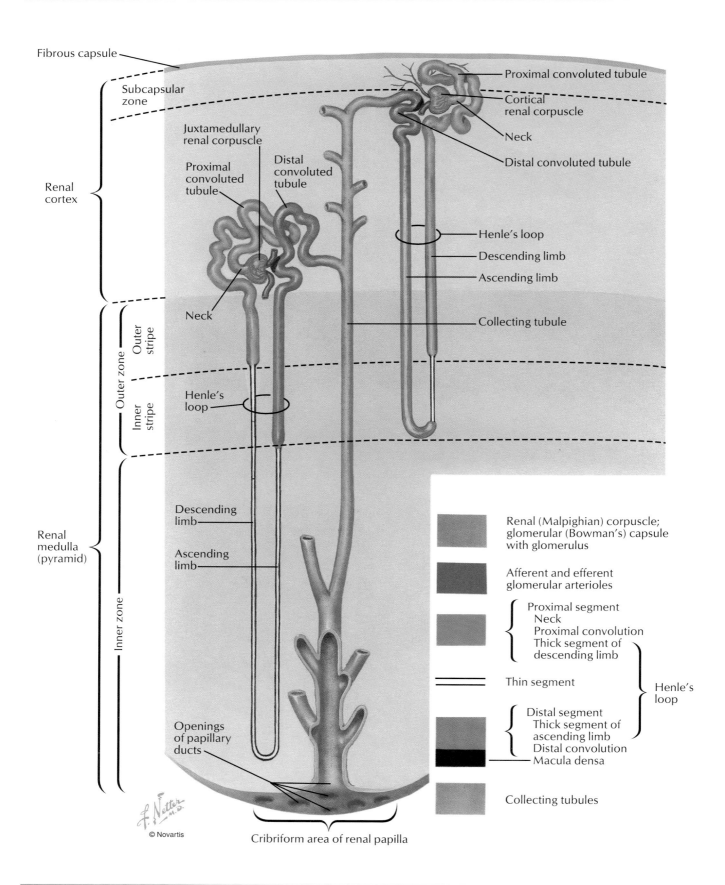

Fibrous capsule

Subcapsular zone

Renal cortex

Juxtamedullary renal corpuscle

Proximal convoluted tubule

Distal convoluted tubule

Neck

Outer zone — Outer stripe

Inner stripe — Henle's loop

Renal medulla (pyramid)

Inner zone

Descending limb

Ascending limb

Openings of papillary ducts

Proximal convoluted tubule

Cortical renal corpuscle

Neck

Distal convoluted tubule

Henle's loop

Descending limb

Ascending limb

Collecting tubule

Renal (Malpighian) corpuscle; glomerular (Bowman's) capsule with glomerulus

Afferent and efferent glomerular arterioles

Proximal segment
Neck
Proximal convolution
Thick segment of descending limb

Thin segment

Henle's loop

Distal segment
Thick segment of ascending limb
Distal convolution
Macula densa

Collecting tubules

Cribriform area of renal papilla

© Novartis

**PLATE 317**

**ABDOMEN**

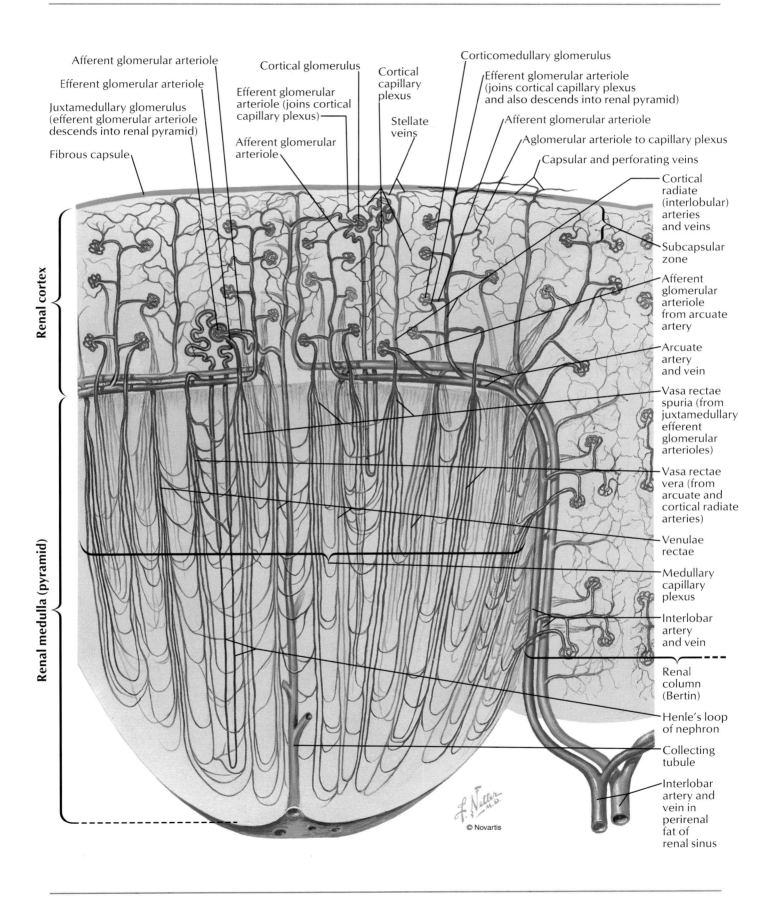

Afferent glomerular arteriole

Efferent glomerular arteriole

Juxtamedullary glomerulus (efferent glomerular arteriole descends into renal pyramid)

Fibrous capsule

Cortical glomerulus

Efferent glomerular arteriole (joins cortical capillary plexus)

Afferent glomerular arteriole

Cortical capillary plexus

Stellate veins

Corticomedullary glomerulus

Efferent glomerular arteriole (joins cortical capillary plexus and also descends into renal pyramid)

Afferent glomerular arteriole

Aglomerular arteriole to capillary plexus

Capsular and perforating veins

Cortical radiate (interlobular) arteries and veins

Subcapsular zone

Afferent glomerular arteriole from arcuate artery

Arcuate artery and vein

Vasa rectae spuria (from juxtamedullary efferent glomerular arterioles)

Vasa rectae vera (from arcuate and cortical radiate arteries)

Venulae rectae

Medullary capillary plexus

Interlobar artery and vein

Renal column (Bertin)

Henle's loop of nephron

Collecting tubule

Interlobar artery and vein in perirenal fat of renal sinus

Renal cortex

Renal medulla (pyramid)

© Novartis

# *Ureters*

*SEE ALSO PLATES 339, 340, 344*

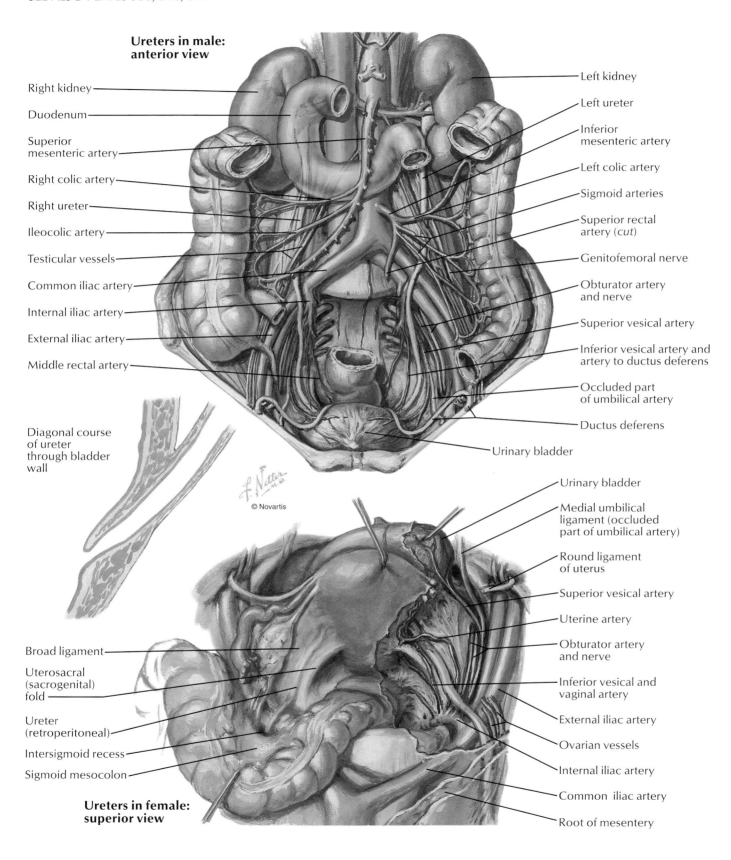

**Ureters in male: anterior view**

Right kidney

Duodenum

Superior mesenteric artery

Right colic artery

Right ureter

Ileocolic artery

Testicular vessels

Common iliac artery

Internal iliac artery

External iliac artery

Middle rectal artery

Left kidney

Left ureter

Inferior mesenteric artery

Left colic artery

Sigmoid arteries

Superior rectal artery (*cut*)

Genitofemoral nerve

Obturator artery and nerve

Superior vesical artery

Inferior vesical artery and artery to ductus deferens

Occluded part of umbilical artery

Ductus deferens

Urinary bladder

Diagonal course of ureter through bladder wall

© Novartis

Urinary bladder

Medial umbilical ligament (occluded part of umbilical artery)

Round ligament of uterus

Superior vesical artery

Uterine artery

Obturator artery and nerve

Inferior vesical and vaginal artery

External iliac artery

Ovarian vessels

Internal iliac artery

Common iliac artery

Root of mesentery

Broad ligament

Uterosacral (sacrogenital) fold

Ureter (retroperitoneal)

Intersigmoid recess

Sigmoid mesocolon

**Ureters in female: superior view**

*PLATE 319*

**ABDOMEN**

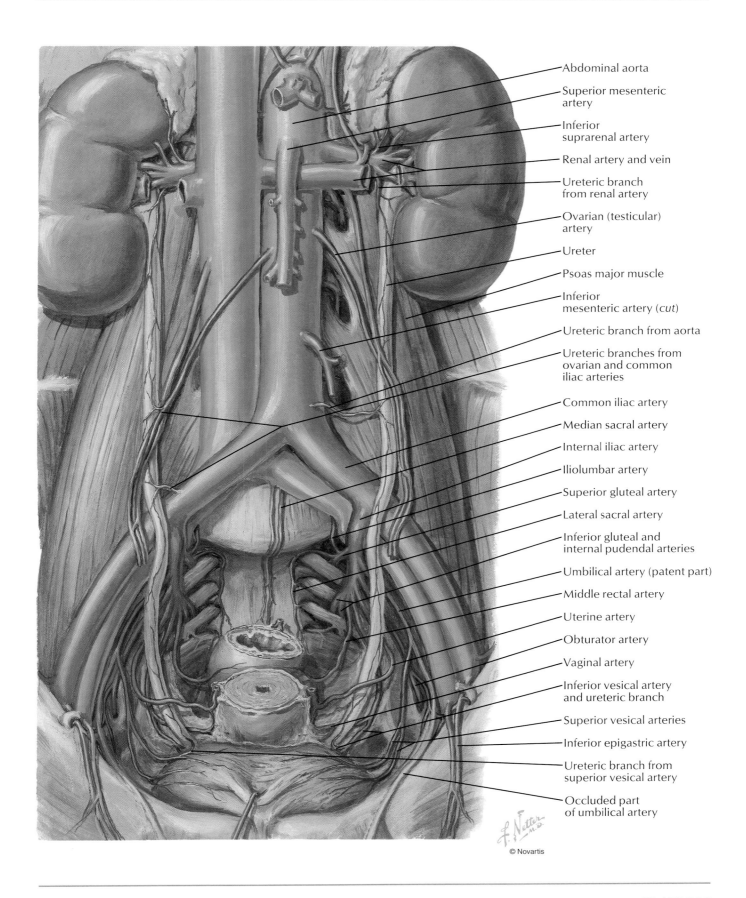

Abdominal aorta

Superior mesenteric artery

Inferior suprarenal artery

Renal artery and vein

Ureteric branch from renal artery

Ovarian (testicular) artery

Ureter

Psoas major muscle

Inferior mesenteric artery (*cut*)

Ureteric branch from aorta

Ureteric branches from ovarian and common iliac arteries

Common iliac artery

Median sacral artery

Internal iliac artery

Iliolumbar artery

Superior gluteal artery

Lateral sacral artery

Inferior gluteal and internal pudendal arteries

Umbilical artery (patent part)

Middle rectal artery

Uterine artery

Obturator artery

Vaginal artery

Inferior vesical artery and ureteric branch

Superior vesical arteries

Inferior epigastric artery

Ureteric branch from superior vesical artery

Occluded part of umbilical artery

© Novartis

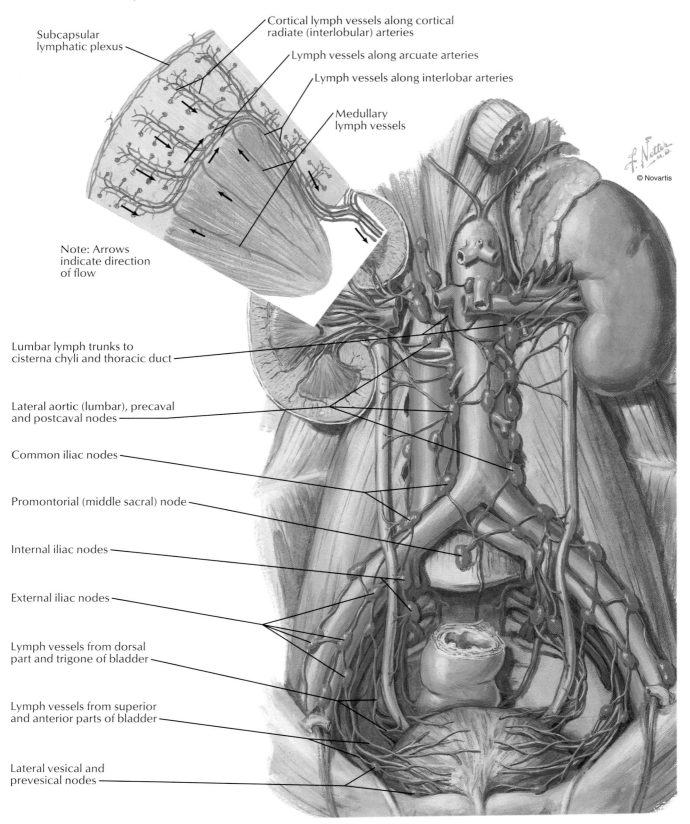

Subcapsular lymphatic plexus

Cortical lymph vessels along cortical radiate (interlobular) arteries

Lymph vessels along arcuate arteries

Lymph vessels along interlobar arteries

Medullary lymph vessels

Note: Arrows indicate direction of flow

Lumbar lymph trunks to cisterna chyli and thoracic duct

Lateral aortic (lumbar), precaval and postcaval nodes

Common iliac nodes

Promontorial (middle sacral) node

Internal iliac nodes

External iliac nodes

Lymph vessels from dorsal part and trigone of bladder

Lymph vessels from superior and anterior parts of bladder

Lateral vesical and prevesical nodes

© Novartis

**PLATE 321**

**ABDOMEN**

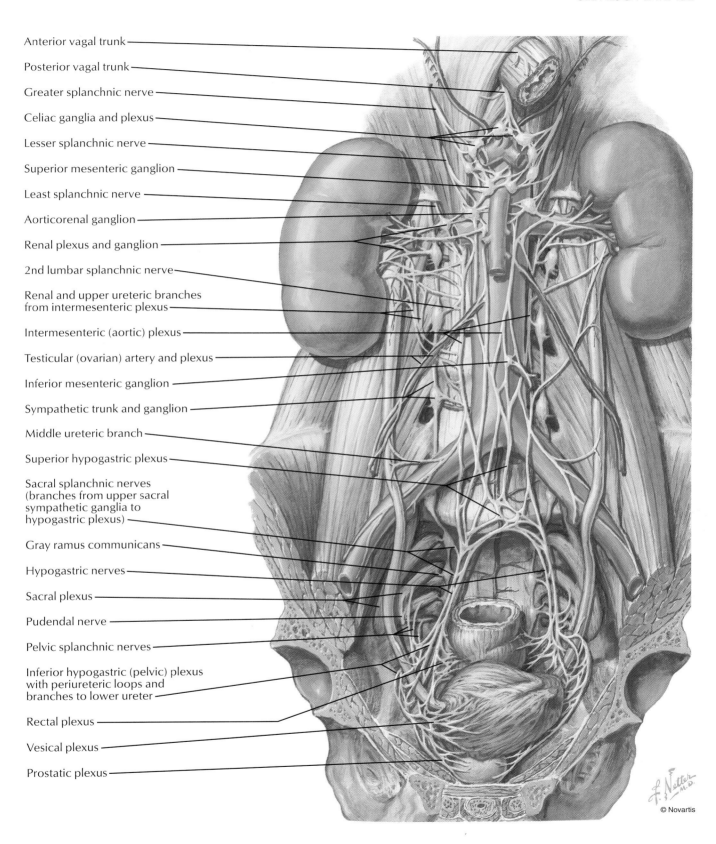

Anterior vagal trunk

Posterior vagal trunk

Greater splanchnic nerve

Celiac ganglia and plexus

Lesser splanchnic nerve

Superior mesenteric ganglion

Least splanchnic nerve

Aorticorenal ganglion

Renal plexus and ganglion

2nd lumbar splanchnic nerve

Renal and upper ureteric branches from intermesenteric plexus

Intermesenteric (aortic) plexus

Testicular (ovarian) artery and plexus

Inferior mesenteric ganglion

Sympathetic trunk and ganglion

Middle ureteric branch

Superior hypogastric plexus

Sacral splanchnic nerves (branches from upper sacral sympathetic ganglia to hypogastric plexus)

Gray ramus communicans

Hypogastric nerves

Sacral plexus

Pudendal nerve

Pelvic splanchnic nerves

Inferior hypogastric (pelvic) plexus with periureteric loops and branches to lower ureter

Rectal plexus

Vesical plexus

Prostatic plexus

© Novartis

SEE ALSO PLATES 153, 388

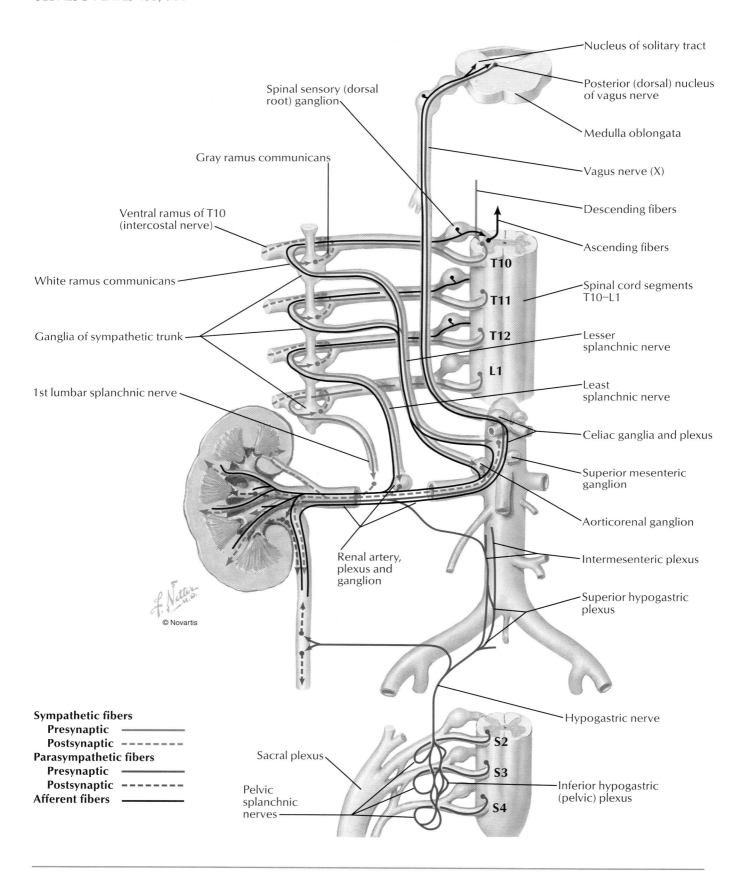

Nucleus of solitary tract

Posterior (dorsal) nucleus of vagus nerve

Spinal sensory (dorsal root) ganglion

Medulla oblongata

Vagus nerve (X)

Gray ramus communicans

Descending fibers

Ventral ramus of T10 (intercostal nerve)

Ascending fibers

**T10**

White ramus communicans

Spinal cord segments T10–L1

**T11**

**T12**

Lesser splanchnic nerve

Ganglia of sympathetic trunk

**L1**

1st lumbar splanchnic nerve

Least splanchnic nerve

Celiac ganglia and plexus

Superior mesenteric ganglion

Aorticorenal ganglion

Renal artery, plexus and ganglion

Intermesenteric plexus

Superior hypogastric plexus

Hypogastric nerve

**Sympathetic fibers**
   Presynaptic ————
   Postsynaptic –––––––
**Parasympathetic fibers**
   Presynaptic ————
   Postsynaptic –––––––
**Afferent fibers** ————

Sacral plexus

**S2**

**S3**

Pelvic splanchnic nerves

Inferior hypogastric (pelvic) plexus

**S4**

F. Netter
© Novartis

**PLATE 323**

**ABDOMEN**

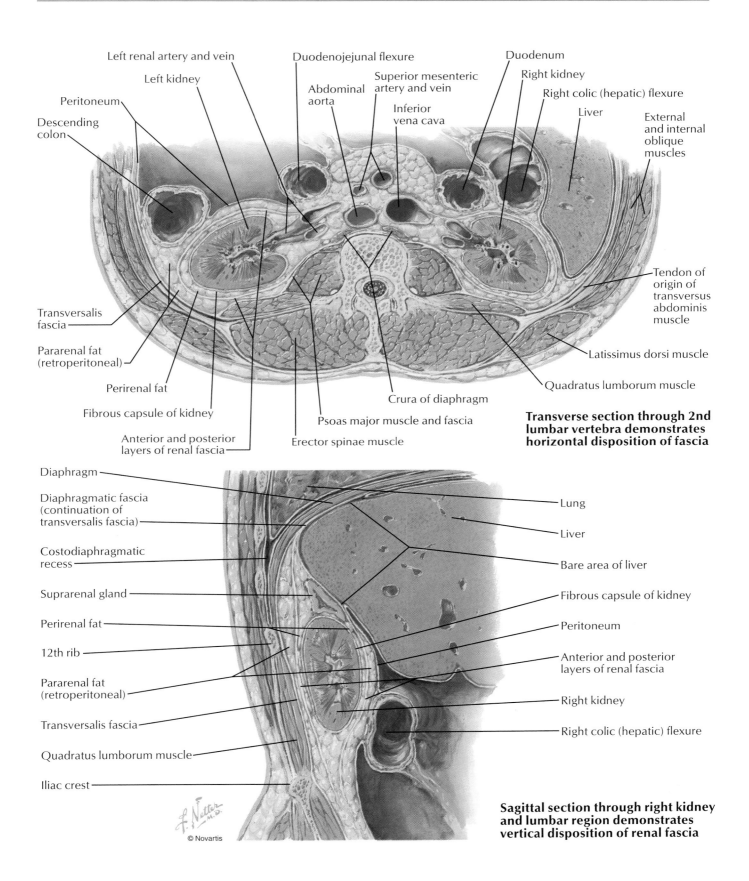

Left renal artery and vein

Left kidney

Peritoneum

Descending colon

Duodenojejunal flexure

Superior mesenteric artery and vein

Abdominal aorta

Inferior vena cava

Duodenum

Right kidney

Right colic (hepatic) flexure

Liver

External and internal oblique muscles

Transversalis fascia

Pararenal fat (retroperitoneal)

Perirenal fat

Fibrous capsule of kidney

Anterior and posterior layers of renal fascia

Erector spinae muscle

Psoas major muscle and fascia

Crura of diaphragm

Tendon of origin of transversus abdominis muscle

Latissimus dorsi muscle

Quadratus lumborum muscle

**Transverse section through 2nd lumbar vertebra demonstrates horizontal disposition of fascia**

Diaphragm

Diaphragmatic fascia (continuation of transversalis fascia)

Costodiaphragmatic recess

Suprarenal gland

Perirenal fat

12th rib

Pararenal fat (retroperitoneal)

Transversalis fascia

Quadratus lumborum muscle

Iliac crest

Lung

Liver

Bare area of liver

Fibrous capsule of kidney

Peritoneum

Anterior and posterior layers of renal fascia

Right kidney

Right colic (hepatic) flexure

**Sagittal section through right kidney and lumbar region demonstrates vertical disposition of renal fascia**

© Novartis

# Arteries and Veins of Suprarenal Glands In Situ

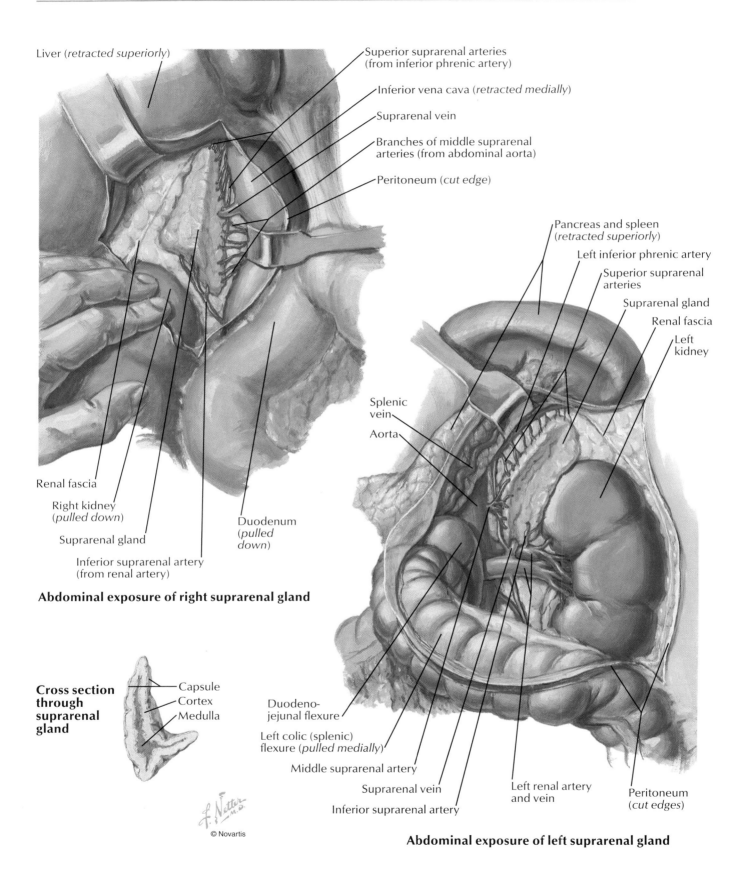

Liver (*retracted superiorly*)

Superior suprarenal arteries (from inferior phrenic artery)

Inferior vena cava (*retracted medially*)

Suprarenal vein

Branches of middle suprarenal arteries (from abdominal aorta)

Peritoneum (*cut edge*)

Pancreas and spleen (*retracted superiorly*)

Left inferior phrenic artery

Superior suprarenal arteries

Suprarenal gland

Renal fascia

Left kidney

Splenic vein

Aorta

Renal fascia

Right kidney (*pulled down*)

Suprarenal gland

Inferior suprarenal artery (from renal artery)

Duodenum (*pulled down*)

**Abdominal exposure of right suprarenal gland**

**Cross section through suprarenal gland**

Capsule

Cortex

Medulla

Duodeno-jejunal flexure

Left colic (splenic) flexure (*pulled medially*)

Middle suprarenal artery

Suprarenal vein

Inferior suprarenal artery

Left renal artery and vein

Peritoneum (*cut edges*)

**Abdominal exposure of left suprarenal gland**

© Novartis

**PLATE 325**

**ABDOMEN**

*SEE ALSO PLATES 152, 153*

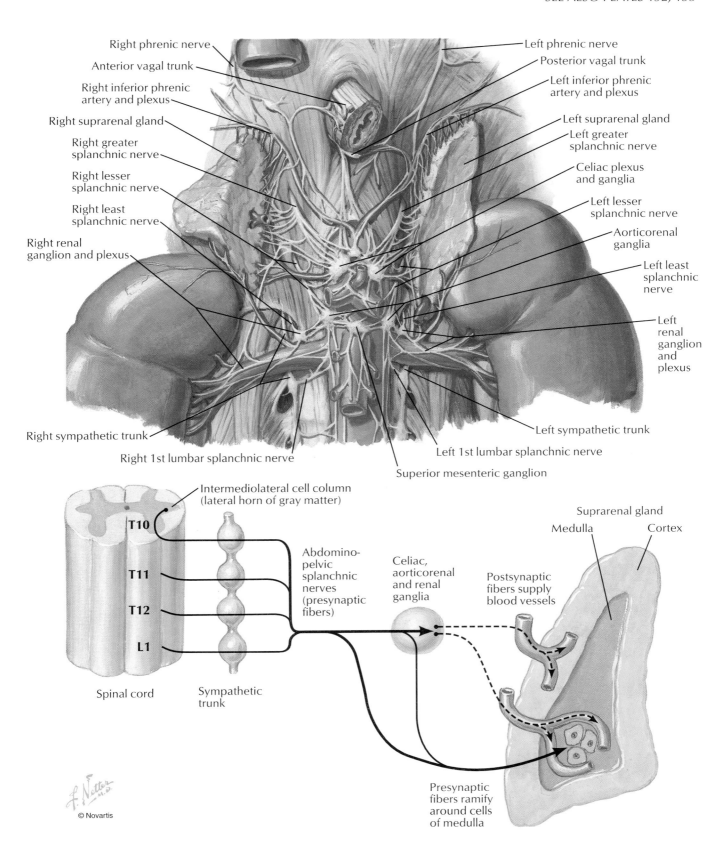

Right phrenic nerve

Anterior vagal trunk

Right inferior phrenic artery and plexus

Right suprarenal gland

Right greater splanchnic nerve

Right lesser splanchnic nerve

Right least splanchnic nerve

Right renal ganglion and plexus

Right sympathetic trunk

Right 1st lumbar splanchnic nerve

Left phrenic nerve

Posterior vagal trunk

Left inferior phrenic artery and plexus

Left suprarenal gland

Left greater splanchnic nerve

Celiac plexus and ganglia

Left lesser splanchnic nerve

Aorticorenal ganglia

Left least splanchnic nerve

Left renal ganglion and plexus

Left sympathetic trunk

Left 1st lumbar splanchnic nerve

Superior mesenteric ganglion

Intermediolateral cell column (lateral horn of gray matter)

T10

T11

T12

L1

Spinal cord

Sympathetic trunk

Abdomino-pelvic splanchnic nerves (presynaptic fibers)

Celiac, aorticorenal and renal ganglia

Postsynaptic fibers supply blood vessels

Suprarenal gland

Medulla

Cortex

Presynaptic fibers ramify around cells of medulla

© Novartis

# Schematic Cross Section of Abdomen at T12 (Superior View)

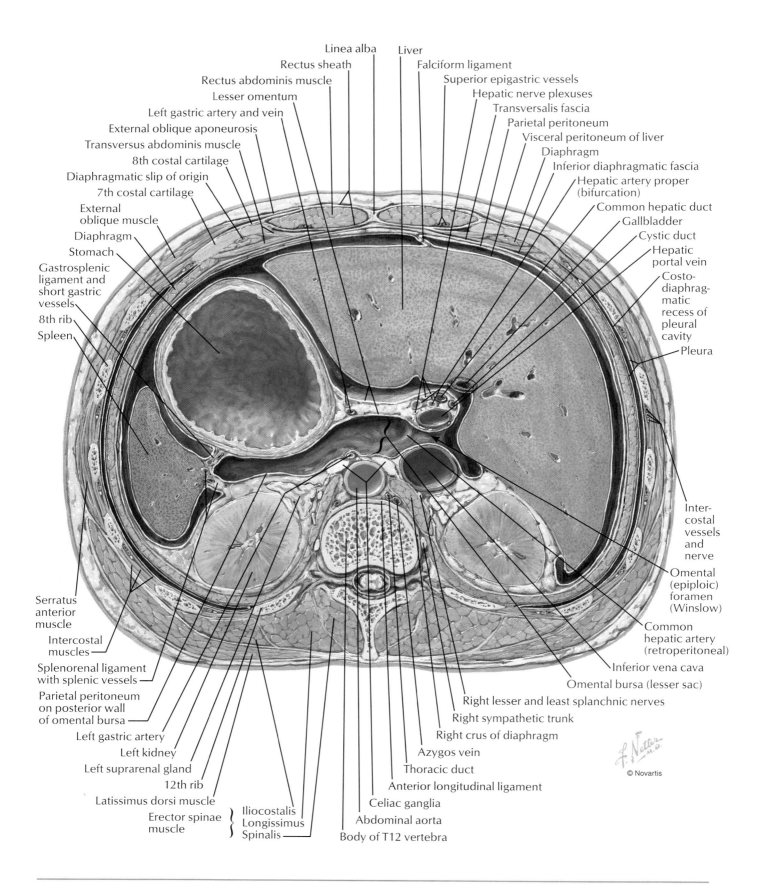

Linea alba
Rectus sheath
Rectus abdominis muscle
Lesser omentum
Left gastric artery and vein
External oblique aponeurosis
Transversus abdominis muscle
8th costal cartilage
Diaphragmatic slip of origin
7th costal cartilage
External oblique muscle
Diaphragm
Stomach
Gastrosplenic ligament and short gastric vessels
8th rib
Spleen

Liver
Falciform ligament
Superior epigastric vessels
Hepatic nerve plexuses
Transversalis fascia
Parietal peritoneum
Visceral peritoneum of liver
Diaphragm
Inferior diaphragmatic fascia
Hepatic artery proper (bifurcation)
Common hepatic duct
Gallbladder
Cystic duct
Hepatic portal vein
Costo-diaphrag-matic recess of pleural cavity
Pleura

Serratus anterior muscle
Intercostal muscles
Splenorenal ligament with splenic vessels
Parietal peritoneum on posterior wall of omental bursa
Left gastric artery
Left kidney
Left suprarenal gland
12th rib
Latissimus dorsi muscle
Erector spinae muscle
Iliocostalis
Longissimus
Spinalis

Body of T12 vertebra
Abdominal aorta
Celiac ganglia
Anterior longitudinal ligament
Thoracic duct
Azygos vein
Right crus of diaphragm
Right sympathetic trunk
Right lesser and least splanchnic nerves
Omental bursa (lesser sac)
Inferior vena cava
Common hepatic artery (retroperitoneal)
Omental (epiploic) foramen (Winslow)
Inter-costal vessels and nerve

© Novartis

**PLATE 327**                                                                **ABDOMEN**

# Schematic Cross Section of Abdomen at L2,3 (Superior View)

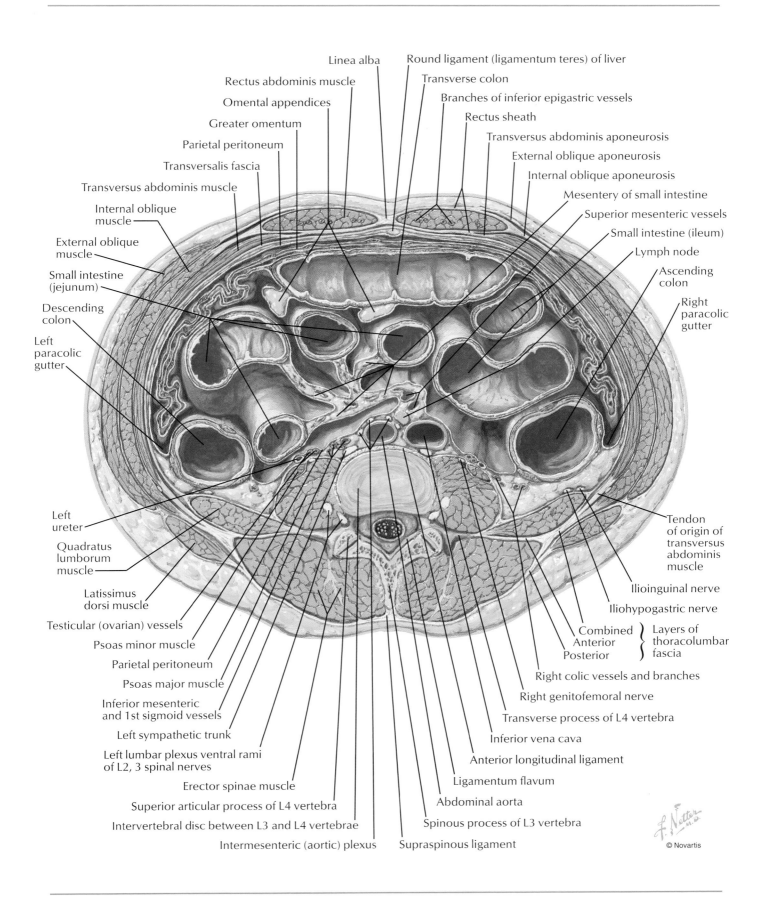

Linea alba

Rectus abdominis muscle

Omental appendices

Greater omentum

Parietal peritoneum

Transversalis fascia

Transversus abdominis muscle

Internal oblique muscle

External oblique muscle

Small intestine (jejunum)

Descending colon

Left paracolic gutter

Left ureter

Quadratus lumborum muscle

Latissimus dorsi muscle

Testicular (ovarian) vessels

Psoas minor muscle

Parietal peritoneum

Psoas major muscle

Inferior mesenteric and 1st sigmoid vessels

Left sympathetic trunk

Left lumbar plexus ventral rami of L2, 3 spinal nerves

Erector spinae muscle

Superior articular process of L4 vertebra

Intervertebral disc between L3 and L4 vertebrae

Intermesenteric (aortic) plexus

Round ligament (ligamentum teres) of liver

Transverse colon

Branches of inferior epigastric vessels

Rectus sheath

Transversus abdominis aponeurosis

External oblique aponeurosis

Internal oblique aponeurosis

Mesentery of small intestine

Superior mesenteric vessels

Small intestine (ileum)

Lymph node

Ascending colon

Right paracolic gutter

Tendon of origin of transversus abdominis muscle

Ilioinguinal nerve

Iliohypogastric nerve

Combined Anterior Posterior } Layers of thoracolumbar fascia

Right colic vessels and branches

Right genitofemoral nerve

Transverse process of L4 vertebra

Inferior vena cava

Anterior longitudinal ligament

Ligamentum flavum

Abdominal aorta

Spinous process of L3 vertebra

Supraspinous ligament

*f. Netter m.s.*

© Novartis

---

**KIDNEYS AND SUPRARENAL GLANDS**

*PLATE 328*

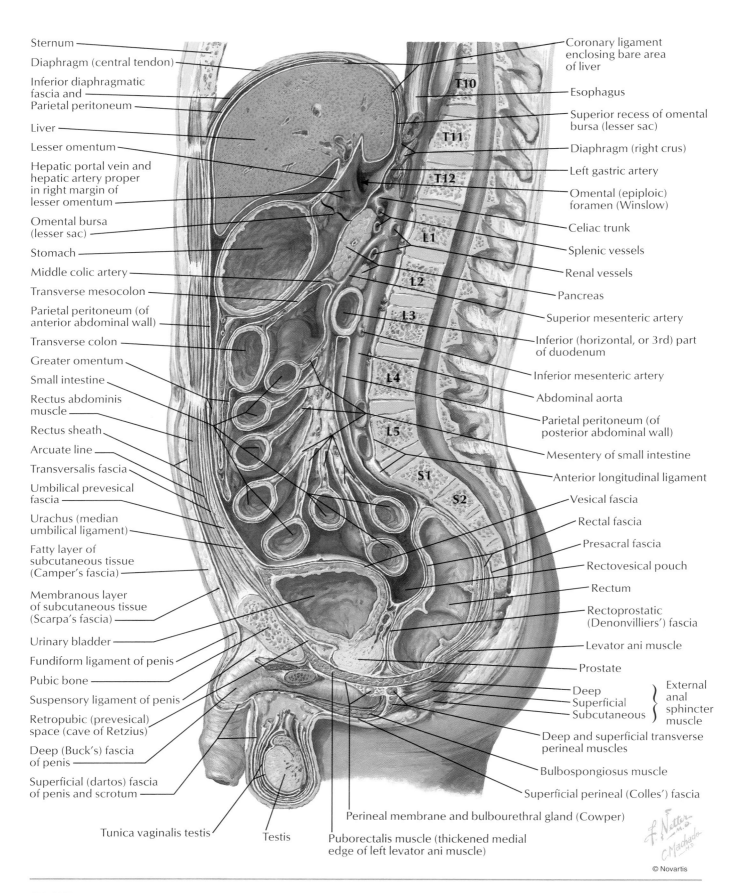

Sternum

Diaphragm (central tendon)

Inferior diaphragmatic fascia and Parietal peritoneum

Liver

Lesser omentum

Hepatic portal vein and hepatic artery proper in right margin of lesser omentum

Omental bursa (lesser sac)

Stomach

Middle colic artery

Transverse mesocolon

Parietal peritoneum (of anterior abdominal wall)

Transverse colon

Greater omentum

Small intestine

Rectus abdominis muscle

Rectus sheath

Arcuate line

Transversalis fascia

Umbilical prevesical fascia

Urachus (median umbilical ligament)

Fatty layer of subcutaneous tissue (Camper's fascia)

Membranous layer of subcutaneous tissue (Scarpa's fascia)

Urinary bladder

Fundiform ligament of penis

Pubic bone

Suspensory ligament of penis

Retropubic (prevesical) space (cave of Retzius)

Deep (Buck's) fascia of penis

Superficial (dartos) fascia of penis and scrotum

Tunica vaginalis testis

Testis

Puborectalis muscle (thickened medial edge of left levator ani muscle)

Perineal membrane and bulbourethral gland (Cowper)

T10

T11

T12

L1

L2

L3

L4

L5

S1

S2

Coronary ligament enclosing bare area of liver

Esophagus

Superior recess of omental bursa (lesser sac)

Diaphragm (right crus)

Left gastric artery

Omental (epiploic) foramen (Winslow)

Celiac trunk

Splenic vessels

Renal vessels

Pancreas

Superior mesenteric artery

Inferior (horizontal, or 3rd) part of duodenum

Inferior mesenteric artery

Abdominal aorta

Parietal peritoneum (of posterior abdominal wall)

Mesentery of small intestine

Anterior longitudinal ligament

Vesical fascia

Rectal fascia

Presacral fascia

Rectovesical pouch

Rectum

Rectoprostatic (Denonvilliers') fascia

Levator ani muscle

Prostate

Deep — 
Superficial — External anal sphincter muscle
Subcutaneous — 

Deep and superficial transverse perineal muscles

Bulbospongiosus muscle

Superficial perineal (Colles') fascia

© Novartis

**PLATE 329**        **ABDOMEN**

# Section V
# PELVIS AND PERINEUM

**BONES AND LIGAMENTS**
*Plates 330 − 332*

330. Bones and Ligaments of Pelvis
331. Bones and Ligaments of Pelvis
   (*continued*)
332. Sex Differences of Pelvis:
   Measurements

**PELVIC FLOOR AND CONTENTS**
*Plates 333 − 343*

333. Pelvic Diaphragm: Female
334. Pelvic Diaphragm: Female
   (*continued*)
335. Pelvic Diaphragm: Male
336. Pelvic Diaphragm: Male
   (*continued*)
337. Pelvic Viscera and Perineum:
   Female
338. Pelvic Viscera and Perineum: Male
339. Pelvic Contents: Female

340. Pelvic Contents: Male
341. Endopelvic Fascia and Potential Spaces
342. Urinary Bladder: Orientation and
   Supports
343. Urinary Bladder: Female and Male

**FEMALE STRUCTURES**
*Plates 344 − 353*

344. Pelvic Viscera
345. Uterus, Vagina and Supporting
   Structures
346. Uterus and Adnexa
347. Uterus: Age Changes and
   Muscle Pattern
348. Uterus: Variations in Position
349. Ovary, Ova and Follicles
350. Perineum and External
   Genitalia (Pudendum or Vulva)
351. Perineum (Superficial
   Dissection)

352. Perineum and Deep Perineum
353. Urethra

**MALE STRUCTURES**
*Plates 354 – 362*
354. Perineum and External Genitalia
(Superficial Dissection)
355. Perineum and External Genitalia
(Deeper Dissection)
356. Penis
357. Perineal Spaces
358. Prostate and Seminal Vesicles
359. Urethra
360. Descent of Testis
361. Scrotum and Contents
362. Testis, Epididymis and
Ductus Deferens

**RECTUM**
*Plates 363 – 368*
363. Rectum In Situ: Female and Male
364. Ischioanal Fossae
365. Rectum and Anal Canal
366. Anorectal Musculature
367. External Anal Sphincter Muscle:
Perineal Views
368. Actual and Potential Perineopelvic
Spaces

**VASCULATURE**
*Plates 369 – 379*
369. Arteries of Rectum and Anal Canal
370. Veins of Rectum and Anal Canal

371. Arteries and Veins of Pelvic Organs:
Female
372. Arteries and Veins of Testis
373. Arteries and Veins of Pelvis: Female
374. Arteries and Veins of Pelvis: Male
375. Arteries and Veins of Perineum
and Uterus
376. Arteries and Veins of Perineum: Male
377. Lymph Vessels and Nodes of Pelvis
and Genitalia: Female
378. Lymph Vessels and Nodes of
Perineum: Female
379. Lymph Vessels and Nodes of Pelvis
and Genitalia: Male

**INNERVATION**
*Plates 380 – 390*
380. Nerves of External Genitalia: Male
381. Nerves of Pelvic Viscera: Male
382. Nerves of Perineum: Male
383. Nerves of Pelvic Viscera: Female
384. Nerves of Perineum and External
Genitalia: Female
385. Neuropathways in Parturition
386. Innervation of Female Reproductive
Organs: Schema
387. Innervation of Male Reproductive
Organs: Schema
388. Innervation of Urinary Bladder and
Lower Ureter: Schema
389. Homologues of External Genitalia
390. Homologues of Internal Genitalia

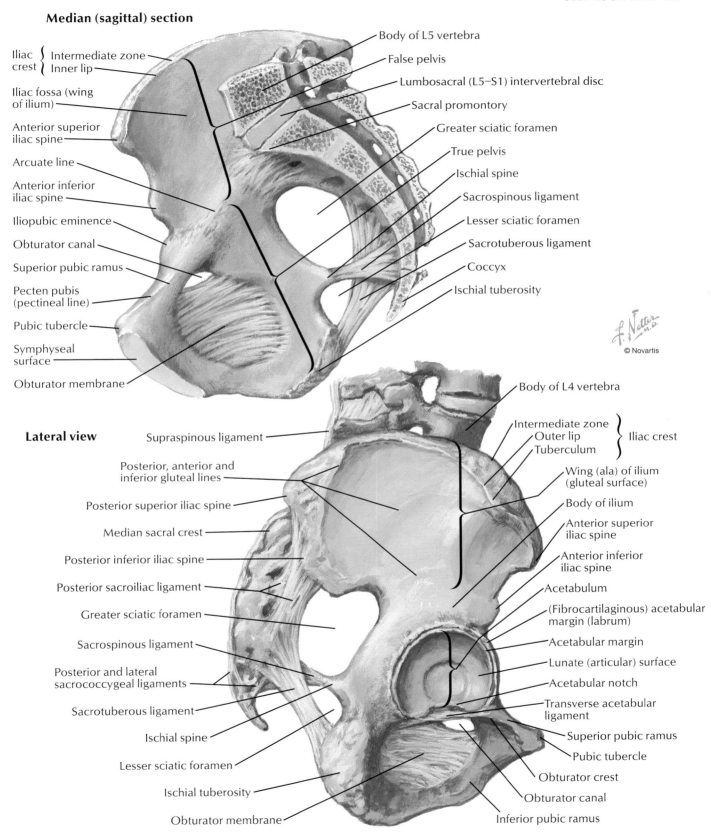

**Median (sagittal) section**

Iliac crest { Intermediate zone
Iliac crest { Inner lip

Iliac fossa (wing of ilium)

Anterior superior iliac spine

Arcuate line

Anterior inferior iliac spine

Iliopubic eminence

Obturator canal

Superior pubic ramus

Pecten pubis (pectineal line)

Pubic tubercle

Symphyseal surface

Obturator membrane

Body of L5 vertebra

False pelvis

Lumbosacral (L5–S1) intervertebral disc

Sacral promontory

Greater sciatic foramen

True pelvis

Ischial spine

Sacrospinous ligament

Lesser sciatic foramen

Sacrotuberous ligament

Coccyx

Ischial tuberosity

**Lateral view**

Supraspinous ligament

Posterior, anterior and inferior gluteal lines

Posterior superior iliac spine

Median sacral crest

Posterior inferior iliac spine

Posterior sacroiliac ligament

Greater sciatic foramen

Sacrospinous ligament

Posterior and lateral sacrococcygeal ligaments

Sacrotuberous ligament

Ischial spine

Lesser sciatic foramen

Ischial tuberosity

Obturator membrane

Body of L4 vertebra

Intermediate zone } 
Outer lip } Iliac crest
Tuberculum }

Wing (ala) of ilium (gluteal surface)

Body of ilium

Anterior superior iliac spine

Anterior inferior iliac spine

Acetabulum

(Fibrocartilaginous) acetabular margin (labrum)

Acetabular margin

Lunate (articular) surface

Acetabular notch

Transverse acetabular ligament

Superior pubic ramus

Pubic tubercle

Obturator crest

Obturator canal

Inferior pubic ramus

# Bones and Ligaments of Pelvis (continued)

SEE ALSO PLATE 145

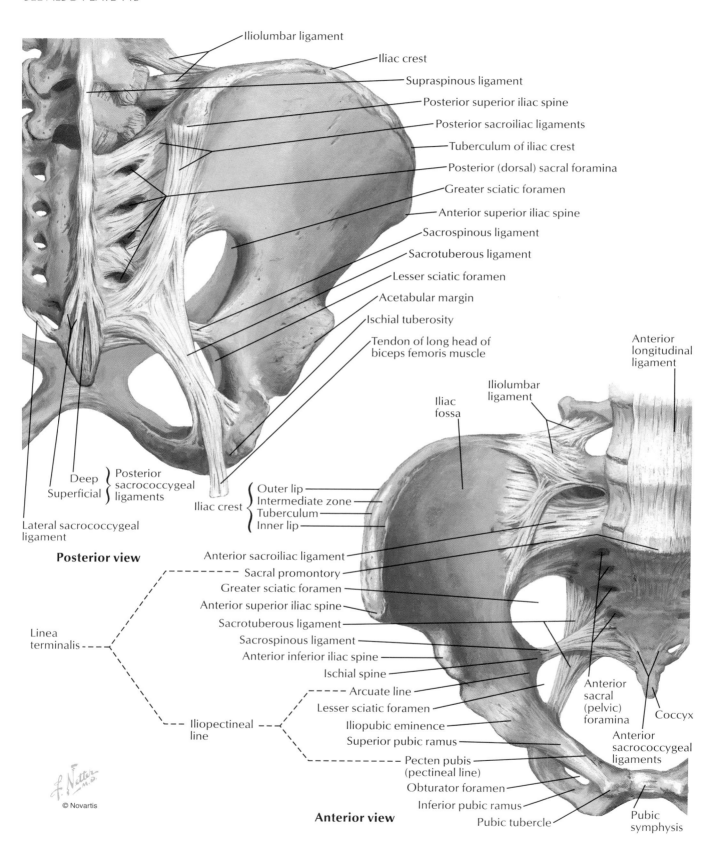

Iliolumbar ligament

Iliac crest

Supraspinous ligament

Posterior superior iliac spine

Posterior sacroiliac ligaments

Tuberculum of iliac crest

Posterior (dorsal) sacral foramina

Greater sciatic foramen

Anterior superior iliac spine

Sacrospinous ligament

Sacrotuberous ligament

Lesser sciatic foramen

Acetabular margin

Ischial tuberosity

Tendon of long head of biceps femoris muscle

Deep
Superficial } Posterior sacrococcygeal ligaments

Lateral sacrococcygeal ligament

**Posterior view**

Iliac crest {
Outer lip
Intermediate zone
Tuberculum
Inner lip

Anterior longitudinal ligament

Iliolumbar ligament

Iliac fossa

Anterior sacroiliac ligament

Sacral promontory

Greater sciatic foramen

Anterior superior iliac spine

Sacrotuberous ligament

Sacrospinous ligament

Anterior inferior iliac spine

Ischial spine

Arcuate line

Lesser sciatic foramen

Iliopubic eminence

Superior pubic ramus

Pecten pubis (pectineal line)

Obturator foramen

Inferior pubic ramus

Pubic tubercle

Anterior sacral (pelvic) foramina

Coccyx

Anterior sacrococcygeal ligaments

Pubic symphysis

Linea terminalis

Iliopectineal line

**Anterior view**

© Novartis

**PLATE 331**                                                           **PELVIS AND PERINEUM**

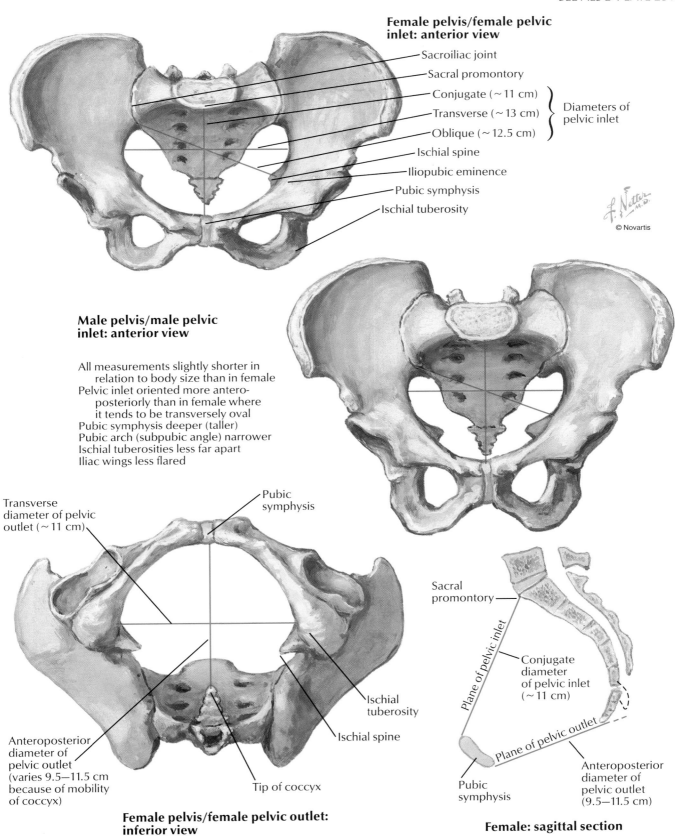

**Female pelvis/female pelvic inlet: anterior view**

- Sacroiliac joint
- Sacral promontory
- Conjugate (~11 cm)
- Transverse (~13 cm) — Diameters of pelvic inlet
- Oblique (~12.5 cm)
- Ischial spine
- Iliopubic eminence
- Pubic symphysis
- Ischial tuberosity

© Novartis

**Male pelvis/male pelvic inlet: anterior view**

All measurements slightly shorter in relation to body size than in female
Pelvic inlet oriented more antero-posteriorly than in female where it tends to be transversely oval
Pubic symphysis deeper (taller)
Pubic arch (subpubic angle) narrower
Ischial tuberosities less far apart
Iliac wings less flared

Transverse diameter of pelvic outlet (~11 cm)

Pubic symphysis

Anteroposterior diameter of pelvic outlet (varies 9.5—11.5 cm because of mobility of coccyx)

Tip of coccyx

Ischial tuberosity

Ischial spine

**Female pelvis/female pelvic outlet: inferior view**

Sacral promontory

Conjugate diameter of pelvic inlet (~11 cm)

Plane of pelvic inlet

Plane of pelvic outlet

Anteroposterior diameter of pelvic outlet (9.5—11.5 cm)

Pubic symphysis

**Female: sagittal section**

# Pelvic Diaphragm: Female

SEE ALSO PLATES 246, 343, 345, 364

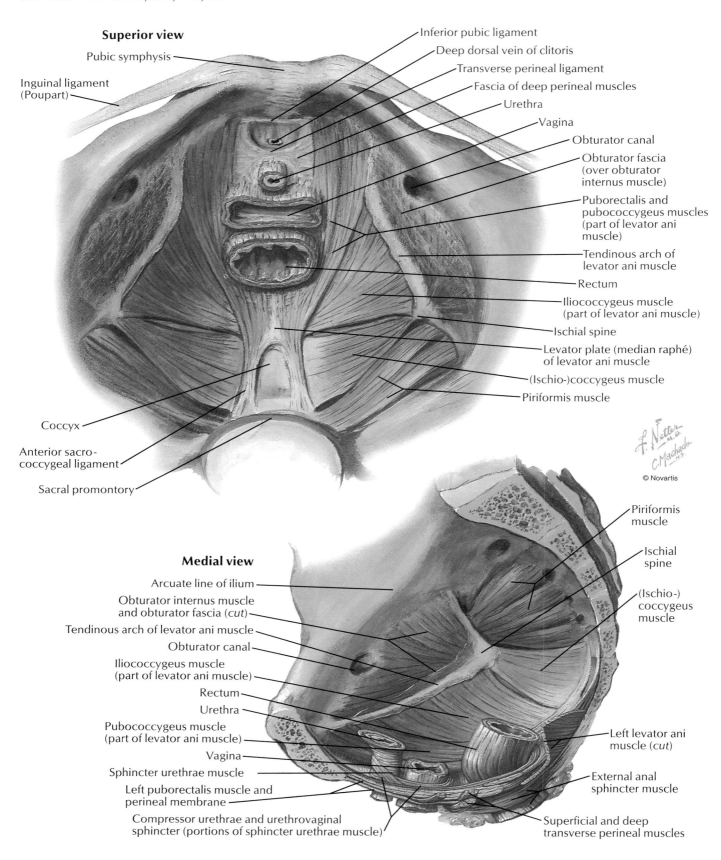

**Superior view**

Pubic symphysis

Inguinal ligament
(Poupart)

Inferior pubic ligament

Deep dorsal vein of clitoris

Transverse perineal ligament

Fascia of deep perineal muscles

Urethra

Vagina

Obturator canal

Obturator fascia
(over obturator
internus muscle)

Puborectalis and
pubococcygeus muscles
(part of levator ani
muscle)

Tendinous arch of
levator ani muscle

Rectum

Iliococcygeus muscle
(part of levator ani muscle)

Ischial spine

Levator plate (median raphé)
of levator ani muscle

(Ischio-)coccygeus muscle

Piriformis muscle

Coccyx

Anterior sacro-
coccygeal ligament

Sacral promontory

**Medial view**

Arcuate line of ilium

Obturator internus muscle
and obturator fascia (cut)

Tendinous arch of levator ani muscle

Obturator canal

Iliococcygeus muscle
(part of levator ani muscle)

Rectum

Urethra

Pubococcygeus muscle
(part of levator ani muscle)

Vagina

Sphincter urethrae muscle

Left puborectalis muscle and
perineal membrane

Compressor urethrae and urethrovaginal
sphincter (portions of sphincter urethrae muscle)

Piriformis
muscle

Ischial
spine

(Ischio-)
coccygeus
muscle

Left levator ani
muscle (cut)

External anal
sphincter muscle

Superficial and deep
transverse perineal muscles

**PLATE 333**

**PELVIS AND PERINEUM**

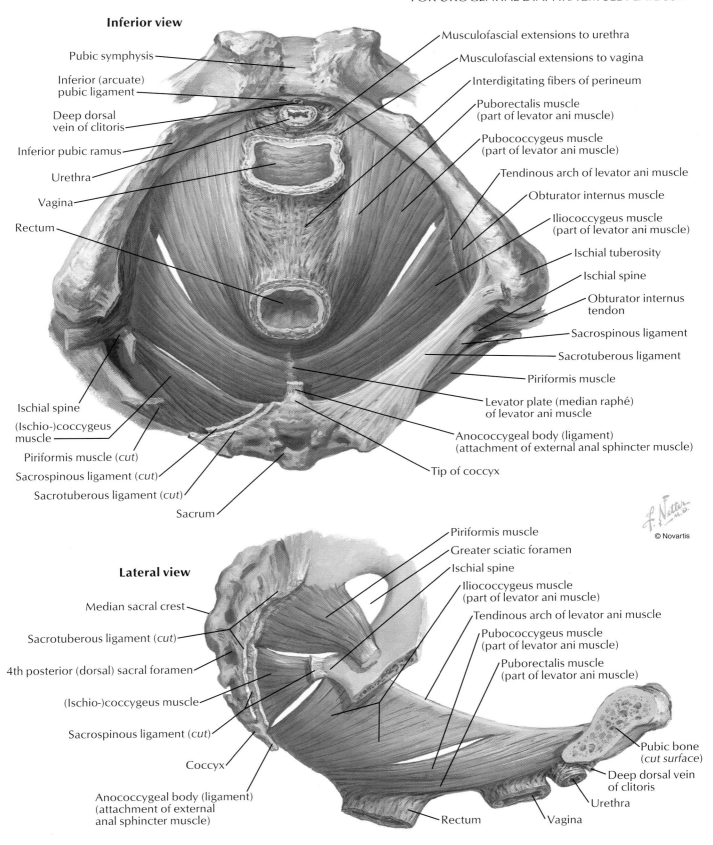

**Inferior view**

Pubic symphysis

Inferior (arcuate) pubic ligament

Deep dorsal vein of clitoris

Inferior pubic ramus

Urethra

Vagina

Rectum

Ischial spine

(Ischio-)coccygeus muscle

Piriformis muscle (*cut*)

Sacrospinous ligament (*cut*)

Sacrotuberous ligament (*cut*)

Sacrum

Musculofascial extensions to urethra

Musculofascial extensions to vagina

Interdigitating fibers of perineum

Puborectalis muscle (part of levator ani muscle)

Pubococcygeus muscle (part of levator ani muscle)

Tendinous arch of levator ani muscle

Obturator internus muscle

Iliococcygeus muscle (part of levator ani muscle)

Ischial tuberosity

Ischial spine

Obturator internus tendon

Sacrospinous ligament

Sacrotuberous ligament

Piriformis muscle

Levator plate (median raphé) of levator ani muscle

Anococcygeal body (ligament) (attachment of external anal sphincter muscle)

Tip of coccyx

**Lateral view**

Median sacral crest

Sacrotuberous ligament (*cut*)

4th posterior (dorsal) sacral foramen

(Ischio-)coccygeus muscle

Sacrospinous ligament (*cut*)

Coccyx

Anococcygeal body (ligament) (attachment of external anal sphincter muscle)

Piriformis muscle

Greater sciatic foramen

Ischial spine

Iliococcygeus muscle (part of levator ani muscle)

Tendinous arch of levator ani muscle

Pubococcygeus muscle (part of levator ani muscle)

Puborectalis muscle (part of levator ani muscle)

Pubic bone (*cut surface*)

Deep dorsal vein of clitoris

Urethra

Vagina

Rectum

© Novartis

**Superior view**
(**viscera removed**)

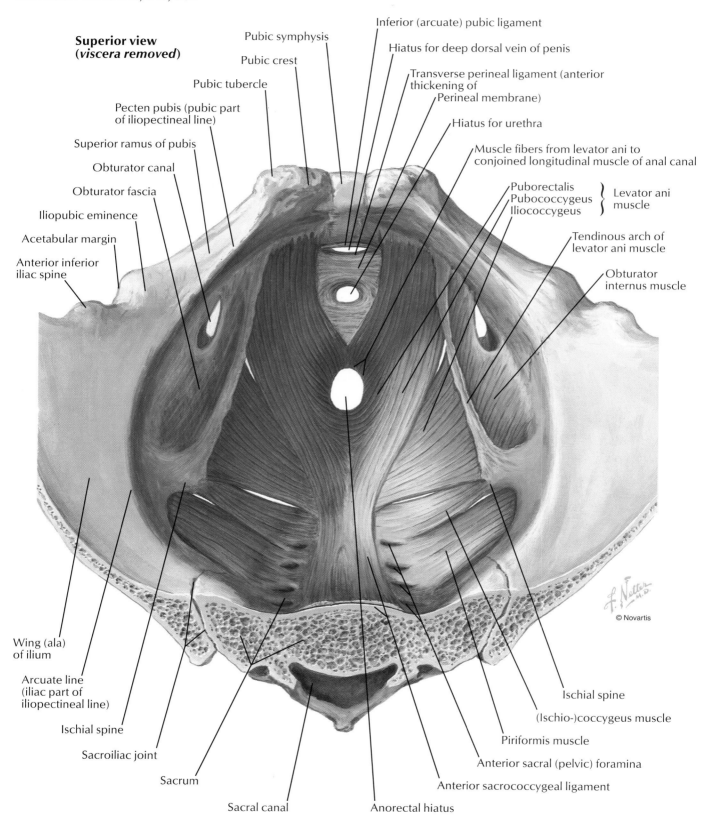

Pubic symphysis

Pubic crest

Pubic tubercle

Pecten pubis (pubic part of iliopectineal line)

Superior ramus of pubis

Obturator canal

Obturator fascia

Iliopubic eminence

Acetabular margin

Anterior inferior iliac spine

Inferior (arcuate) pubic ligament

Hiatus for deep dorsal vein of penis

Transverse perineal ligament (anterior thickening of Perineal membrane)

Hiatus for urethra

Muscle fibers from levator ani to conjoined longitudinal muscle of anal canal

Puborectalis
Pubococcygeus
Iliococcygeus
} Levator ani muscle

Tendinous arch of levator ani muscle

Obturator internus muscle

Wing (ala) of ilium

Arcuate line (iliac part of iliopectineal line)

Ischial spine

Sacroiliac joint

Sacrum

Sacral canal

Anorectal hiatus

Anterior sacrococcygeal ligament

Anterior sacral (pelvic) foramina

Piriformis muscle

(Ischio-)coccygeus muscle

Ischial spine

© Novartis

**PLATE 335**

**PELVIS AND PERINEUM**

**Inferior view**

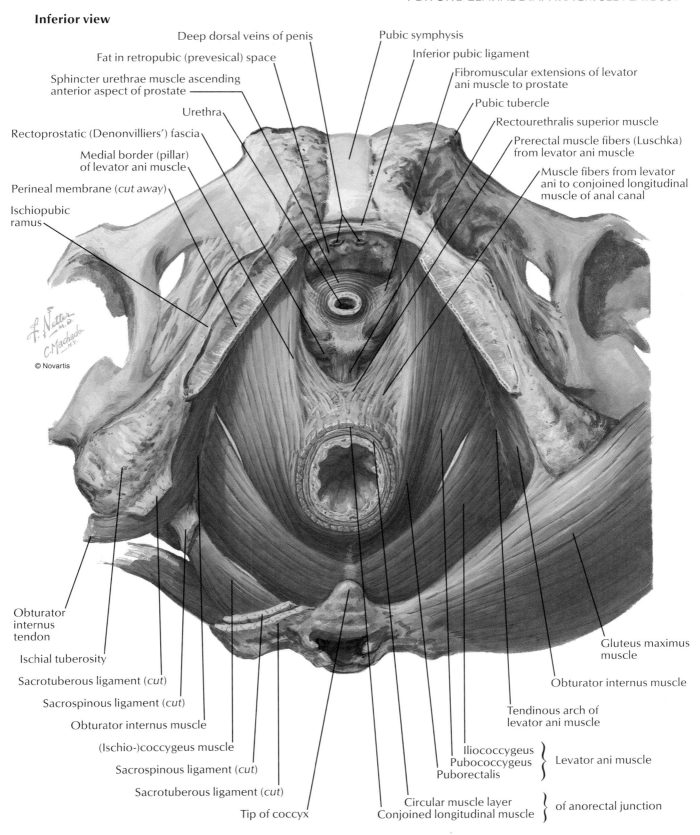

Deep dorsal veins of penis

Fat in retropubic (prevesical) space

Sphincter urethrae muscle ascending anterior aspect of prostate

Urethra

Rectoprostatic (Denonvilliers') fascia

Medial border (pillar) of levator ani muscle

Perineal membrane (*cut away*)

Ischiopubic ramus

Pubic symphysis

Inferior pubic ligament

Fibromuscular extensions of levator ani muscle to prostate

Pubic tubercle

Rectourethralis superior muscle

Prerectal muscle fibers (Luschka) from levator ani muscle

Muscle fibers from levator ani to conjoined longitudinal muscle of anal canal

Obturator internus tendon

Ischial tuberosity

Sacrotuberous ligament (*cut*)

Sacrospinous ligament (*cut*)

Obturator internus muscle

(Ischio-)coccygeus muscle

Sacrospinous ligament (*cut*)

Sacrotuberous ligament (*cut*)

Tip of coccyx

Gluteus maximus muscle

Obturator internus muscle

Tendinous arch of levator ani muscle

Iliococcygeus
Pubococcygeus } Levator ani muscle
Puborectalis

Circular muscle layer } of anorectal junction
Conjoined longitudinal muscle

© Novartis

# Pelvic Viscera and Perineum: Female

## Median (sagittal) section

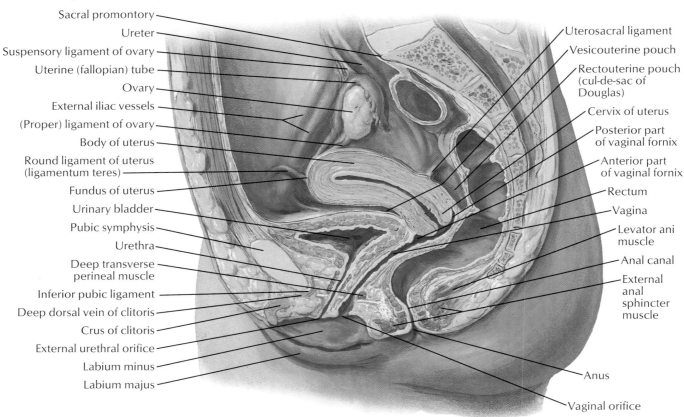

Sacral promontory
Ureter
Suspensory ligament of ovary
Uterine (fallopian) tube
Ovary
External iliac vessels
(Proper) ligament of ovary
Body of uterus
Round ligament of uterus (ligamentum teres)
Fundus of uterus
Urinary bladder
Pubic symphysis
Urethra
Deep transverse perineal muscle
Inferior pubic ligament
Deep dorsal vein of clitoris
Crus of clitoris
External urethral orifice
Labium minus
Labium majus

Uterosacral ligament
Vesicouterine pouch
Rectouterine pouch (cul-de-sac of Douglas)
Cervix of uterus
Posterior part of vaginal fornix
Anterior part of vaginal fornix
Rectum
Vagina
Levator ani muscle
Anal canal
External anal sphincter muscle
Anus
Vaginal orifice

## Paramedian (sagittal) dissection

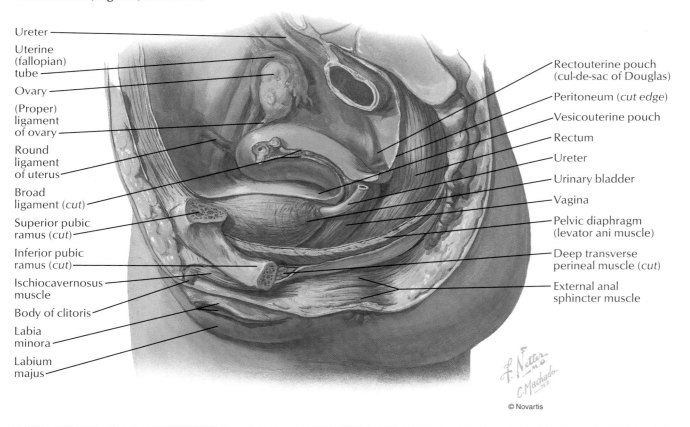

Ureter
Uterine (fallopian) tube
Ovary
(Proper) ligament of ovary
Round ligament of uterus
Broad ligament (cut)
Superior pubic ramus (cut)
Inferior pubic ramus (cut)
Ischiocavernosus muscle
Body of clitoris
Labia minora
Labium majus

Rectouterine pouch (cul-de-sac of Douglas)
Peritoneum (cut edge)
Vesicouterine pouch
Rectum
Ureter
Urinary bladder
Vagina
Pelvic diaphragm (levator ani muscle)
Deep transverse perineal muscle (cut)
External anal sphincter muscle

© Novartis

**PLATE 337**　　　　　　**PELVIS AND PERINEUM**

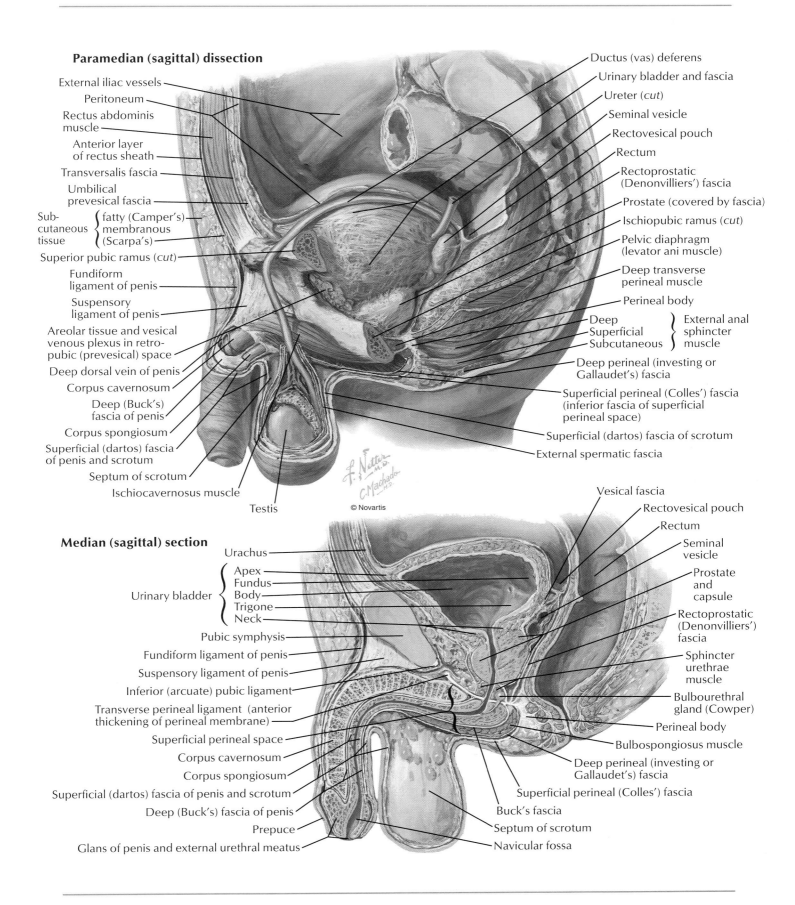

**Paramedian (sagittal) dissection**

External iliac vessels

Peritoneum

Rectus abdominis muscle

Anterior layer of rectus sheath

Transversalis fascia

Umbilical prevesical fascia

Sub-cutaneous tissue { fatty (Camper's) membranous (Scarpa's)

Superior pubic ramus (*cut*)

Fundiform ligament of penis

Suspensory ligament of penis

Areolar tissue and vesical venous plexus in retro-pubic (prevesical) space

Deep dorsal vein of penis

Corpus cavernosum

Deep (Buck's) fascia of penis

Corpus spongiosum

Superficial (dartos) fascia of penis and scrotum

Septum of scrotum

Ischiocavernosus muscle

Testis

Ductus (vas) deferens

Urinary bladder and fascia

Ureter (*cut*)

Seminal vesicle

Rectovesical pouch

Rectum

Rectoprostatic (Denonvilliers') fascia

Prostate (covered by fascia)

Ischiopubic ramus (*cut*)

Pelvic diaphragm (levator ani muscle)

Deep transverse perineal muscle

Perineal body

Deep, Superficial, Subcutaneous } External anal sphincter muscle

Deep perineal (investing or Gallaudet's) fascia

Superficial perineal (Colles') fascia (inferior fascia of superficial perineal space)

Superficial (dartos) fascia of scrotum

External spermatic fascia

*F. Netter M.D.*
*C. Machado M.D.*
© Novartis

**Median (sagittal) section**

Urachus

Urinary bladder { Apex, Fundus, Body, Trigone, Neck

Pubic symphysis

Fundiform ligament of penis

Suspensory ligament of penis

Inferior (arcuate) pubic ligament

Transverse perineal ligament (anterior thickening of perineal membrane)

Superficial perineal space

Corpus cavernosum

Corpus spongiosum

Superficial (dartos) fascia of penis and scrotum

Deep (Buck's) fascia of penis

Prepuce

Glans of penis and external urethral meatus

Vesical fascia

Rectovesical pouch

Rectum

Seminal vesicle

Prostate and capsule

Rectoprostatic (Denonvilliers') fascia

Sphincter urethrae muscle

Bulbourethral gland (Cowper)

Perineal body

Bulbospongiosus muscle

Deep perineal (investing or Gallaudet's) fascia

Superficial perineal (Colles') fascia

Buck's fascia

Septum of scrotum

Navicular fossa

# Pelvic Contents: Female

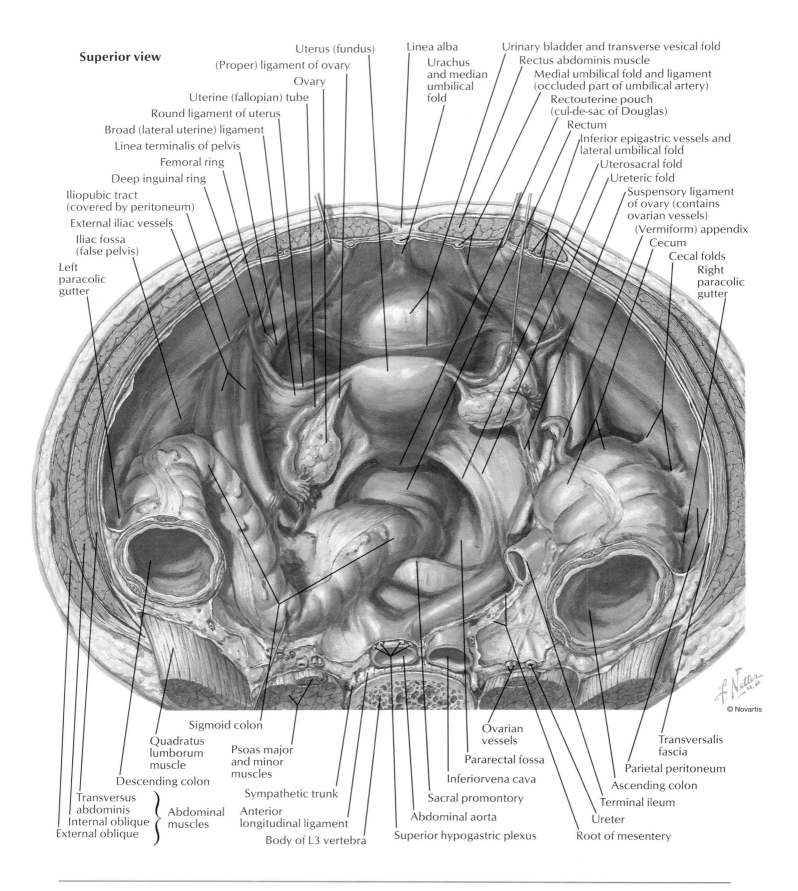

Uterus (fundus)

(Proper) ligament of ovary

Ovary

Uterine (fallopian) tube

Round ligament of uterus

Broad (lateral uterine) ligament

Linea terminalis of pelvis

Femoral ring

Deep inguinal ring

Iliopubic tract (covered by peritoneum)

External iliac vessels

Iliac fossa (false pelvis)

Left paracolic gutter

Linea alba

Urachus and median umbilical fold

Urinary bladder and transverse vesical fold

Rectus abdominis muscle

Medial umbilical fold and ligament (occluded part of umbilical artery)

Rectouterine pouch (cul-de-sac of Douglas)

Rectum

Inferior epigastric vessels and lateral umbilical fold

Uterosacral fold

Ureteric fold

Suspensory ligament of ovary (contains ovarian vessels)

(Vermiform) appendix

Cecum

Cecal folds

Right paracolic gutter

Sigmoid colon

Quadratus lumborum muscle

Descending colon

Transversus abdominis

Internal oblique

External oblique

} Abdominal muscles

Psoas major and minor muscles

Sympathetic trunk

Anterior longitudinal ligament

Body of L3 vertebra

Ovarian vessels

Pararectal fossa

Inferiorvena cava

Sacral promontory

Abdominal aorta

Superior hypogastric plexus

Transversalis fascia

Parietal peritoneum

Ascending colon

Terminal ileum

Ureter

Root of mesentery

*F. Netter M.D.*

© Novartis

**PLATE 339**

**Superior view**

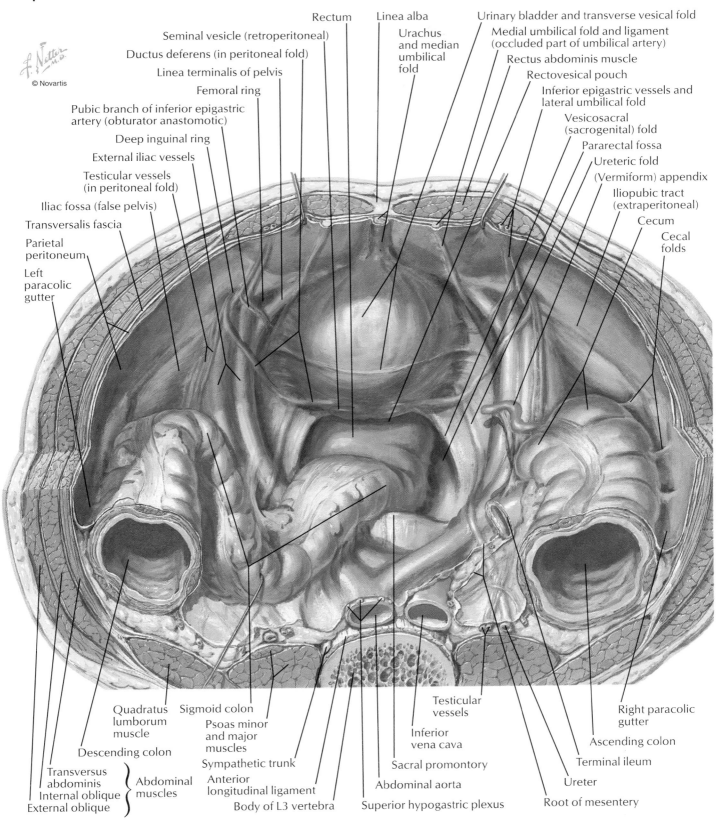

Rectum

Seminal vesicle (retroperitoneal)

Ductus deferens (in peritoneal fold)

Linea terminalis of pelvis

Femoral ring

Pubic branch of inferior epigastric artery (obturator anastomotic)

Deep inguinal ring

External iliac vessels

Testicular vessels (in peritoneal fold)

Iliac fossa (false pelvis)

Transversalis fascia

Parietal peritoneum

Left paracolic gutter

Linea alba

Urachus and median umbilical fold

Urinary bladder and transverse vesical fold

Medial umbilical fold and ligament (occluded part of umbilical artery)

Rectus abdominis muscle

Rectovesical pouch

Inferior epigastric vessels and lateral umbilical fold

Vesicosacral (sacrogenital) fold

Pararectal fossa

Ureteric fold

(Vermiform) appendix

Iliopubic tract (extraperitoneal)

Cecum

Cecal folds

Quadratus lumborum muscle

Sigmoid colon

Descending colon

Psoas minor and major muscles

Transversus abdominis
Internal oblique
External oblique } Abdominal muscles

Anterior longitudinal ligament

Sympathetic trunk

Body of L3 vertebra

Sacral promontory

Abdominal aorta

Superior hypogastric plexus

Inferior vena cava

Testicular vessels

Right paracolic gutter

Ascending colon

Terminal ileum

Ureter

Root of mesentery

**Female: superior view (peritoneum and loose areolar tissue removed)**

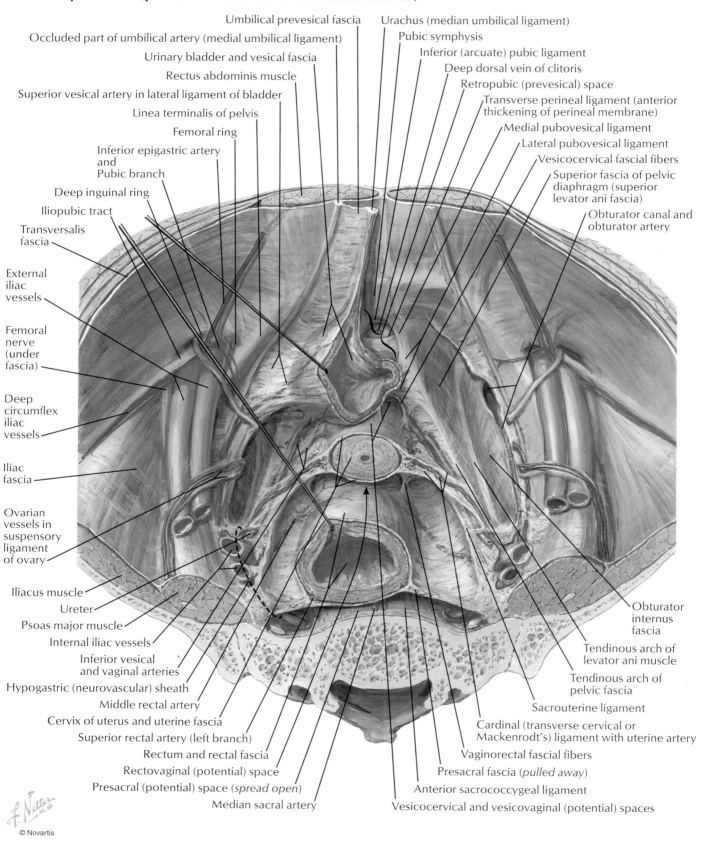

Umbilical prevesical fascia

Occluded part of umbilical artery (medial umbilical ligament)

Urinary bladder and vesical fascia

Rectus abdominis muscle

Superior vesical artery in lateral ligament of bladder

Linea terminalis of pelvis

Femoral ring

Inferior epigastric artery and Pubic branch

Deep inguinal ring

Iliopubic tract

Transversalis fascia

External iliac vessels

Femoral nerve (under fascia)

Deep circumflex iliac vessels

Iliac fascia

Ovarian vessels in suspensory ligament of ovary

Iliacus muscle

Ureter

Psoas major muscle

Internal iliac vessels

Inferior vesical and vaginal arteries

Hypogastric (neurovascular) sheath

Middle rectal artery

Cervix of uterus and uterine fascia

Superior rectal artery (left branch)

Rectum and rectal fascia

Rectovaginal (potential) space

Presacral (potential) space (*spread open*)

Median sacral artery

Urachus (median umbilical ligament)

Pubic symphysis

Inferior (arcuate) pubic ligament

Deep dorsal vein of clitoris

Retropubic (prevesical) space

Transverse perineal ligament (anterior thickening of perineal membrane)

Medial pubovesical ligament

Lateral pubovesical ligament

Vesicocervical fascial fibers

Superior fascia of pelvic diaphragm (superior levator ani fascia)

Obturator canal and obturator artery

Obturator internus fascia

Tendinous arch of levator ani muscle

Tendinous arch of pelvic fascia

Sacrouterine ligament

Cardinal (transverse cervical or Mackenrodt's) ligament with uterine artery

Vaginorectal fascial fibers

Presacral fascia (*pulled away*)

Anterior sacrococcygeal ligament

Vesicocervical and vesicovaginal (potential) spaces

*f. Netter M.D.*

© Novartis

**PLATE 341**

**Female: midsagittal section**

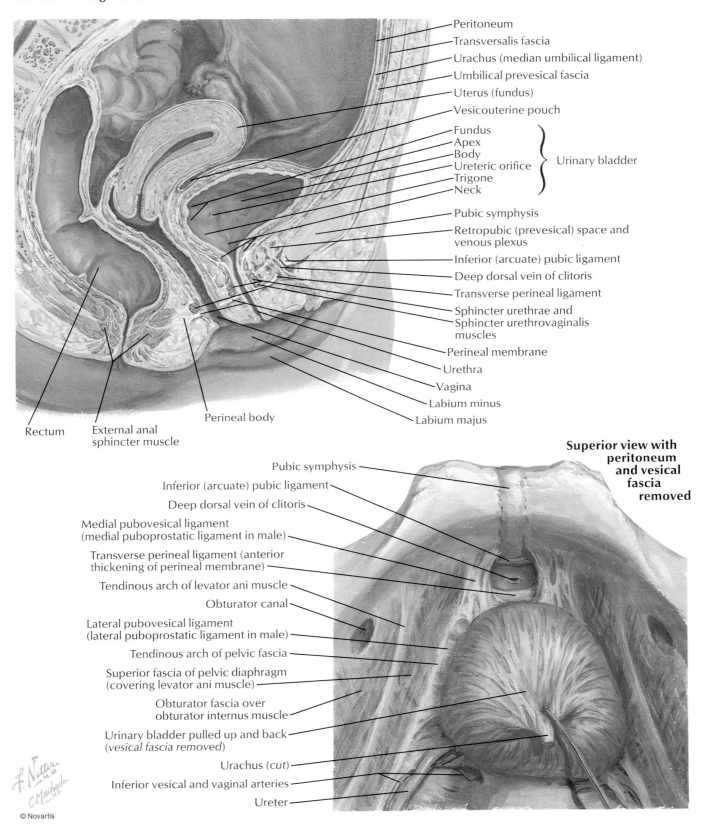

Peritoneum

Transversalis fascia

Urachus (median umbilical ligament)

Umbilical prevesical fascia

Uterus (fundus)

Vesicouterine pouch

Fundus
Apex
Body
Ureteric orifice
Trigone
Neck

Urinary bladder

Pubic symphysis

Retropubic (prevesical) space and venous plexus

Inferior (arcuate) pubic ligament

Deep dorsal vein of clitoris

Transverse perineal ligament

Sphincter urethrae and Sphincter urethrovaginalis muscles

Perineal membrane

Urethra

Vagina

Labium minus

Labium majus

Rectum

External anal sphincter muscle

Perineal body

**Superior view with peritoneum and vesical fascia removed**

Pubic symphysis

Inferior (arcuate) pubic ligament

Deep dorsal vein of clitoris

Medial pubovesical ligament (medial puboprostatic ligament in male)

Transverse perineal ligament (anterior thickening of perineal membrane)

Tendinous arch of levator ani muscle

Obturator canal

Lateral pubovesical ligament (lateral puboprostatic ligament in male)

Tendinous arch of pelvic fascia

Superior fascia of pelvic diaphragm (covering levator ani muscle)

Obturator fascia over obturator internus muscle

Urinary bladder pulled up and back (vesical fascia removed)

Urachus (cut)

Inferior vesical and vaginal arteries

Ureter

© Novartis

# Urinary Bladder: Female and Male

SEE ALSO PLATES 321, 337, 338, 342, 371, 373, 374, 388

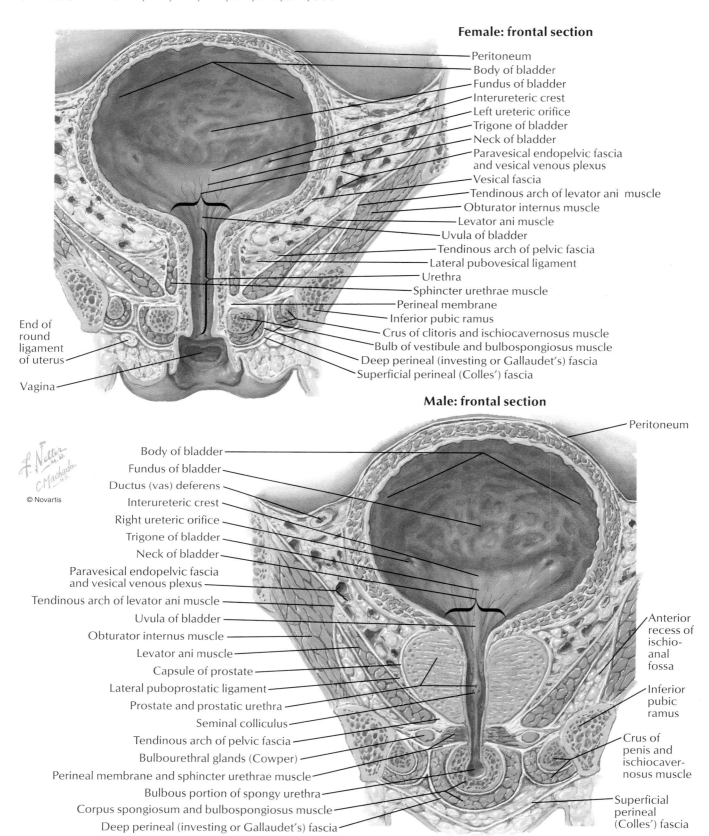

**Female: frontal section**

Peritoneum
Body of bladder
Fundus of bladder
Interureteric crest
Left ureteric orifice
Trigone of bladder
Neck of bladder
Paravesical endopelvic fascia and vesical venous plexus
Vesical fascia
Tendinous arch of levator ani muscle
Obturator internus muscle
Levator ani muscle
Uvula of bladder
Tendinous arch of pelvic fascia
Lateral pubovesical ligament
Urethra
Sphincter urethrae muscle
Perineal membrane
Inferior pubic ramus
Crus of clitoris and ischiocavernosus muscle
Bulb of vestibule and bulbospongiosus muscle
Deep perineal (investing or Gallaudet's) fascia
Superficial perineal (Colles') fascia

End of round ligament of uterus

Vagina

**Male: frontal section**

Peritoneum

Body of bladder
Fundus of bladder
Ductus (vas) deferens
Interureteric crest
Right ureteric orifice
Trigone of bladder
Neck of bladder
Paravesical endopelvic fascia and vesical venous plexus
Tendinous arch of levator ani muscle
Uvula of bladder
Obturator internus muscle
Levator ani muscle
Capsule of prostate
Lateral puboprostatic ligament
Prostate and prostatic urethra
Seminal colliculus
Tendinous arch of pelvic fascia
Bulbourethral glands (Cowper)
Perineal membrane and sphincter urethrae muscle
Bulbous portion of spongy urethra
Corpus spongiosum and bulbospongiosus muscle
Deep perineal (investing or Gallaudet's) fascia

Anterior recess of ischio-anal fossa

Inferior pubic ramus

Crus of penis and ischiocavernosus muscle

Superficial perineal (Colles') fascia

© Novartis

**PLATE 343**

**PELVIS AND PERINEUM**

**Superior view with peritoneum intact**

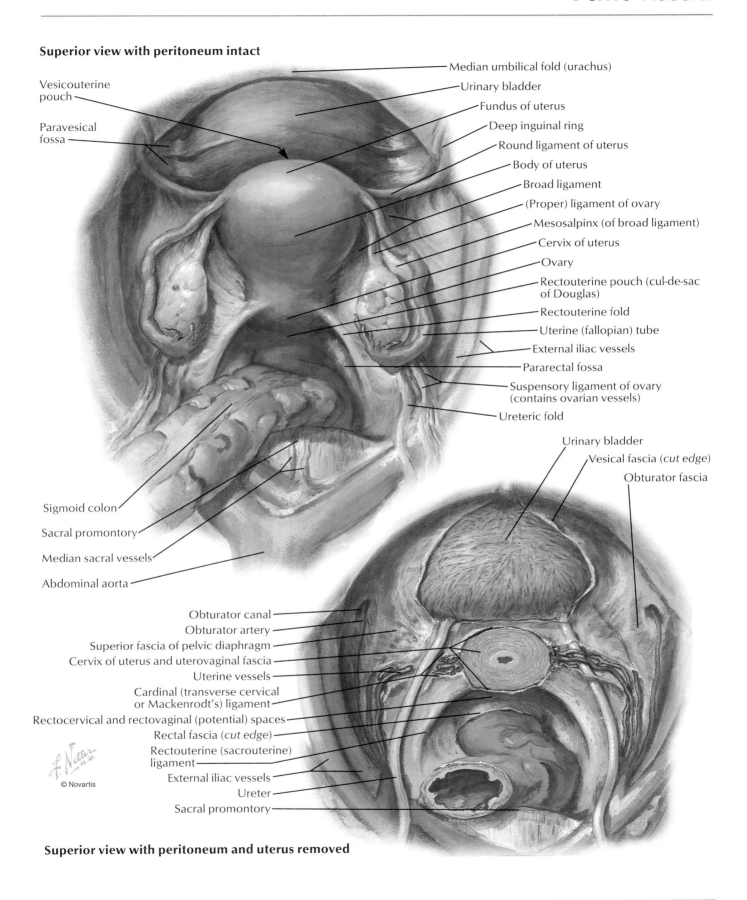

Median umbilical fold (urachus)

Urinary bladder

Fundus of uterus

Deep inguinal ring

Round ligament of uterus

Body of uterus

Broad ligament

(Proper) ligament of ovary

Mesosalpinx (of broad ligament)

Cervix of uterus

Ovary

Rectouterine pouch (cul-de-sac of Douglas)

Rectouterine fold

Uterine (fallopian) tube

External iliac vessels

Pararectal fossa

Suspensory ligament of ovary (contains ovarian vessels)

Ureteric fold

Vesicouterine pouch

Paravesical fossa

Sigmoid colon

Sacral promontory

Median sacral vessels

Abdominal aorta

Urinary bladder

Vesical fascia (*cut edge*)

Obturator fascia

Obturator canal

Obturator artery

Superior fascia of pelvic diaphragm

Cervix of uterus and uterovaginal fascia

Uterine vessels

Cardinal (transverse cervical or Mackenrodt's) ligament

Rectocervical and rectovaginal (potential) spaces

Rectal fascia (*cut edge*)

Rectouterine (sacrouterine) ligament

External iliac vessels

Ureter

Sacral promontory

F. Netter M.D.

© Novartis

**Superior view with peritoneum and uterus removed**

**FEMALE STRUCTURES**

*PLATE 344*

# Uterus, Vagina and Supporting Structures

*SEE ALSO PLATES 371, 373, 375, 377, 383, 385, 386*

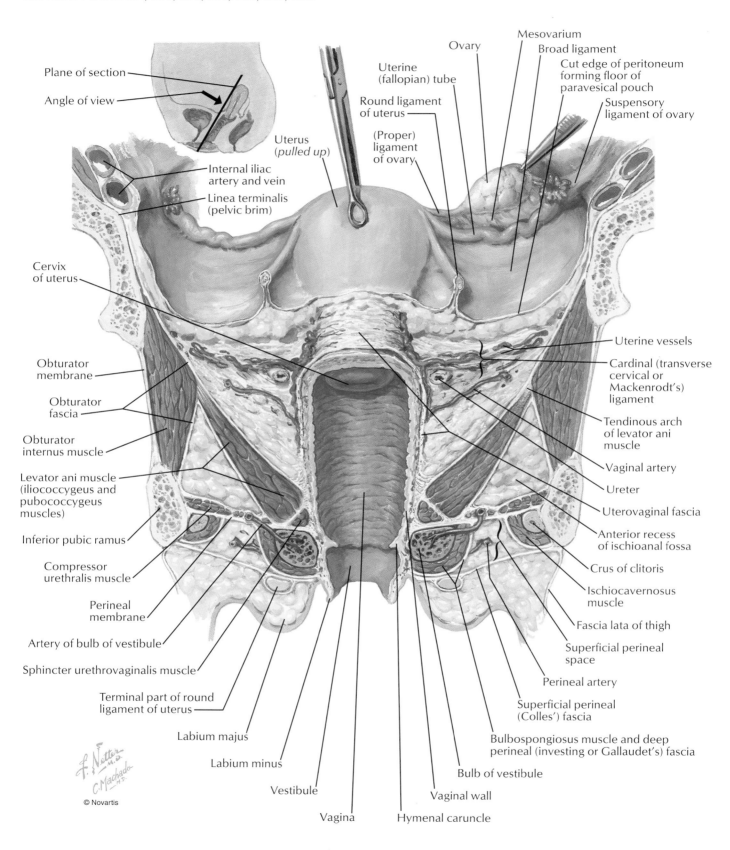

Plane of section

Angle of view

Uterus (*pulled up*)

Internal iliac artery and vein

Linea terminalis (pelvic brim)

Cervix of uterus

Obturator membrane

Obturator fascia

Obturator internus muscle

Levator ani muscle (iliococcygeus and pubococcygeus muscles)

Inferior pubic ramus

Compressor urethralis muscle

Perineal membrane

Artery of bulb of vestibule

Sphincter urethrovaginalis muscle

Terminal part of round ligament of uterus

Labium majus

Labium minus

Vestibule

Vagina

Hymenal caruncle

Vaginal wall

Bulb of vestibule

Bulbospongiosus muscle and deep perineal (investing or Gallaudet's) fascia

Superficial perineal (Colles') fascia

Perineal artery

Superficial perineal space

Fascia lata of thigh

Ischiocavernosus muscle

Crus of clitoris

Anterior recess of ischioanal fossa

Uterovaginal fascia

Ureter

Vaginal artery

Tendinous arch of levator ani muscle

Cardinal (transverse cervical or Mackenrodt's) ligament

Uterine vessels

Ovary

Mesovarium

Broad ligament

Cut edge of peritoneum forming floor of paravesical pouch

Suspensory ligament of ovary

Uterine (fallopian) tube

Round ligament of uterus

(Proper) ligament of ovary

© Novartis

**PLATE 345**

**PELVIS AND PERINEUM**

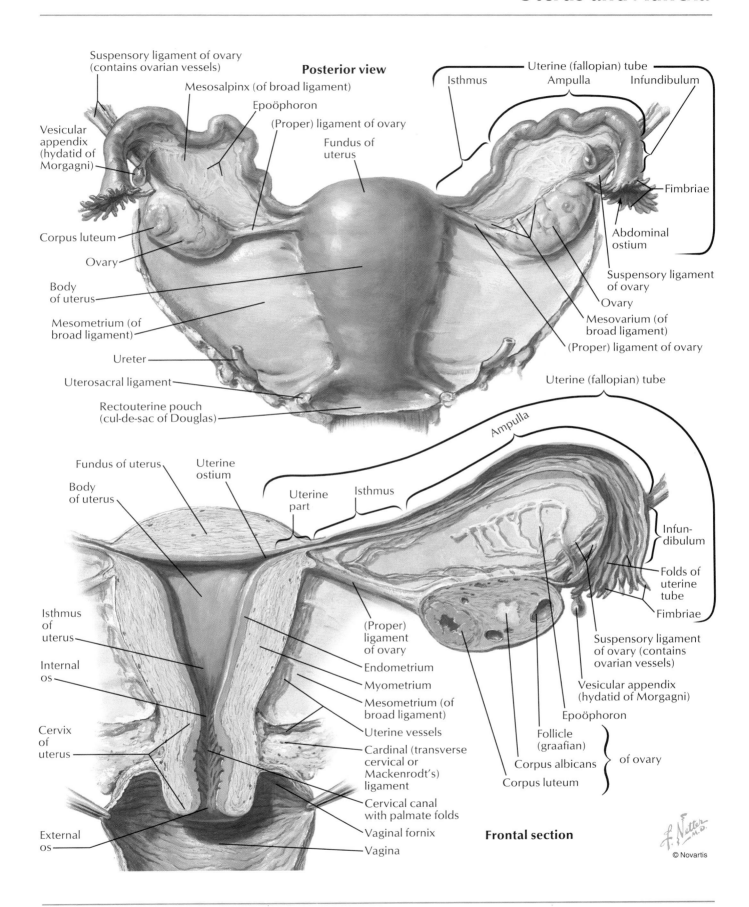

Suspensory ligament of ovary (contains ovarian vessels)

**Posterior view**

Mesosalpinx (of broad ligament)

Epoöphoron

(Proper) ligament of ovary

Fundus of uterus

Vesicular appendix (hydatid of Morgagni)

Corpus luteum

Ovary

Body of uterus

Mesometrium (of broad ligament)

Ureter

Uterosacral ligament

Rectouterine pouch (cul-de-sac of Douglas)

Uterine (fallopian) tube

Isthmus

Ampulla

Infundibulum

Fimbriae

Abdominal ostium

Suspensory ligament of ovary

Ovary

Mesovarium (of broad ligament)

(Proper) ligament of ovary

Uterine (fallopian) tube

Fundus of uterus

Body of uterus

Uterine ostium

Uterine part

Isthmus

Ampulla

Infundibulum

Folds of uterine tube

Fimbriae

Isthmus of uterus

Internal os

Cervix of uterus

External os

(Proper) ligament of ovary

Endometrium

Myometrium

Mesometrium (of broad ligament)

Uterine vessels

Cardinal (transverse cervical or Mackenrodt's) ligament

Cervical canal with palmate folds

Vaginal fornix

Vagina

Suspensory ligament of ovary (contains ovarian vessels)

Vesicular appendix (hydatid of Morgagni)

Epoöphoron

Follicle (graafian)

Corpus albicans

Corpus luteum

} of ovary

**Frontal section**

© Novartis

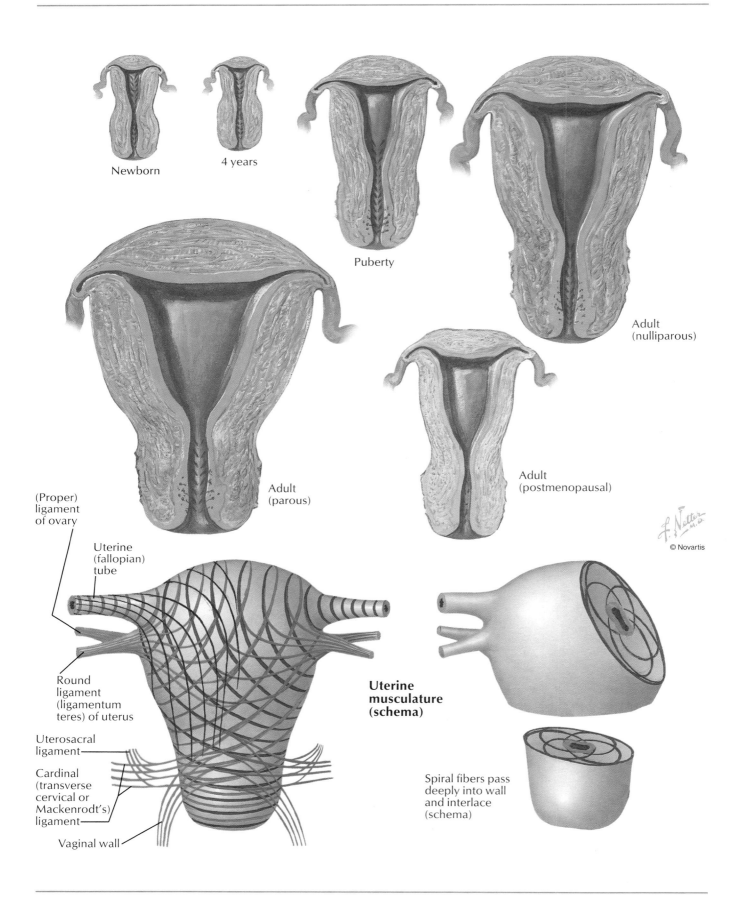

Newborn

4 years

Puberty

Adult (nulliparous)

Adult (parous)

Adult (postmenopausal)

(Proper) ligament of ovary

Uterine (fallopian) tube

Round ligament (ligamentum teres) of uterus

Uterosacral ligament

Cardinal (transverse cervical or Mackenrodt's) ligament

Vaginal wall

**Uterine musculature (schema)**

Spiral fibers pass deeply into wall and interlace (schema)

© Novartis

**PLATE 347**

**PELVIS AND PERINEUM**

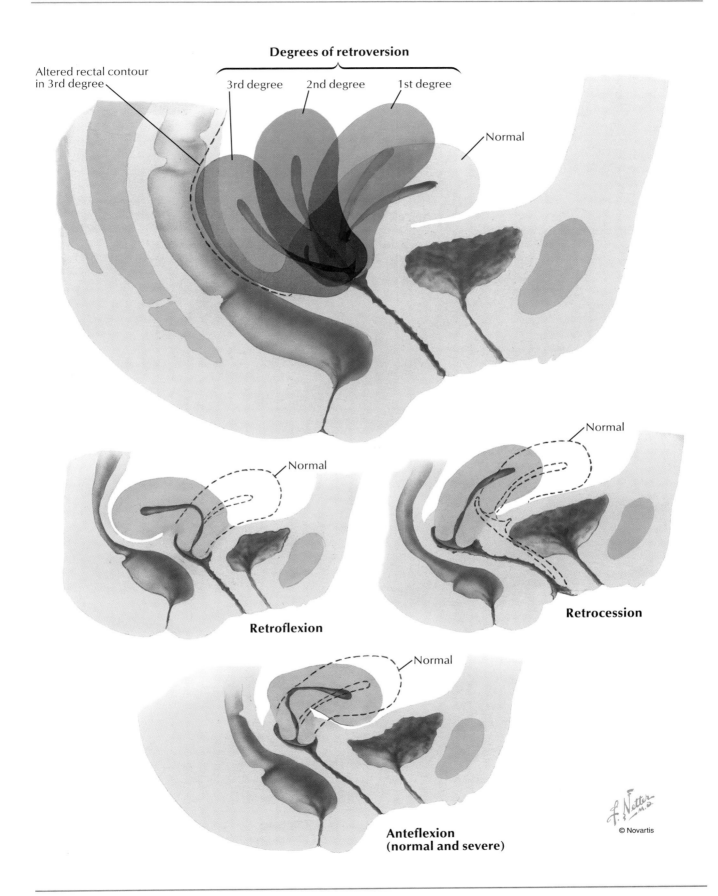

**Degrees of retroversion**

Altered rectal contour in 3rd degree

3rd degree    2nd degree    1st degree

Normal

Normal

**Retroflexion**

Normal

**Retrocession**

Normal

**Anteflexion
(normal and severe)**

© Novartis

# *Ovary, Ova and Follicles*

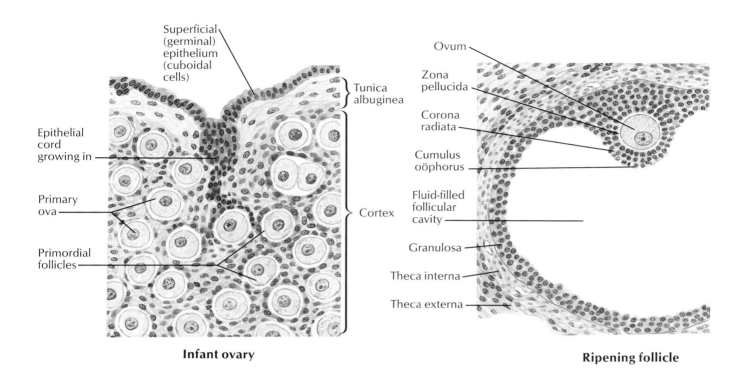

**Infant ovary**

Superficial (germinal) epithelium (cuboidal cells)

Tunica albuginea

Epithelial cord growing in

Primary ova

Primordial follicles

Cortex

**Ripening follicle**

Ovum

Zona pellucida

Corona radiata

Cumulus oöphorus

Fluid-filled follicular cavity

Granulosa

Theca interna

Theca externa

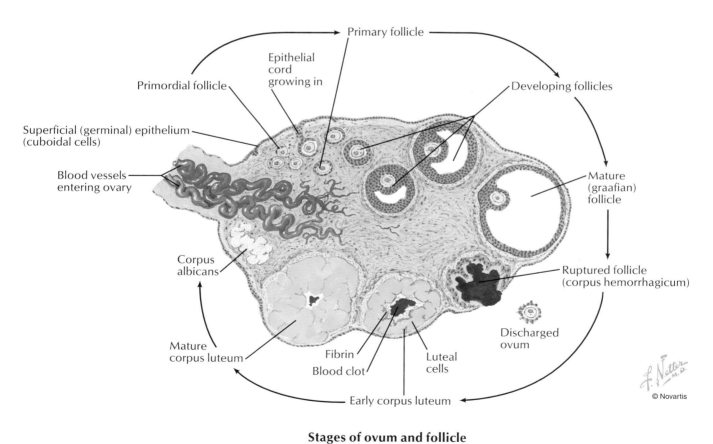

Primary follicle

Epithelial cord growing in

Primordial follicle

Developing follicles

Superficial (germinal) epithelium (cuboidal cells)

Blood vessels entering ovary

Mature (graafian) follicle

Corpus albicans

Ruptured follicle (corpus hemorrhagicum)

Mature corpus luteum

Fibrin

Blood clot

Luteal cells

Discharged ovum

Early corpus luteum

**Stages of ovum and follicle**

**PLATE 349**

**PELVIS AND PERINEUM**

*SEE ALSO PLATES 375, 377, 378, 384*

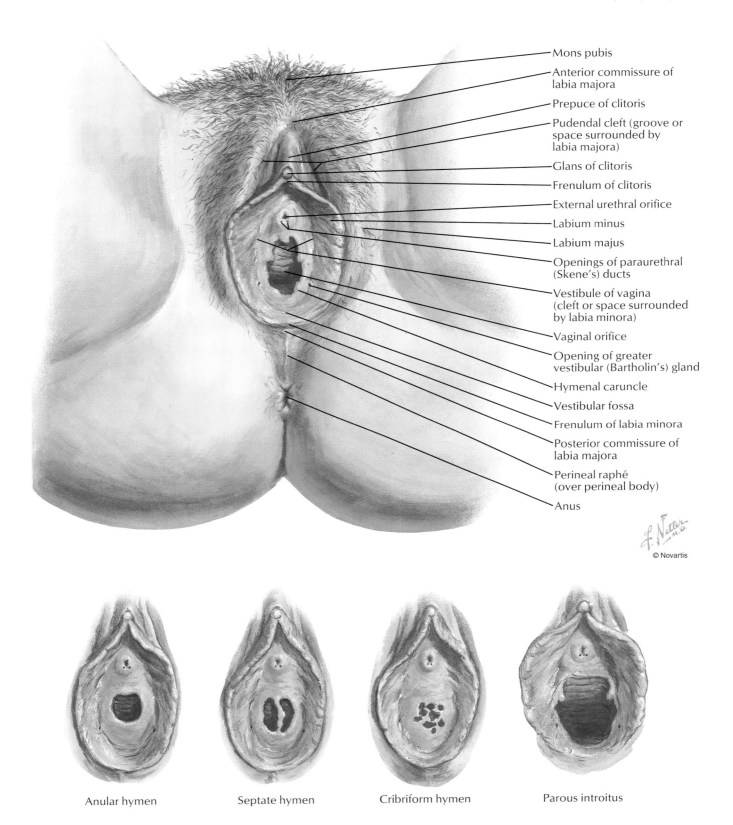

Mons pubis

Anterior commissure of labia majora

Prepuce of clitoris

Pudendal cleft (groove or space surrounded by labia majora)

Glans of clitoris

Frenulum of clitoris

External urethral orifice

Labium minus

Labium majus

Openings of paraurethral (Skene's) ducts

Vestibule of vagina (cleft or space surrounded by labia minora)

Vaginal orifice

Opening of greater vestibular (Bartholin's) gland

Hymenal caruncle

Vestibular fossa

Frenulum of labia minora

Posterior commissure of labia majora

Perineal raphé (over perineal body)

Anus

© Novartis

Anular hymen     Septate hymen     Cribriform hymen     Parous introitus

**FEMALE STRUCTURES**                                                              *PLATE 350*

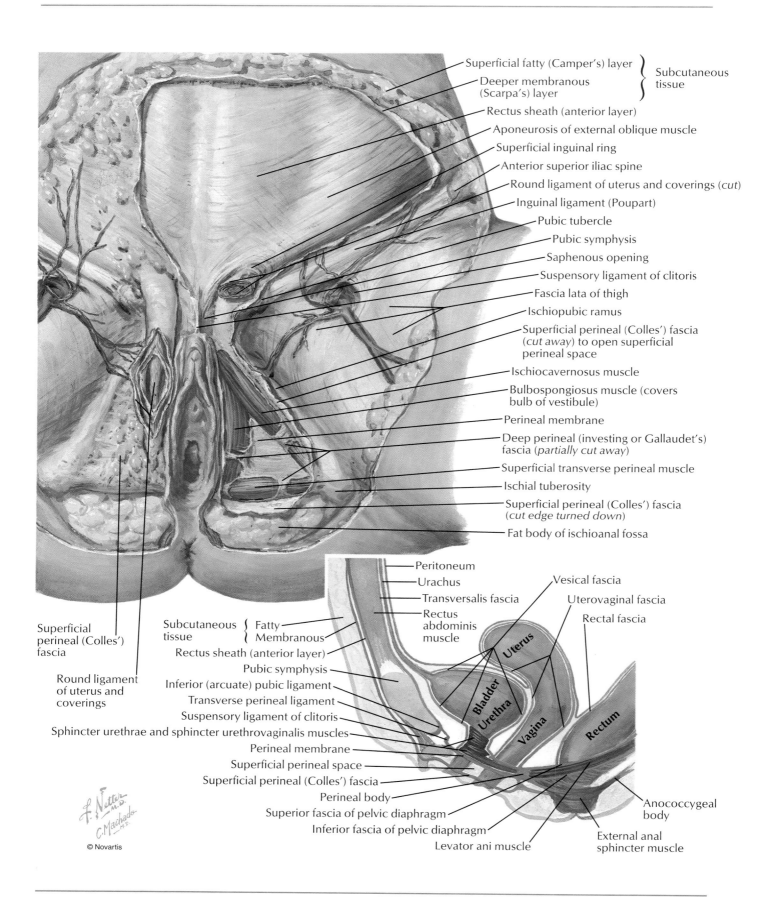

Superficial fatty (Camper's) layer

Deeper membranous (Scarpa's) layer

Subcutaneous tissue

Rectus sheath (anterior layer)

Aponeurosis of external oblique muscle

Superficial inguinal ring

Anterior superior iliac spine

Round ligament of uterus and coverings (*cut*)

Inguinal ligament (Poupart)

Pubic tubercle

Pubic symphysis

Saphenous opening

Suspensory ligament of clitoris

Fascia lata of thigh

Ischiopubic ramus

Superficial perineal (Colles') fascia (*cut away*) to open superficial perineal space

Ischiocavernosus muscle

Bulbospongiosus muscle (covers bulb of vestibule)

Perineal membrane

Deep perineal (investing or Gallaudet's) fascia (*partially cut away*)

Superficial transverse perineal muscle

Ischial tuberosity

Superficial perineal (Colles') fascia (*cut edge turned down*)

Fat body of ischioanal fossa

Superficial perineal (Colles') fascia

Round ligament of uterus and coverings

Subcutaneous tissue { Fatty / Membranous }

Rectus sheath (anterior layer)

Pubic symphysis

Inferior (arcuate) pubic ligament

Transverse perineal ligament

Suspensory ligament of clitoris

Sphincter urethrae and sphincter urethrovaginalis muscles

Perineal membrane

Superficial perineal space

Superficial perineal (Colles') fascia

Perineal body

Superior fascia of pelvic diaphragm

Inferior fascia of pelvic diaphragm

Levator ani muscle

Peritoneum

Urachus

Transversalis fascia

Rectus abdominis muscle

Vesical fascia

Uterovaginal fascia

Rectal fascia

Uterus

Bladder

Urethra

Vagina

Rectum

Anococcygeal body

External anal sphincter muscle

*F. Netter M.D.*

*C. Machado M.D.*

© Novartis

**PLATE 351**　　　　　　　　　　　　　　　　　　　　**PELVIS AND PERINEUM**

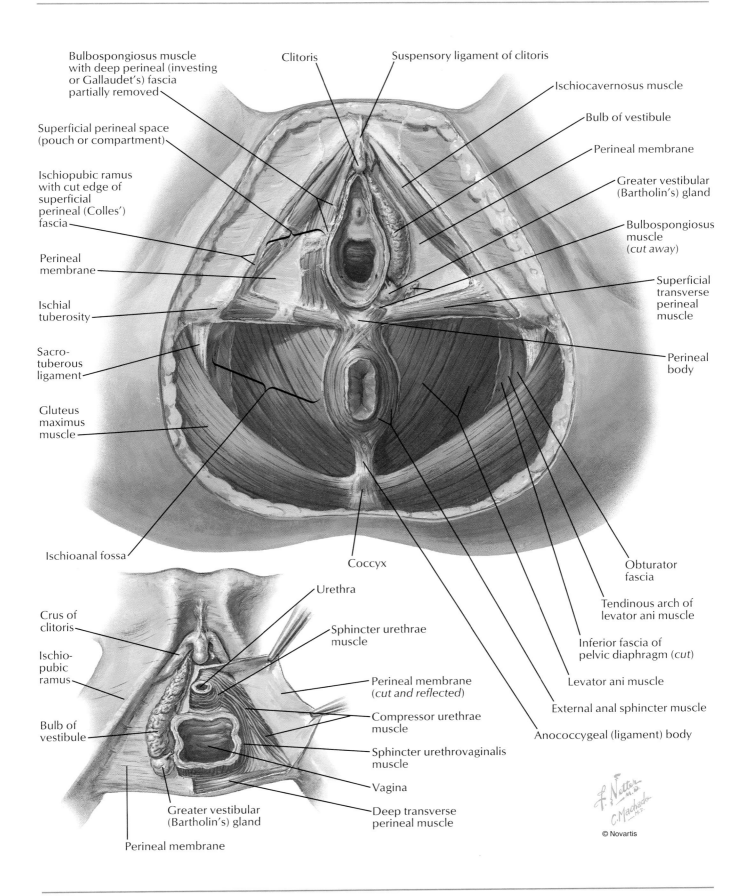

Bulbospongiosus muscle with deep perineal (investing or Gallaudet's) fascia partially removed

Superficial perineal space (pouch or compartment)

Ischiopubic ramus with cut edge of superficial perineal (Colles') fascia

Perineal membrane

Ischial tuberosity

Sacro-tuberous ligament

Gluteus maximus muscle

Ischioanal fossa

Clitoris

Suspensory ligament of clitoris

Ischiocavernosus muscle

Bulb of vestibule

Perineal membrane

Greater vestibular (Bartholin's) gland

Bulbospongiosus muscle (*cut away*)

Superficial transverse perineal muscle

Perineal body

Coccyx

Obturator fascia

Tendinous arch of levator ani muscle

Inferior fascia of pelvic diaphragm (*cut*)

Levator ani muscle

External anal sphincter muscle

Anococcygeal (ligament) body

Crus of clitoris

Ischio-pubic ramus

Bulb of vestibule

Urethra

Sphincter urethrae muscle

Perineal membrane (*cut and reflected*)

Compressor urethrae muscle

Sphincter urethrovaginalis muscle

Vagina

Deep transverse perineal muscle

Greater vestibular (Bartholin's) gland

Perineal membrane

**FEMALE STRUCTURES**

**PLATE 352**

© Novartis

# *Urethra*

SEE ALSO PLATES 337, 342

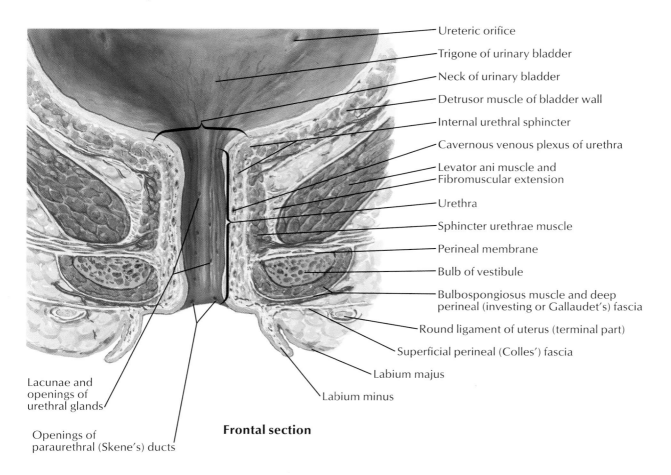

Ureteric orifice

Trigone of urinary bladder

Neck of urinary bladder

Detrusor muscle of bladder wall

Internal urethral sphincter

Cavernous venous plexus of urethra

Levator ani muscle and
Fibromuscular extension

Urethra

Sphincter urethrae muscle

Perineal membrane

Bulb of vestibule

Bulbospongiosus muscle and deep
perineal (investing or Gallaudet's) fascia

Round ligament of uterus (terminal part)

Superficial perineal (Colles') fascia

Labium majus

Labium minus

Lacunae and
openings of
urethral glands

Openings of
paraurethral (Skene's) ducts

**Frontal section**

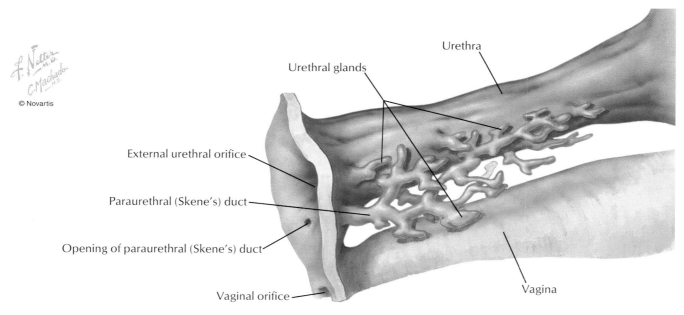

Urethra

Urethral glands

External urethral orifice

Paraurethral (Skene's) duct

Opening of paraurethral (Skene's) duct

Vaginal orifice

Vagina

**Schematic reconstruction**

© Novartis

*PLATE 353*                                                                                           **PELVIS AND PERINEUM**

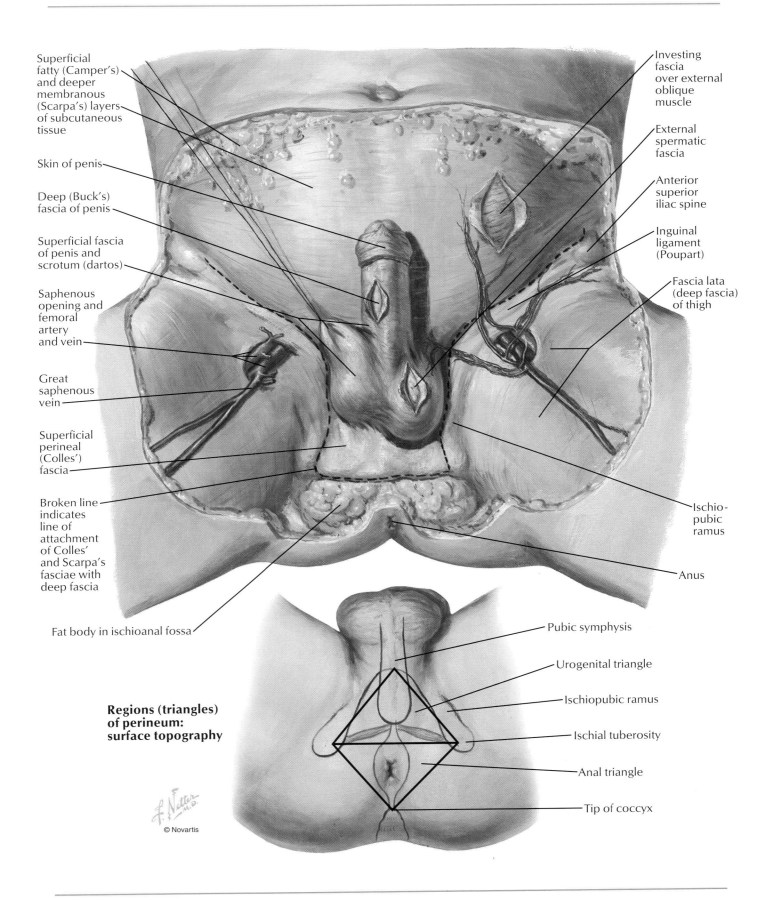

Superficial fatty (Camper's) and deeper membranous (Scarpa's) layers of subcutaneous tissue

Skin of penis

Deep (Buck's) fascia of penis

Superficial fascia of penis and scrotum (dartos)

Saphenous opening and femoral artery and vein

Great saphenous vein

Superficial perineal (Colles') fascia

Broken line indicates line of attachment of Colles' and Scarpa's fasciae with deep fascia

Fat body in ischioanal fossa

Investing fascia over external oblique muscle

External spermatic fascia

Anterior superior iliac spine

Inguinal ligament (Poupart)

Fascia lata (deep fascia) of thigh

Ischio-pubic ramus

Anus

**Regions (triangles) of perineum: surface topography**

Pubic symphysis

Urogenital triangle

Ischiopubic ramus

Ischial tuberosity

Anal triangle

Tip of coccyx

© Novartis

SEE ALSO PLATES 374, 376, 379, 380, 381, 382, 387

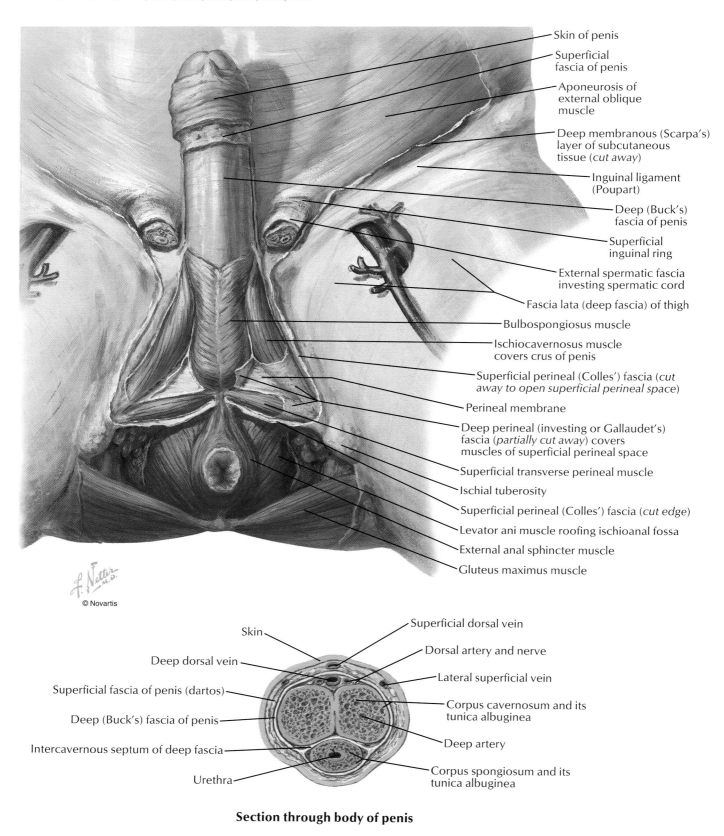

Skin of penis

Superficial fascia of penis

Aponeurosis of external oblique muscle

Deep membranous (Scarpa's) layer of subcutaneous tissue (*cut away*)

Inguinal ligament (Poupart)

Deep (Buck's) fascia of penis

Superficial inguinal ring

External spermatic fascia investing spermatic cord

Fascia lata (deep fascia) of thigh

Bulbospongiosus muscle

Ischiocavernosus muscle covers crus of penis

Superficial perineal (Colles') fascia (*cut away to open superficial perineal space*)

Perineal membrane

Deep perineal (investing or Gallaudet's) fascia (*partially cut away*) covers muscles of superficial perineal space

Superficial transverse perineal muscle

Ischial tuberosity

Superficial perineal (Colles') fascia (*cut edge*)

Levator ani muscle roofing ischioanal fossa

External anal sphincter muscle

Gluteus maximus muscle

© Novartis

Skin

Superficial dorsal vein

Deep dorsal vein

Dorsal artery and nerve

Superficial fascia of penis (dartos)

Lateral superficial vein

Deep (Buck's) fascia of penis

Corpus cavernosum and its tunica albuginea

Intercavernous septum of deep fascia

Deep artery

Urethra

Corpus spongiosum and its tunica albuginea

**Section through body of penis**

**PLATE 355**

**PELVIS AND PERINEUM**

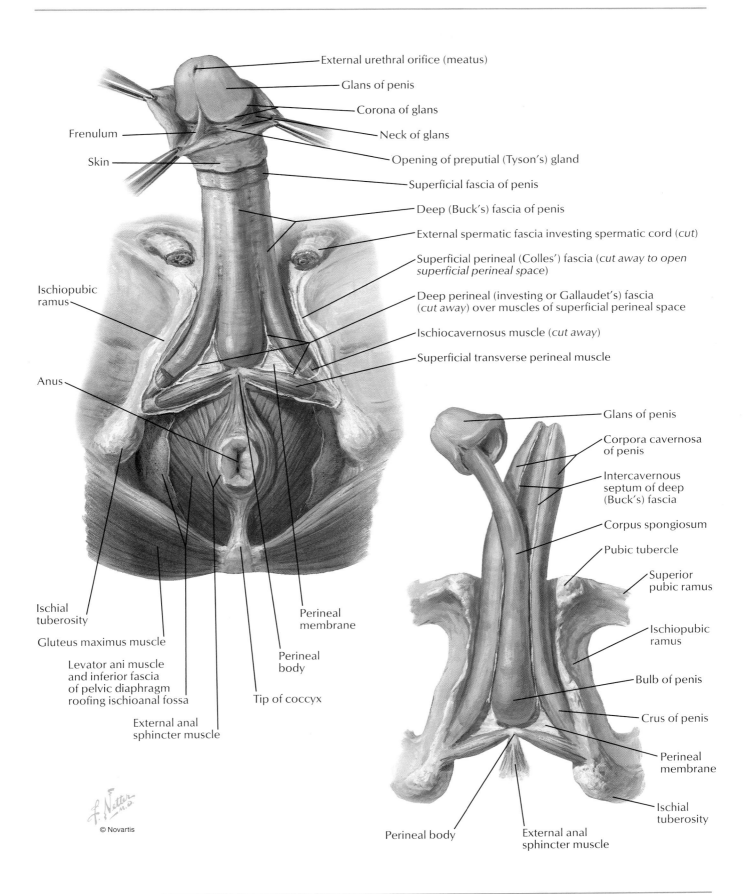

External urethral orifice (meatus)

Glans of penis

Corona of glans

Frenulum

Neck of glans

Skin

Opening of preputial (Tyson's) gland

Superficial fascia of penis

Deep (Buck's) fascia of penis

External spermatic fascia investing spermatic cord (*cut*)

Superficial perineal (Colles') fascia (*cut away to open superficial perineal space*)

Deep perineal (investing or Gallaudet's) fascia (*cut away*) over muscles of superficial perineal space

Ischiocavernosus muscle (*cut away*)

Ischiopubic ramus

Superficial transverse perineal muscle

Anus

Glans of penis

Corpora cavernosa of penis

Intercavernous septum of deep (Buck's) fascia

Corpus spongiosum

Pubic tubercle

Superior pubic ramus

Ischiopubic ramus

Ischial tuberosity

Gluteus maximus muscle

Bulb of penis

Levator ani muscle and inferior fascia of pelvic diaphragm roofing ischioanal fossa

Crus of penis

Perineal membrane

Perineal body

External anal sphincter muscle

Perineal body

Tip of coccyx

Perineal membrane

Ischial tuberosity

External anal sphincter muscle

*f. Netter*
© Novartis

# *Perineal Spaces*

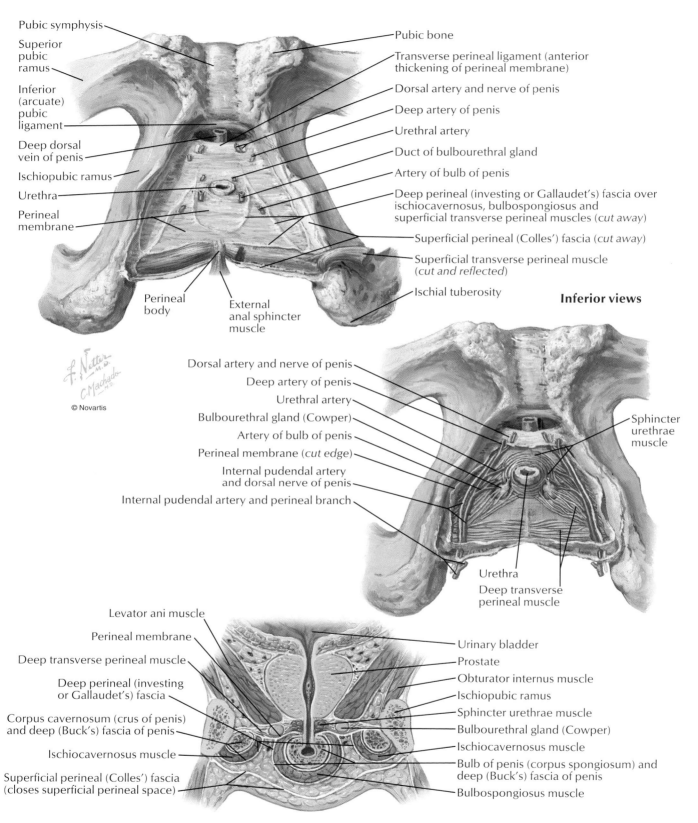

Pubic symphysis
Superior pubic ramus
Inferior (arcuate) pubic ligament
Deep dorsal vein of penis
Ischiopubic ramus
Urethra
Perineal membrane

Pubic bone
Transverse perineal ligament (anterior thickening of perineal membrane)
Dorsal artery and nerve of penis
Deep artery of penis
Urethral artery
Duct of bulbourethral gland
Artery of bulb of penis
Deep perineal (investing or Gallaudet's) fascia over ischiocavernosus, bulbospongiosus and superficial transverse perineal muscles (*cut away*)
Superficial perineal (Colles') fascia (*cut away*)
Superficial transverse perineal muscle (*cut and reflected*)
Ischial tuberosity

Perineal body
External anal sphincter muscle

**Inferior views**

Dorsal artery and nerve of penis
Deep artery of penis
Urethral artery
Bulbourethral gland (Cowper)
Artery of bulb of penis
Perineal membrane (*cut edge*)
Internal pudendal artery and dorsal nerve of penis
Internal pudendal artery and perineal branch

Sphincter urethrae muscle

Urethra
Deep transverse perineal muscle

Levator ani muscle
Perineal membrane
Deep transverse perineal muscle
Deep perineal (investing or Gallaudet's) fascia
Corpus cavernosum (crus of penis) and deep (Buck's) fascia of penis
Ischiocavernosus muscle
Superficial perineal (Colles') fascia (closes superficial perineal space)

Urinary bladder
Prostate
Obturator internus muscle
Ischiopubic ramus
Sphincter urethrae muscle
Bulbourethral gland (Cowper)
Ischiocavernosus muscle
Bulb of penis (corpus spongiosum) and deep (Buck's) fascia of penis
Bulbospongiosus muscle

**Frontal section through perineum and urethra: schema**

*PLATE 357*

**PELVIS AND PERINEUM**

*SEE ALSO PLATES 338, 340, 343, 374, 381*

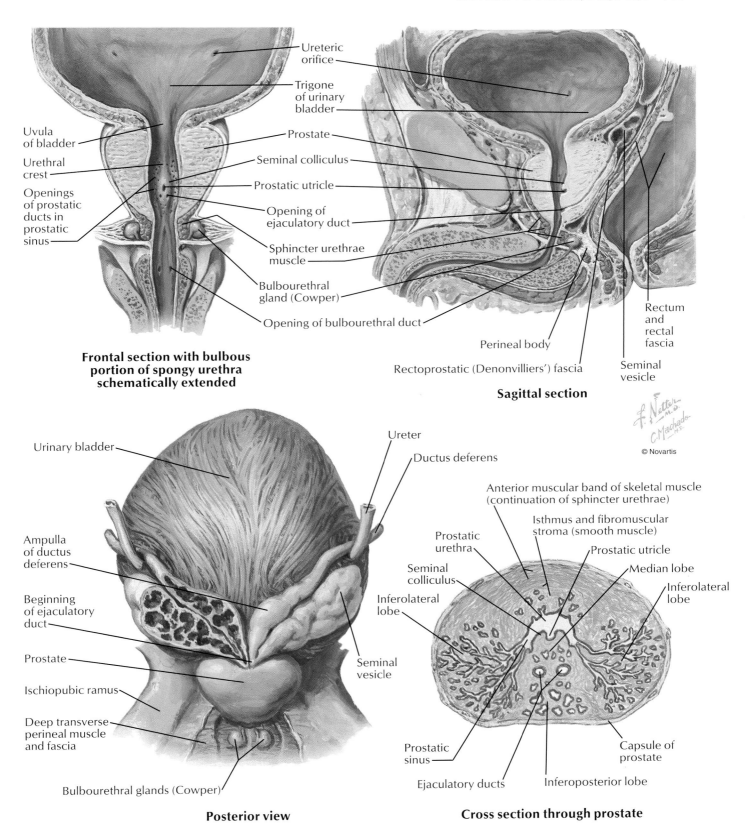

Ureteric orifice

Trigone of urinary bladder

Uvula of bladder

Urethral crest

Openings of prostatic ducts in prostatic sinus

Prostate

Seminal colliculus

Prostatic utricle

Opening of ejaculatory duct

Sphincter urethrae muscle

Bulbourethral gland (Cowper)

Opening of bulbourethral duct

**Frontal section with bulbous portion of spongy urethra schematically extended**

Perineal body

Rectoprostatic (Denonvilliers') fascia

Rectum and rectal fascia

Seminal vesicle

**Sagittal section**

© Novartis

Urinary bladder

Ureter

Ductus deferens

Ampulla of ductus deferens

Beginning of ejaculatory duct

Prostate

Ischiopubic ramus

Deep transverse perineal muscle and fascia

Bulbourethral glands (Cowper)

Seminal vesicle

**Posterior view**

Anterior muscular band of skeletal muscle (continuation of sphincter urethrae)

Isthmus and fibromuscular stroma (smooth muscle)

Prostatic urethra

Seminal colliculus

Inferolateral lobe

Prostatic utricle

Median lobe

Inferolateral lobe

Prostatic sinus

Ejaculatory ducts

Inferoposterior lobe

Capsule of prostate

**Cross section through prostate**

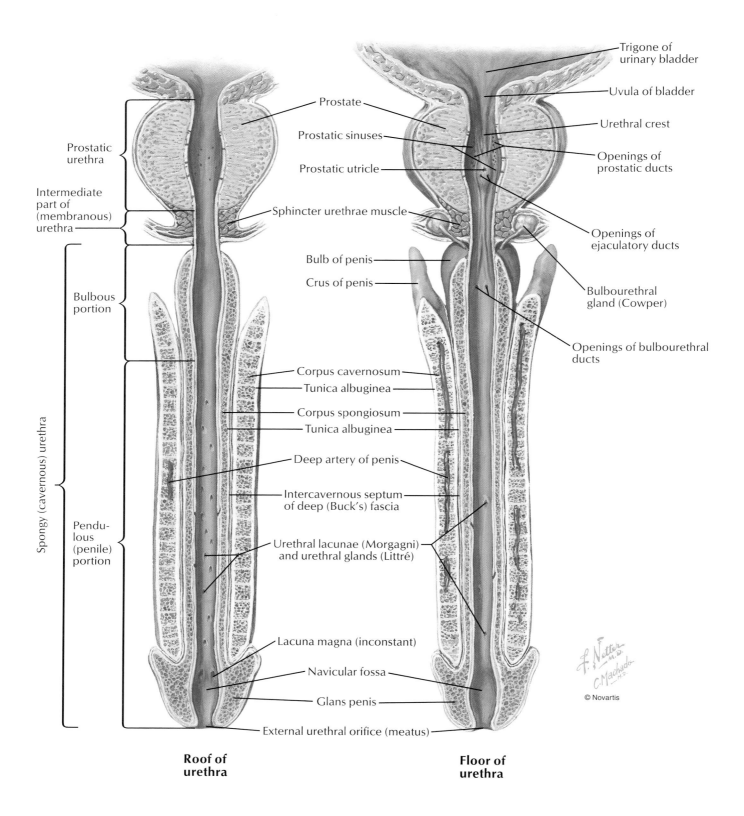

Prostatic urethra

Intermediate part of (membranous) urethra

Bulbous portion

Spongy (cavernous) urethra

Pendulous (penile) portion

Prostate

Prostatic sinuses

Prostatic utricle

Sphincter urethrae muscle

Bulb of penis

Crus of penis

Corpus cavernosum

Tunica albuginea

Corpus spongiosum

Tunica albuginea

Deep artery of penis

Intercavernous septum of deep (Buck's) fascia

Urethral lacunae (Morgagni) and urethral glands (Littré)

Lacuna magna (inconstant)

Navicular fossa

Glans penis

External urethral orifice (meatus)

Trigone of urinary bladder

Uvula of bladder

Urethral crest

Openings of prostatic ducts

Openings of ejaculatory ducts

Bulbourethral gland (Cowper)

Openings of bulbourethral ducts

**Roof of urethra**

**Floor of urethra**

© Novartis

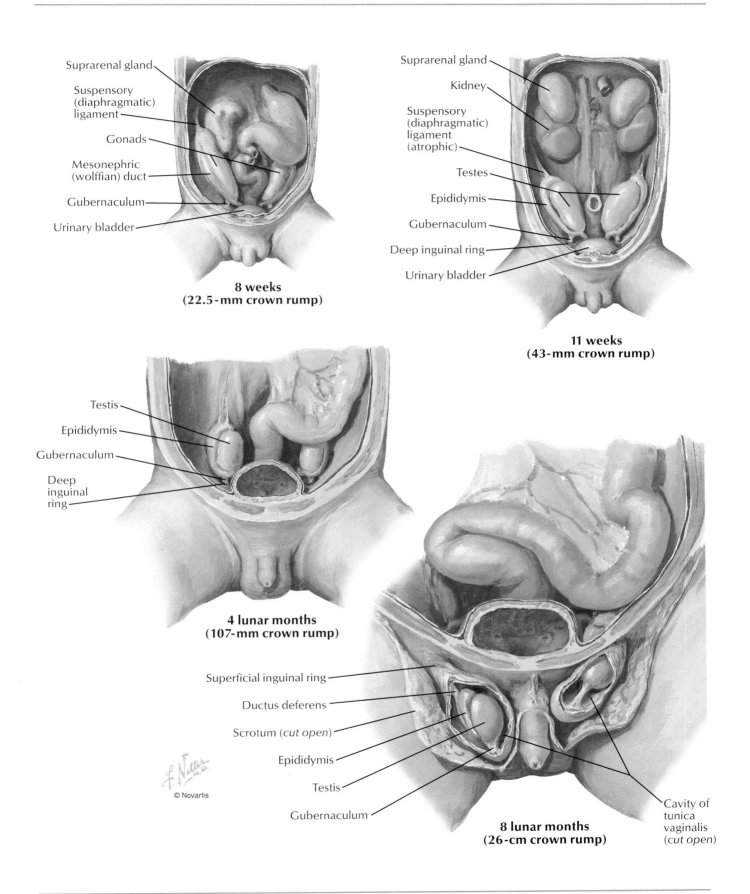

Suprarenal gland

Suspensory (diaphragmatic) ligament

Gonads

Mesonephric (wolffian) duct

Gubernaculum

Urinary bladder

**8 weeks (22.5-mm crown rump)**

Suprarenal gland

Kidney

Suspensory (diaphragmatic) ligament (atrophic)

Testes

Epididymis

Gubernaculum

Deep inguinal ring

Urinary bladder

**11 weeks (43-mm crown rump)**

Testis

Epididymis

Gubernaculum

Deep inguinal ring

**4 lunar months (107-mm crown rump)**

Superficial inguinal ring

Ductus deferens

Scrotum (*cut open*)

Epididymis

Testis

Gubernaculum

**8 lunar months (26-cm crown rump)**

Cavity of tunica vaginalis (*cut open*)

© Novartis

# Scrotum and Contents

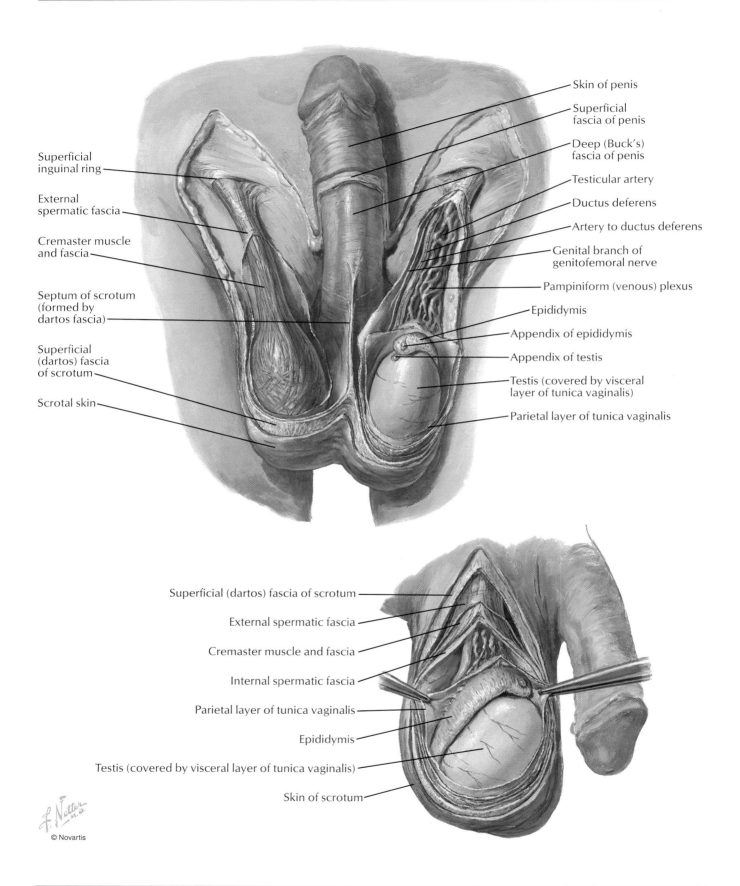

Skin of penis

Superficial fascia of penis

Deep (Buck's) fascia of penis

Testicular artery

Ductus deferens

Artery to ductus deferens

Genital branch of genitofemoral nerve

Pampiniform (venous) plexus

Epididymis

Appendix of epididymis

Appendix of testis

Testis (covered by visceral layer of tunica vaginalis)

Parietal layer of tunica vaginalis

Superficial inguinal ring

External spermatic fascia

Cremaster muscle and fascia

Septum of scrotum (formed by dartos fascia)

Superficial (dartos) fascia of scrotum

Scrotal skin

Superficial (dartos) fascia of scrotum

External spermatic fascia

Cremaster muscle and fascia

Internal spermatic fascia

Parietal layer of tunica vaginalis

Epididymis

Testis (covered by visceral layer of tunica vaginalis)

Skin of scrotum

© Novartis

**PLATE 361**　　　　　　　　　　　　**PELVIS AND PERINEUM**

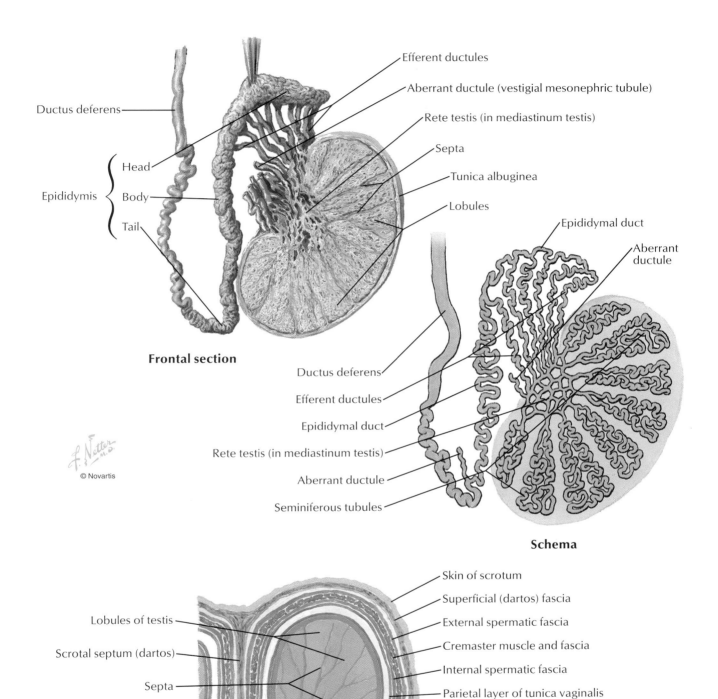

**Frontal section**

Ductus deferens

Epididymis
- Head
- Body
- Tail

Efferent ductules

Aberrant ductule (vestigial mesonephric tubule)

Rete testis (in mediastinum testis)

Septa

Tunica albuginea

Lobules

**Schema**

Epididymal duct

Aberrant ductule

Ductus deferens

Efferent ductules

Epididymal duct

Rete testis (in mediastinum testis)

Aberrant ductule

Seminiferous tubules

f. Netter
© Novartis

**Cross section through scrotum and testis**

Lobules of testis

Scrotal septum (dartos)

Septa

Rete testis (in mediastinum testis)

Ductus deferens

Skin of scrotum

Superficial (dartos) fascia

External spermatic fascia

Cremaster muscle and fascia

Internal spermatic fascia

Parietal layer of tunica vaginalis

Visceral layer of tunica vaginalis

Tunica albuginea of testis

Sinus of epididymis

Epididymis

# Rectum In Situ: Female and Male

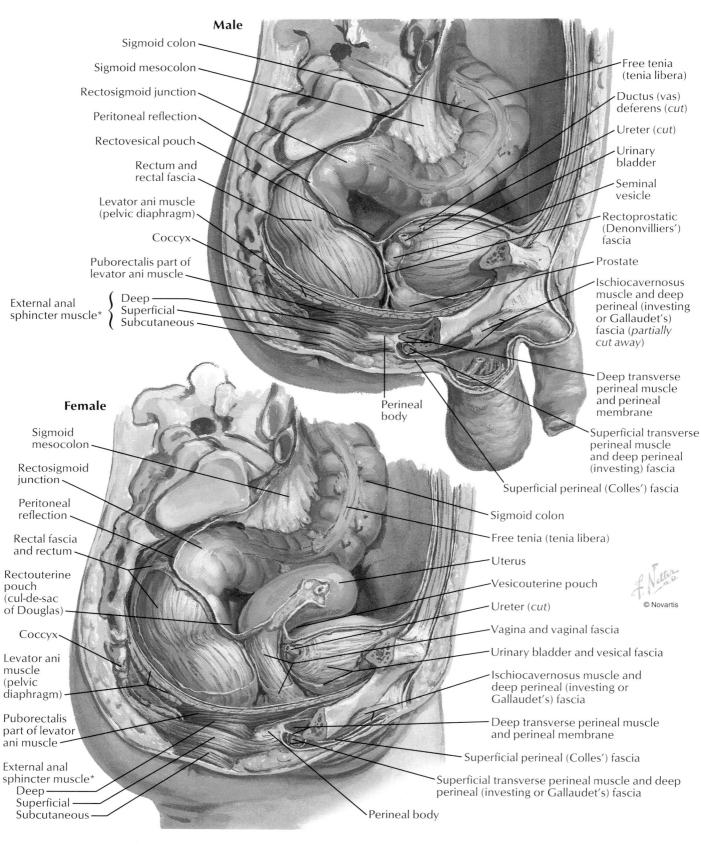

**Male**

Sigmoid colon

Sigmoid mesocolon

Rectosigmoid junction

Peritoneal reflection

Rectovesical pouch

Rectum and rectal fascia

Levator ani muscle (pelvic diaphragm)

Coccyx

Puborectalis part of levator ani muscle

External anal sphincter muscle*
{ Deep
Superficial
Subcutaneous

Free tenia (tenia libera)

Ductus (vas) deferens (cut)

Ureter (cut)

Urinary bladder

Seminal vesicle

Rectoprostatic (Denonvilliers') fascia

Prostate

Ischiocavernosus muscle and deep perineal (investing or Gallaudet's) fascia (partially cut away)

Deep transverse perineal muscle and perineal membrane

Superficial transverse perineal muscle and deep perineal (investing) fascia

Superficial perineal (Colles') fascia

Perineal body

**Female**

Sigmoid mesocolon

Rectosigmoid junction

Peritoneal reflection

Rectal fascia and rectum

Rectouterine pouch (cul-de-sac of Douglas)

Coccyx

Levator ani muscle (pelvic diaphragm)

Puborectalis part of levator ani muscle

External anal sphincter muscle*
Deep
Superficial
Subcutaneous

Sigmoid colon

Free tenia (tenia libera)

Uterus

Vesicouterine pouch

Ureter (cut)

Vagina and vaginal fascia

Urinary bladder and vesical fascia

Ischiocavernosus muscle and deep perineal (investing or Gallaudet's) fascia

Deep transverse perineal muscle and perineal membrane

Superficial perineal (Colles') fascia

Superficial transverse perineal muscle and deep perineal (investing or Gallaudet's) fascia

Perineal body

*Parts variable and often indistinct

f. Netter
© Novartis

**PLATE 363**

**PELVIS AND PERINEUM**

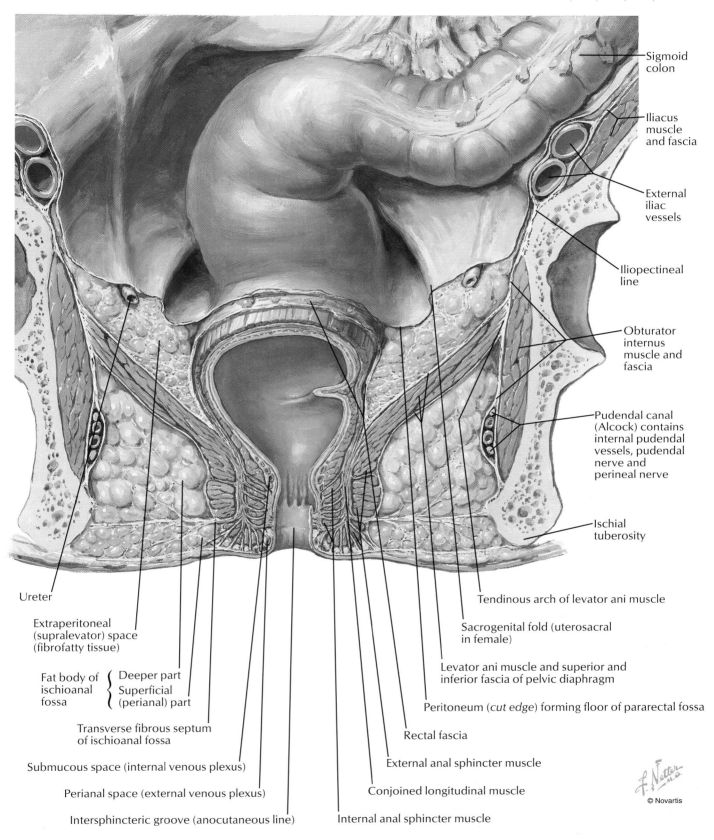

Sigmoid colon

Iliacus muscle and fascia

External iliac vessels

Iliopectineal line

Obturator internus muscle and fascia

Pudendal canal (Alcock) contains internal pudendal vessels, pudendal nerve and perineal nerve

Ischial tuberosity

Ureter

Extraperitoneal (supralevator) space (fibrofatty tissue)

Fat body of ischioanal fossa { Deeper part / Superficial (perianal) part

Transverse fibrous septum of ischioanal fossa

Submucous space (internal venous plexus)

Perianal space (external venous plexus)

Intersphincteric groove (anocutaneous line)

Tendinous arch of levator ani muscle

Sacrogenital fold (uterosacral in female)

Levator ani muscle and superior and inferior fascia of pelvic diaphragm

Peritoneum (*cut edge*) forming floor of pararectal fossa

Rectal fascia

External anal sphincter muscle

Conjoined longitudinal muscle

Internal anal sphincter muscle

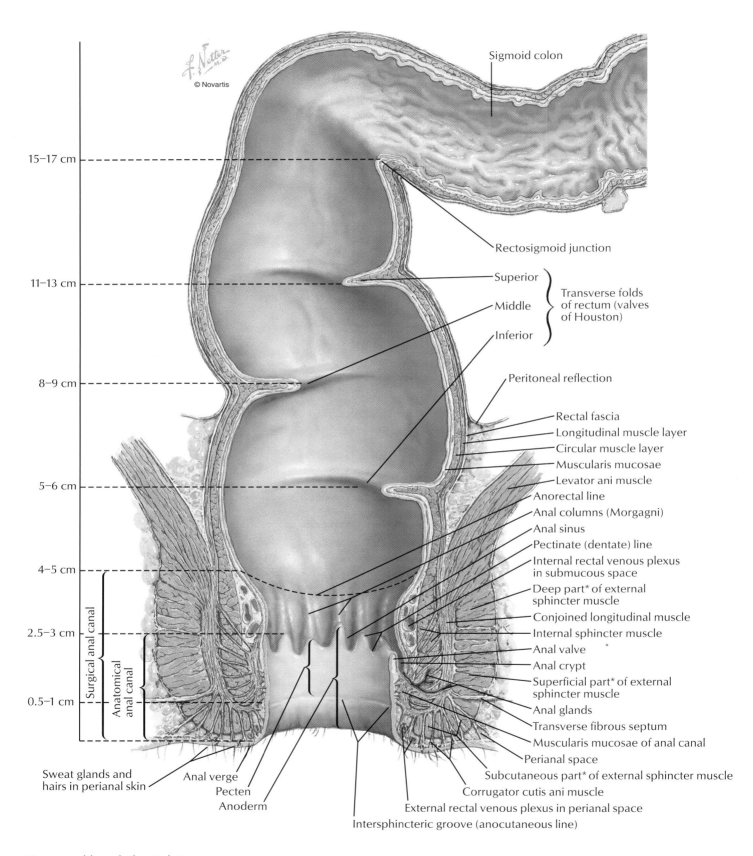

Sigmoid colon

15–17 cm

Rectosigmoid junction

11–13 cm

Superior

Middle

Inferior

Transverse folds of rectum (valves of Houston)

8–9 cm

Peritoneal reflection

Rectal fascia

Longitudinal muscle layer

Circular muscle layer

Muscularis mucosae

5–6 cm

Levator ani muscle

Anorectal line

Anal columns (Morgagni)

Anal sinus

Pectinate (dentate) line

Internal rectal venous plexus in submucous space

4–5 cm

Deep part* of external sphincter muscle

Conjoined longitudinal muscle

Surgical anal canal

2.5–3 cm

Internal sphincter muscle

Anal valve

Anal crypt

Anatomical anal canal

Superficial part* of external sphincter muscle

0.5–1 cm

Anal glands

Transverse fibrous septum

Muscularis mucosae of anal canal

Perianal space

Sweat glands and hairs in perianal skin

Anal verge

Pecten

Anoderm

Subcutaneous part* of external sphincter muscle

Corrugator cutis ani muscle

External rectal venous plexus in perianal space

Intersphincteric groove (anocutaneous line)

*Parts variable and often indistinct

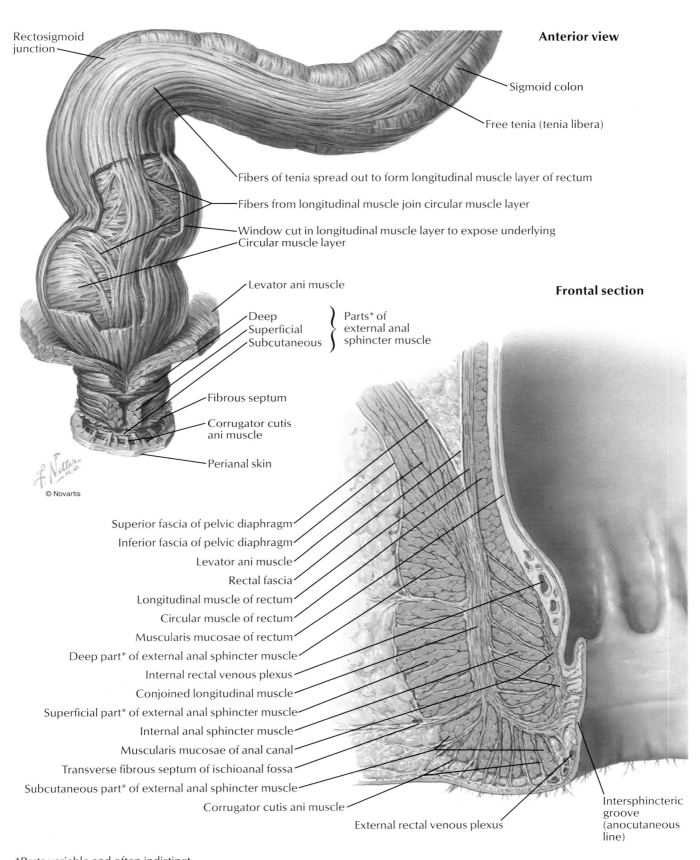

**Anterior view**

Rectosigmoid junction

Sigmoid colon

Free tenia (tenia libera)

Fibers of tenia spread out to form longitudinal muscle layer of rectum

Fibers from longitudinal muscle join circular muscle layer

Window cut in longitudinal muscle layer to expose underlying
Circular muscle layer

Levator ani muscle

Deep
Superficial    } Parts* of
Subcutaneous } external anal
              sphincter muscle

**Frontal section**

Fibrous septum

Corrugator cutis ani muscle

Perianal skin

Superior fascia of pelvic diaphragm

Inferior fascia of pelvic diaphragm

Levator ani muscle

Rectal fascia

Longitudinal muscle of rectum

Circular muscle of rectum

Muscularis mucosae of rectum

Deep part* of external anal sphincter muscle

Internal rectal venous plexus

Conjoined longitudinal muscle

Superficial part* of external anal sphincter muscle

Internal anal sphincter muscle

Muscularis mucosae of anal canal

Transverse fibrous septum of ischioanal fossa

Subcutaneous part* of external anal sphincter muscle

Corrugator cutis ani muscle

External rectal venous plexus

Intersphincteric groove (anocutaneous line)

*Parts variable and often indistinct

# External Anal Sphincter Muscle: Perineal Views

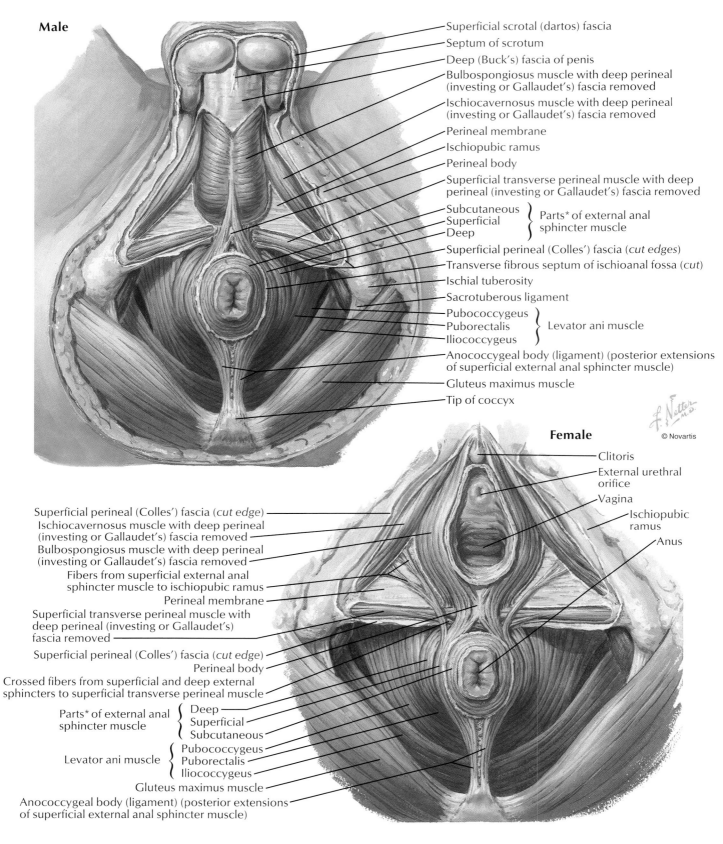

**Male**

- Superficial scrotal (dartos) fascia
- Septum of scrotum
- Deep (Buck's) fascia of penis
- Bulbospongiosus muscle with deep perineal (investing or Gallaudet's) fascia removed
- Ischiocavernosus muscle with deep perineal (investing or Gallaudet's) fascia removed
- Perineal membrane
- Ischiopubic ramus
- Perineal body
- Superficial transverse perineal muscle with deep perineal (investing or Gallaudet's) fascia removed
- Subcutaneous ⎫
- Superficial ⎬ Parts* of external anal sphincter muscle
- Deep ⎭
- Superficial perineal (Colles') fascia (*cut edges*)
- Transverse fibrous septum of ischioanal fossa (*cut*)
- Ischial tuberosity
- Sacrotuberous ligament
- Pubococcygeus ⎫
- Puborectalis ⎬ Levator ani muscle
- Iliococcygeus ⎭
- Anococcygeal body (ligament) (posterior extensions of superficial external anal sphincter muscle)
- Gluteus maximus muscle
- Tip of coccyx

**Female**

- Clitoris
- External urethral orifice
- Vagina
- Ischiopubic ramus
- Anus

- Superficial perineal (Colles') fascia (*cut edge*)
- Ischiocavernosus muscle with deep perineal (investing or Gallaudet's) fascia removed
- Bulbospongiosus muscle with deep perineal (investing or Gallaudet's) fascia removed
- Fibers from superficial external anal sphincter muscle to ischiopubic ramus
- Perineal membrane
- Superficial transverse perineal muscle with deep perineal (investing or Gallaudet's) fascia removed
- Superficial perineal (Colles') fascia (*cut edge*)
- Perineal body
- Crossed fibers from superficial and deep external sphincters to superficial transverse perineal muscle
- Parts* of external anal sphincter muscle ⎰ Deep / Superficial / Subcutaneous
- Levator ani muscle ⎰ Pubococcygeus / Puborectalis / Iliococcygeus
- Gluteus maximus muscle
- Anococcygeal body (ligament) (posterior extensions of superficial external anal sphincter muscle)

*Parts variable and often indistinct

**PLATE 367**

**PELVIS AND PERINEUM**

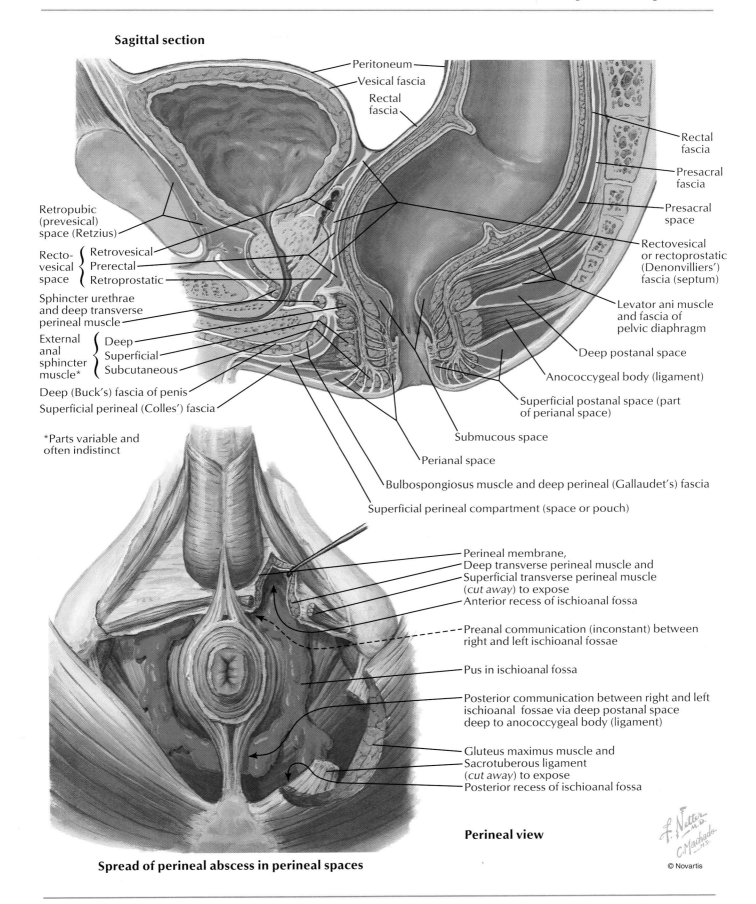

**Sagittal section**

Peritoneum

Vesical fascia

Rectal fascia

Rectal fascia

Presacral fascia

Presacral space

Retropubic (prevesical) space (Retzius)

Recto-vesical space { Retrovesical / Prerectal / Retroprostatic

Rectovesical or rectoprostatic (Denonvilliers') fascia (septum)

Sphincter urethrae and deep transverse perineal muscle

Levator ani muscle and fascia of pelvic diaphragm

External anal sphincter muscle* { Deep / Superficial / Subcutaneous

Deep postanal space

Anococcygeal body (ligament)

Deep (Buck's) fascia of penis

Superficial postanal space (part of perianal space)

Superficial perineal (Colles') fascia

Submucous space

*Parts variable and often indistinct

Perianal space

Bulbospongiosus muscle and deep perineal (Gallaudet's) fascia

Superficial perineal compartment (space or pouch)

Perineal membrane, Deep transverse perineal muscle and Superficial transverse perineal muscle (*cut away*) to expose Anterior recess of ischioanal fossa

Preanal communication (inconstant) between right and left ischioanal fossae

Pus in ischioanal fossa

Posterior communication between right and left ischioanal fossae via deep postanal space deep to anococcygeal body (ligament)

Gluteus maximus muscle and Sacrotuberous ligament (*cut away*) to expose Posterior recess of ischioanal fossa

**Perineal view**

**Spread of perineal abscess in perineal spaces**

© Novartis

# Arteries of Rectum and Anal Canal

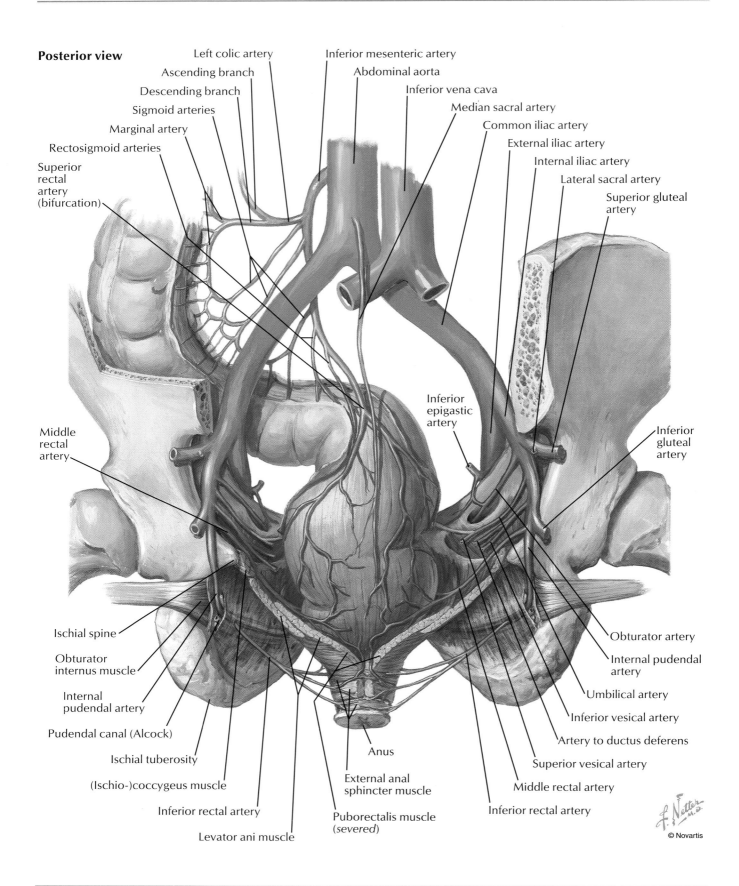

**Posterior view**

Left colic artery

Ascending branch

Descending branch

Sigmoid arteries

Marginal artery

Rectosigmoid arteries

Superior rectal artery (bifurcation)

Inferior mesenteric artery

Abdominal aorta

Inferior vena cava

Median sacral artery

Common iliac artery

External iliac artery

Internal iliac artery

Lateral sacral artery

Superior gluteal artery

Inferior epigastic artery

Inferior gluteal artery

Middle rectal artery

Obturator artery

Internal pudendal artery

Umbilical artery

Inferior vesical artery

Artery to ductus deferens

Superior vesical artery

Middle rectal artery

Inferior rectal artery

Ischial spine

Obturator internus muscle

Internal pudendal artery

Pudendal canal (Alcock)

Ischial tuberosity

(Ischio-)coccygeus muscle

Inferior rectal artery

Levator ani muscle

Anus

External anal sphincter muscle

Puborectalis muscle (*severed*)

© Novartis

**PLATE 369**

**PELVIS AND PERINEUM**

**Anterior view**

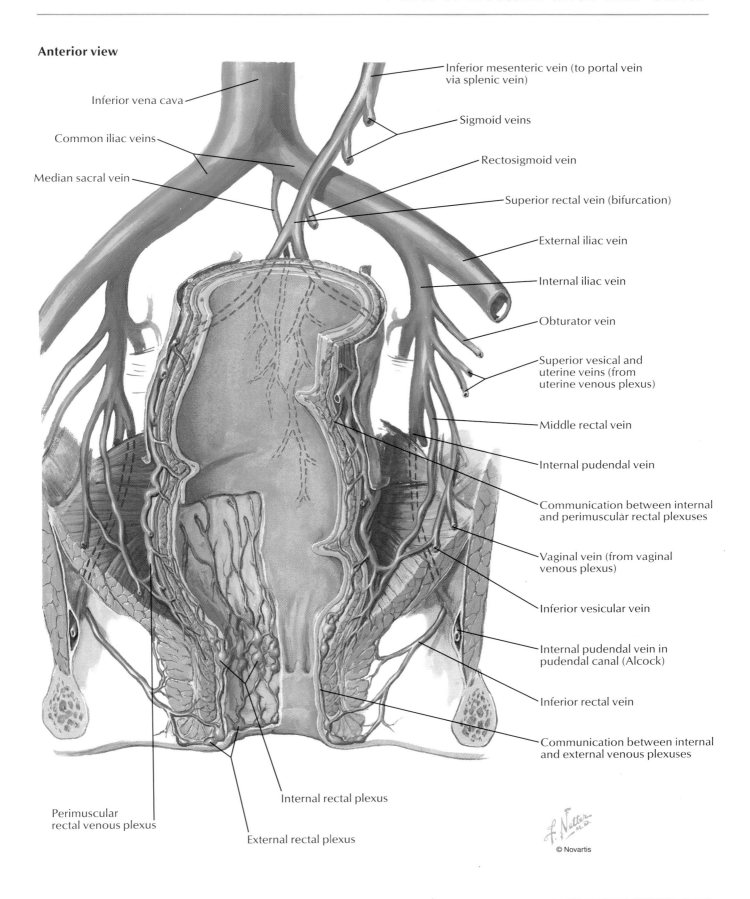

Inferior vena cava

Common iliac veins

Median sacral vein

Inferior mesenteric vein (to portal vein via splenic vein)

Sigmoid veins

Rectosigmoid vein

Superior rectal vein (bifurcation)

External iliac vein

Internal iliac vein

Obturator vein

Superior vesical and uterine veins (from uterine venous plexus)

Middle rectal vein

Internal pudendal vein

Communication between internal and perimuscular rectal plexuses

Vaginal vein (from vaginal venous plexus)

Inferior vesicular vein

Internal pudendal vein in pudendal canal (Alcock)

Inferior rectal vein

Communication between internal and external venous plexuses

Internal rectal plexus

Perimuscular rectal venous plexus

External rectal plexus

© Novartis

**Anterior view**

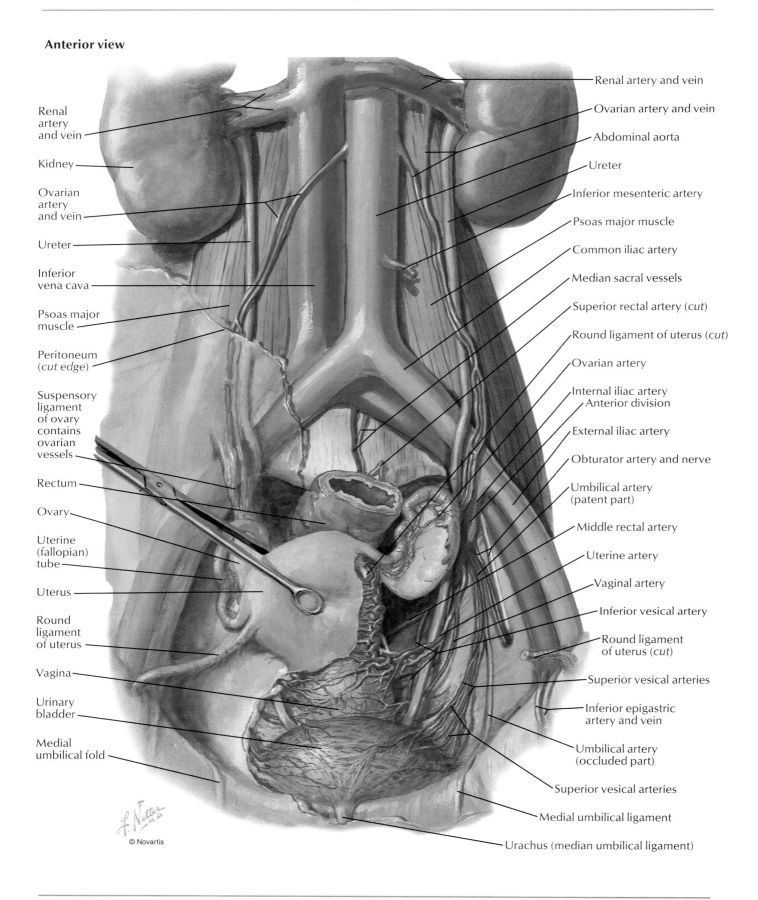

Renal artery and vein

Kidney

Ovarian artery and vein

Ureter

Inferior vena cava

Psoas major muscle

Peritoneum (*cut edge*)

Suspensory ligament of ovary contains ovarian vessels

Rectum

Ovary

Uterine (fallopian) tube

Uterus

Round ligament of uterus

Vagina

Urinary bladder

Medial umbilical fold

Renal artery and vein

Ovarian artery and vein

Abdominal aorta

Ureter

Inferior mesenteric artery

Psoas major muscle

Common iliac artery

Median sacral vessels

Superior rectal artery (*cut*)

Round ligament of uterus (*cut*)

Ovarian artery

Internal iliac artery Anterior division

External iliac artery

Obturator artery and nerve

Umbilical artery (patent part)

Middle rectal artery

Uterine artery

Vaginal artery

Inferior vesical artery

Round ligament of uterus (*cut*)

Superior vesical arteries

Inferior epigastric artery and vein

Umbilical artery (occluded part)

Superior vesical arteries

Medial umbilical ligament

Urachus (median umbilical ligament)

© Novartis

**PLATE 371**

**PELVIS AND PERINEUM**

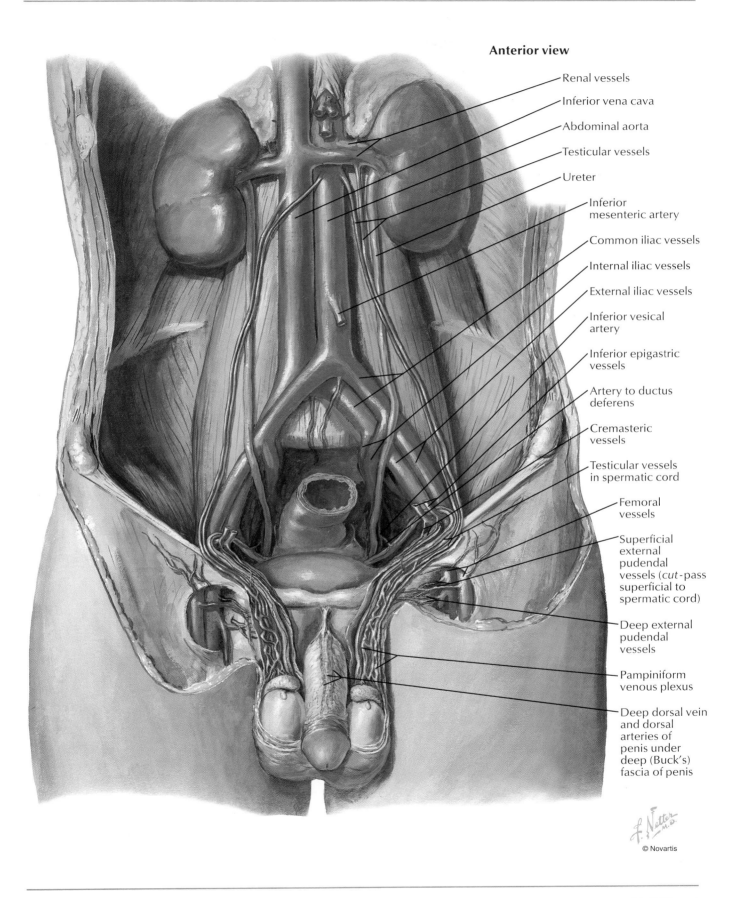

**Anterior view**

Renal vessels

Inferior vena cava

Abdominal aorta

Testicular vessels

Ureter

Inferior mesenteric artery

Common iliac vessels

Internal iliac vessels

External iliac vessels

Inferior vesical artery

Inferior epigastric vessels

Artery to ductus deferens

Cremasteric vessels

Testicular vessels in spermatic cord

Femoral vessels

Superficial external pudendal vessels (*cut*-pass superficial to spermatic cord)

Deep external pudendal vessels

Pampiniform venous plexus

Deep dorsal vein and dorsal arteries of penis under deep (Buck's) fascia of penis

© Novartis

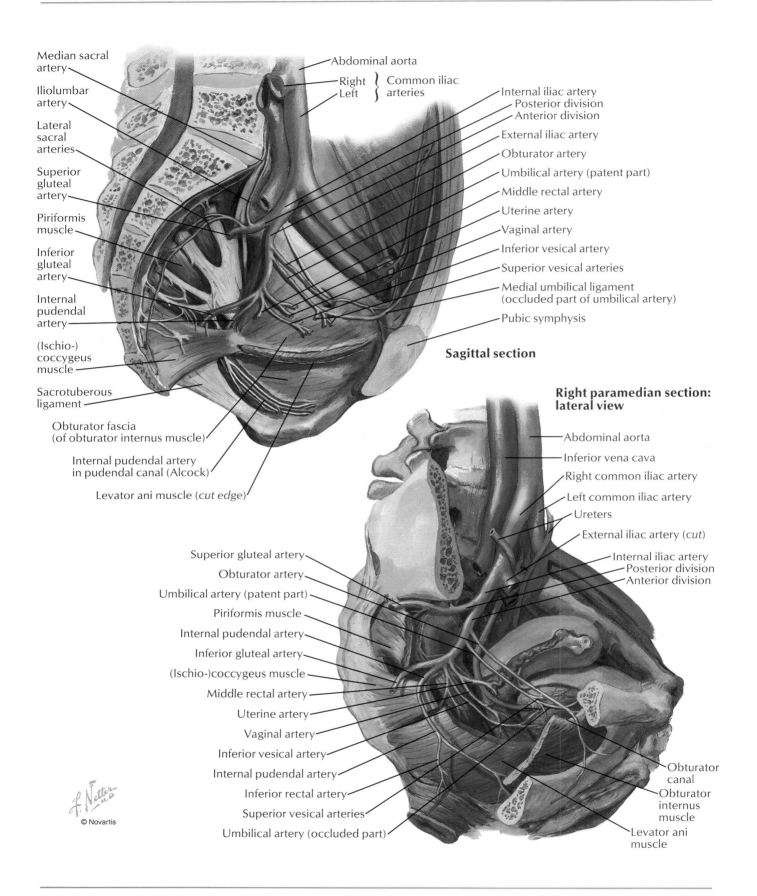

Median sacral artery

Iliolumbar artery

Lateral sacral arteries

Superior gluteal artery

Piriformis muscle

Inferior gluteal artery

Internal pudendal artery

(Ischio-)coccygeus muscle

Sacrotuberous ligament

Obturator fascia (of obturator internus muscle)

Internal pudendal artery in pudendal canal (Alcock)

Levator ani muscle (*cut edge*)

Abdominal aorta

Right ⎱ Common iliac
Left  ⎰ arteries

Internal iliac artery
Posterior division
Anterior division

External iliac artery

Obturator artery

Umbilical artery (patent part)

Middle rectal artery

Uterine artery

Vaginal artery

Inferior vesical artery

Superior vesical arteries

Medial umbilical ligament (occluded part of umbilical artery)

Pubic symphysis

**Sagittal section**

**Right paramedian section: lateral view**

Abdominal aorta

Inferior vena cava

Right common iliac artery

Left common iliac artery

Ureters

External iliac artery (*cut*)

Internal iliac artery
Posterior division
Anterior division

Superior gluteal artery

Obturator artery

Umbilical artery (patent part)

Piriformis muscle

Internal pudendal artery

Inferior gluteal artery

(Ischio-)coccygeus muscle

Middle rectal artery

Uterine artery

Vaginal artery

Inferior vesical artery

Internal pudendal artery

Inferior rectal artery

Superior vesical arteries

Umbilical artery (occluded part)

Obturator canal

Obturator internus muscle

Levator ani muscle

© Novartis

**PLATE 373**

**PELVIS AND PERINEUM**

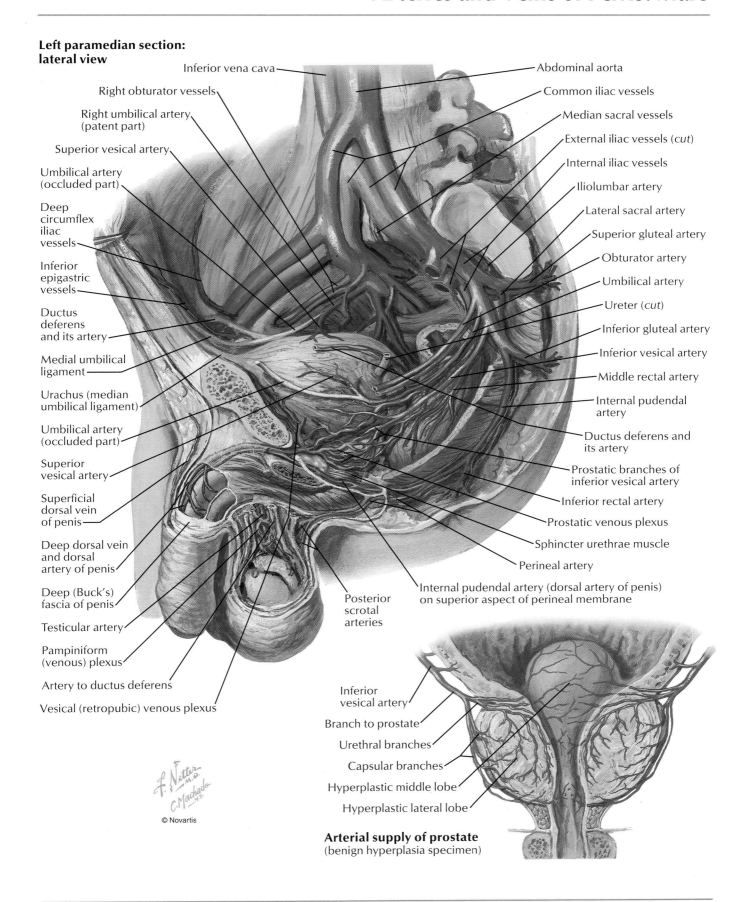

**Left paramedian section:
lateral view**

Inferior vena cava

Right obturator vessels

Right umbilical artery
(patent part)

Superior vesical artery

Umbilical artery
(occluded part)

Deep
circumflex
iliac
vessels

Inferior
epigastric
vessels

Ductus
deferens
and its artery

Medial umbilical
ligament

Urachus (median
umbilical ligament)

Umbilical artery
(occluded part)

Superior
vesical artery

Superficial
dorsal vein
of penis

Deep dorsal vein
and dorsal
artery of penis

Deep (Buck's)
fascia of penis

Testicular artery

Pampiniform
(venous) plexus

Artery to ductus deferens

Vesical (retropubic) venous plexus

Abdominal aorta

Common iliac vessels

Median sacral vessels

External iliac vessels (*cut*)

Internal iliac vessels

Iliolumbar artery

Lateral sacral artery

Superior gluteal artery

Obturator artery

Umbilical artery

Ureter (*cut*)

Inferior gluteal artery

Inferior vesical artery

Middle rectal artery

Internal pudendal
artery

Ductus deferens and
its artery

Prostatic branches of
inferior vesical artery

Inferior rectal artery

Prostatic venous plexus

Sphincter urethrae muscle

Perineal artery

Internal pudendal artery (dorsal artery of penis)
on superior aspect of perineal membrane

Posterior
scrotal
arteries

Inferior
vesical artery

Branch to prostate

Urethral branches

Capsular branches

Hyperplastic middle lobe

Hyperplastic lateral lobe

**Arterial supply of prostate**
(benign hyperplasia specimen)

© Novartis

# Arteries and Veins of Perineum and Uterus

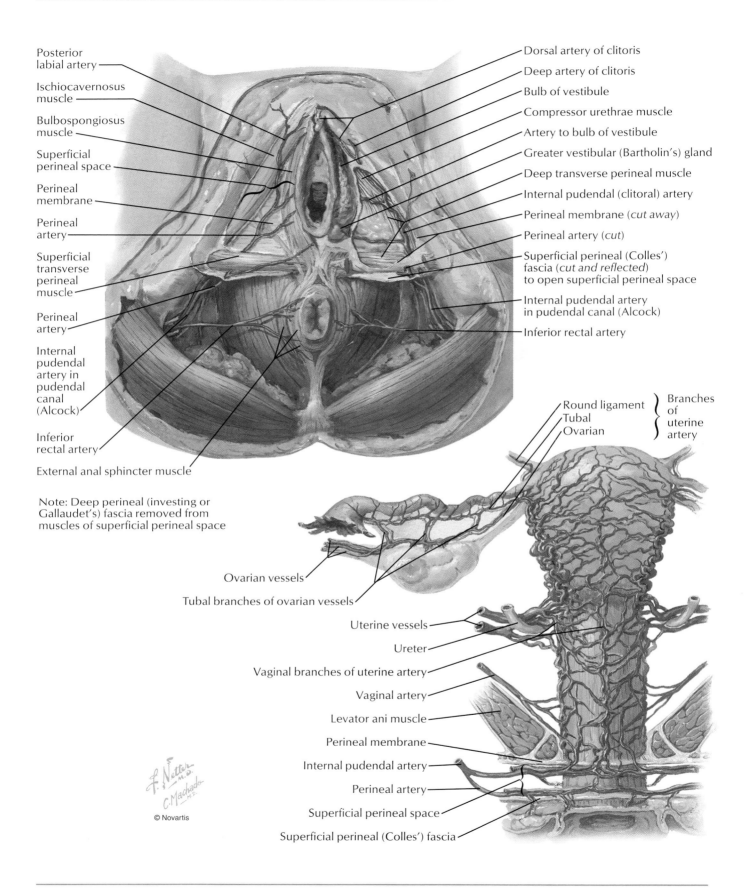

Posterior labial artery

Ischiocavernosus muscle

Bulbospongiosus muscle

Superficial perineal space

Perineal membrane

Perineal artery

Superficial transverse perineal muscle

Perineal artery

Internal pudendal artery in pudendal canal (Alcock)

Inferior rectal artery

External anal sphincter muscle

Note: Deep perineal (investing or Gallaudet's) fascia removed from muscles of superficial perineal space

Dorsal artery of clitoris

Deep artery of clitoris

Bulb of vestibule

Compressor urethrae muscle

Artery to bulb of vestibule

Greater vestibular (Bartholin's) gland

Deep transverse perineal muscle

Internal pudendal (clitoral) artery

Perineal membrane (cut away)

Perineal artery (cut)

Superficial perineal (Colles') fascia (cut and reflected) to open superficial perineal space

Internal pudendal artery in pudendal canal (Alcock)

Inferior rectal artery

Round ligament } Branches of uterine artery
Tubal
Ovarian

Ovarian vessels

Tubal branches of ovarian vessels

Uterine vessels

Ureter

Vaginal branches of uterine artery

Vaginal artery

Levator ani muscle

Perineal membrane

Internal pudendal artery

Perineal artery

Superficial perineal space

Superficial perineal (Colles') fascia

© Novartis

**PLATE 375**

**PELVIS AND PERINEUM**

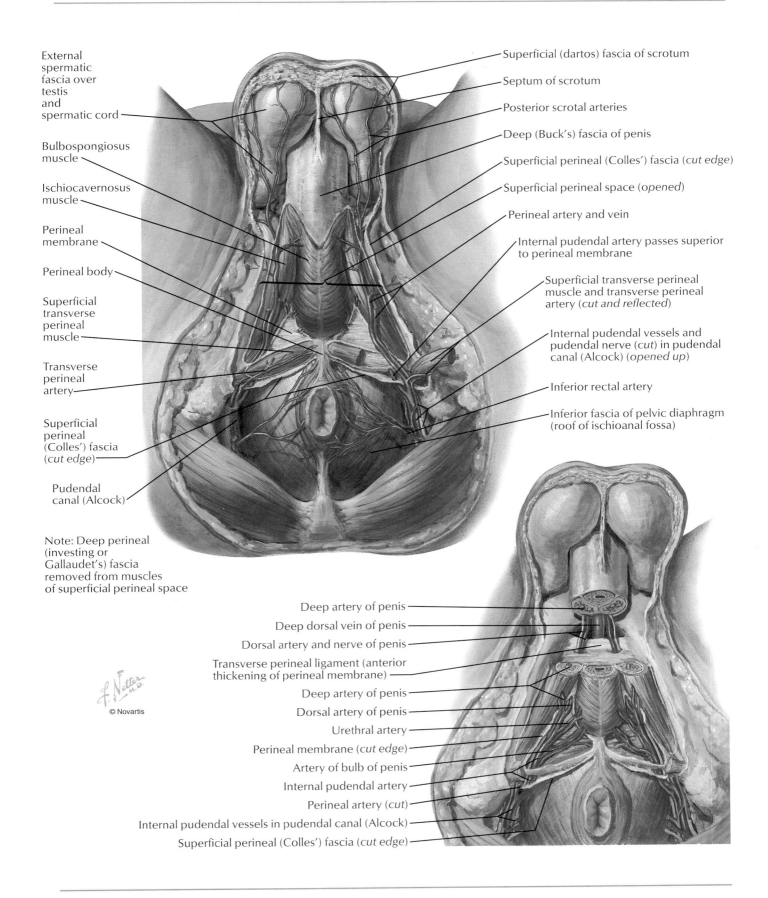

External spermatic fascia over testis and spermatic cord

Bulbospongiosus muscle

Ischiocavernosus muscle

Perineal membrane

Perineal body

Superficial transverse perineal muscle

Transverse perineal artery

Superficial perineal (Colles') fascia (cut edge)

Pudendal canal (Alcock)

Note: Deep perineal (investing or Gallaudet's) fascia removed from muscles of superficial perineal space

Superficial (dartos) fascia of scrotum

Septum of scrotum

Posterior scrotal arteries

Deep (Buck's) fascia of penis

Superficial perineal (Colles') fascia (cut edge)

Superficial perineal space (opened)

Perineal artery and vein

Internal pudendal artery passes superior to perineal membrane

Superficial transverse perineal muscle and transverse perineal artery (cut and reflected)

Internal pudendal vessels and pudendal nerve (cut) in pudendal canal (Alcock) (opened up)

Inferior rectal artery

Inferior fascia of pelvic diaphragm (roof of ischioanal fossa)

Deep artery of penis

Deep dorsal vein of penis

Dorsal artery and nerve of penis

Transverse perineal ligament (anterior thickening of perineal membrane)

Deep artery of penis

Dorsal artery of penis

Urethral artery

Perineal membrane (cut edge)

Artery of bulb of penis

Internal pudendal artery

Perineal artery (cut)

Internal pudendal vessels in pudendal canal (Alcock)

Superficial perineal (Colles') fascia (cut edge)

*F. Netter M.D.*

© Novartis

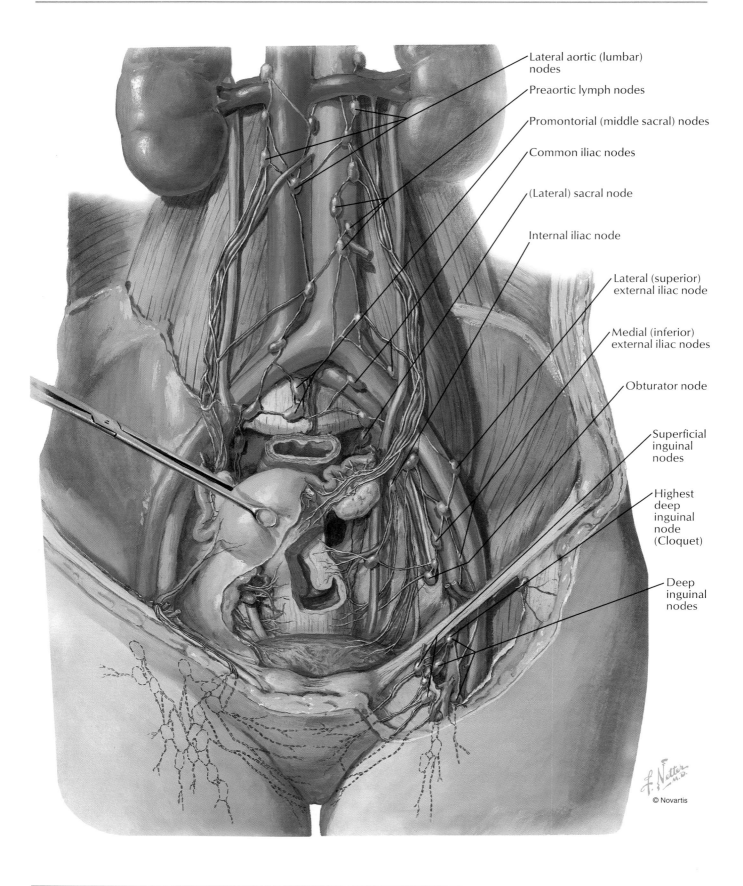

Lateral aortic (lumbar) nodes

Preaortic lymph nodes

Promontorial (middle sacral) nodes

Common iliac nodes

(Lateral) sacral node

Internal iliac node

Lateral (superior) external iliac node

Medial (inferior) external iliac nodes

Obturator node

Superficial inguinal nodes

Highest deep inguinal node (Cloquet)

Deep inguinal nodes

**PLATE 377**

**PELVIS AND PERINEUM**

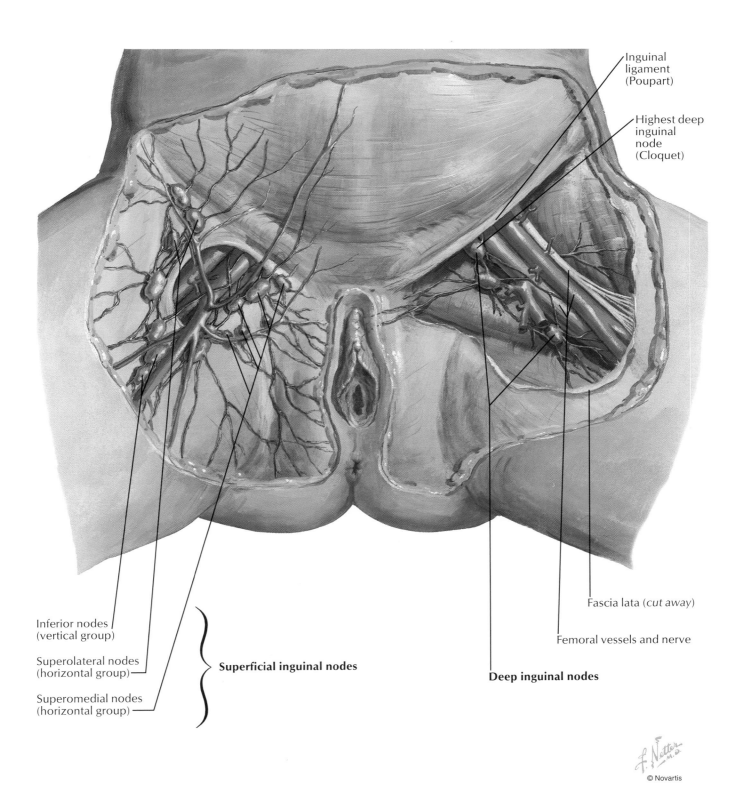

Inguinal ligament (Poupart)

Highest deep inguinal node (Cloquet)

Fascia lata (*cut away*)

Femoral vessels and nerve

**Deep inguinal nodes**

Inferior nodes (vertical group)

Superolateral nodes (horizontal group)

Superomedial nodes (horizontal group)

**Superficial inguinal nodes**

© Novartis

# Lymph Vessels and Nodes of Pelvis and Genitalia: Male

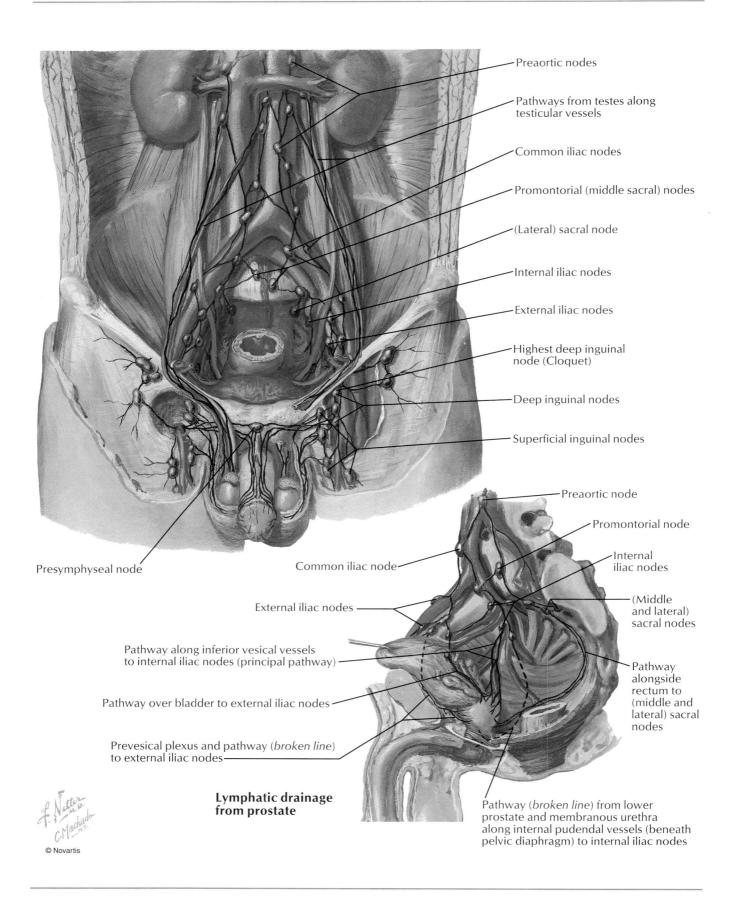

Preaortic nodes

Pathways from testes along testicular vessels

Common iliac nodes

Promontorial (middle sacral) nodes

(Lateral) sacral node

Internal iliac nodes

External iliac nodes

Highest deep inguinal node (Cloquet)

Deep inguinal nodes

Superficial inguinal nodes

Presymphyseal node

Preaortic node

Promontorial node

Internal iliac nodes

Common iliac node

External iliac nodes

(Middle and lateral) sacral nodes

Pathway along inferior vesical vessels to internal iliac nodes (principal pathway)

Pathway over bladder to external iliac nodes

Pathway alongside rectum to (middle and lateral) sacral nodes

Prevesical plexus and pathway (*broken line*) to external iliac nodes

**Lymphatic drainage from prostate**

Pathway (*broken line*) from lower prostate and membranous urethra along internal pudendal vessels (beneath pelvic diaphragm) to internal iliac nodes

© Novartis

**PLATE 379**

**PELVIS AND PERINEUM**

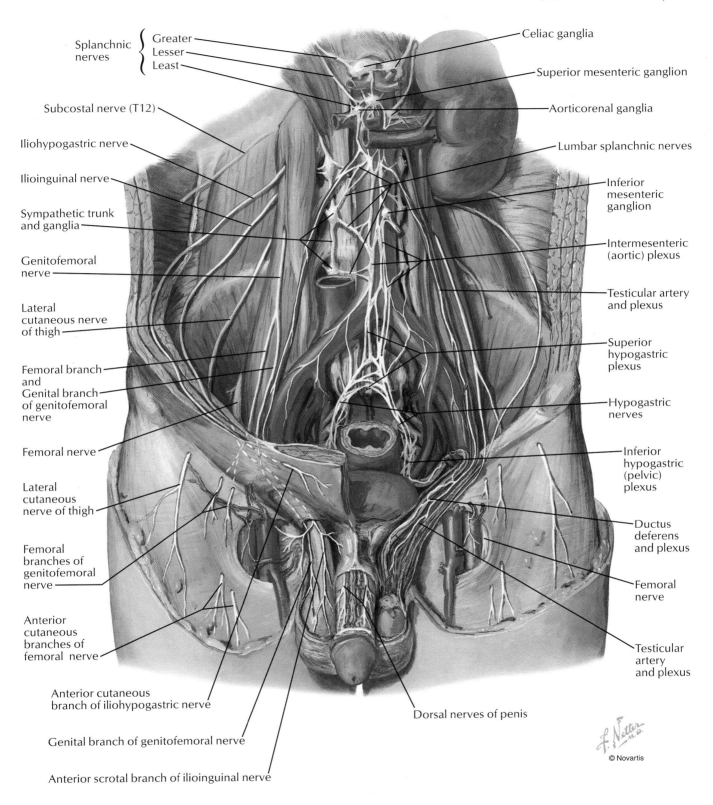

Splanchnic nerves { Greater — Celiac ganglia

Lesser — Superior mesenteric ganglion

Least —

Subcostal nerve (T12) — Aorticorenal ganglia

Iliohypogastric nerve — Lumbar splanchnic nerves

Ilioinguinal nerve — Inferior mesenteric ganglion

Sympathetic trunk and ganglia — Intermesenteric (aortic) plexus

Genitofemoral nerve — Testicular artery and plexus

Lateral cutaneous nerve of thigh — Superior hypogastric plexus

Femoral branch and Genital branch of genitofemoral nerve — Hypogastric nerves

Femoral nerve — Inferior hypogastric (pelvic) plexus

Lateral cutaneous nerve of thigh — Ductus deferens and plexus

Femoral branches of genitofemoral nerve — Femoral nerve

Anterior cutaneous branches of femoral nerve — Testicular artery and plexus

Anterior cutaneous branch of iliohypogastric nerve

Genital branch of genitofemoral nerve — Dorsal nerves of penis

Anterior scrotal branch of ilioinguinal nerve

© Novartis

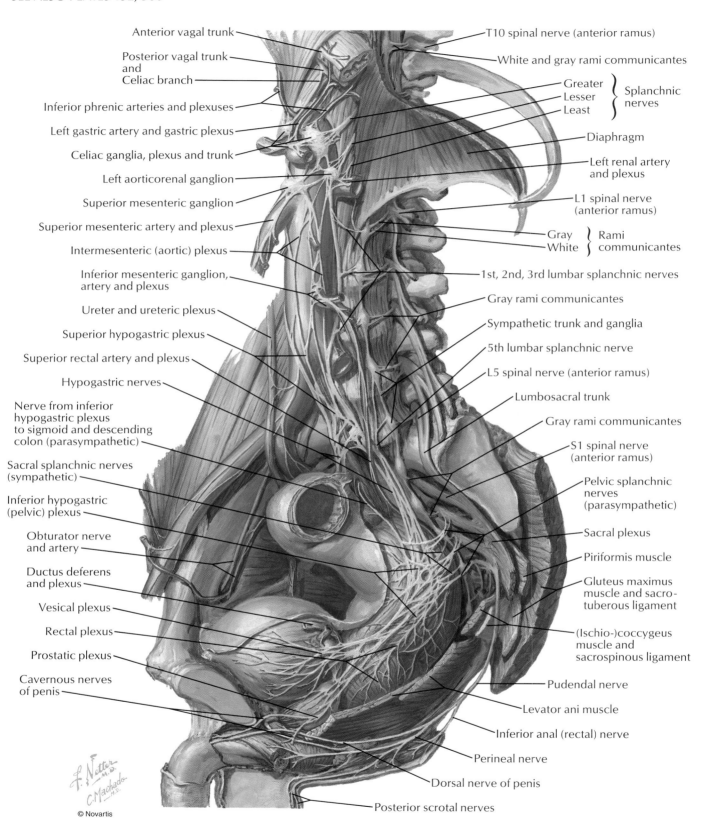

Anterior vagal trunk

Posterior vagal trunk
and
Celiac branch

Inferior phrenic arteries and plexuses

Left gastric artery and gastric plexus

Celiac ganglia, plexus and trunk

Left aorticorenal ganglion

Superior mesenteric ganglion

Superior mesenteric artery and plexus

Intermesenteric (aortic) plexus

Inferior mesenteric ganglion,
artery and plexus

Ureter and ureteric plexus

Superior hypogastric plexus

Superior rectal artery and plexus

Hypogastric nerves

Nerve from inferior
hypogastric plexus
to sigmoid and descending
colon (parasympathetic)

Sacral splanchnic nerves
(sympathetic)

Inferior hypogastric
(pelvic) plexus

Obturator nerve
and artery

Ductus deferens
and plexus

Vesical plexus

Rectal plexus

Prostatic plexus

Cavernous nerves
of penis

T10 spinal nerve (anterior ramus)

White and gray rami communicantes

Greater
Lesser   } Splanchnic
Least    }   nerves

Diaphragm

Left renal artery
and plexus

L1 spinal nerve
(anterior ramus)

Gray   } Rami
White  } communicantes

1st, 2nd, 3rd lumbar splanchnic nerves

Gray rami communicantes

Sympathetic trunk and ganglia

5th lumbar splanchnic nerve

L5 spinal nerve (anterior ramus)

Lumbosacral trunk

Gray rami communicantes

S1 spinal nerve
(anterior ramus)

Pelvic splanchnic
nerves
(parasympathetic)

Sacral plexus

Piriformis muscle

Gluteus maximus
muscle and sacro-
tuberous ligament

(Ischio-)coccygeus
muscle and
sacrospinous ligament

Pudendal nerve

Levator ani muscle

Inferior anal (rectal) nerve

Perineal nerve

Dorsal nerve of penis

Posterior scrotal nerves

**PLATE 381**                                    **PELVIS AND PERINEUM**

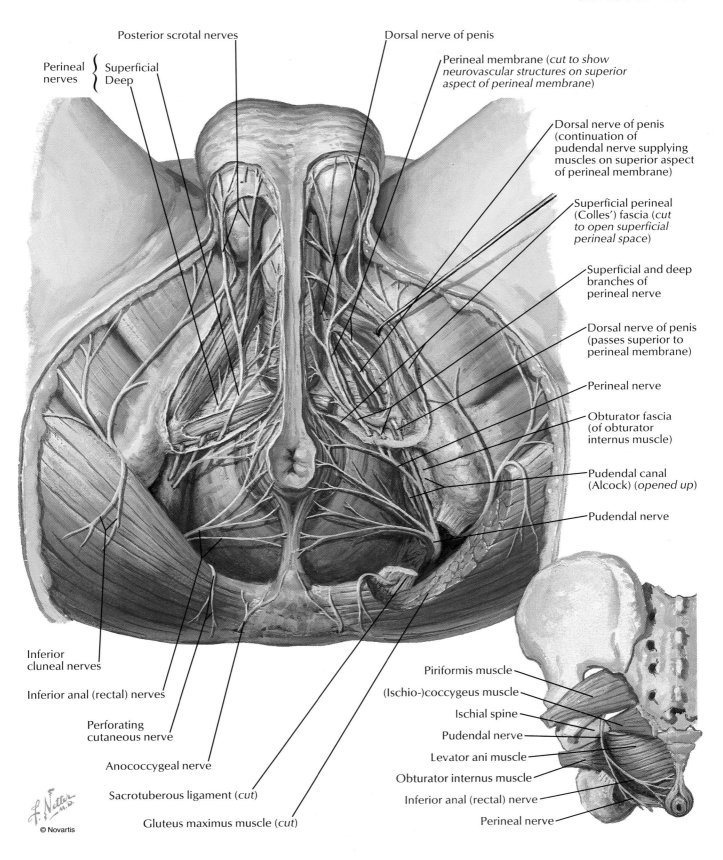

Posterior scrotal nerves

Dorsal nerve of penis

Perineal nerves { Superficial / Deep }

Perineal membrane (*cut to show neurovascular structures on superior aspect of perineal membrane*)

Dorsal nerve of penis (continuation of pudendal nerve supplying muscles on superior aspect of perineal membrane)

Superficial perineal (Colles') fascia (*cut to open superficial perineal space*)

Superficial and deep branches of perineal nerve

Dorsal nerve of penis (passes superior to perineal membrane)

Perineal nerve

Obturator fascia (of obturator internus muscle)

Pudendal canal (Alcock) (*opened up*)

Pudendal nerve

Inferior cluneal nerves

Inferior anal (rectal) nerves

Perforating cutaneous nerve

Anococcygeal nerve

Sacrotuberous ligament (*cut*)

Gluteus maximus muscle (*cut*)

Piriformis muscle

(Ischio-)coccygeus muscle

Ischial spine

Pudendal nerve

Levator ani muscle

Obturator internus muscle

Inferior anal (rectal) nerve

Perineal nerve

*f. Netter* M.D.
© Novartis

**INNERVATION**

**PLATE 382**

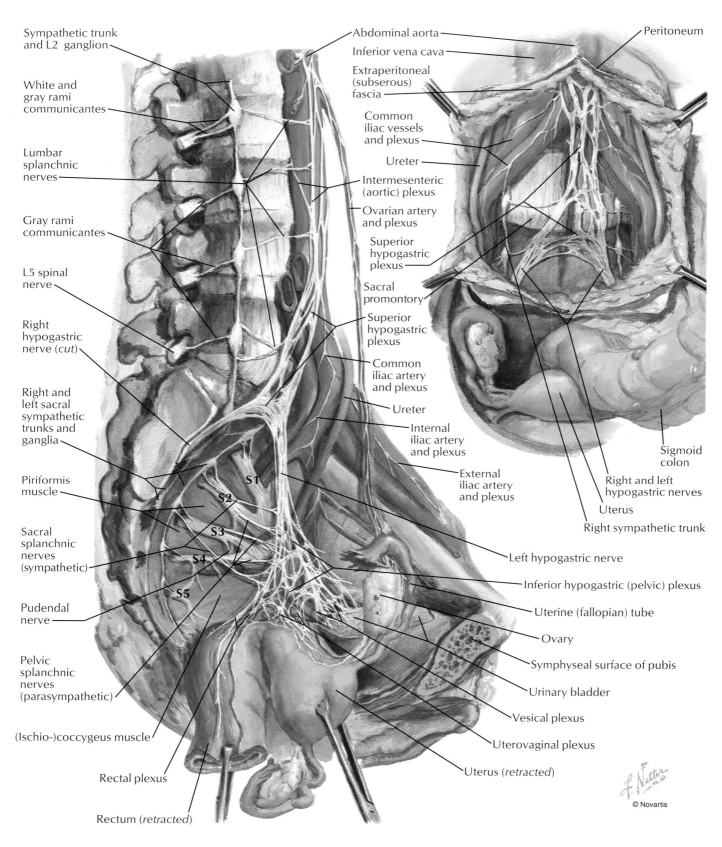

Sympathetic trunk and L2 ganglion

White and gray rami communicantes

Lumbar splanchnic nerves

Gray rami communicantes

L5 spinal nerve

Right hypogastric nerve (cut)

Right and left sacral sympathetic trunks and ganglia

Piriformis muscle

Sacral splanchnic nerves (sympathetic)

Pudendal nerve

Pelvic splanchnic nerves (parasympathetic)

(Ischio-)coccygeus muscle

Rectal plexus

Rectum (retracted)

Abdominal aorta

Inferior vena cava

Extraperitoneal (subserous) fascia

Common iliac vessels and plexus

Ureter

Intermesenteric (aortic) plexus

Ovarian artery and plexus

Superior hypogastric plexus

Sacral promontory

Superior hypogastric plexus

Common iliac artery and plexus

Ureter

Internal iliac artery and plexus

External iliac artery and plexus

Peritoneum

Sigmoid colon

Right and left hypogastric nerves

Uterus

Right sympathetic trunk

Left hypogastric nerve

Inferior hypogastric (pelvic) plexus

Uterine (fallopian) tube

Ovary

Symphyseal surface of pubis

Urinary bladder

Vesical plexus

Uterovaginal plexus

Uterus (retracted)

S1
S2
S3
S4
S5

© Novartis

**PLATE 383**

**PELVIS AND PERINEUM**

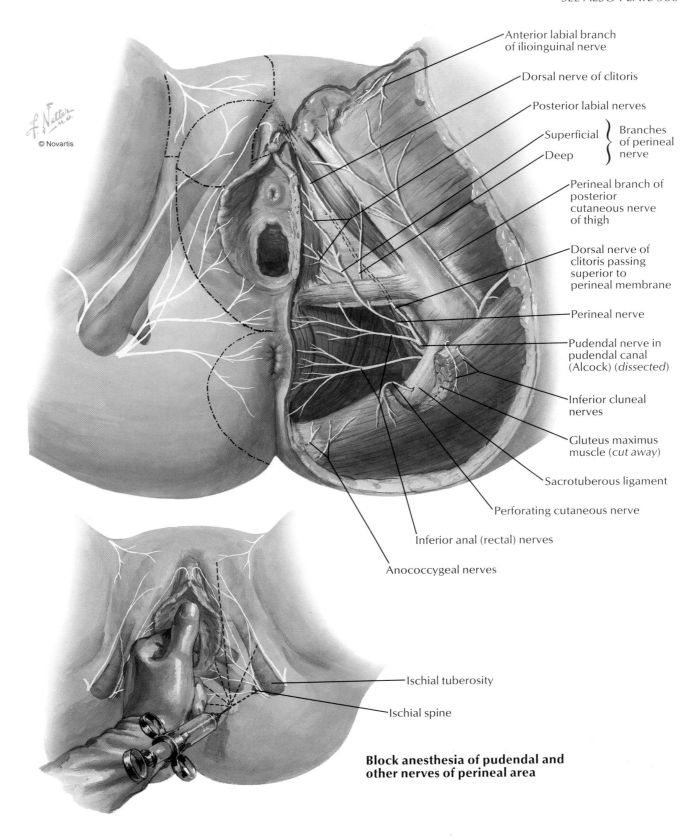

Anterior labial branch of ilioinguinal nerve

Dorsal nerve of clitoris

Posterior labial nerves

Superficial } Branches of perineal nerve

Deep }

Perineal branch of posterior cutaneous nerve of thigh

Dorsal nerve of clitoris passing superior to perineal membrane

Perineal nerve

Pudendal nerve in pudendal canal (Alcock) (*dissected*)

Inferior cluneal nerves

Gluteus maximus muscle (*cut away*)

Sacrotuberous ligament

Perforating cutaneous nerve

Inferior anal (rectal) nerves

Anococcygeal nerves

Ischial tuberosity

Ischial spine

**Block anesthesia of pudendal and other nerves of perineal area**

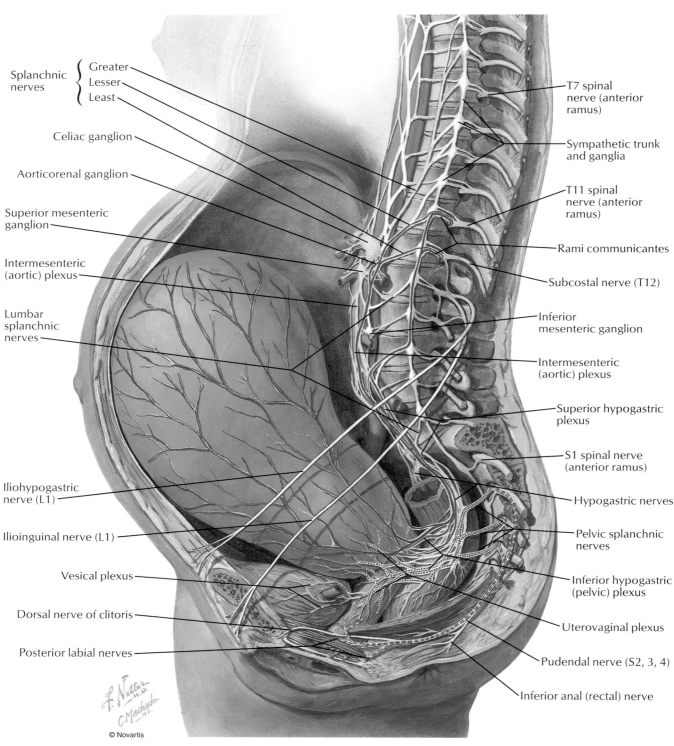

Splanchnic nerves { Greater / Lesser / Least }

Celiac ganglion

Aorticorenal ganglion

Superior mesenteric ganglion

Intermesenteric (aortic) plexus

Lumbar splanchnic nerves

Iliohypogastric nerve (L1)

Ilioinguinal nerve (L1)

Vesical plexus

Dorsal nerve of clitoris

Posterior labial nerves

T7 spinal nerve (anterior ramus)

Sympathetic trunk and ganglia

T11 spinal nerve (anterior ramus)

Rami communicantes

Subcostal nerve (T12)

Inferior mesenteric ganglion

Intermesenteric (aortic) plexus

Superior hypogastric plexus

S1 spinal nerve (anterior ramus)

Hypogastric nerves

Pelvic splanchnic nerves

Inferior hypogastric (pelvic) plexus

Uterovaginal plexus

Pudendal nerve (S2, 3, 4)

Inferior anal (rectal) nerve

© Novartis

—— Sensory fibers from uterine body and fundus accompany sympathetic fibers via hypogastric plexuses to T11, 12 (L1?)

—— Motor fibers to uterine body and fundus (sympathetic)

········· Sensory fibers from cervix and upper vagina accompany pelvic splanchnic nerves (parasympathetic) to S2, 3, 4

··········· Motor fibers to lower uterine segment, cervix and upper vagina (parasympathetic)

‑ ‑ ‑ Sensory fibers from lower vagina and perineum accompany somatic fibers via pudendal nerve to S2, 3, 4

‑ ‑ ‑ ‑ Motor fibers to lower vagina and perineum via pudendal nerve (somatic)

**PLATE 385**

**PELVIS AND PERINEUM**

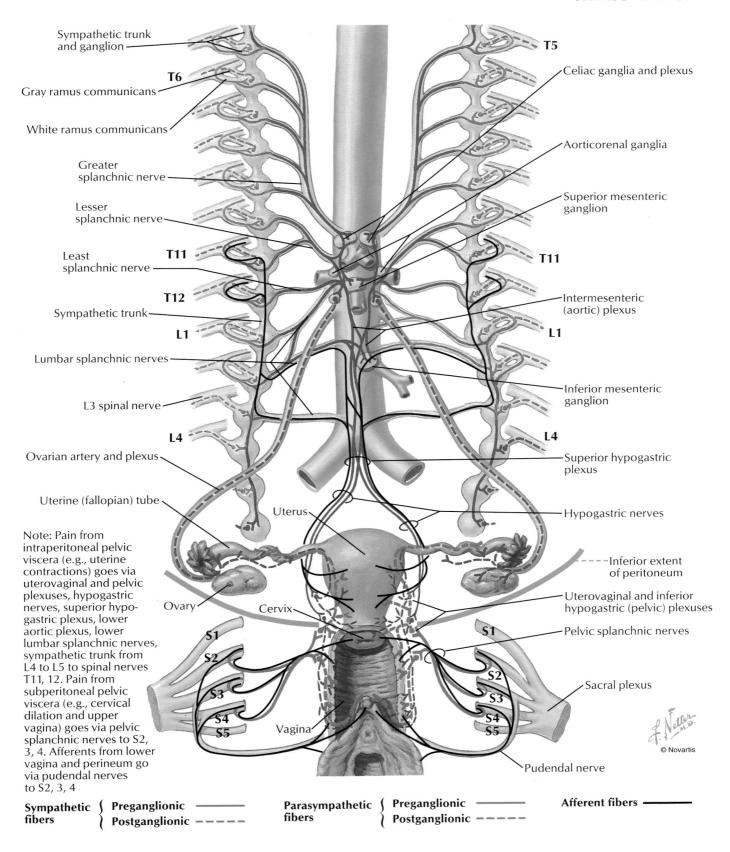

Sympathetic trunk and ganglion

T6

Gray ramus communicans

White ramus communicans

Greater splanchnic nerve

Lesser splanchnic nerve

T11

Least splanchnic nerve

T12

Sympathetic trunk

L1

Lumbar splanchnic nerves

L3 spinal nerve

L4

Ovarian artery and plexus

Uterine (fallopian) tube

Note: Pain from intraperitoneal pelvic viscera (e.g., uterine contractions) goes via uterovaginal and pelvic plexuses, hypogastric nerves, superior hypogastric plexus, lower aortic plexus, lower lumbar splanchnic nerves, sympathetic trunk from L4 to L5 to spinal nerves T11, 12. Pain from subperitoneal pelvic viscera (e.g., cervical dilation and upper vagina) goes via pelvic splanchnic nerves to S2, 3, 4. Afferents from lower vagina and perineum go via pudendal nerves to S2, 3, 4

T5

Celiac ganglia and plexus

Aorticorenal ganglia

Superior mesenteric ganglion

T11

Intermesenteric (aortic) plexus

L1

Inferior mesenteric ganglion

L4

Superior hypogastric plexus

Hypogastric nerves

Uterus

Ovary

Cervix

S1

S2

S3

S4

S5

Vagina

Inferior extent of peritoneum

Uterovaginal and inferior hypogastric (pelvic) plexuses

Pelvic splanchnic nerves

S1

S2

S3

S4

S5

Sacral plexus

Pudendal nerve

**Sympathetic fibers** { Preganglionic ———  Postganglionic - - - - -

**Parasympathetic fibers** { Preganglionic ———  Postganglionic - - - - -

**Afferent fibers** ———

© Novartis

# Innervation of Male Reproductive Organs: Schema

SEE ALSO PLATE 153

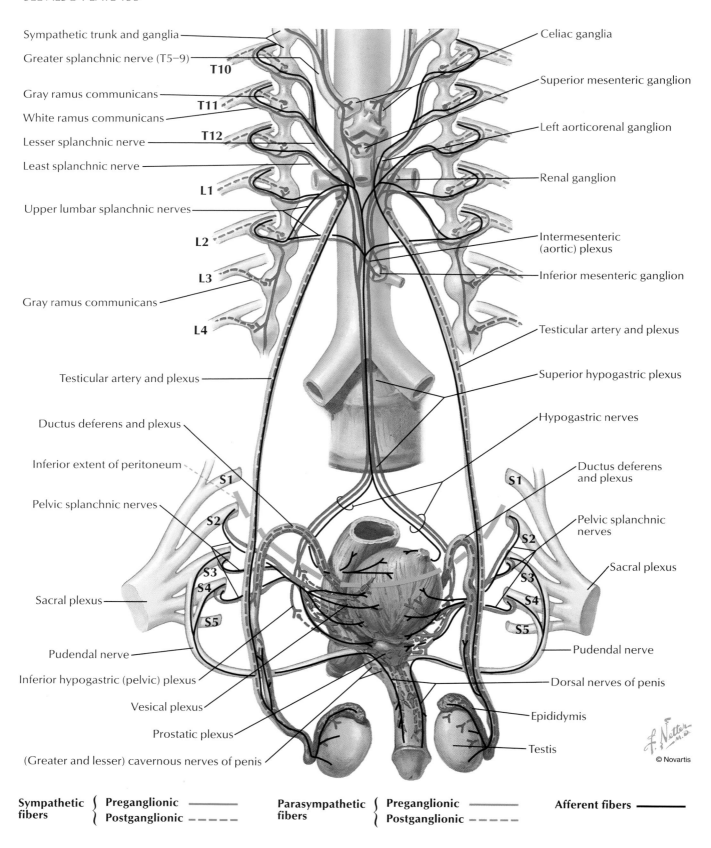

Sympathetic trunk and ganglia

Greater splanchnic nerve (T5–9)    **T10**

Gray ramus communicans

White ramus communicans    **T11**

Lesser splanchnic nerve    **T12**

Least splanchnic nerve

**L1**

Upper lumbar splanchnic nerves

**L2**

**L3**

Gray ramus communicans

**L4**

Testicular artery and plexus

Ductus deferens and plexus

Inferior extent of peritoneum    **S1**

Pelvic splanchnic nerves    **S2**

**S3**
**S4**

Sacral plexus    **S5**

Pudendal nerve

Inferior hypogastric (pelvic) plexus

Vesical plexus

Prostatic plexus

(Greater and lesser) cavernous nerves of penis

Celiac ganglia

Superior mesenteric ganglion

Left aorticorenal ganglion

Renal ganglion

Intermesenteric (aortic) plexus

Inferior mesenteric ganglion

Testicular artery and plexus

Superior hypogastric plexus

Hypogastric nerves

Ductus deferens and plexus    **S1**

Pelvic splanchnic nerves    **S2**

Sacral plexus    **S3**
**S4**

Pudendal nerve    **S5**

Dorsal nerves of penis

Epididymis

Testis

© Novartis

| Sympathetic fibers | Preganglionic ———  Postganglionic – – – – | Parasympathetic fibers | Preganglionic ———  Postganglionic – – – – | Afferent fibers ——— |

**PLATE 387**    **PELVIS AND PERINEUM**

SEE ALSO PLATE 153

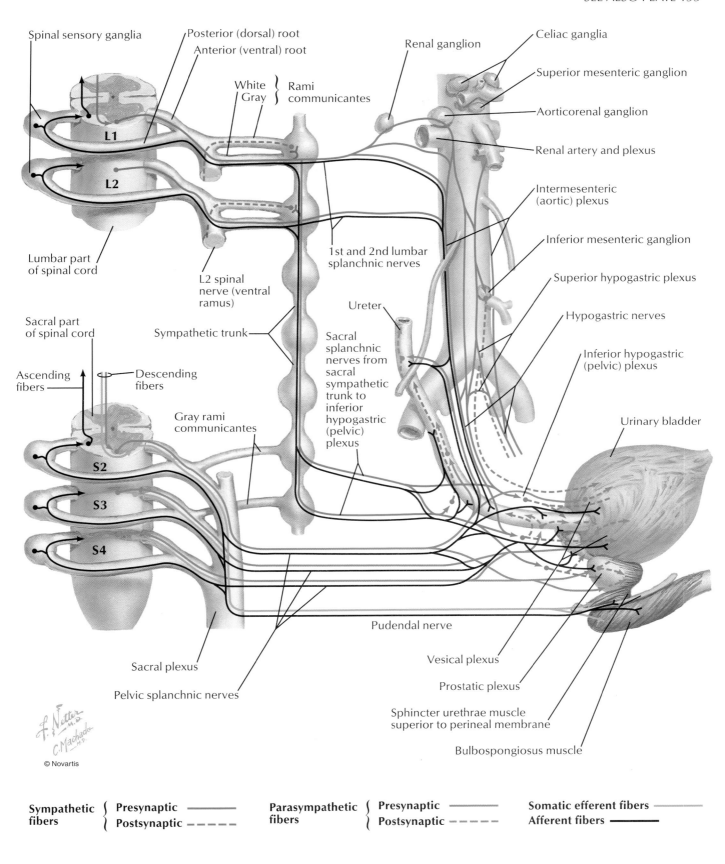

Spinal sensory ganglia

Posterior (dorsal) root
Anterior (ventral) root

Renal ganglion

Celiac ganglia

Superior mesenteric ganglion

White
Gray } Rami communicantes

Aorticorenal ganglion

L1

Renal artery and plexus

L2

Intermesenteric (aortic) plexus

Lumbar part of spinal cord

1st and 2nd lumbar splanchnic nerves

Inferior mesenteric ganglion

L2 spinal nerve (ventral ramus)

Superior hypogastric plexus

Ureter

Hypogastric nerves

Sympathetic trunk

Inferior hypogastric (pelvic) plexus

Sacral part of spinal cord

Sacral splanchnic nerves from sacral sympathetic trunk to inferior hypogastric (pelvic) plexus

Ascending fibers

Descending fibers

Gray rami communicantes

Urinary bladder

S2

S3

S4

Sacral plexus

Pudendal nerve

Pelvic splanchnic nerves

Vesical plexus

Prostatic plexus

Sphincter urethrae muscle superior to perineal membrane

Bulbospongiosus muscle

f. Netter
C. Machado

© Novartis

| Sympathetic fibers | Presynaptic ——— | Parasympathetic fibers | Presynaptic ——— | Somatic efferent fibers ——— |
| | Postsynaptic - - - - | | Postsynaptic - - - - | Afferent fibers ——— |

# Homologues of External Genitalia

**Undifferentiated**

Glans area
Epithelial tag
Urogenital fold
Urogenital groove
Lateral buttress
Anal tubercle
Anal pit

Genital tubercle

**Male**

45–50 mm
(~10 weeks)

**Female**

45–50 mm
(~10 weeks)

Glans
Epithelial tag
Coronal sulcus
Site of future origin of prepuce
Urethral fold
Urogenital groove
Lateral buttress
(corpus, or shaft)
Labioscrotal swelling
Urethral folds partly
fused (urethral raphé)
Anal tubercle
Anus

External urethral orifice
Glans penis
Prepuce
Body (shaft)
of penis
Raphé
of penis
Scrotum

**Fully developed**

**Fully developed**

Body of
clitoris
Prepuce
Glans of
clitoris
External
urethral
orifice
Labium
minus
Labium
majus
Vaginal
orifice
Posterior
commissure

Perineal raphé
Perianal tissues
(including external
anal sphincter
muscle)

© Novartis

*PLATE 389*

**PELVIS AND PERINEUM**

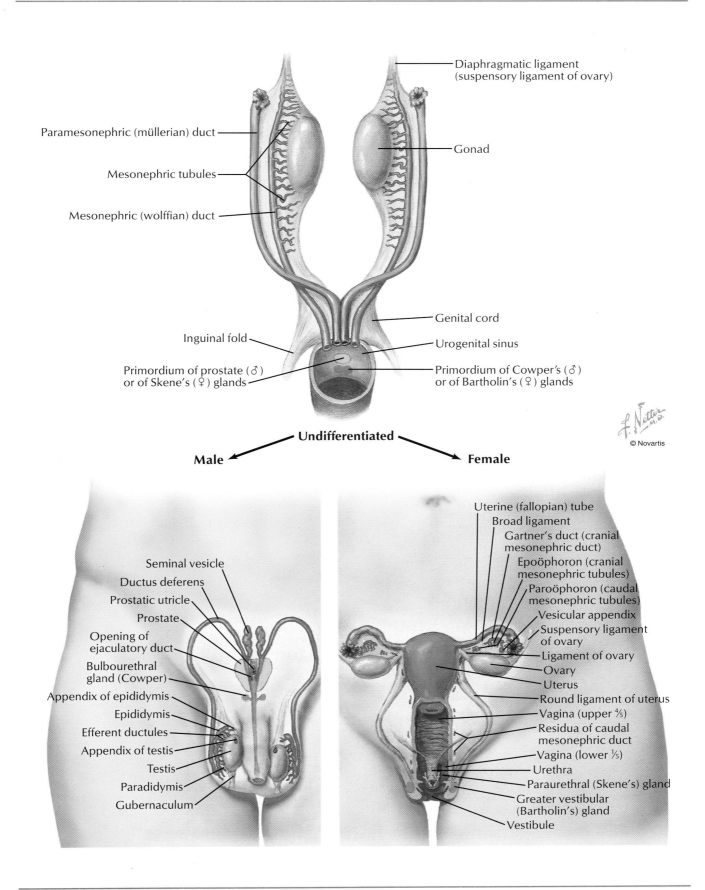

Diaphragmatic ligament (suspensory ligament of ovary)

Paramesonephric (müllerian) duct

Mesonephric tubules

Mesonephric (wolffian) duct

Gonad

Genital cord

Inguinal fold

Urogenital sinus

Primordium of prostate (♂) or of Skene's (♀) glands

Primordium of Cowper's (♂) or of Bartholin's (♀) glands

© Novartis

**Undifferentiated**

**Male**

**Female**

Seminal vesicle

Ductus deferens

Prostatic utricle

Prostate

Opening of ejaculatory duct

Bulbourethral gland (Cowper)

Appendix of epididymis

Epididymis

Efferent ductules

Appendix of testis

Testis

Paradidymis

Gubernaculum

Uterine (fallopian) tube

Broad ligament

Gartner's duct (cranial mesonephric duct)

Epoöphoron (cranial mesonephric tubules)

Paroöphoron (caudal mesonephric tubules)

Vesicular appendix

Suspensory ligament of ovary

Ligament of ovary

Ovary

Uterus

Round ligament of uterus

Vagina (upper ⅘)

Residua of caudal mesonephric duct

Vagina (lower ⅕)

Urethra

Paraurethral (Skene's) gland

Greater vestibular (Bartholin's) gland

Vestibule

# Section VI
# UPPER LIMB

**SHOULDER AND AXILLA**
*Plates 391 – 401*

391. Clavicle and Sternoclavicular Joint
392. Humerus and Scapula: Anterior Views
393. Humerus and Scapula:
     Posterior Views
394. Shoulder (Glenohumeral) Joint
395. Muscles of Shoulder
396. Muscles of Rotator Cuff
397. Scapulohumeral Dissection
398. Axillary Artery and
     Anastomoses Around Scapula
399. Pectoral, Clavipectoral
     and Axillary Fasciae
400. Axilla (Dissection):
     Anterior View
401. Brachial Plexus: Schema

**ARM**
*Plates 402 – 406*

402. Muscles of Arm: Anterior Views

403. Muscles of Arm: Posterior Views
404. Brachial Artery In Situ
405. Brachial Artery and Anastomoses
     Around Elbow
406. Arm: Serial Cross Sections

**ELBOW AND FOREARM**
*Plates 407 – 421*

407. Bones of Elbow
408. Ligaments of Elbow
409. Bones of Forearm
410. Individual Muscles of Forearm:
     Rotators of Radius
411. Individual Muscles of Forearm:
     Extensors of Wrist and Digits
412. Individual Muscles of Forearm:
     Flexors of Wrist
413. Individual Muscles of Forearm:
     Flexors of Digits
414. Muscles of Forearm (Superficial
     Layer): Posterior View

415. Muscles of Forearm (Deep Layer): Posterior View
416. Muscles of Forearm (Superficial Layer): Anterior View
417. Muscles of Forearm (Intermediate Layer): Anterior View
418. Muscles of Forearm (Deep Layer): Anterior View
419. Forearm: Serial Cross Sections
420. Attachments of Muscles of Forearm: Anterior View
421 Attachments of Muscles of Forearm: Posterior View

**WRIST AND HAND**
*Plates 422 – 440*

422. Carpal Bones
423. Movements of Wrist
424. Ligaments of Wrist
425. Ligaments of Wrist (*continued*)
426. Bones of Wrist and Hand
427. Metacarpophalangeal and Interphalangeal Ligaments
428. Wrist and Hand: Superficial Palmar Dissections
429. Wrist and Hand: Deeper Palmar Dissections
430. Flexor Tendons, Arteries and Nerves at Wrist
431. Bursae, Spaces and Tendon Sheaths of Hand
432. Lumbrical Muscles and Bursae, Spaces and Sheaths: Schema

433. Flexor and Extensor Tendons in Fingers
434. Intrinsic Muscles of Hand
435. Arteries and Nerves of Hand: Palmar Views
436. Wrist and Hand: Superficial Radial Dissection
437. Wrist and Hand: Superficial Dorsal Dissection
438. Wrist and Hand: Deep Dorsal Dissection
439. Extensor Tendons at Wrist
440. Fingers

**NEUROVASCULATURE**
*Plates 441 – 452*

441. Cutaneous Innervation of Wrist and Hand
442. Arteries and Nerves of Upper Limb
443. Musculocutaneous Nerve
444. Median Nerve
445. Ulnar Nerve
446. Radial Nerve in Arm and Nerves of Posterior Shoulder
447. Radial Nerve in Forearm
448. Cutaneous Nerves and Superficial Veins of Shoulder and Arm
449. Cutaneous Nerves and Superficial Veins of Forearm
450. Cutaneous Innervation of Upper Limb
451. Dermatomes of Upper Limb
452. Lymph Vessels and Nodes of Upper Limb

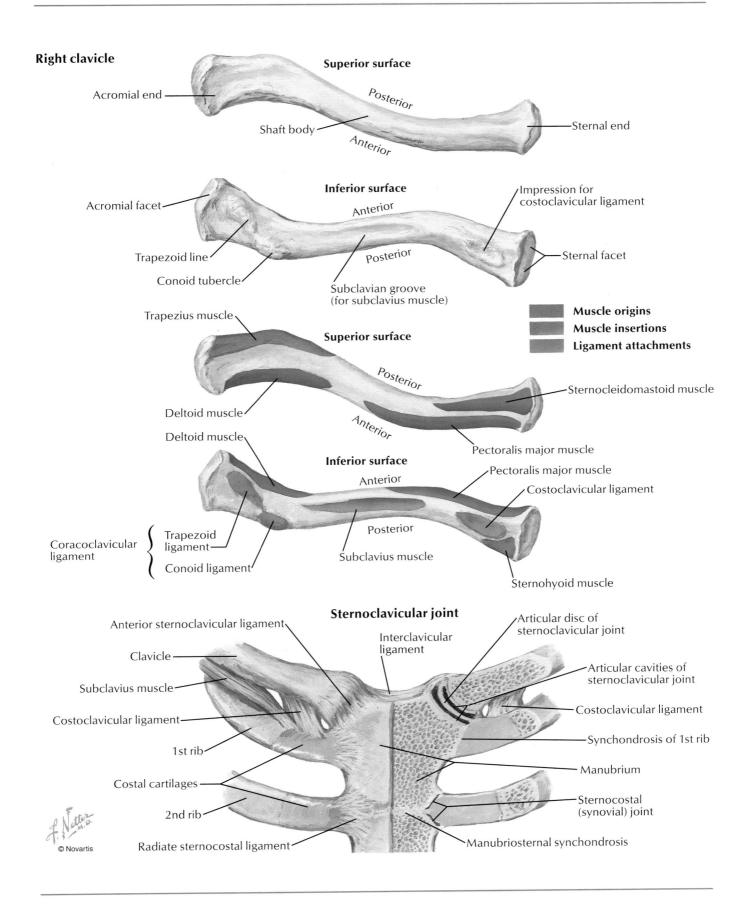

**Right clavicle**

**Superior surface**

Acromial end

Posterior

Shaft body

Anterior

Sternal end

**Inferior surface**

Acromial facet

Anterior

Impression for costoclavicular ligament

Trapezoid line

Posterior

Conoid tubercle

Sternal facet

Subclavian groove (for subclavius muscle)

Trapezius muscle

**Superior surface**

Posterior

Deltoid muscle

Anterior

Sternocleidomastoid muscle

Deltoid muscle

Pectoralis major muscle

**Inferior surface**

Anterior

Pectoralis major muscle

Costoclavicular ligament

Coracoclavicular ligament

Trapezoid ligament

Posterior

Conoid ligament

Subclavius muscle

Sternohyoid muscle

Muscle origins
Muscle insertions
Ligament attachments

**Sternoclavicular joint**

Anterior sternoclavicular ligament

Interclavicular ligament

Articular disc of sternoclavicular joint

Clavicle

Articular cavities of sternoclavicular joint

Subclavius muscle

Costoclavicular ligament

Costoclavicular ligament

Synchondrosis of 1st rib

1st rib

Manubrium

Costal cartilages

Sternocostal (synovial) joint

2nd rib

Radiate sternocostal ligament

Manubriosternal synchondrosis

F. Netter M.D.
© Novartis

# Humerus and Scapula: Anterior Views

SEE ALSO PLATE 170

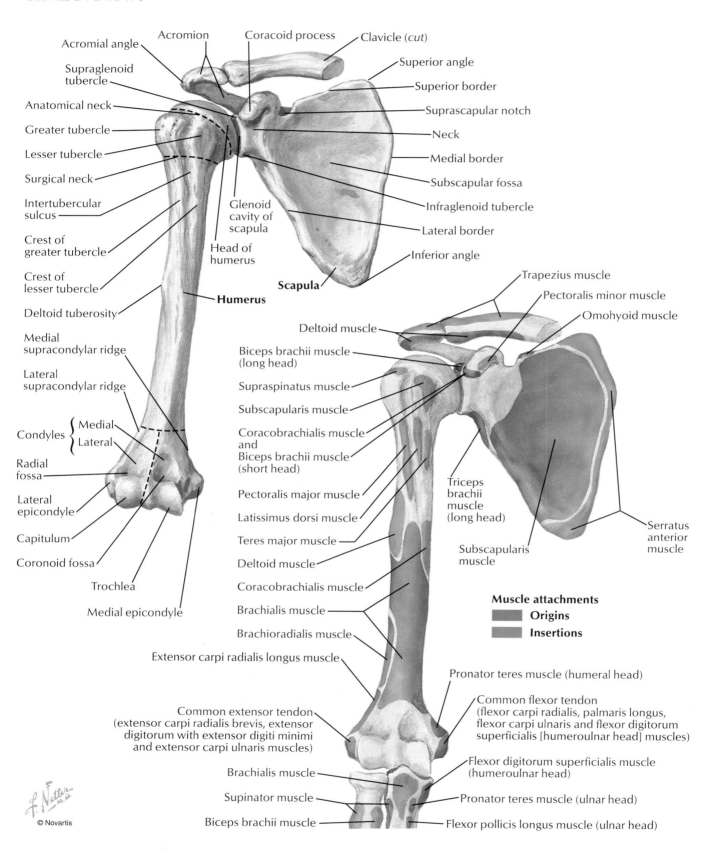

Acromial angle
Acromion
Coracoid process
Clavicle (cut)
Supraglenoid tubercle
Anatomical neck
Greater tubercle
Lesser tubercle
Surgical neck
Intertubercular sulcus
Crest of greater tubercle
Crest of lesser tubercle
Deltoid tuberosity
Medial supracondylar ridge
Lateral supracondylar ridge
Condyles { Medial / Lateral }
Radial fossa
Lateral epicondyle
Capitulum
Coronoid fossa
Trochlea
Medial epicondyle

Superior angle
Superior border
Suprascapular notch
Neck
Medial border
Subscapular fossa
Infraglenoid tubercle
Lateral border
Inferior angle
Glenoid cavity of scapula
Head of humerus
**Scapula**
**Humerus**

Trapezius muscle
Pectoralis minor muscle
Omohyoid muscle
Deltoid muscle
Biceps brachii muscle (long head)
Supraspinatus muscle
Subscapularis muscle
Coracobrachialis muscle and Biceps brachii muscle (short head)
Pectoralis major muscle
Latissimus dorsi muscle
Teres major muscle
Deltoid muscle
Coracobrachialis muscle
Brachialis muscle
Brachioradialis muscle
Extensor carpi radialis longus muscle
Triceps brachii muscle (long head)
Subscapularis muscle
Serratus anterior muscle

**Muscle attachments**
■ **Origins**
■ **Insertions**

Common extensor tendon (extensor carpi radialis brevis, extensor digitorum with extensor digiti minimi and extensor carpi ulnaris muscles)
Brachialis muscle
Supinator muscle
Biceps brachii muscle

Pronator teres muscle (humeral head)
Common flexor tendon (flexor carpi radialis, palmaris longus, flexor carpi ulnaris and flexor digitorum superficialis [humeroulnar head] muscles)
Flexor digitorum superficialis muscle (humeroulnar head)
Pronator teres muscle (ulnar head)
Flexor pollicis longus muscle (ulnar head)

f. Netter
© Novartis

**PLATE 392**

**UPPER LIMB**

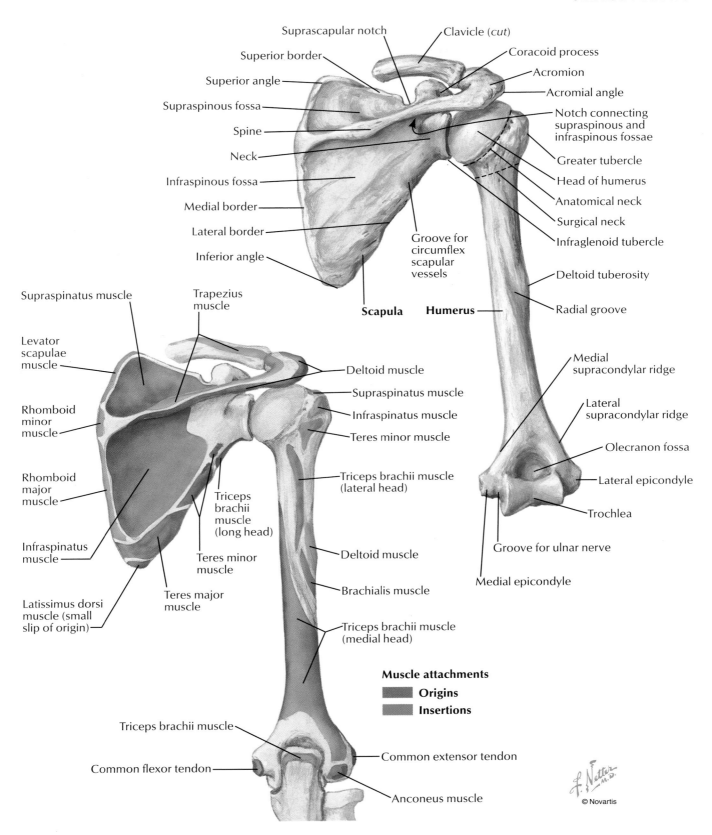

Suprascapular notch

Clavicle (*cut*)

Superior border

Coracoid process

Acromion

Superior angle

Acromial angle

Supraspinous fossa

Notch connecting supraspinous and infraspinous fossae

Spine

Greater tubercle

Neck

Head of humerus

Infraspinous fossa

Anatomical neck

Medial border

Surgical neck

Lateral border

Infraglenoid tubercle

Inferior angle

Groove for circumflex scapular vessels

Deltoid tuberosity

**Scapula**     **Humerus**

Radial groove

Supraspinatus muscle

Trapezius muscle

Medial supracondylar ridge

Levator scapulae muscle

Deltoid muscle

Lateral supracondylar ridge

Supraspinatus muscle

Rhomboid minor muscle

Infraspinatus muscle

Olecranon fossa

Teres minor muscle

Lateral epicondyle

Rhomboid major muscle

Triceps brachii muscle (lateral head)

Trochlea

Triceps brachii muscle (long head)

Infraspinatus muscle

Teres minor muscle

Deltoid muscle

Groove for ulnar nerve

Latissimus dorsi muscle (small slip of origin)

Teres major muscle

Medial epicondyle

Brachialis muscle

Triceps brachii muscle (medial head)

**Muscle attachments**

**Origins**

**Insertions**

Triceps brachii muscle

Common extensor tendon

Common flexor tendon

Anconeus muscle

© Novartis

# Shoulder (Glenohumeral) Joint

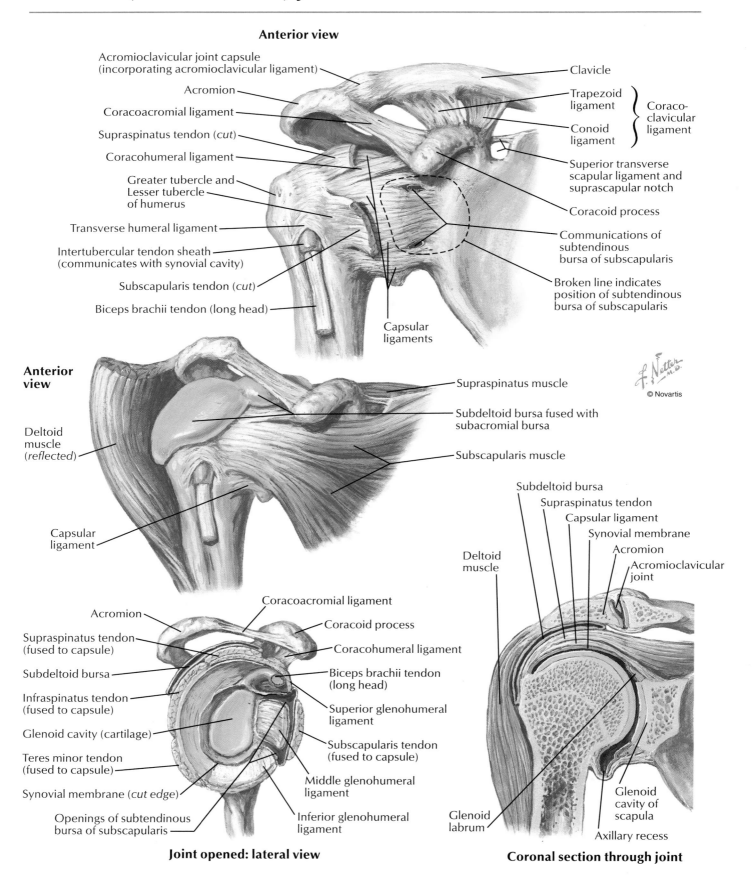

**Anterior view**

Acromioclavicular joint capsule (incorporating acromioclavicular ligament)

Acromion

Coracoacromial ligament

Supraspinatus tendon (*cut*)

Coracohumeral ligament

Greater tubercle and Lesser tubercle of humerus

Transverse humeral ligament

Intertubercular tendon sheath (communicates with synovial cavity)

Subscapularis tendon (*cut*)

Biceps brachii tendon (long head)

Clavicle

Trapezoid ligament

Conoid ligament

} Coraco-clavicular ligament

Superior transverse scapular ligament and suprascapular notch

Coracoid process

Communications of subtendinous bursa of subscapularis

Broken line indicates position of subtendinous bursa of subscapularis

Capsular ligaments

**Anterior view**

Deltoid muscle (*reflected*)

Capsular ligament

Supraspinatus muscle

Subdeltoid bursa fused with subacromial bursa

Subscapularis muscle

Deltoid muscle

Subdeltoid bursa

Supraspinatus tendon

Capsular ligament

Synovial membrane

Acromion

Acromioclavicular joint

Glenoid labrum

Glenoid cavity of scapula

Axillary recess

Acromion

Supraspinatus tendon (fused to capsule)

Subdeltoid bursa

Infraspinatus tendon (fused to capsule)

Glenoid cavity (cartilage)

Teres minor tendon (fused to capsule)

Synovial membrane (*cut edge*)

Openings of subtendinous bursa of subscapularis

Coracoacromial ligament

Coracoid process

Coracohumeral ligament

Biceps brachii tendon (long head)

Superior glenohumeral ligament

Subscapularis tendon (fused to capsule)

Middle glenohumeral ligament

Inferior glenohumeral ligament

**Joint opened: lateral view**

**Coronal section through joint**

**PLATE 394**

**UPPER LIMB**

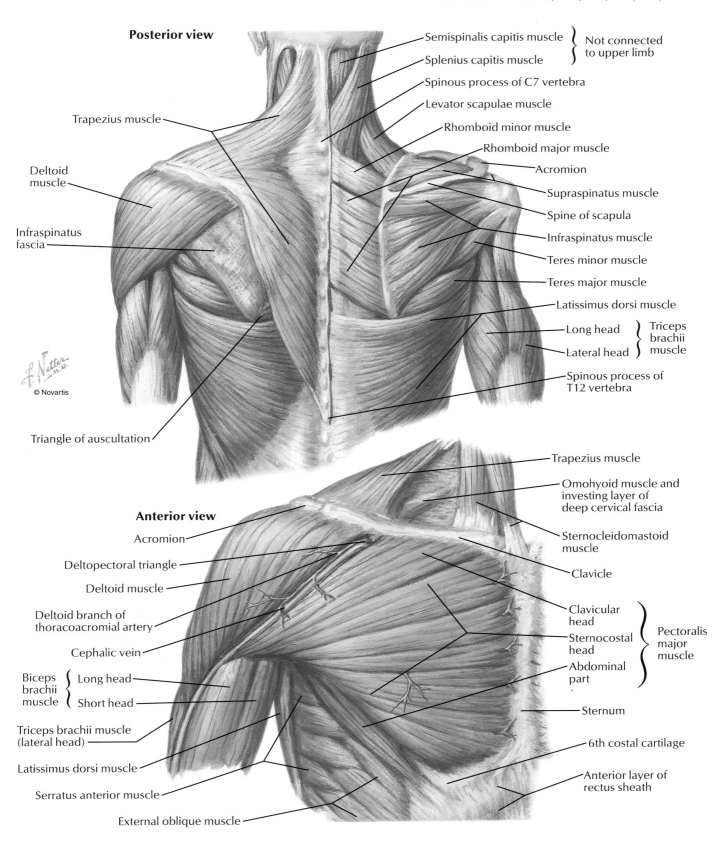

**Posterior view**

Semispinalis capitis muscle ⎫ Not connected
Splenius capitis muscle ⎭ to upper limb

Spinous process of C7 vertebra

Levator scapulae muscle

Rhomboid minor muscle

Rhomboid major muscle

Acromion

Supraspinatus muscle

Spine of scapula

Infraspinatus muscle

Teres minor muscle

Teres major muscle

Latissimus dorsi muscle

Long head ⎫ Triceps
Lateral head ⎭ brachii muscle

Spinous process of T12 vertebra

Trapezius muscle

Deltoid muscle

Infraspinatus fascia

Triangle of auscultation

Trapezius muscle

Omohyoid muscle and investing layer of deep cervical fascia

Sternocleidomastoid muscle

Clavicle

Clavicular head ⎫
Sternocostal head ⎬ Pectoralis major muscle
Abdominal part ⎭

Sternum

6th costal cartilage

Anterior layer of rectus sheath

**Anterior view**

Acromion

Deltopectoral triangle

Deltoid muscle

Deltoid branch of thoracoacromial artery

Cephalic vein

Biceps brachii muscle ⎰ Long head
⎱ Short head

Triceps brachii muscle (lateral head)

Latissimus dorsi muscle

Serratus anterior muscle

External oblique muscle

# Muscles of Rotator Cuff

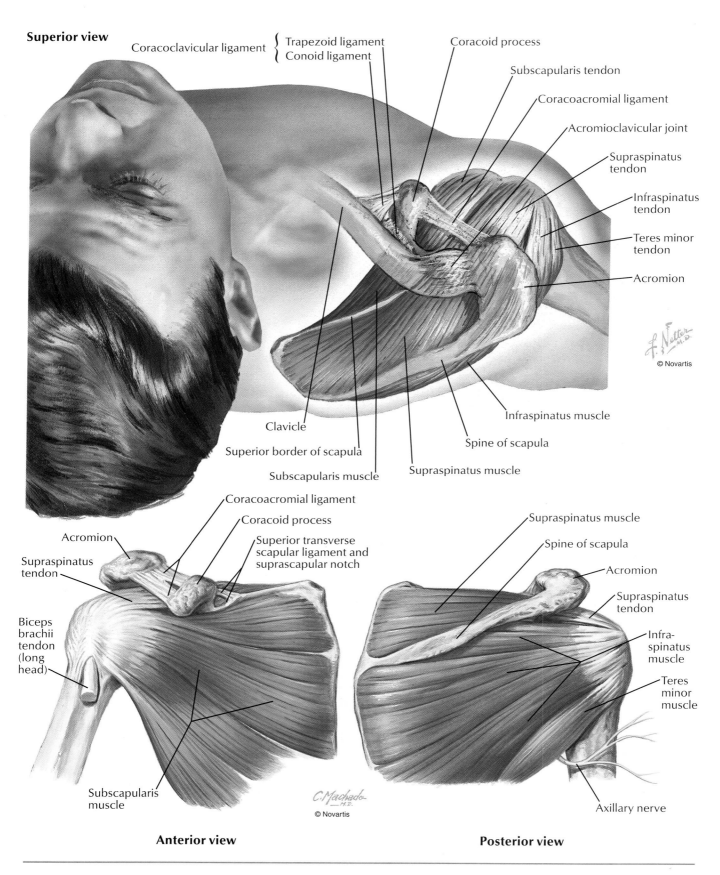

**Superior view**

Coracoclavicular ligament { Trapezoid ligament / Conoid ligament

Coracoid process

Subscapularis tendon

Coracoacromial ligament

Acromioclavicular joint

Supraspinatus tendon

Infraspinatus tendon

Teres minor tendon

Acromion

Infraspinatus muscle

Spine of scapula

Supraspinatus muscle

Subscapularis muscle

Superior border of scapula

Clavicle

Coracoacromial ligament

Coracoid process

Acromion

Superior transverse scapular ligament and suprascapular notch

Supraspinatus tendon

Biceps brachii tendon (long head)

Subscapularis muscle

**Anterior view**

Supraspinatus muscle

Spine of scapula

Acromion

Supraspinatus tendon

Infra-spinatus muscle

Teres minor muscle

Axillary nerve

**Posterior view**

**PLATE 396**

**UPPER LIMB**

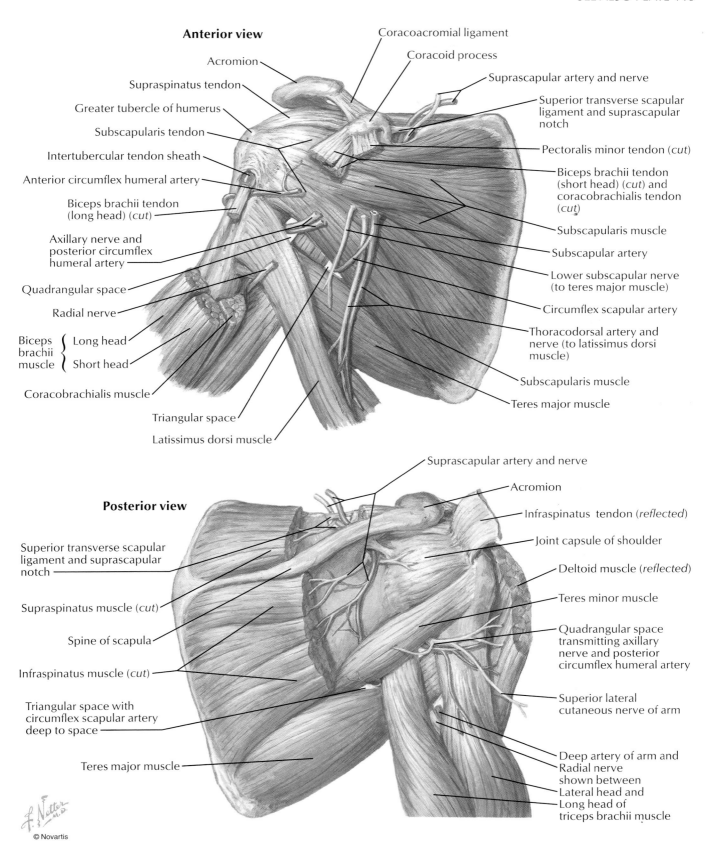

**Anterior view**

Acromion

Supraspinatus tendon

Greater tubercle of humerus

Subscapularis tendon

Intertubercular tendon sheath

Anterior circumflex humeral artery

Biceps brachii tendon (long head) (*cut*)

Axillary nerve and posterior circumflex humeral artery

Quadrangular space

Radial nerve

Biceps brachii muscle { Long head / Short head

Coracobrachialis muscle

Triangular space

Latissimus dorsi muscle

Coracoacromial ligament

Coracoid process

Suprascapular artery and nerve

Superior transverse scapular ligament and suprascapular notch

Pectoralis minor tendon (*cut*)

Biceps brachii tendon (short head) (*cut*) and coracobrachialis tendon (*cut*)

Subscapularis muscle

Subscapular artery

Lower subscapular nerve (to teres major muscle)

Circumflex scapular artery

Thoracodorsal artery and nerve (to latissimus dorsi muscle)

Subscapularis muscle

Teres major muscle

**Posterior view**

Superior transverse scapular ligament and suprascapular notch

Supraspinatus muscle (*cut*)

Spine of scapula

Infraspinatus muscle (*cut*)

Triangular space with circumflex scapular artery deep to space

Teres major muscle

Suprascapular artery and nerve

Acromion

Infraspinatus tendon (*reflected*)

Joint capsule of shoulder

Deltoid muscle (*reflected*)

Teres minor muscle

Quadrangular space transmitting axillary nerve and posterior circumflex humeral artery

Superior lateral cutaneous nerve of arm

Deep artery of arm and Radial nerve shown between Lateral head and Long head of triceps brachii muscle

© Novartis

# Axillary Artery and Anastomoses Around Scapula

SEE ALSO PLATES 28, 405

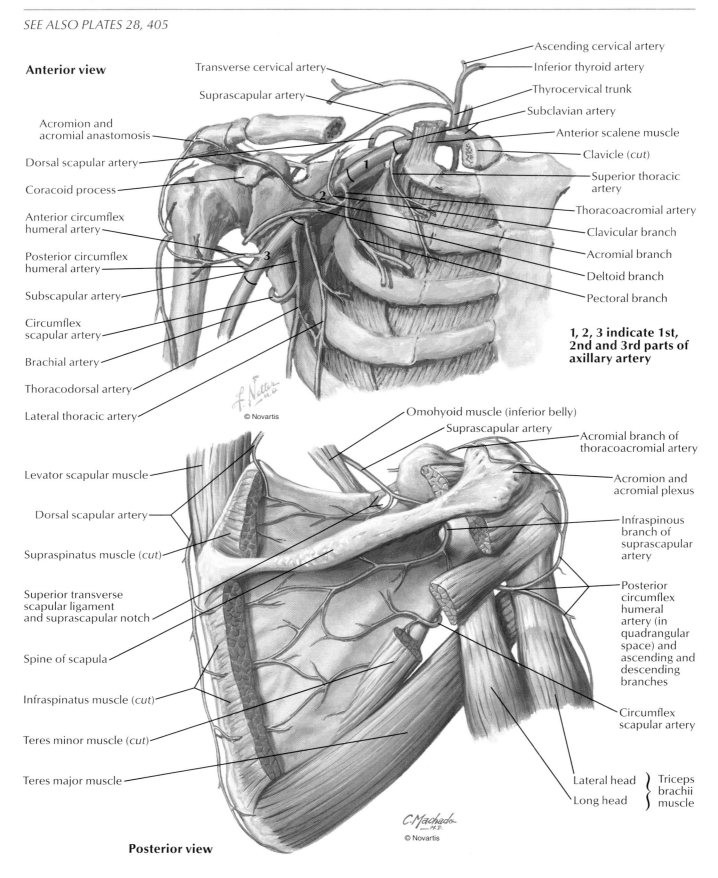

**Anterior view**

Transverse cervical artery

Suprascapular artery

Ascending cervical artery

Inferior thyroid artery

Thyrocervical trunk

Subclavian artery

Anterior scalene muscle

Clavicle (*cut*)

Superior thoracic artery

Thoracoacromial artery

Clavicular branch

Acromial branch

Deltoid branch

Pectoral branch

Acromion and acromial anastomosis

Dorsal scapular artery

Coracoid process

Anterior circumflex humeral artery

Posterior circumflex humeral artery

Subscapular artery

Circumflex scapular artery

Brachial artery

Thoracodorsal artery

Lateral thoracic artery

**1, 2, 3 indicate 1st, 2nd and 3rd parts of axillary artery**

Omohyoid muscle (inferior belly)

Suprascapular artery

Acromial branch of thoracoacromial artery

Acromion and acromial plexus

Infraspinous branch of suprascapular artery

Posterior circumflex humeral artery (in quadrangular space) and ascending and descending branches

Circumflex scapular artery

Levator scapular muscle

Dorsal scapular artery

Supraspinatus muscle (*cut*)

Superior transverse scapular ligament and suprascapular notch

Spine of scapula

Infraspinatus muscle (*cut*)

Teres minor muscle (*cut*)

Teres major muscle

Lateral head

Long head

} Triceps brachii muscle

**Posterior view**

**PLATE 398**

**UPPER LIMB**

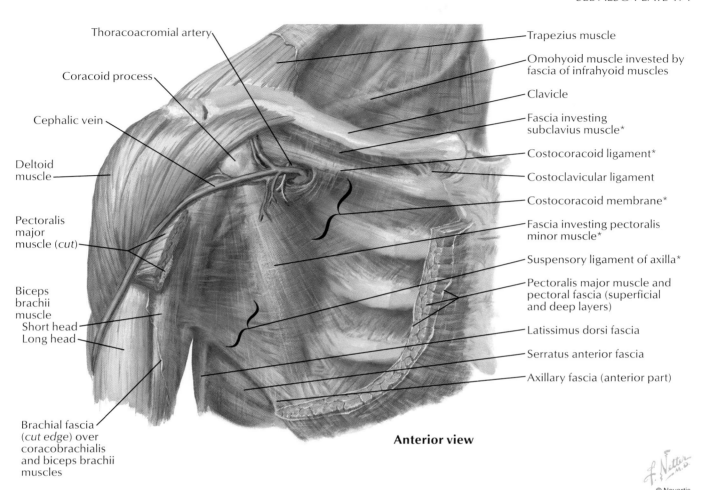

Thoracoacromial artery

Coracoid process

Cephalic vein

Deltoid muscle

Pectoralis major muscle (*cut*)

Biceps brachii muscle
Short head
Long head

Brachial fascia (*cut edge*) over coracobrachialis and biceps brachii muscles

Trapezius muscle

Omohyoid muscle invested by fascia of infrahyoid muscles

Clavicle

Fascia investing subclavius muscle*

Costocoracoid ligament*

Costoclavicular ligament

Costocoracoid membrane*

Fascia investing pectoralis minor muscle*

Suspensory ligament of axilla*

Pectoralis major muscle and pectoral fascia (superficial and deep layers)

Latissimus dorsi fascia

Serratus anterior fascia

Axillary fascia (anterior part)

**Anterior view**

© Novartis

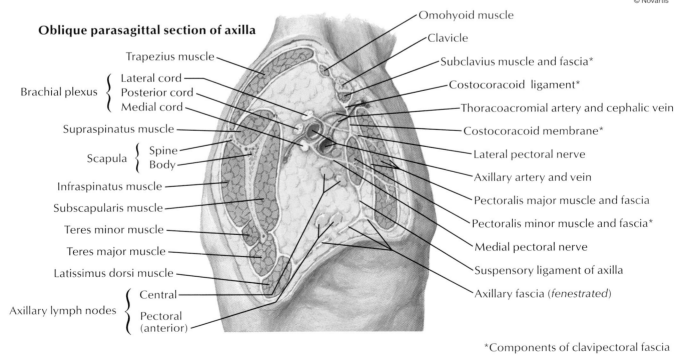

**Oblique parasagittal section of axilla**

Trapezius muscle

Brachial plexus {
Lateral cord
Posterior cord
Medial cord

Supraspinatus muscle

Scapula { Spine
Body

Infraspinatus muscle

Subscapularis muscle

Teres minor muscle

Teres major muscle

Latissimus dorsi muscle

Axillary lymph nodes { Central
Pectoral (anterior)

Omohyoid muscle

Clavicle

Subclavius muscle and fascia*

Costocoracoid ligament*

Thoracoacromial artery and cephalic vein

Costocoracoid membrane*

Lateral pectoral nerve

Axillary artery and vein

Pectoralis major muscle and fascia

Pectoralis minor muscle and fascia*

Medial pectoral nerve

Suspensory ligament of axilla

Axillary fascia (*fenestrated*)

*Components of clavipectoral fascia

# Axilla (Dissection): Anterior View

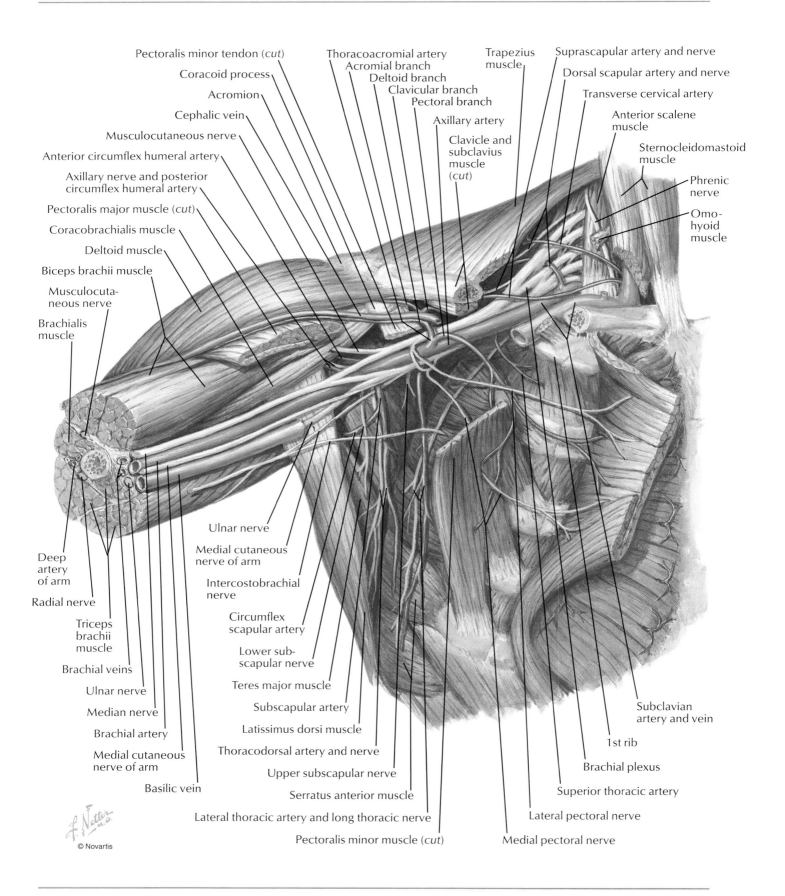

Pectoralis minor tendon (*cut*)
Coracoid process
Acromion
Cephalic vein
Musculocutaneous nerve
Anterior circumflex humeral artery
Axillary nerve and posterior circumflex humeral artery
Pectoralis major muscle (*cut*)
Coracobrachialis muscle
Deltoid muscle
Biceps brachii muscle
Musculocuta-neous nerve
Brachialis muscle

Thoracoacromial artery
Acromial branch
Deltoid branch
Clavicular branch
Pectoral branch
Axillary artery
Clavicle and subclavius muscle (*cut*)

Trapezius muscle

Suprascapular artery and nerve
Dorsal scapular artery and nerve
Transverse cervical artery
Anterior scalene muscle
Sternocleidomastoid muscle
Phrenic nerve
Omo-hyoid muscle

Deep artery of arm
Radial nerve
Triceps brachii muscle
Brachial veins
Ulnar nerve
Median nerve
Brachial artery
Medial cutaneous nerve of arm
Basilic vein

Ulnar nerve
Medial cutaneous nerve of arm
Intercostobrachial nerve
Circumflex scapular artery
Lower sub-scapular nerve
Teres major muscle
Subscapular artery
Latissimus dorsi muscle
Thoracodorsal artery and nerve
Upper subscapular nerve
Serratus anterior muscle
Lateral thoracic artery and long thoracic nerve
Pectoralis minor muscle (*cut*)

Subclavian artery and vein
1st rib
Brachial plexus
Superior thoracic artery
Lateral pectoral nerve
Medial pectoral nerve

f. Netter
© Novartis

**PLATE 400**

**UPPER LIMB**

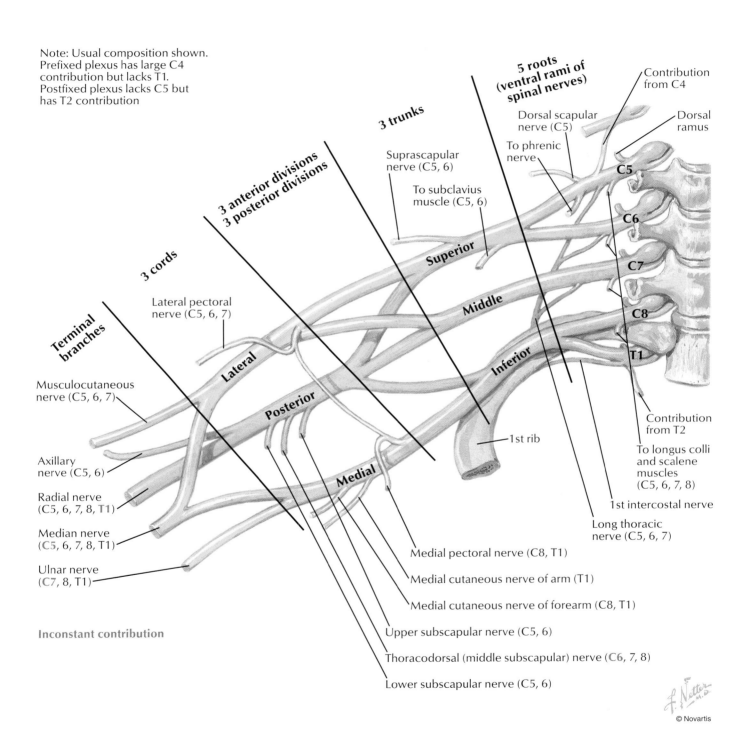

Note: Usual composition shown.
Prefixed plexus has large C4
contribution but lacks T1.
Postfixed plexus lacks C5 but
has T2 contribution

5 roots
(ventral rami of
spinal nerves)

3 trunks

3 anterior divisions
3 posterior divisions

3 cords

Terminal
branches

Contribution
from C4

Dorsal scapular
nerve (C5)

Dorsal
ramus

Suprascapular
nerve (C5, 6)

To phrenic
nerve

C5

To subclavius
muscle (C5, 6)

C6

Superior

C7

Middle

C8

Lateral pectoral
nerve (C5, 6, 7)

T1

Lateral

Inferior

Superior

Musculocutaneous
nerve (C5, 6, 7)

Posterior

Contribution
from T2

Axillary
nerve (C5, 6)

1st rib

To longus colli
and scalene
muscles
(C5, 6, 7, 8)

Radial nerve
(C5, 6, 7, 8, T1)

Medial

1st intercostal nerve

Median nerve
(C5, 6, 7, 8, T1)

Long thoracic
nerve (C5, 6, 7)

Ulnar nerve
(C7, 8, T1)

Medial pectoral nerve (C8, T1)

Medial cutaneous nerve of arm (T1)

Medial cutaneous nerve of forearm (C8, T1)

**Inconstant contribution**

Upper subscapular nerve (C5, 6)

Thoracodorsal (middle subscapular) nerve (C6, 7, 8)

Lower subscapular nerve (C5, 6)

*SEE ALSO PLATE 443*

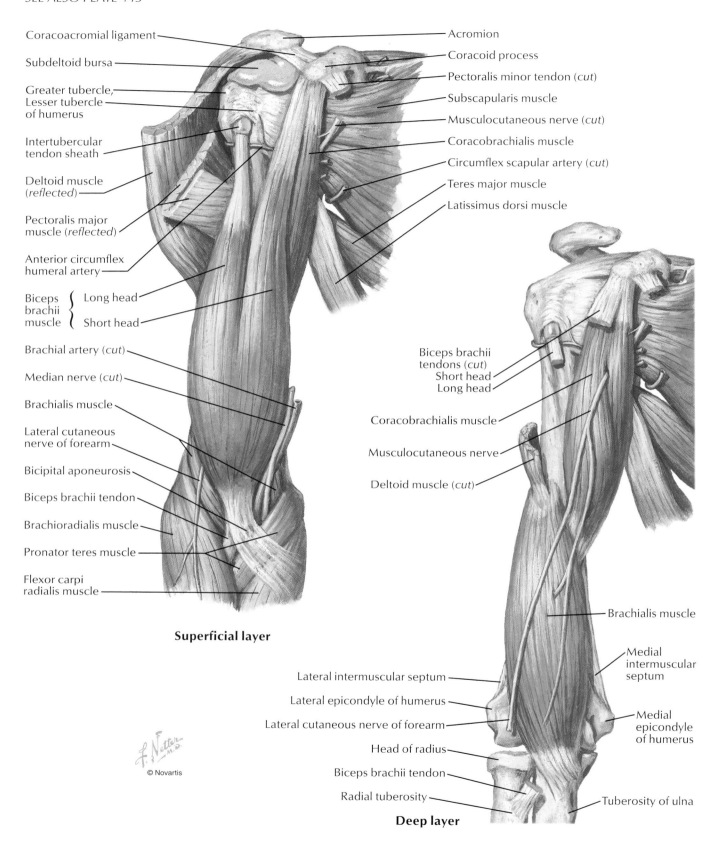

Coracoacromial ligament

Subdeltoid bursa

Greater tubercle,
Lesser tubercle
of humerus

Intertubercular
tendon sheath

Deltoid muscle
(*reflected*)

Pectoralis major
muscle (*reflected*)

Anterior circumflex
humeral artery

Biceps { Long head
brachii {
muscle { Short head

Brachial artery (*cut*)

Median nerve (*cut*)

Brachialis muscle

Lateral cutaneous
nerve of forearm

Bicipital aponeurosis

Biceps brachii tendon

Brachioradialis muscle

Pronator teres muscle

Flexor carpi
radialis muscle

Acromion

Coracoid process

Pectoralis minor tendon (*cut*)

Subscapularis muscle

Musculocutaneous nerve (*cut*)

Coracobrachialis muscle

Circumflex scapular artery (*cut*)

Teres major muscle

Latissimus dorsi muscle

**Superficial layer**

Biceps brachii
tendons (*cut*)
Short head
Long head

Coracobrachialis muscle

Musculocutaneous nerve

Deltoid muscle (*cut*)

Brachialis muscle

Medial
intermuscular
septum

Lateral intermuscular septum

Lateral epicondyle of humerus

Lateral cutaneous nerve of forearm

Head of radius

Biceps brachii tendon

Radial tuberosity

Medial
epicondyle
of humerus

Tuberosity of ulna

**Deep layer**

© Novartis

**PLATE 402**

**UPPER LIMB**

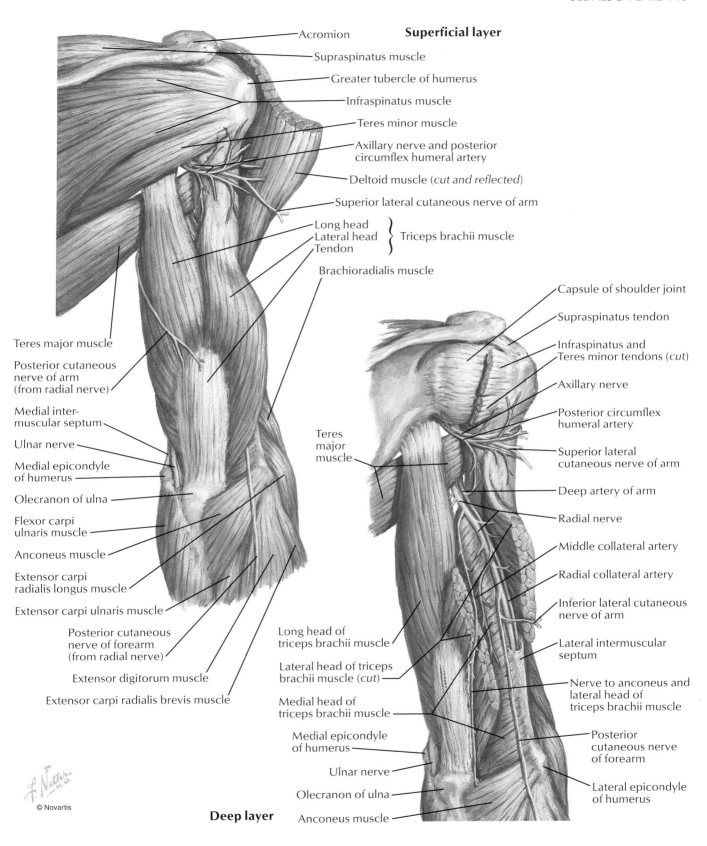

**Superficial layer**

Acromion

Supraspinatus muscle

Greater tubercle of humerus

Infraspinatus muscle

Teres minor muscle

Axillary nerve and posterior circumflex humeral artery

Deltoid muscle (*cut and reflected*)

Superior lateral cutaneous nerve of arm

Long head
Lateral head } Triceps brachii muscle
Tendon

Brachioradialis muscle

Teres major muscle

Posterior cutaneous nerve of arm (from radial nerve)

Medial inter-muscular septum

Ulnar nerve

Medial epicondyle of humerus

Olecranon of ulna

Flexor carpi ulnaris muscle

Anconeus muscle

Extensor carpi radialis longus muscle

Extensor carpi ulnaris muscle

Posterior cutaneous nerve of forearm (from radial nerve)

Extensor digitorum muscle

Extensor carpi radialis brevis muscle

Teres major muscle

Long head of triceps brachii muscle

Lateral head of triceps brachii muscle (*cut*)

Medial head of triceps brachii muscle

Medial epicondyle of humerus

Ulnar nerve

Olecranon of ulna

Anconeus muscle

Capsule of shoulder joint

Supraspinatus tendon

Infraspinatus and Teres minor tendons (*cut*)

Axillary nerve

Posterior circumflex humeral artery

Superior lateral cutaneous nerve of arm

Deep artery of arm

Radial nerve

Middle collateral artery

Radial collateral artery

Inferior lateral cutaneous nerve of arm

Lateral intermuscular septum

Nerve to anconeus and lateral head of triceps brachii muscle

Posterior cutaneous nerve of forearm

Lateral epicondyle of humerus

**Deep layer**

© Novartis

# Brachial Artery In Situ

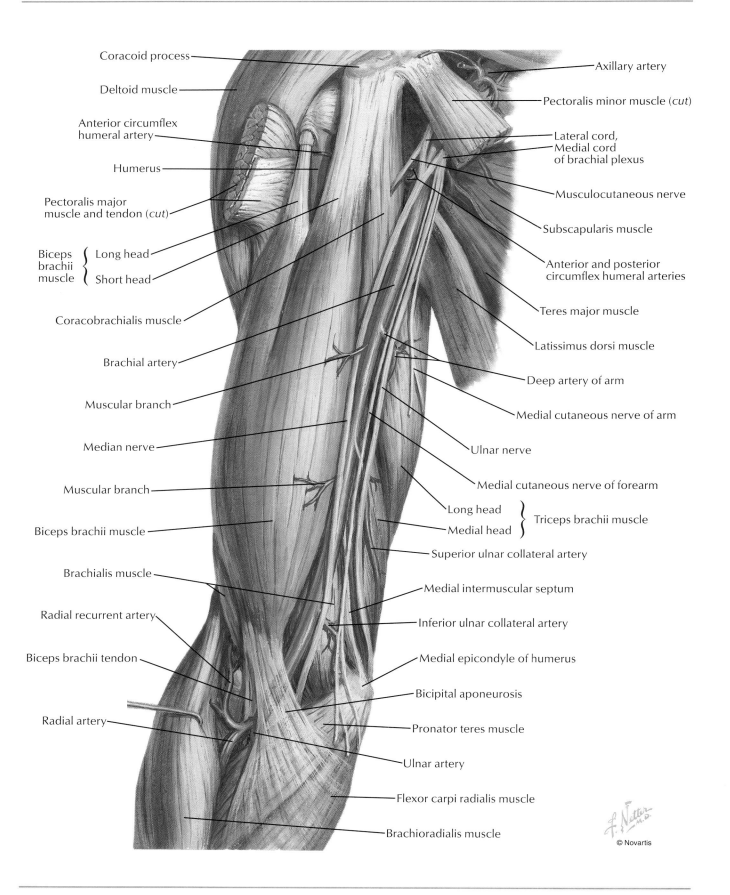

Coracoid process

Deltoid muscle

Anterior circumflex humeral artery

Humerus

Pectoralis major muscle and tendon (cut)

Biceps brachii muscle { Long head / Short head }

Coracobrachialis muscle

Brachial artery

Muscular branch

Median nerve

Muscular branch

Biceps brachii muscle

Brachialis muscle

Radial recurrent artery

Biceps brachii tendon

Radial artery

Axillary artery

Pectoralis minor muscle (cut)

Lateral cord, Medial cord of brachial plexus

Musculocutaneous nerve

Subscapularis muscle

Anterior and posterior circumflex humeral arteries

Teres major muscle

Latissimus dorsi muscle

Deep artery of arm

Medial cutaneous nerve of arm

Ulnar nerve

Medial cutaneous nerve of forearm

Long head / Medial head } Triceps brachii muscle

Superior ulnar collateral artery

Medial intermuscular septum

Inferior ulnar collateral artery

Medial epicondyle of humerus

Bicipital aponeurosis

Pronator teres muscle

Ulnar artery

Flexor carpi radialis muscle

Brachioradialis muscle

© Novartis

**PLATE 404**

**UPPER LIMB**

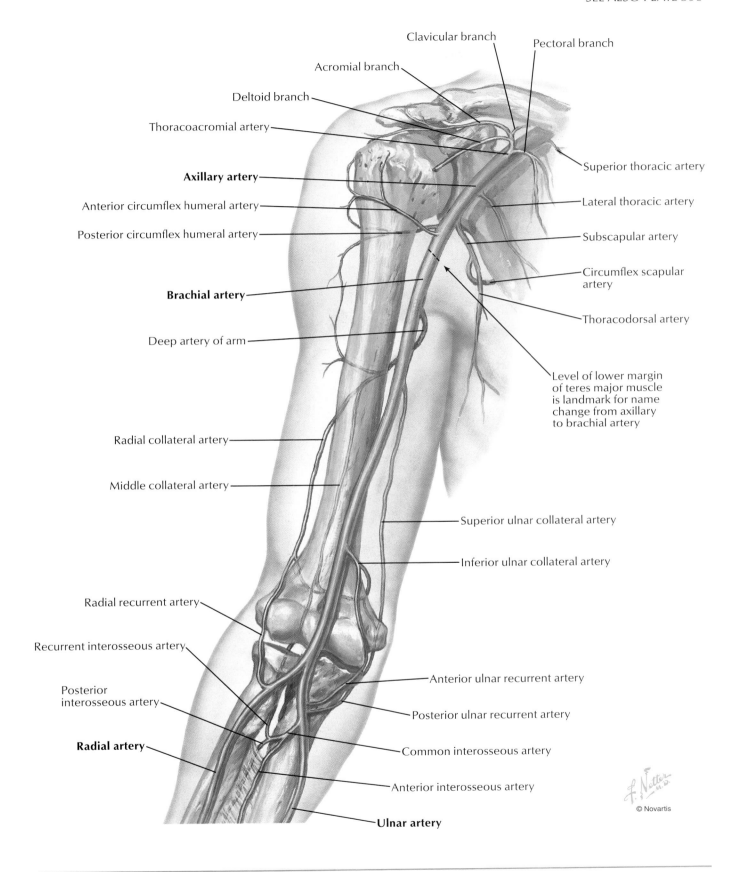

Clavicular branch

Pectoral branch

Acromial branch

Deltoid branch

Thoracoacromial artery

Axillary artery

Anterior circumflex humeral artery

Posterior circumflex humeral artery

Brachial artery

Deep artery of arm

Radial collateral artery

Middle collateral artery

Radial recurrent artery

Recurrent interosseous artery

Posterior interosseous artery

Radial artery

Superior thoracic artery

Lateral thoracic artery

Subscapular artery

Circumflex scapular artery

Thoracodorsal artery

Level of lower margin of teres major muscle is landmark for name change from axillary to brachial artery

Superior ulnar collateral artery

Inferior ulnar collateral artery

Anterior ulnar recurrent artery

Posterior ulnar recurrent artery

Common interosseous artery

Anterior interosseous artery

Ulnar artery

© Novartis

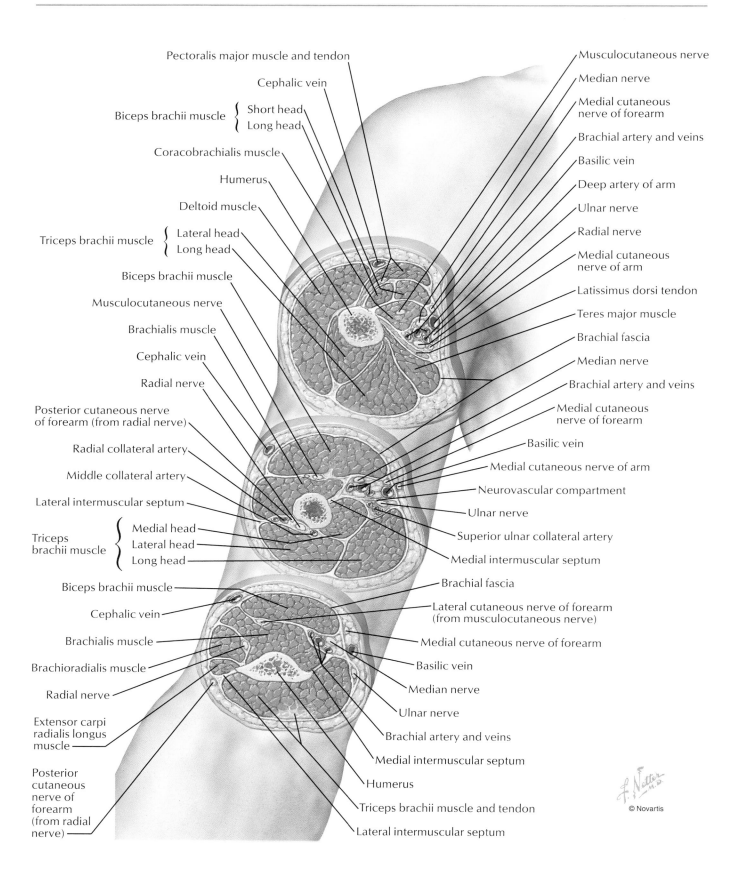

Pectoralis major muscle and tendon

Cephalic vein

Biceps brachii muscle { Short head / Long head }

Coracobrachialis muscle

Humerus

Deltoid muscle

Triceps brachii muscle { Lateral head / Long head }

Biceps brachii muscle

Musculocutaneous nerve

Brachialis muscle

Cephalic vein

Radial nerve

Posterior cutaneous nerve of forearm (from radial nerve)

Radial collateral artery

Middle collateral artery

Lateral intermuscular septum

Triceps brachii muscle { Medial head / Lateral head / Long head }

Biceps brachii muscle

Cephalic vein

Brachialis muscle

Brachioradialis muscle

Radial nerve

Extensor carpi radialis longus muscle

Posterior cutaneous nerve of forearm (from radial nerve)

Musculocutaneous nerve

Median nerve

Medial cutaneous nerve of forearm

Brachial artery and veins

Basilic vein

Deep artery of arm

Ulnar nerve

Radial nerve

Medial cutaneous nerve of arm

Latissimus dorsi tendon

Teres major muscle

Brachial fascia

Median nerve

Brachial artery and veins

Medial cutaneous nerve of forearm

Basilic vein

Medial cutaneous nerve of arm

Neurovascular compartment

Ulnar nerve

Superior ulnar collateral artery

Medial intermuscular septum

Brachial fascia

Lateral cutaneous nerve of forearm (from musculocutaneous nerve)

Medial cutaneous nerve of forearm

Basilic vein

Median nerve

Ulnar nerve

Brachial artery and veins

Medial intermuscular septum

Humerus

Triceps brachii muscle and tendon

Lateral intermuscular septum

© Novartis

**PLATE 406**       **UPPER LIMB**

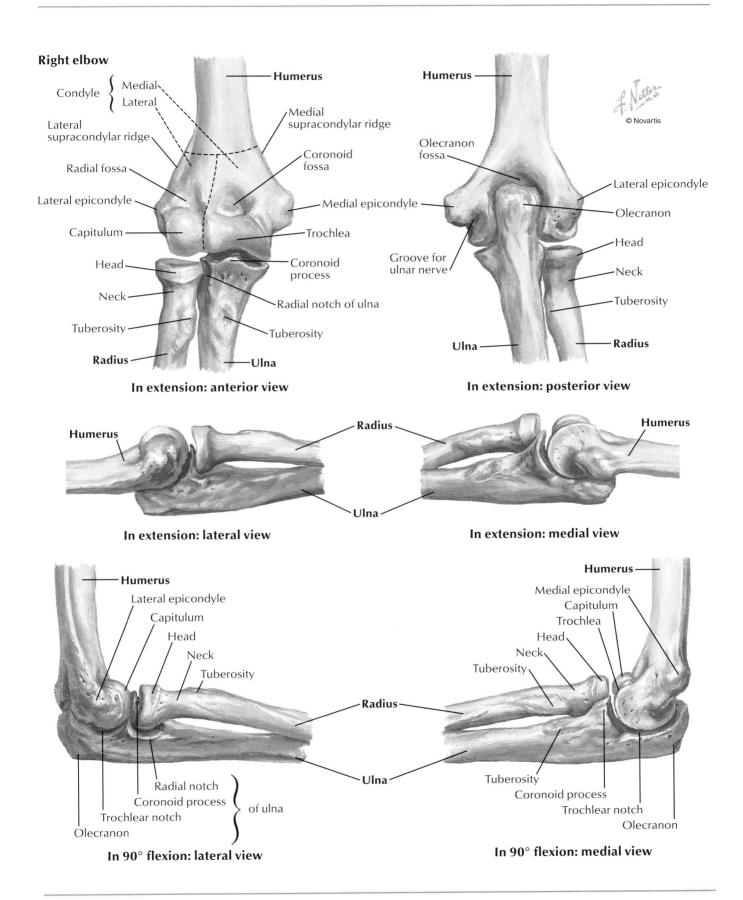

**Right elbow**

Condyle { Medial
Lateral

Lateral
supracondylar ridge

Radial fossa

Lateral epicondyle

Capitulum

Head

Neck

Tuberosity

**Radius**

Humerus

Medial
supracondylar ridge

Coronoid
fossa

Medial epicondyle

Trochlea

Coronoid
process

Radial notch of ulna

Tuberosity

**Ulna**

**In extension: anterior view**

Humerus

Olecranon
fossa

Groove for
ulnar nerve

**Ulna**

Lateral epicondyle

Olecranon

Head

Neck

Tuberosity

**Radius**

**In extension: posterior view**

**Humerus**

**Radius**

**Ulna**

**In extension: lateral view**

**Radius**

**Humerus**

**Ulna**

**In extension: medial view**

**Humerus**

Lateral epicondyle

Capitulum

Head

Neck

Tuberosity

**Radius**

Radial notch
Coronoid process } of ulna
Trochlear notch

Olecranon

**Ulna**

**In 90° flexion: lateral view**

**Humerus**

Medial epicondyle

Capitulum

Trochlea

Head

Neck

Tuberosity

**Radius**

Tuberosity

Coronoid process

Trochlear notch

Olecranon

**Ulna**

**In 90° flexion: medial view**

# Ligaments of Elbow

**Right elbow**

## Anterior view

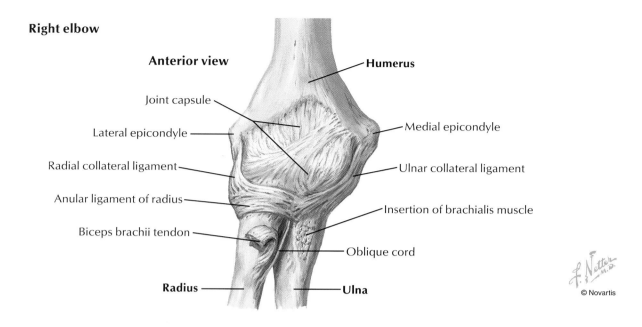

Joint capsule

Lateral epicondyle

Radial collateral ligament

Anular ligament of radius

Biceps brachii tendon

**Radius**

Humerus

Medial epicondyle

Ulnar collateral ligament

Insertion of brachialis muscle

Oblique cord

**Ulna**

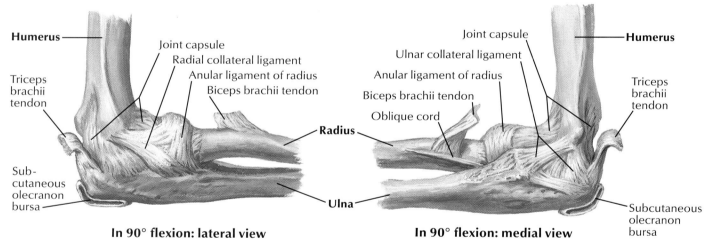

**Humerus**

Triceps brachii tendon

Sub-cutaneous olecranon bursa

Joint capsule

Radial collateral ligament

Anular ligament of radius

Biceps brachii tendon

**Radius**

**Ulna**

**In 90° flexion: lateral view**

Joint capsule

Ulnar collateral ligament

Anular ligament of radius

Biceps brachii tendon

Oblique cord

**Humerus**

Triceps brachii tendon

Subcutaneous olecranon bursa

**In 90° flexion: medial view**

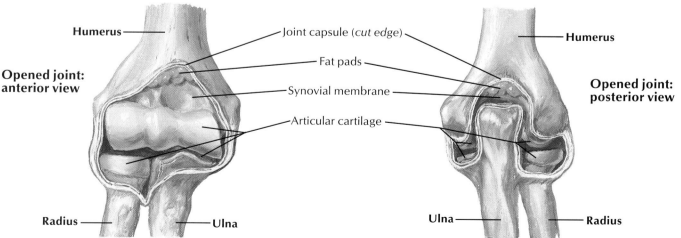

**Humerus**

**Opened joint: anterior view**

**Radius**

**Ulna**

Joint capsule (*cut edge*)

Fat pads

Synovial membrane

Articular cartilage

**Humerus**

**Opened joint: posterior view**

**Ulna**

**Radius**

*PLATE 408*

**UPPER LIMB**

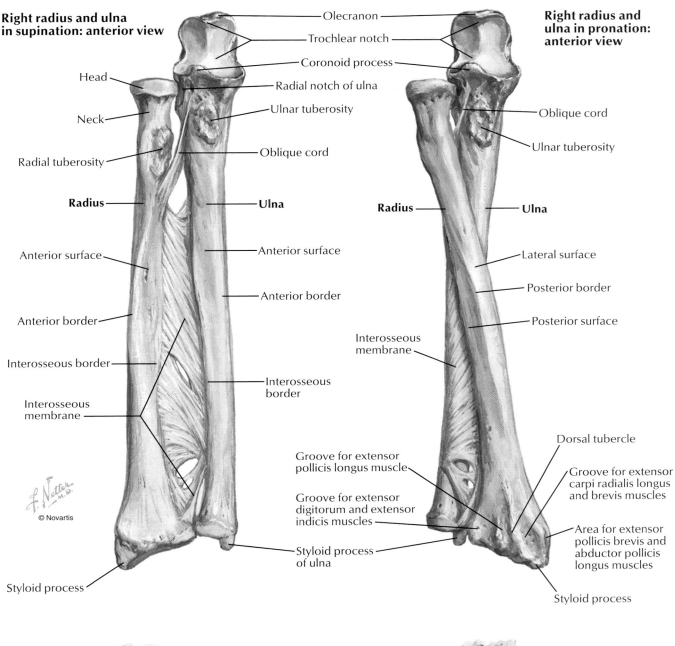

**Right radius and ulna in supination: anterior view**

Olecranon

Trochlear notch

Coronoid process

Head

Radial notch of ulna

Neck

Ulnar tuberosity

Radial tuberosity

Oblique cord

**Radius**

**Ulna**

Anterior surface

Anterior surface

Anterior border

Anterior border

Interosseous border

Interosseous border

Interosseous membrane

Interosseous membrane

Groove for extensor pollicis longus muscle

Groove for extensor digitorum and extensor indicis muscles

Styloid process of ulna

Styloid process

**Right radius and ulna in pronation: anterior view**

Oblique cord

Ulnar tuberosity

**Radius**

**Ulna**

Lateral surface

Posterior border

Posterior surface

Interosseous membrane

Dorsal tubercle

Groove for extensor carpi radialis longus and brevis muscles

Area for extensor pollicis brevis and abductor pollicis longus muscles

Styloid process

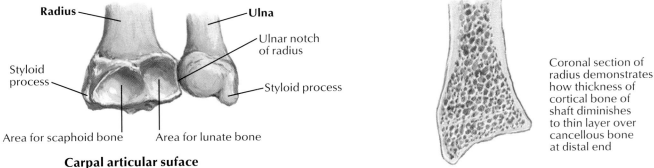

**Radius**

**Ulna**

Ulnar notch of radius

Styloid process

Styloid process

Area for scaphoid bone

Area for lunate bone

**Carpal articular suface**

Coronal section of radius demonstrates how thickness of cortical bone of shaft diminishes to thin layer over cancellous bone at distal end

# Individual Muscles of Forearm: Rotators of Radius

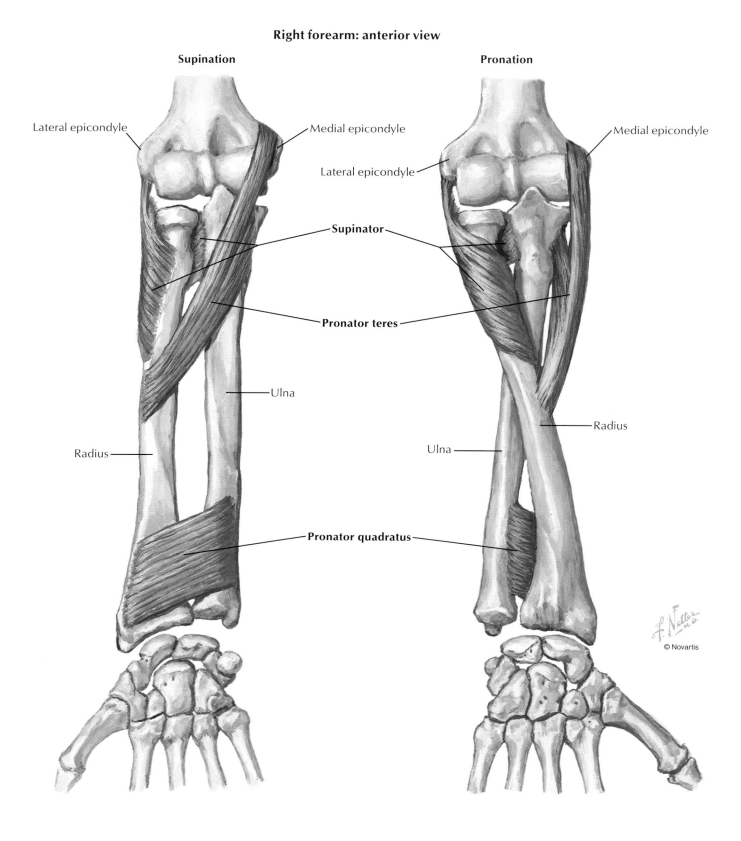

**Right forearm: anterior view**

Supination

Pronation

Lateral epicondyle

Medial epicondyle

Medial epicondyle

Lateral epicondyle

**Supinator**

**Pronator teres**

Ulna

Radius

Radius

Ulna

**Pronator quadratus**

© Novartis

*PLATE 410*

**UPPER LIMB**

# Individual Muscles of Forearm: Extensors of Wrist and Digits

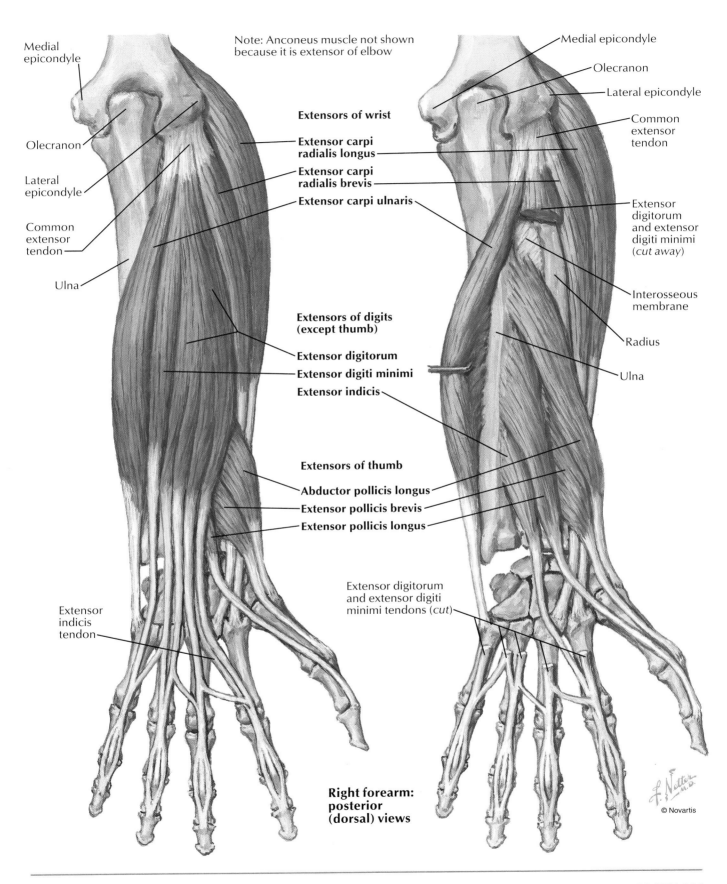

Medial epicondyle

Olecranon

Lateral epicondyle

Common extensor tendon

Ulna

Extensor indicis tendon

Note: Anconeus muscle not shown because it is extensor of elbow

**Extensors of wrist**

**Extensor carpi radialis longus**

**Extensor carpi radialis brevis**

**Extensor carpi ulnaris**

**Extensors of digits (except thumb)**

**Extensor digitorum**

**Extensor digiti minimi**

**Extensor indicis**

**Extensors of thumb**

**Abductor pollicis longus**

**Extensor pollicis brevis**

**Extensor pollicis longus**

Extensor digitorum and extensor digiti minimi tendons (*cut*)

**Right forearm: posterior (dorsal) views**

Medial epicondyle

Olecranon

Lateral epicondyle

Common extensor tendon

Extensor digitorum and extensor digiti minimi (*cut away*)

Interosseous membrane

Radius

Ulna

**ELBOW AND FOREARM**

**PLATE 411**

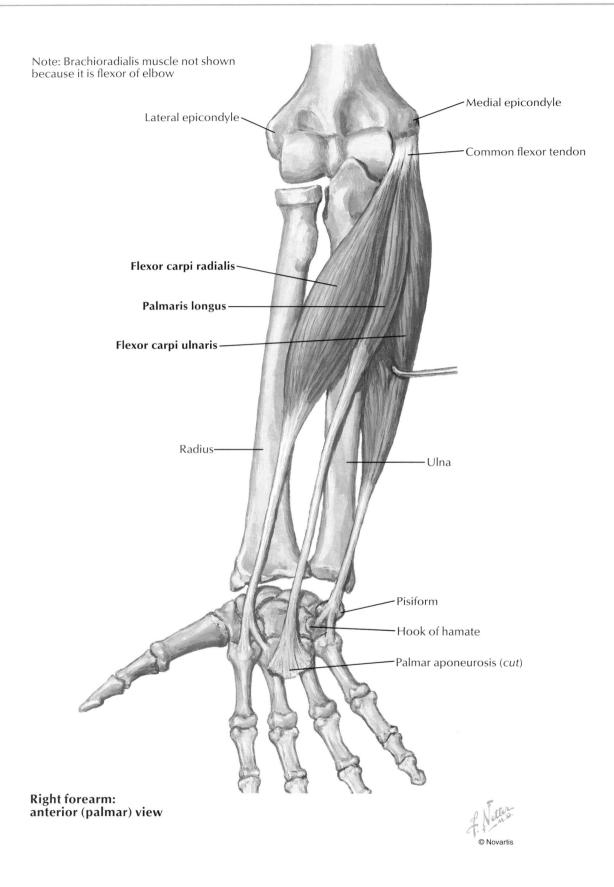

Note: Brachioradialis muscle not shown
because it is flexor of elbow

Lateral epicondyle

Medial epicondyle

Common flexor tendon

**Flexor carpi radialis**

**Palmaris longus**

**Flexor carpi ulnaris**

Radius

Ulna

Pisiform

Hook of hamate

Palmar aponeurosis (*cut*)

**Right forearm:
anterior (palmar) view**

*F. Netter*
*M.D.*

© Novartis

**PLATE 412**

**UPPER LIMB**

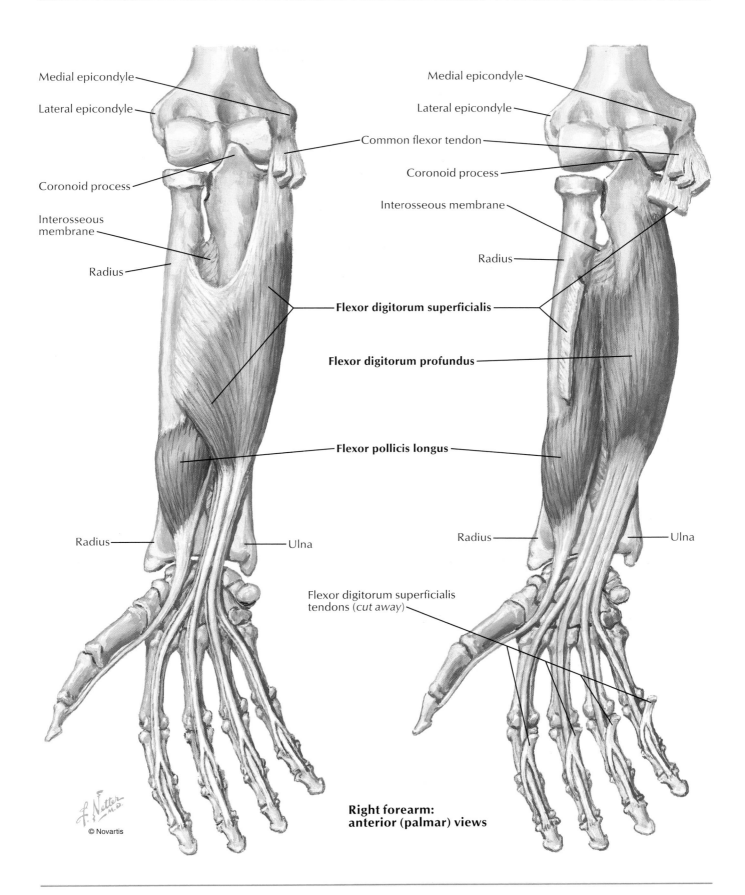

Medial epicondyle

Lateral epicondyle

Coronoid process

Interosseous membrane

Radius

Medial epicondyle

Lateral epicondyle

Common flexor tendon

Coronoid process

Interosseous membrane

Radius

**Flexor digitorum superficialis**

**Flexor digitorum profundus**

**Flexor pollicis longus**

Radius

Ulna

Radius

Ulna

Flexor digitorum superficialis tendons (*cut away*)

**Right forearm:
anterior (palmar) views**

© Novartis

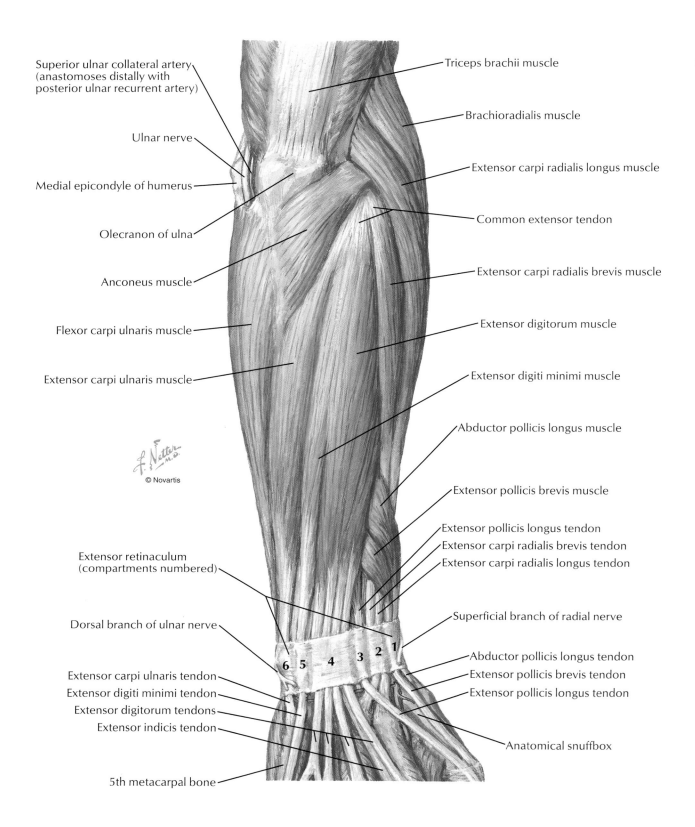

Superior ulnar collateral artery (anastomoses distally with posterior ulnar recurrent artery)

Ulnar nerve

Medial epicondyle of humerus

Olecranon of ulna

Anconeus muscle

Flexor carpi ulnaris muscle

Extensor carpi ulnaris muscle

Extensor retinaculum (compartments numbered)

Dorsal branch of ulnar nerve

Extensor carpi ulnaris tendon

Extensor digiti minimi tendon

Extensor digitorum tendons

Extensor indicis tendon

5th metacarpal bone

Triceps brachii muscle

Brachioradialis muscle

Extensor carpi radialis longus muscle

Common extensor tendon

Extensor carpi radialis brevis muscle

Extensor digitorum muscle

Extensor digiti minimi muscle

Abductor pollicis longus muscle

Extensor pollicis brevis muscle

Extensor pollicis longus tendon

Extensor carpi radialis brevis tendon

Extensor carpi radialis longus tendon

Superficial branch of radial nerve

Abductor pollicis longus tendon

Extensor pollicis brevis tendon

Extensor pollicis longus tendon

Anatomical snuffbox

6 5 4 3 2 1

© Novartis

**PLATE 414**

**UPPER LIMB**

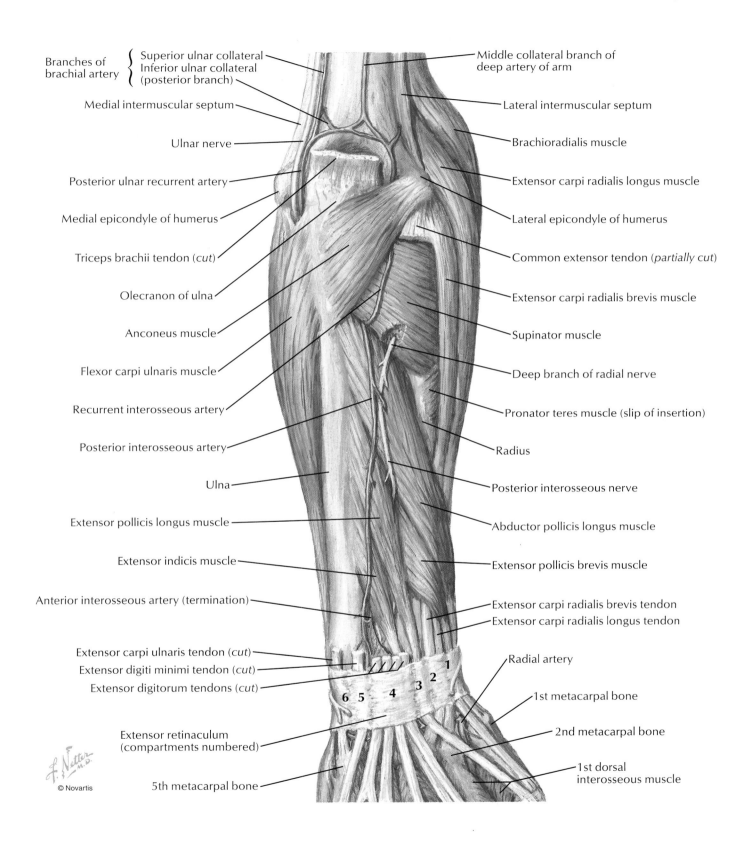

Branches of brachial artery { Superior ulnar collateral
Inferior ulnar collateral (posterior branch)

Medial intermuscular septum

Ulnar nerve

Posterior ulnar recurrent artery

Medial epicondyle of humerus

Triceps brachii tendon (cut)

Olecranon of ulna

Anconeus muscle

Flexor carpi ulnaris muscle

Recurrent interosseous artery

Posterior interosseous artery

Ulna

Extensor pollicis longus muscle

Extensor indicis muscle

Anterior interosseous artery (termination)

Extensor carpi ulnaris tendon (cut)
Extensor digiti minimi tendon (cut)
Extensor digitorum tendons (cut)

Extensor retinaculum (compartments numbered)

5th metacarpal bone

Middle collateral branch of deep artery of arm

Lateral intermuscular septum

Brachioradialis muscle

Extensor carpi radialis longus muscle

Lateral epicondyle of humerus

Common extensor tendon (partially cut)

Extensor carpi radialis brevis muscle

Supinator muscle

Deep branch of radial nerve

Pronator teres muscle (slip of insertion)

Radius

Posterior interosseous nerve

Abductor pollicis longus muscle

Extensor pollicis brevis muscle

Extensor carpi radialis brevis tendon
Extensor carpi radialis longus tendon

Radial artery

1st metacarpal bone

2nd metacarpal bone

1st dorsal interosseous muscle

© Novartis

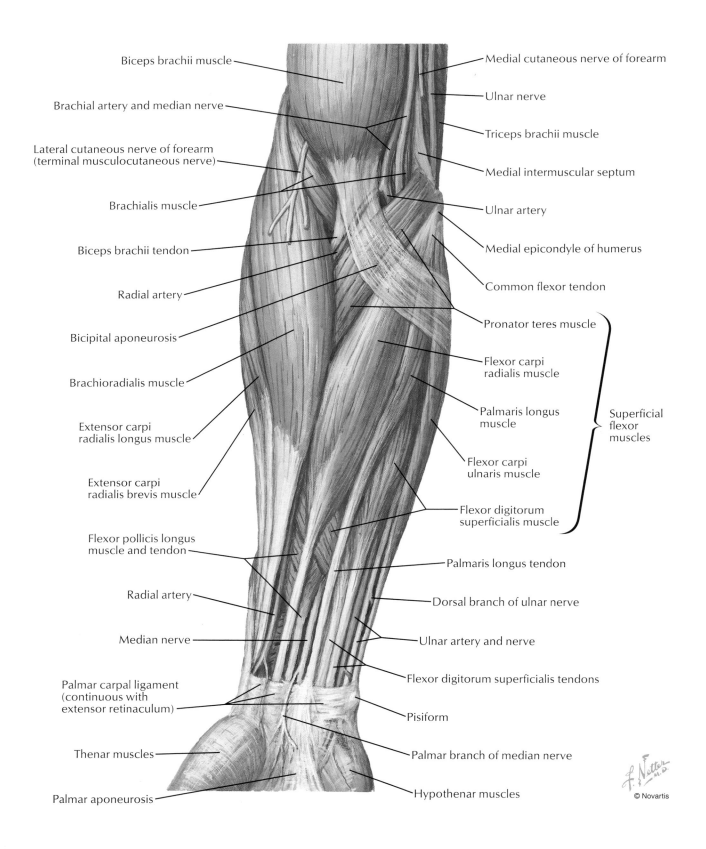

Biceps brachii muscle

Brachial artery and median nerve

Lateral cutaneous nerve of forearm (terminal musculocutaneous nerve)

Brachialis muscle

Biceps brachii tendon

Radial artery

Bicipital aponeurosis

Brachioradialis muscle

Extensor carpi radialis longus muscle

Extensor carpi radialis brevis muscle

Flexor pollicis longus muscle and tendon

Radial artery

Median nerve

Palmar carpal ligament (continuous with extensor retinaculum)

Thenar muscles

Palmar aponeurosis

Medial cutaneous nerve of forearm

Ulnar nerve

Triceps brachii muscle

Medial intermuscular septum

Ulnar artery

Medial epicondyle of humerus

Common flexor tendon

Pronator teres muscle

Flexor carpi radialis muscle

Palmaris longus muscle

Flexor carpi ulnaris muscle

Flexor digitorum superficialis muscle

Superficial flexor muscles

Palmaris longus tendon

Dorsal branch of ulnar nerve

Ulnar artery and nerve

Flexor digitorum superficialis tendons

Pisiform

Palmar branch of median nerve

Hypothenar muscles

© Novartis

**PLATE 416**

**UPPER LIMB**

# Muscles of Forearm (Intermediate Layer): Anterior View

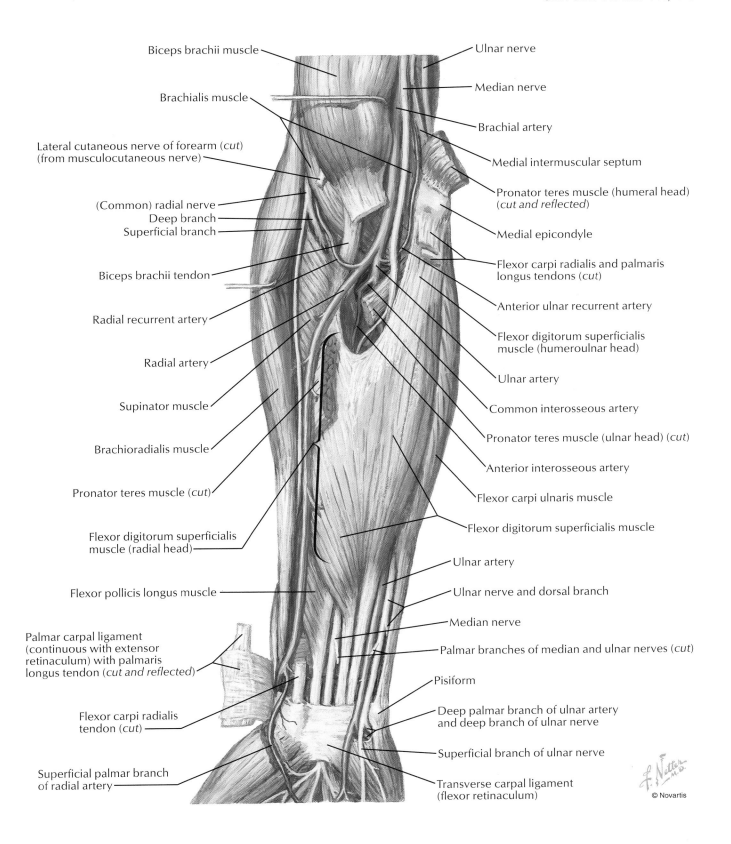

Biceps brachii muscle

Brachialis muscle

Lateral cutaneous nerve of forearm (cut)
(from musculocutaneous nerve)

(Common) radial nerve
Deep branch
Superficial branch

Biceps brachii tendon

Radial recurrent artery

Radial artery

Supinator muscle

Brachioradialis muscle

Pronator teres muscle (cut)

Flexor digitorum superficialis
muscle (radial head)

Flexor pollicis longus muscle

Palmar carpal ligament
(continuous with extensor
retinaculum) with palmaris
longus tendon (cut and reflected)

Flexor carpi radialis
tendon (cut)

Superficial palmar branch
of radial artery

Ulnar nerve

Median nerve

Brachial artery

Medial intermuscular septum

Pronator teres muscle (humeral head)
(cut and reflected)

Medial epicondyle

Flexor carpi radialis and palmaris
longus tendons (cut)

Anterior ulnar recurrent artery

Flexor digitorum superficialis
muscle (humeroulnar head)

Ulnar artery

Common interosseous artery

Pronator teres muscle (ulnar head) (cut)

Anterior interosseous artery

Flexor carpi ulnaris muscle

Flexor digitorum superficialis muscle

Ulnar artery

Ulnar nerve and dorsal branch

Median nerve

Palmar branches of median and ulnar nerves (cut)

Pisiform

Deep palmar branch of ulnar artery
and deep branch of ulnar nerve

Superficial branch of ulnar nerve

Transverse carpal ligament
(flexor retinaculum)

F. Netter M.D.

© Novartis

**ELBOW AND FOREARM**

**PLATE 417**

*SEE ALSO PLATES 444, 445*

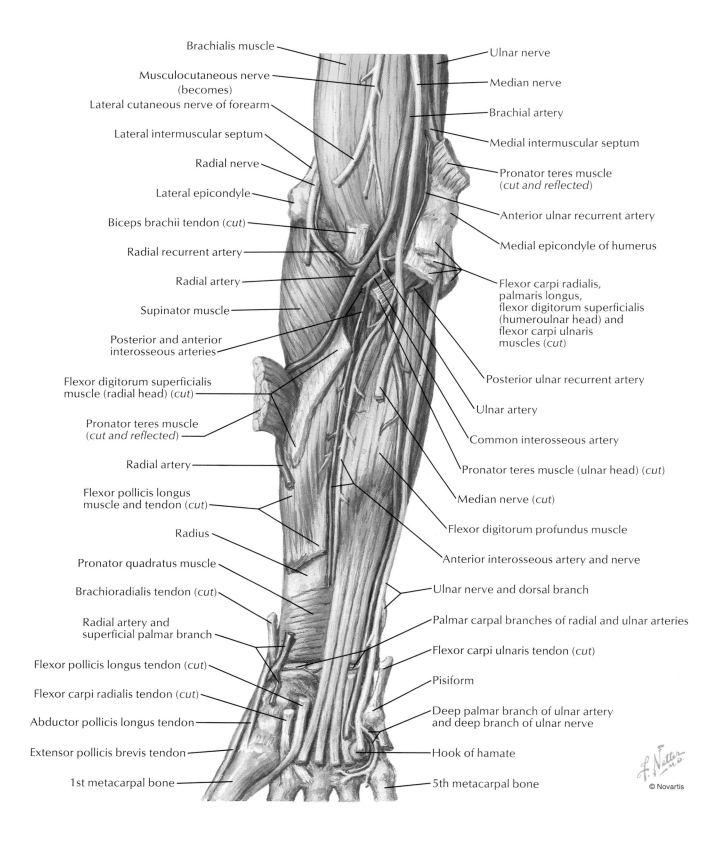

Brachialis muscle

Musculocutaneous nerve (becomes)

Lateral cutaneous nerve of forearm

Lateral intermuscular septum

Radial nerve

Lateral epicondyle

Biceps brachii tendon (*cut*)

Radial recurrent artery

Radial artery

Supinator muscle

Posterior and anterior interosseous arteries

Flexor digitorum superficialis muscle (radial head) (*cut*)

Pronator teres muscle (*cut and reflected*)

Radial artery

Flexor pollicis longus muscle and tendon (*cut*)

Radius

Pronator quadratus muscle

Brachioradialis tendon (*cut*)

Radial artery and superficial palmar branch

Flexor pollicis longus tendon (*cut*)

Flexor carpi radialis tendon (*cut*)

Abductor pollicis longus tendon

Extensor pollicis brevis tendon

1st metacarpal bone

Ulnar nerve

Median nerve

Brachial artery

Medial intermuscular septum

Pronator teres muscle (*cut and reflected*)

Anterior ulnar recurrent artery

Medial epicondyle of humerus

Flexor carpi radialis, palmaris longus, flexor digitorum superficialis (humeroulnar head) and flexor carpi ulnaris muscles (*cut*)

Posterior ulnar recurrent artery

Ulnar artery

Common interosseous artery

Pronator teres muscle (ulnar head) (*cut*)

Median nerve (*cut*)

Flexor digitorum profundus muscle

Anterior interosseous artery and nerve

Ulnar nerve and dorsal branch

Palmar carpal branches of radial and ulnar arteries

Flexor carpi ulnaris tendon (*cut*)

Pisiform

Deep palmar branch of ulnar artery and deep branch of ulnar nerve

Hook of hamate

5th metacarpal bone

*f. Netter M.D.*

© Novartis

**PLATE 418**

**UPPER LIMB**

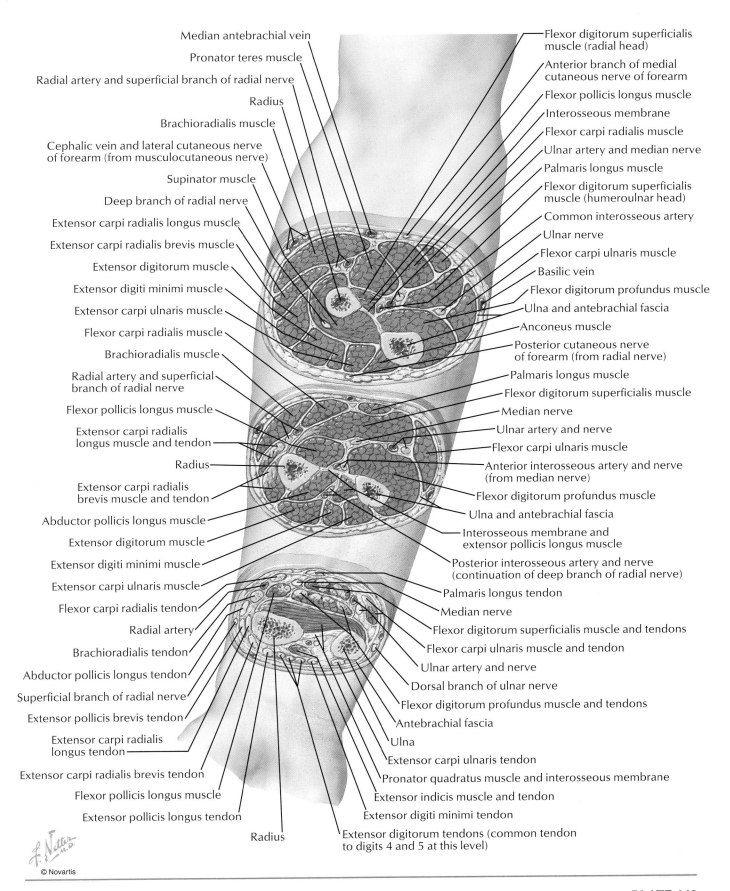

Median antebrachial vein

Pronator teres muscle

Radial artery and superficial branch of radial nerve

Radius

Brachioradialis muscle

Cephalic vein and lateral cutaneous nerve of forearm (from musculocutaneous nerve)

Supinator muscle

Deep branch of radial nerve

Extensor carpi radialis longus muscle

Extensor carpi radialis brevis muscle

Extensor digitorum muscle

Extensor digiti minimi muscle

Extensor carpi ulnaris muscle

Flexor carpi radialis muscle

Brachioradialis muscle

Radial artery and superficial branch of radial nerve

Flexor pollicis longus muscle

Extensor carpi radialis longus muscle and tendon

Radius

Extensor carpi radialis brevis muscle and tendon

Abductor pollicis longus muscle

Extensor digitorum muscle

Extensor digiti minimi muscle

Extensor carpi ulnaris muscle

Flexor carpi radialis tendon

Radial artery

Brachioradialis tendon

Abductor pollicis longus tendon

Superficial branch of radial nerve

Extensor pollicis brevis tendon

Extensor carpi radialis longus tendon

Extensor carpi radialis brevis tendon

Flexor pollicis longus muscle

Extensor pollicis longus tendon

Radius

Flexor digitorum superficialis muscle (radial head)

Anterior branch of medial cutaneous nerve of forearm

Flexor pollicis longus muscle

Interosseous membrane

Flexor carpi radialis muscle

Ulnar artery and median nerve

Palmaris longus muscle

Flexor digitorum superficialis muscle (humeroulnar head)

Common interosseous artery

Ulnar nerve

Flexor carpi ulnaris muscle

Basilic vein

Flexor digitorum profundus muscle

Ulna and antebrachial fascia

Anconeus muscle

Posterior cutaneous nerve of forearm (from radial nerve)

Palmaris longus muscle

Flexor digitorum superficialis muscle

Median nerve

Ulnar artery and nerve

Flexor carpi ulnaris muscle

Anterior interosseous artery and nerve (from median nerve)

Flexor digitorum profundus muscle

Ulna and antebrachial fascia

Interosseous membrane and extensor pollicis longus muscle

Posterior interosseous artery and nerve (continuation of deep branch of radial nerve)

Palmaris longus tendon

Median nerve

Flexor digitorum superficialis muscle and tendons

Flexor carpi ulnaris muscle and tendon

Ulnar artery and nerve

Dorsal branch of ulnar nerve

Flexor digitorum profundus muscle and tendons

Antebrachial fascia

Ulna

Extensor carpi ulnaris tendon

Pronator quadratus muscle and interosseous membrane

Extensor indicis muscle and tendon

Extensor digiti minimi tendon

Extensor digitorum tendons (common tendon to digits 4 and 5 at this level)

**ELBOW AND FOREARM**

*PLATE 419*

# Attachments of Muscles of Forearm: Anterior View

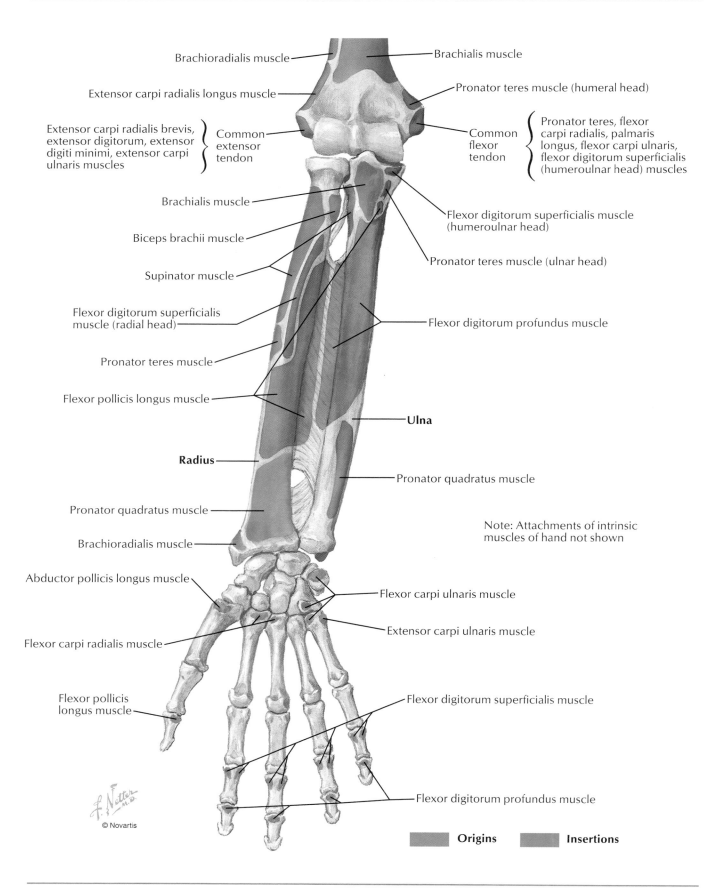

Brachioradialis muscle

Brachialis muscle

Extensor carpi radialis longus muscle

Pronator teres muscle (humeral head)

Extensor carpi radialis brevis, extensor digitorum, extensor digiti minimi, extensor carpi ulnaris muscles } Common extensor tendon

Common flexor tendon } Pronator teres, flexor carpi radialis, palmaris longus, flexor carpi ulnaris, flexor digitorum superficialis (humeroulnar head) muscles

Brachialis muscle

Flexor digitorum superficialis muscle (humeroulnar head)

Biceps brachii muscle

Supinator muscle

Pronator teres muscle (ulnar head)

Flexor digitorum superficialis muscle (radial head)

Flexor digitorum profundus muscle

Pronator teres muscle

Flexor pollicis longus muscle

Ulna

Radius

Pronator quadratus muscle

Pronator quadratus muscle

Note: Attachments of intrinsic muscles of hand not shown

Brachioradialis muscle

Abductor pollicis longus muscle

Flexor carpi ulnaris muscle

Extensor carpi ulnaris muscle

Flexor carpi radialis muscle

Flexor pollicis longus muscle

Flexor digitorum superficialis muscle

Flexor digitorum profundus muscle

© Novartis

Origins       Insertions

**PLATE 420**

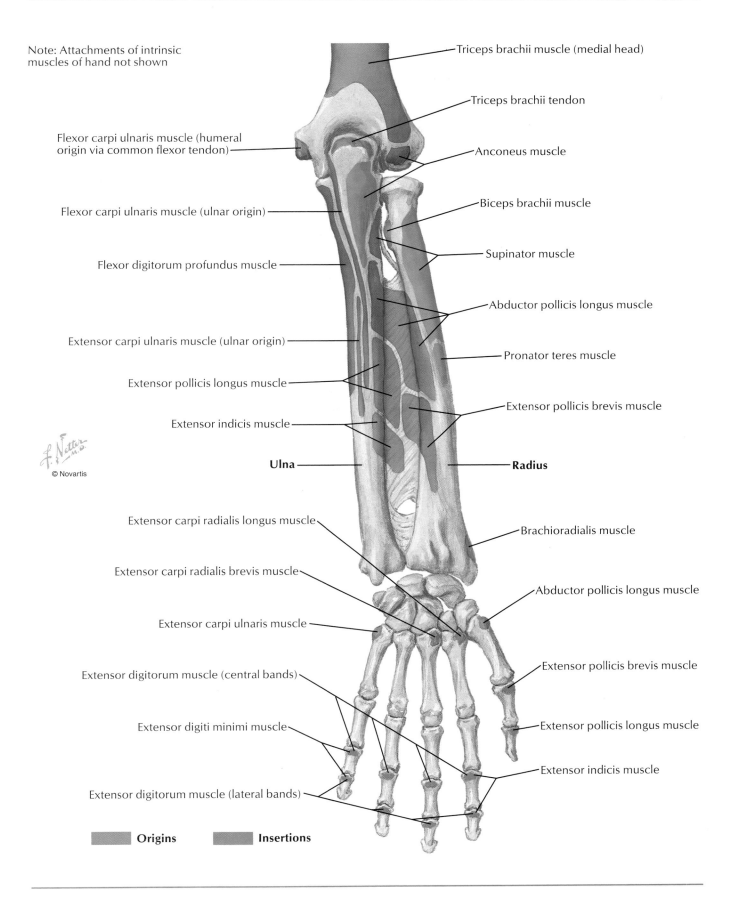

Note: Attachments of intrinsic muscles of hand not shown

Flexor carpi ulnaris muscle (humeral origin via common flexor tendon)

Flexor carpi ulnaris muscle (ulnar origin)

Flexor digitorum profundus muscle

Extensor carpi ulnaris muscle (ulnar origin)

Extensor pollicis longus muscle

Extensor indicis muscle

**Ulna**

Extensor carpi radialis longus muscle

Extensor carpi radialis brevis muscle

Extensor carpi ulnaris muscle

Extensor digitorum muscle (central bands)

Extensor digiti minimi muscle

Extensor digitorum muscle (lateral bands)

Triceps brachii muscle (medial head)

Triceps brachii tendon

Anconeus muscle

Biceps brachii muscle

Supinator muscle

Abductor pollicis longus muscle

Pronator teres muscle

Extensor pollicis brevis muscle

**Radius**

Brachioradialis muscle

Abductor pollicis longus muscle

Extensor pollicis brevis muscle

Extensor pollicis longus muscle

Extensor indicis muscle

**Origins**　**Insertions**

© Novartis

# *Carpal Bones*

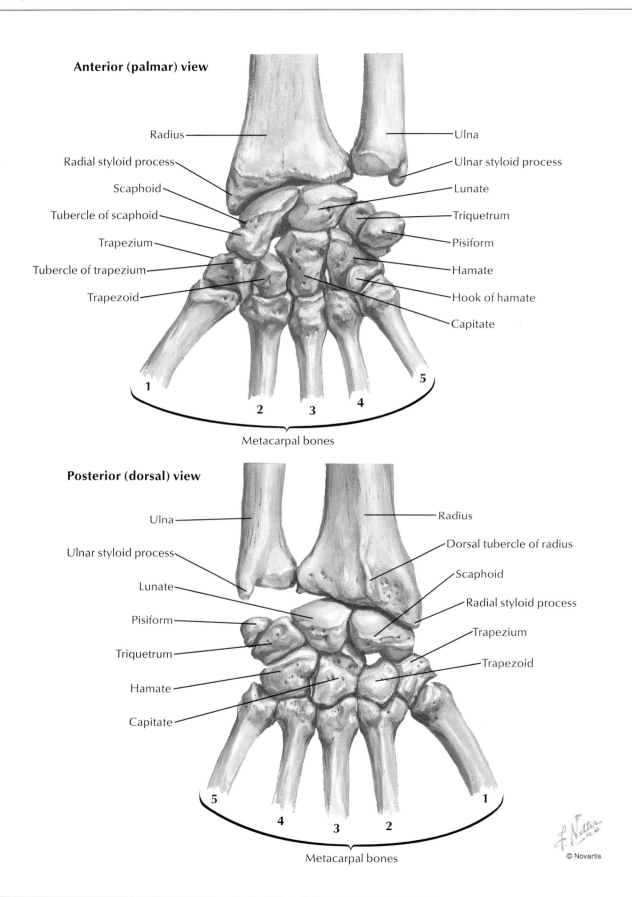

**Anterior (palmar) view**

Radius
Radial styloid process
Scaphoid
Tubercle of scaphoid
Trapezium
Tubercle of trapezium
Trapezoid

Ulna
Ulnar styloid process
Lunate
Triquetrum
Pisiform
Hamate
Hook of hamate
Capitate

Metacarpal bones

**Posterior (dorsal) view**

Ulna
Ulnar styloid process
Lunate
Pisiform
Triquetrum
Hamate
Capitate

Radius
Dorsal tubercle of radius
Scaphoid
Radial styloid process
Trapezium
Trapezoid

Metacarpal bones

*PLATE 422*

**UPPER LIMB**

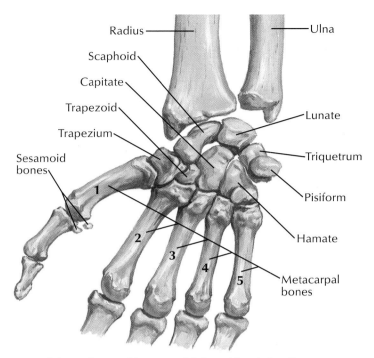

Radius — Ulna

Scaphoid

Capitate

Trapezoid

Trapezium

Sesamoid bones

Lunate

Triquetrum

Pisiform

Hamate

1
2
3
4
5

Metacarpal bones

**Position of carpal bones with hand in abduction: anterior (palmar) view**

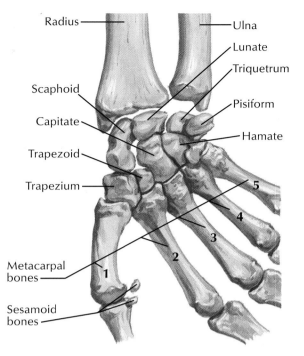

Radius — Ulna

Lunate

Triquetrum

Scaphoid

Pisiform

Capitate

Hamate

Trapezoid

Trapezium

5
4
3
2
1

Metacarpal bones

Sesamoid bones

**Position of carpal bones with hand in adduction: anterior (palmar) view**

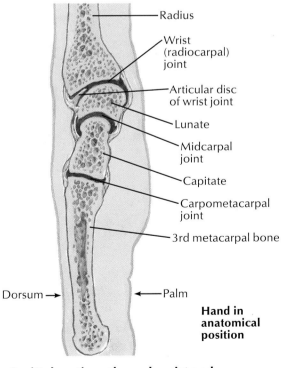

Radius

Wrist (radiocarpal) joint

Articular disc of wrist joint

Lunate

Midcarpal joint

Capitate

Carpometacarpal joint

3rd metacarpal bone

Dorsum ← → Palm

**Hand in anatomical position**

**Sagittal sections through wrist and middle finger**

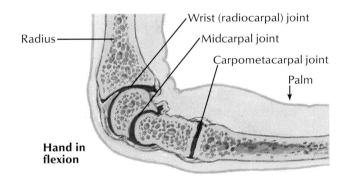

Radius

Wrist (radiocarpal) joint

Midcarpal joint

Carpometacarpal joint

Palm

**Hand in flexion**

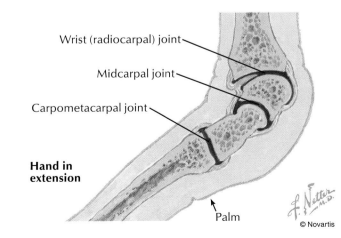

Wrist (radiocarpal) joint

Midcarpal joint

Carpometacarpal joint

**Hand in extension**

Palm

© Novartis

# *Ligaments of Wrist*

## Carpal tunnel: palmar view

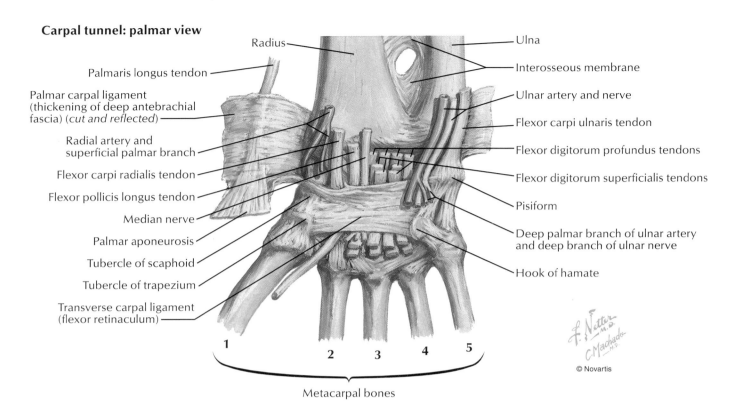

Palmaris longus tendon

Palmar carpal ligament (thickening of deep antebrachial fascia) (*cut and reflected*)

Radial artery and superficial palmar branch

Flexor carpi radialis tendon

Flexor pollicis longus tendon

Median nerve

Palmar aponeurosis

Tubercle of scaphoid

Tubercle of trapezium

Transverse carpal ligament (flexor retinaculum)

Radius

Ulna

Interosseous membrane

Ulnar artery and nerve

Flexor carpi ulnaris tendon

Flexor digitorum profundus tendons

Flexor digitorum superficialis tendons

Pisiform

Deep palmar branch of ulnar artery and deep branch of ulnar nerve

Hook of hamate

1  2  3  4  5

Metacarpal bones

© Novartis

## Flexor retinaculum removed: palmar view

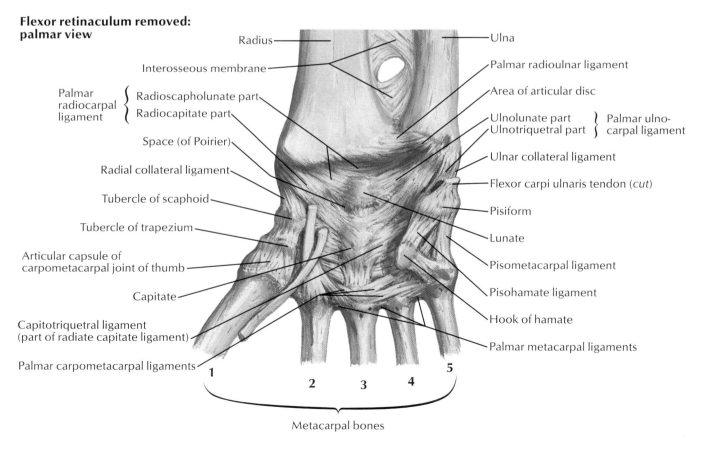

Radius

Interosseous membrane

Palmar radiocarpal ligament
- Radioscapholunate part
- Radiocapitate part

Space (of Poirier)

Radial collateral ligament

Tubercle of scaphoid

Tubercle of trapezium

Articular capsule of carpometacarpal joint of thumb

Capitate

Capitotriquetral ligament (part of radiate capitate ligament)

Palmar carpometacarpal ligaments

Ulna

Palmar radioulnar ligament

Area of articular disc

Ulnolunate part
Ulnotriquetral part
} Palmar ulno-carpal ligament

Ulnar collateral ligament

Flexor carpi ulnaris tendon (*cut*)

Pisiform

Lunate

Pisometacarpal ligament

Pisohamate ligament

Hook of hamate

Palmar metacarpal ligaments

1  2  3  4  5

Metacarpal bones

*PLATE 424*

**UPPER LIMB**

**Posterior (dorsal) view**

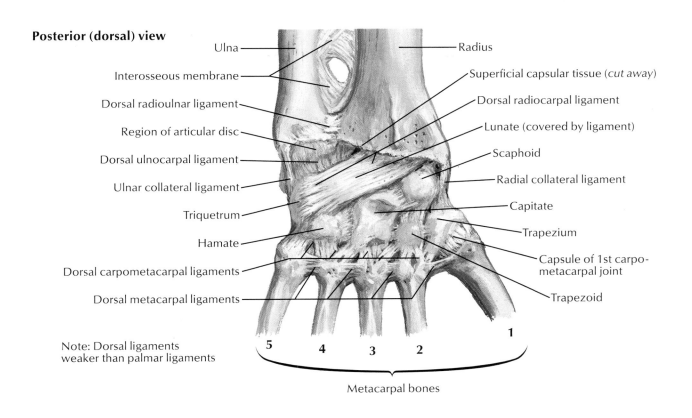

Ulna

Interosseous membrane

Dorsal radioulnar ligament

Region of articular disc

Dorsal ulnocarpal ligament

Ulnar collateral ligament

Triquetrum

Hamate

Dorsal carpometacarpal ligaments

Dorsal metacarpal ligaments

Radius

Superficial capsular tissue (*cut away*)

Dorsal radiocarpal ligament

Lunate (covered by ligament)

Scaphoid

Radial collateral ligament

Capitate

Trapezium

Capsule of 1st carpo-
metacarpal joint

Trapezoid

Note: Dorsal ligaments
weaker than palmar ligaments

5  4  3  2  1

Metacarpal bones

**Coronal section: dorsal view**

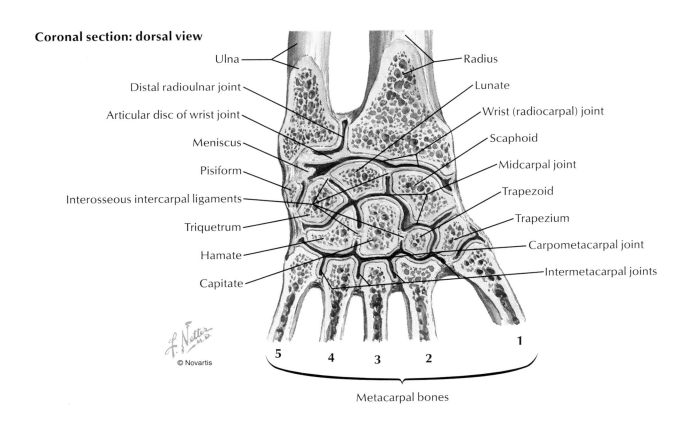

Ulna

Distal radioulnar joint

Articular disc of wrist joint

Meniscus

Pisiform

Interosseous intercarpal ligaments

Triquetrum

Hamate

Capitate

Radius

Lunate

Wrist (radiocarpal) joint

Scaphoid

Midcarpal joint

Trapezoid

Trapezium

Carpometacarpal joint

Intermetacarpal joints

5  4  3  2  1

Metacarpal bones

© Novartis

**WRIST AND HAND**

*PLATE 425*

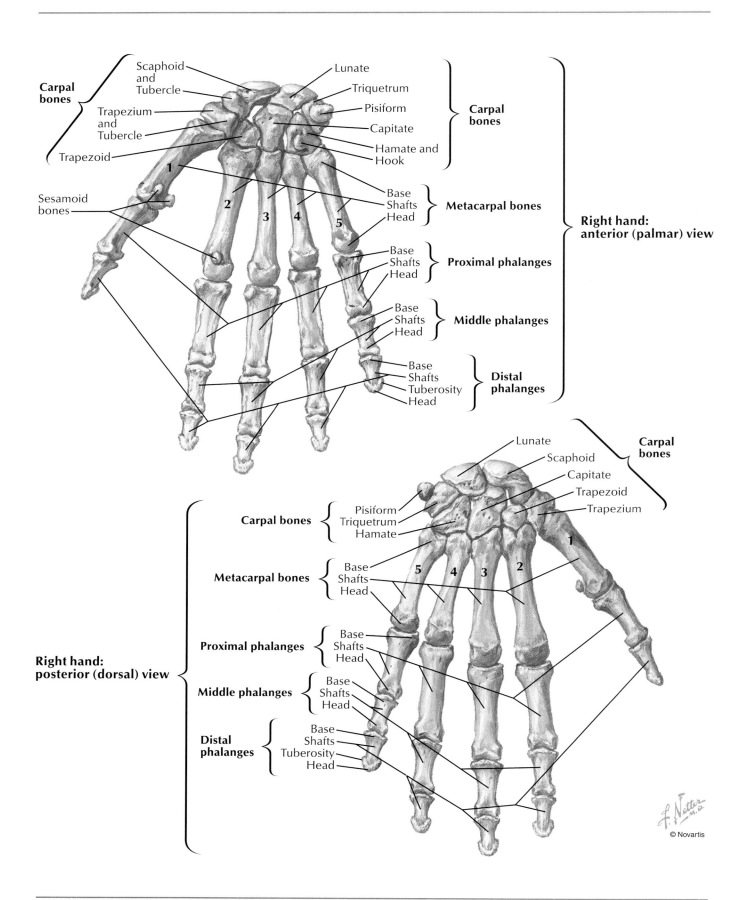

Carpal bones

Scaphoid and Tubercle

Lunate

Trapezium and Tubercle

Triquetrum

Trapezoid

Pisiform

Capitate

Hamate and Hook

Carpal bones

1

2

3

4

5

Sesamoid bones

Base
Shafts
Head — **Metacarpal bones**

Base
Shafts
Head — **Proximal phalanges**

Base
Shafts
Head — **Middle phalanges**

Base
Shafts
Tuberosity
Head — **Distal phalanges**

**Right hand: anterior (palmar) view**

Lunate

Scaphoid

Capitate

Trapezoid

Trapezium

Carpal bones

**Carpal bones**
Pisiform
Triquetrum
Hamate

**Right hand: posterior (dorsal) view**

**Metacarpal bones**
Base
Shafts
Head

5  4  3  2  1

**Proximal phalanges**
Base
Shafts
Head

**Middle phalanges**
Base
Shafts
Head

**Distal phalanges**
Base
Shafts
Tuberosity
Head

© Novartis

**PLATE 426**

**UPPER LIMB**

# Metacarpophalangeal and Interphalangeal Ligaments

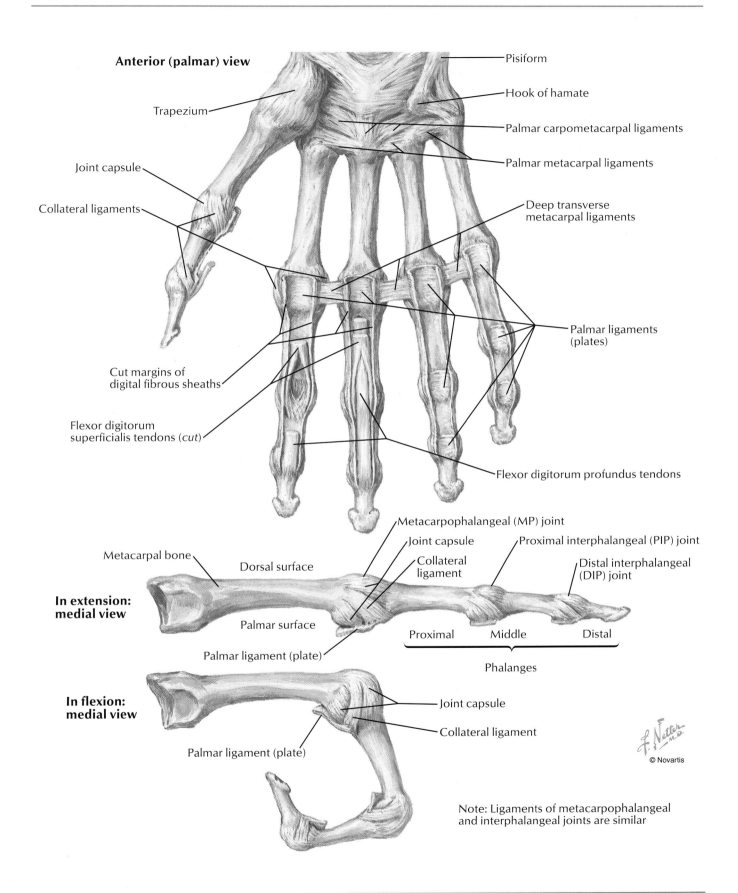

**Anterior (palmar) view**

Pisiform

Hook of hamate

Palmar carpometacarpal ligaments

Palmar metacarpal ligaments

Trapezium

Joint capsule

Collateral ligaments

Deep transverse metacarpal ligaments

Palmar ligaments (plates)

Cut margins of digital fibrous sheaths

Flexor digitorum superficialis tendons (*cut*)

Flexor digitorum profundus tendons

Metacarpophalangeal (MP) joint

Joint capsule

Collateral ligament

Proximal interphalangeal (PIP) joint

Distal interphalangeal (DIP) joint

Metacarpal bone

Dorsal surface

**In extension: medial view**

Palmar surface

Palmar ligament (plate)

Proximal    Middle    Distal

Phalanges

**In flexion: medial view**

Joint capsule

Collateral ligament

Palmar ligament (plate)

Note: Ligaments of metacarpophalangeal and interphalangeal joints are similar

# Wrist and Hand: Superficial Palmar Dissections

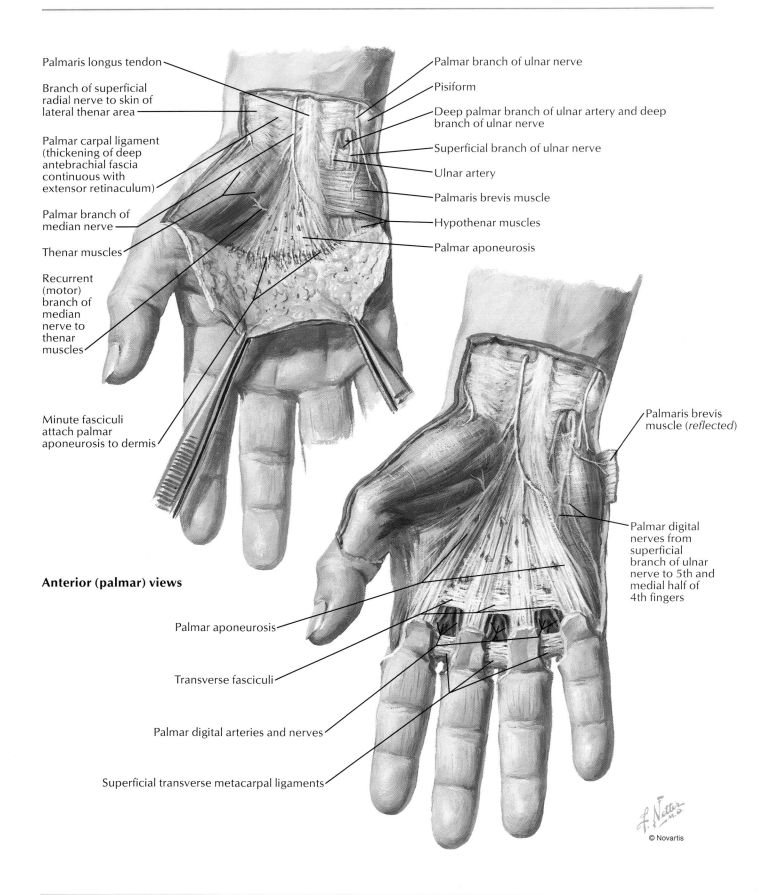

Palmaris longus tendon

Branch of superficial radial nerve to skin of lateral thenar area

Palmar carpal ligament (thickening of deep antebrachial fascia continuous with extensor retinaculum)

Palmar branch of median nerve

Thenar muscles

Recurrent (motor) branch of median nerve to thenar muscles

Minute fasciculi attach palmar aponeurosis to dermis

Palmar branch of ulnar nerve

Pisiform

Deep palmar branch of ulnar artery and deep branch of ulnar nerve

Superficial branch of ulnar nerve

Ulnar artery

Palmaris brevis muscle

Hypothenar muscles

Palmar aponeurosis

Palmaris brevis muscle (reflected)

Palmar digital nerves from superficial branch of ulnar nerve to 5th and medial half of 4th fingers

**Anterior (palmar) views**

Palmar aponeurosis

Transverse fasciculi

Palmar digital arteries and nerves

Superficial transverse metacarpal ligaments

**PLATE 428**

© Novartis

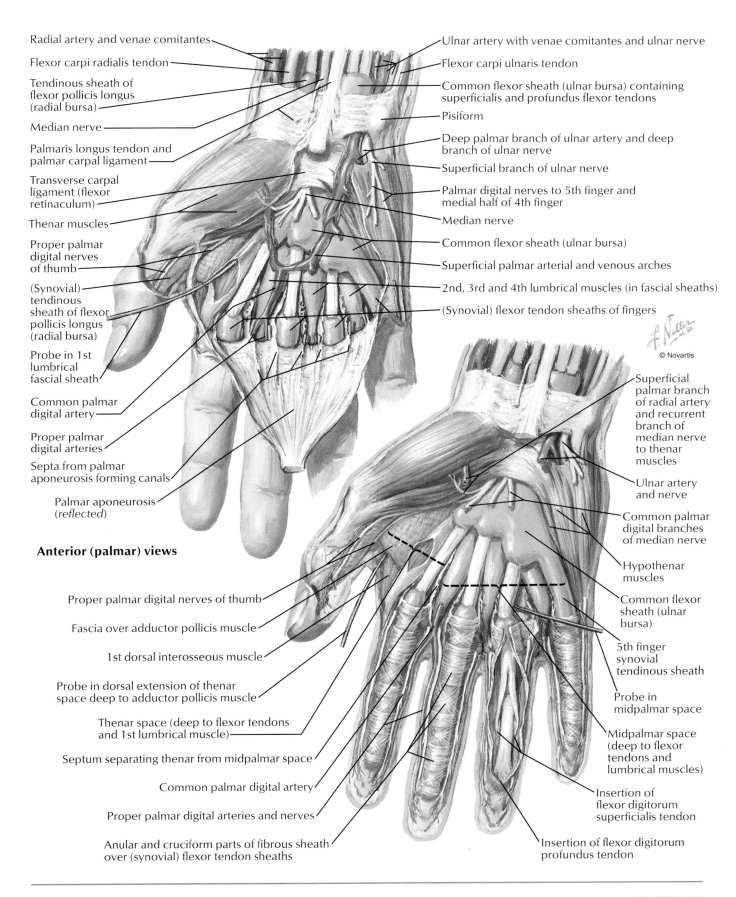

Radial artery and venae comitantes

Flexor carpi radialis tendon

Tendinous sheath of flexor pollicis longus (radial bursa)

Median nerve

Palmaris longus tendon and palmar carpal ligament

Transverse carpal ligament (flexor retinaculum)

Thenar muscles

Proper palmar digital nerves of thumb

(Synovial) tendinous sheath of flexor pollicis longus (radial bursa)

Probe in 1st lumbrical fascial sheath

Common palmar digital artery

Proper palmar digital arteries

Septa from palmar aponeurosis forming canals

Palmar aponeurosis (*reflected*)

**Anterior (palmar) views**

Ulnar artery with venae comitantes and ulnar nerve

Flexor carpi ulnaris tendon

Common flexor sheath (ulnar bursa) containing superficialis and profundus flexor tendons

Pisiform

Deep palmar branch of ulnar artery and deep branch of ulnar nerve

Superficial branch of ulnar nerve

Palmar digital nerves to 5th finger and medial half of 4th finger

Median nerve

Common flexor sheath (ulnar bursa)

Superficial palmar arterial and venous arches

2nd, 3rd and 4th lumbrical muscles (in fascial sheaths)

(Synovial) flexor tendon sheaths of fingers

Superficial palmar branch of radial artery and recurrent branch of median nerve to thenar muscles

Ulnar artery and nerve

Common palmar digital branches of median nerve

Hypothenar muscles

Common flexor sheath (ulnar bursa)

5th finger synovial tendinous sheath

Probe in midpalmar space

Midpalmar space (deep to flexor tendons and lumbrical muscles)

Insertion of flexor digitorum superficialis tendon

Insertion of flexor digitorum profundus tendon

Proper palmar digital nerves of thumb

Fascia over adductor pollicis muscle

1st dorsal interosseous muscle

Probe in dorsal extension of thenar space deep to adductor pollicis muscle

Thenar space (deep to flexor tendons and 1st lumbrical muscle)

Septum separating thenar from midpalmar space

Common palmar digital artery

Proper palmar digital arteries and nerves

Anular and cruciform parts of fibrous sheath over (synovial) flexor tendon sheaths

© Novartis

*f. Netter M.D.*

# Flexor Tendons, Arteries and Nerves at Wrist

**Palmar view**

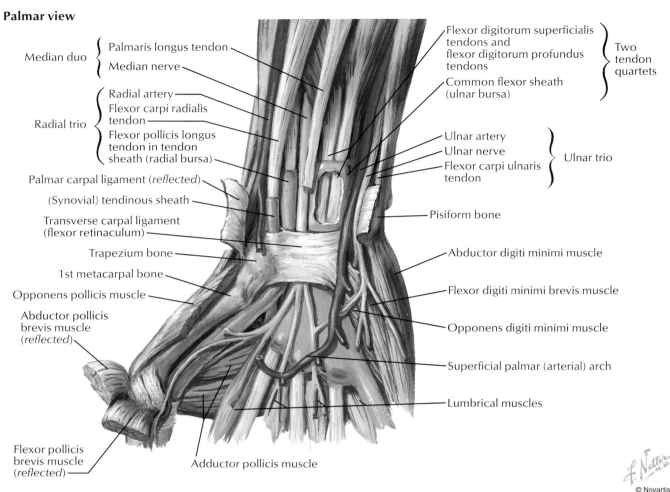

Median duo { Palmaris longus tendon
Median nerve

Radial trio { Radial artery
Flexor carpi radialis tendon
Flexor pollicis longus tendon in tendon sheath (radial bursa)

Palmar carpal ligament (*reflected*)

(Synovial) tendinous sheath

Transverse carpal ligament (flexor retinaculum)

Trapezium bone

1st metacarpal bone

Opponens pollicis muscle

Abductor pollicis brevis muscle (*reflected*)

Flexor pollicis brevis muscle (*reflected*)

Adductor pollicis muscle

Flexor digitorum superficialis tendons and flexor digitorum profundus tendons
Common flexor sheath (ulnar bursa) } Two tendon quartets

Ulnar artery
Ulnar nerve
Flexor carpi ulnaris tendon } Ulnar trio

Pisiform bone

Abductor digiti minimi muscle

Flexor digiti minimi brevis muscle

Opponens digiti minimi muscle

Superficial palmar (arterial) arch

Lumbrical muscles

*F. Netter M.D.*
© Novartis

## Transverse cross section of wrist demonstrating carpal tunnel

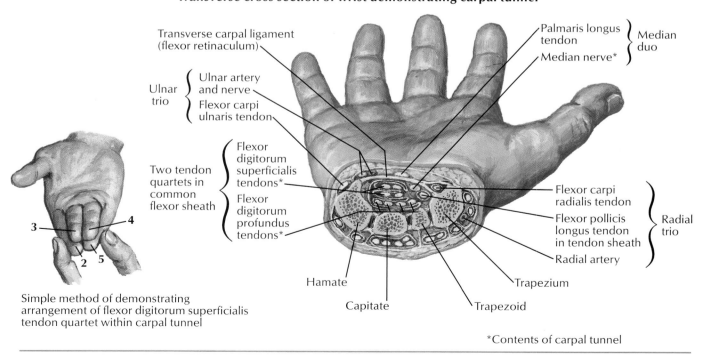

Transverse carpal ligament (flexor retinaculum)

Ulnar trio { Ulnar artery and nerve
Flexor carpi ulnaris tendon

Two tendon quartets in common flexor sheath { Flexor digitorum superficialis tendons*
Flexor digitorum profundus tendons*

3  4
2  5

Simple method of demonstrating arrangement of flexor digitorum superficialis tendon quartet within carpal tunnel

Palmaris longus tendon
Median nerve* } Median duo

Flexor carpi radialis tendon
Flexor pollicis longus tendon in tendon sheath
Radial artery } Radial trio

Hamate
Capitate
Trapezoid
Trapezium

*Contents of carpal tunnel

**PLATE 430**

**UPPER LIMB**

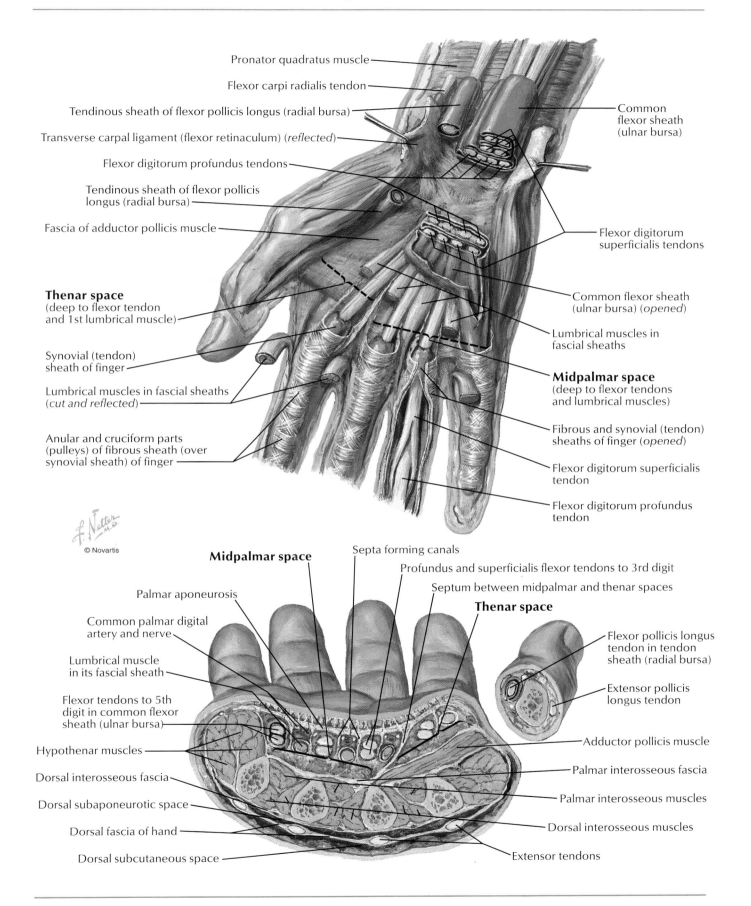

Pronator quadratus muscle

Flexor carpi radialis tendon

Tendinous sheath of flexor pollicis longus (radial bursa)

Transverse carpal ligament (flexor retinaculum) (*reflected*)

Flexor digitorum profundus tendons

Tendinous sheath of flexor pollicis longus (radial bursa)

Fascia of adductor pollicis muscle

**Thenar space**
(deep to flexor tendon
and 1st lumbrical muscle)

Synovial (tendon)
sheath of finger

Lumbrical muscles in fascial sheaths
(*cut and reflected*)

Anular and cruciform parts
(pulleys) of fibrous sheath (over
synovial sheath) of finger

Common
flexor sheath
(ulnar bursa)

Flexor digitorum
superficialis tendons

Common flexor sheath
(ulnar bursa) (*opened*)

Lumbrical muscles in
fascial sheaths

**Midpalmar space**
(deep to flexor tendons
and lumbrical muscles)

Fibrous and synovial (tendon)
sheaths of finger (*opened*)

Flexor digitorum superficialis
tendon

Flexor digitorum profundus
tendon

Septa forming canals

Profundus and superficialis flexor tendons to 3rd digit

Septum between midpalmar and thenar spaces

**Midpalmar space**

Palmar aponeurosis

Common palmar digital
artery and nerve

Lumbrical muscle
in its fascial sheath

Flexor tendons to 5th
digit in common flexor
sheath (ulnar bursa)

Hypothenar muscles

Dorsal interosseous fascia

Dorsal subaponeurotic space

Dorsal fascia of hand

Dorsal subcutaneous space

**Thenar space**

Flexor pollicis longus
tendon in tendon
sheath (radial bursa)

Extensor pollicis
longus tendon

Adductor pollicis muscle

Palmar interosseous fascia

Palmar interosseous muscles

Dorsal interosseous muscles

Extensor tendons

**WRIST AND HAND**

*PLATE 431*

# Lumbrical Muscles and Bursae, Spaces and Sheaths: Schema

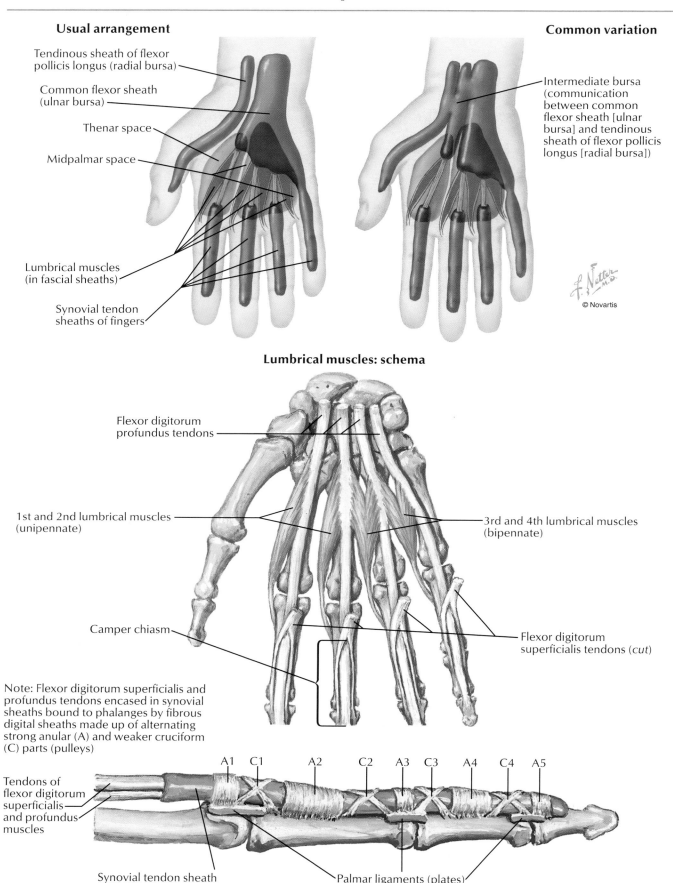

**Usual arrangement**

Tendinous sheath of flexor pollicis longus (radial bursa)

Common flexor sheath (ulnar bursa)

Thenar space

Midpalmar space

Lumbrical muscles (in fascial sheaths)

Synovial tendon sheaths of fingers

**Common variation**

Intermediate bursa (communication between common flexor sheath [ulnar bursa] and tendinous sheath of flexor pollicis longus [radial bursa])

© Novartis

**Lumbrical muscles: schema**

Flexor digitorum profundus tendons

1st and 2nd lumbrical muscles (unipennate)

Camper chiasm

3rd and 4th lumbrical muscles (bipennate)

Flexor digitorum superficialis tendons (*cut*)

Note: Flexor digitorum superficialis and profundus tendons encased in synovial sheaths bound to phalanges by fibrous digital sheaths made up of alternating strong anular (A) and weaker cruciform (C) parts (pulleys)

A1  C1  A2  C2  A3  C3  A4  C4  A5

Tendons of flexor digitorum superficialis and profundus muscles

Synovial tendon sheath

Palmar ligaments (plates)

**PLATE 432**

**UPPER LIMB**

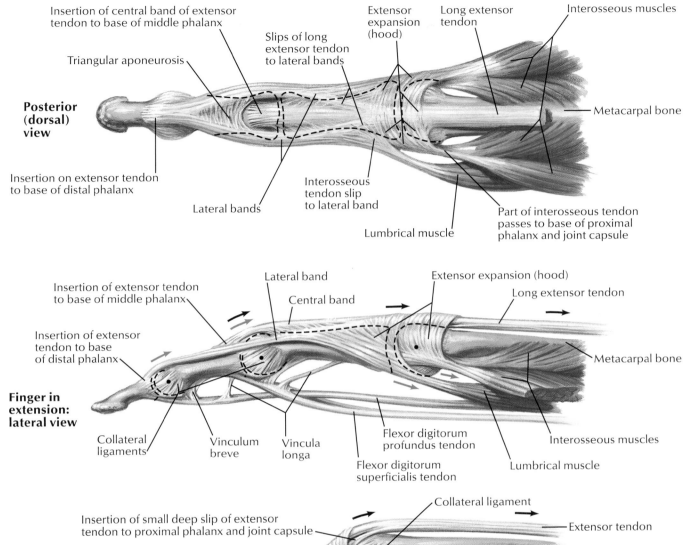

**Posterior (dorsal) view**

Insertion of central band of extensor tendon to base of middle phalanx

Triangular aponeurosis

Slips of long extensor tendon to lateral bands

Extensor expansion (hood)

Long extensor tendon

Interosseous muscles

Metacarpal bone

Insertion on extensor tendon to base of distal phalanx

Lateral bands

Interosseous tendon slip to lateral band

Lumbrical muscle

Part of interosseous tendon passes to base of proximal phalanx and joint capsule

**Finger in extension: lateral view**

Insertion of extensor tendon to base of middle phalanx

Insertion of extensor tendon to base of distal phalanx

Lateral band

Central band

Extensor expansion (hood)

Long extensor tendon

Metacarpal bone

Collateral ligaments

Vinculum breve

Vincula longa

Flexor digitorum profundus tendon

Flexor digitorum superficialis tendon

Interosseous muscles

Lumbrical muscle

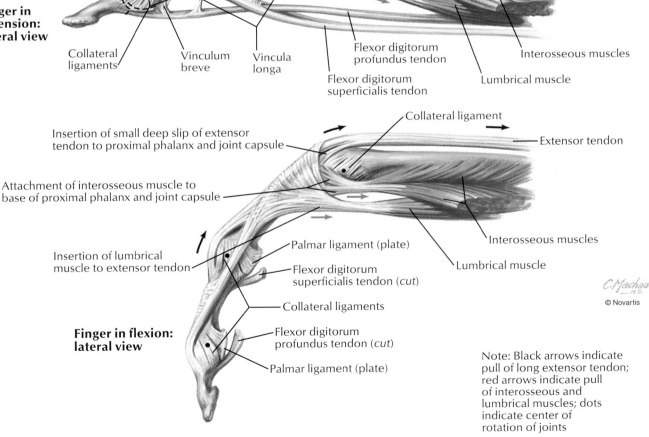

**Finger in flexion: lateral view**

Insertion of small deep slip of extensor tendon to proximal phalanx and joint capsule

Attachment of interosseous muscle to base of proximal phalanx and joint capsule

Insertion of lumbrical muscle to extensor tendon

Collateral ligament

Extensor tendon

Palmar ligament (plate)

Flexor digitorum superficialis tendon (*cut*)

Collateral ligaments

Flexor digitorum profundus tendon (*cut*)

Palmar ligament (plate)

Interosseous muscles

Lumbrical muscle

C. Machado
—M.D.
© Novartis

Note: Black arrows indicate pull of long extensor tendon; red arrows indicate pull of interosseous and lumbrical muscles; dots indicate center of rotation of joints

---

# Intrinsic Muscles of Hand

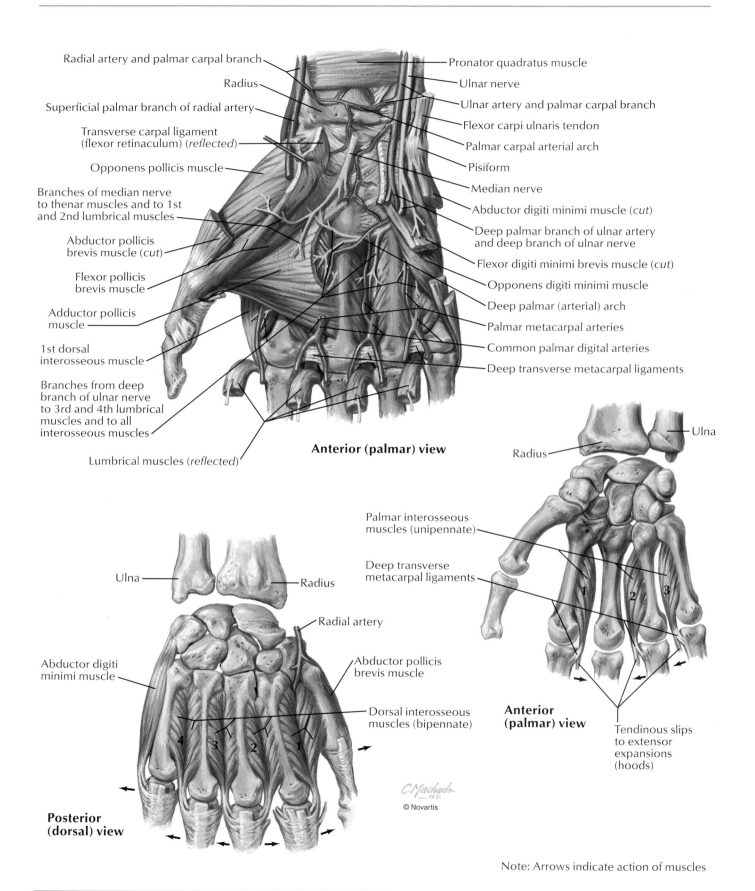

Radial artery and palmar carpal branch

Radius

Superficial palmar branch of radial artery

Transverse carpal ligament (flexor retinaculum) *(reflected)*

Opponens pollicis muscle

Branches of median nerve to thenar muscles and to 1st and 2nd lumbrical muscles

Abductor pollicis brevis muscle *(cut)*

Flexor pollicis brevis muscle

Adductor pollicis muscle

1st dorsal interosseous muscle

Branches from deep branch of ulnar nerve to 3rd and 4th lumbrical muscles and to all interosseous muscles

Lumbrical muscles *(reflected)*

Pronator quadratus muscle

Ulnar nerve

Ulnar artery and palmar carpal branch

Flexor carpi ulnaris tendon

Palmar carpal arterial arch

Pisiform

Median nerve

Abductor digiti minimi muscle *(cut)*

Deep palmar branch of ulnar artery and deep branch of ulnar nerve

Flexor digiti minimi brevis muscle *(cut)*

Opponens digiti minimi muscle

Deep palmar (arterial) arch

Palmar metacarpal arteries

Common palmar digital arteries

Deep transverse metacarpal ligaments

**Anterior (palmar) view**

Palmar interosseous muscles (unipennate)

Deep transverse metacarpal ligaments

Ulna

Radius

**Anterior (palmar) view**

Tendinous slips to extensor expansions (hoods)

Ulna

Radius

Radial artery

Abductor pollicis brevis muscle

Abductor digiti minimi muscle

Dorsal interosseous muscles (bipennate)

**Posterior (dorsal) view**

C. Machado
M.D.
© Novartis

Note: Arrows indicate action of muscles

**PLATE 434**

**UPPER LIMB**

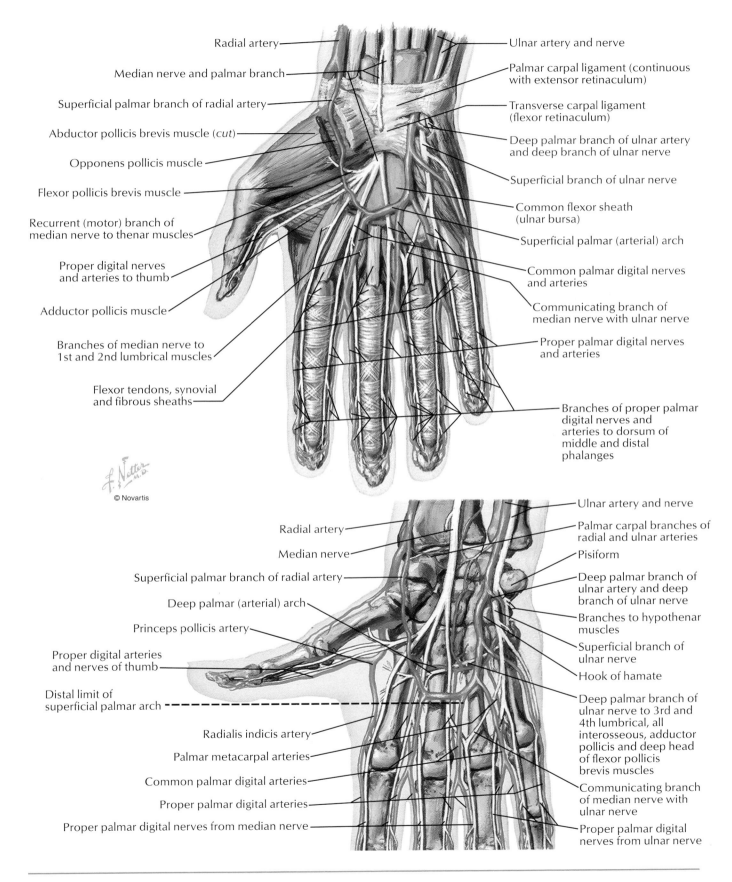

Radial artery

Median nerve and palmar branch

Superficial palmar branch of radial artery

Abductor pollicis brevis muscle (cut)

Opponens pollicis muscle

Flexor pollicis brevis muscle

Recurrent (motor) branch of median nerve to thenar muscles

Proper digital nerves and arteries to thumb

Adductor pollicis muscle

Branches of median nerve to 1st and 2nd lumbrical muscles

Flexor tendons, synovial and fibrous sheaths

© Novartis

Ulnar artery and nerve

Palmar carpal ligament (continuous with extensor retinaculum)

Transverse carpal ligament (flexor retinaculum)

Deep palmar branch of ulnar artery and deep branch of ulnar nerve

Superficial branch of ulnar nerve

Common flexor sheath (ulnar bursa)

Superficial palmar (arterial) arch

Common palmar digital nerves and arteries

Communicating branch of median nerve with ulnar nerve

Proper palmar digital nerves and arteries

Branches of proper palmar digital nerves and arteries to dorsum of middle and distal phalanges

Radial artery

Median nerve

Superficial palmar branch of radial artery

Deep palmar (arterial) arch

Princeps pollicis artery

Proper digital arteries and nerves of thumb

Distal limit of superficial palmar arch

Radialis indicis artery

Palmar metacarpal arteries

Common palmar digital arteries

Proper palmar digital arteries

Proper palmar digital nerves from median nerve

Ulnar artery and nerve

Palmar carpal branches of radial and ulnar arteries

Pisiform

Deep palmar branch of ulnar artery and deep branch of ulnar nerve

Branches to hypothenar muscles

Superficial branch of ulnar nerve

Hook of hamate

Deep palmar branch of ulnar nerve to 3rd and 4th lumbrical, all interosseous, adductor pollicis and deep head of flexor pollicis brevis muscles

Communicating branch of median nerve with ulnar nerve

Proper palmar digital nerves from ulnar nerve

**WRIST AND HAND**

*PLATE 435*

**Lateral (radial) view**

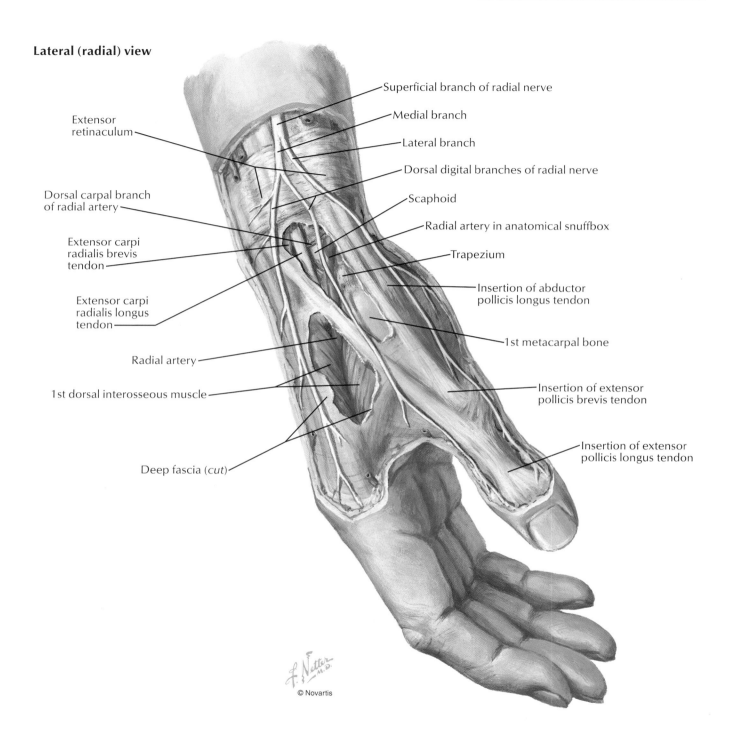

Extensor retinaculum

Dorsal carpal branch of radial artery

Extensor carpi radialis brevis tendon

Extensor carpi radialis longus tendon

Radial artery

1st dorsal interosseous muscle

Deep fascia (*cut*)

Superficial branch of radial nerve

Medial branch

Lateral branch

Dorsal digital branches of radial nerve

Scaphoid

Radial artery in anatomical snuffbox

Trapezium

Insertion of abductor pollicis longus tendon

1st metacarpal bone

Insertion of extensor pollicis brevis tendon

Insertion of extensor pollicis longus tendon

© Novartis

**PLATE 436**

**UPPER LIMB**

**Posterior (dorsal) view**

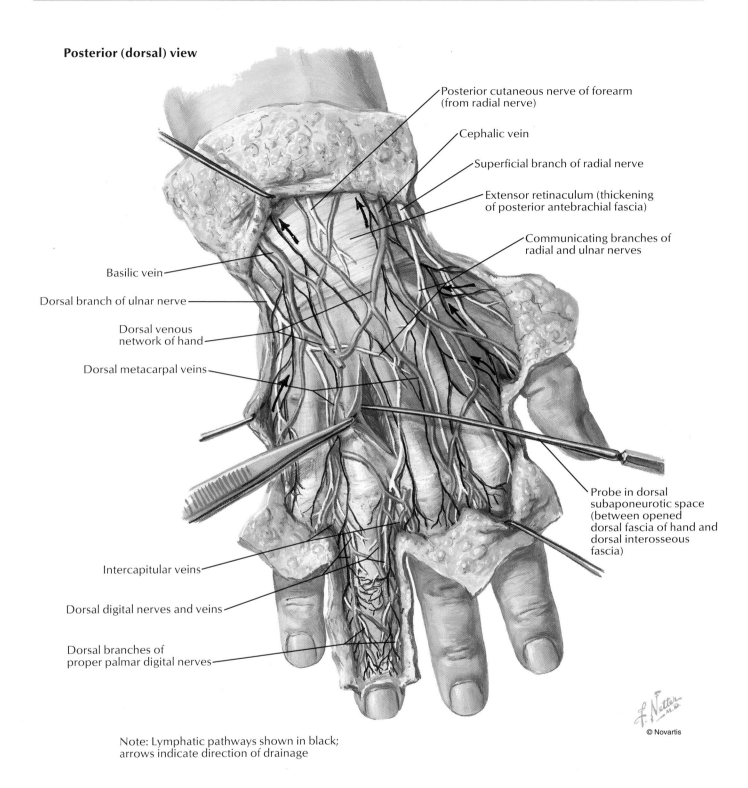

Posterior cutaneous nerve of forearm (from radial nerve)

Cephalic vein

Superficial branch of radial nerve

Extensor retinaculum (thickening of posterior antebrachial fascia)

Communicating branches of radial and ulnar nerves

Basilic vein

Dorsal branch of ulnar nerve

Dorsal venous network of hand

Dorsal metacarpal veins

Probe in dorsal subaponeurotic space (between opened dorsal fascia of hand and dorsal interosseous fascia)

Intercapitular veins

Dorsal digital nerves and veins

Dorsal branches of proper palmar digital nerves

Note: Lymphatic pathways shown in black; arrows indicate direction of drainage

© Novartis

# *Wrist and Hand: Deep Dorsal Dissection*

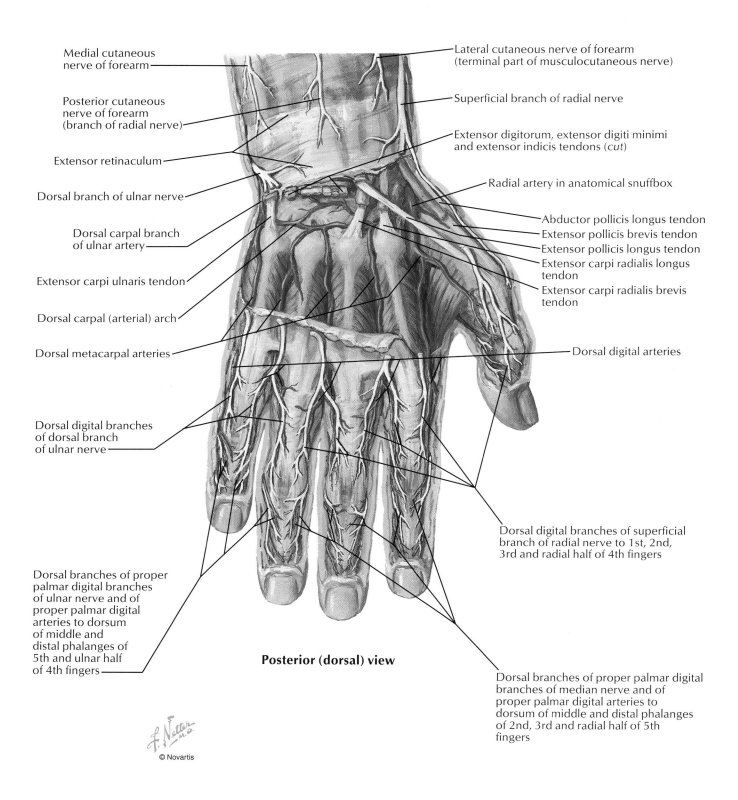

Medial cutaneous nerve of forearm

Posterior cutaneous nerve of forearm (branch of radial nerve)

Extensor retinaculum

Dorsal branch of ulnar nerve

Dorsal carpal branch of ulnar artery

Extensor carpi ulnaris tendon

Dorsal carpal (arterial) arch

Dorsal metacarpal arteries

Dorsal digital branches of dorsal branch of ulnar nerve

Dorsal branches of proper palmar digital branches of ulnar nerve and of proper palmar digital arteries to dorsum of middle and distal phalanges of 5th and ulnar half of 4th fingers

Lateral cutaneous nerve of forearm (terminal part of musculocutaneous nerve)

Superficial branch of radial nerve

Extensor digitorum, extensor digiti minimi and extensor indicis tendons (*cut*)

Radial artery in anatomical snuffbox

Abductor pollicis longus tendon
Extensor pollicis brevis tendon
Extensor pollicis longus tendon
Extensor carpi radialis longus tendon
Extensor carpi radialis brevis tendon

Dorsal digital arteries

Dorsal digital branches of superficial branch of radial nerve to 1st, 2nd, 3rd and radial half of 4th fingers

**Posterior (dorsal) view**

Dorsal branches of proper palmar digital branches of median nerve and of proper palmar digital arteries to dorsum of middle and distal phalanges of 2nd, 3rd and radial half of 5th fingers

© Novartis

**PLATE 438**

**UPPER LIMB**

**Posterior (dorsal) view**

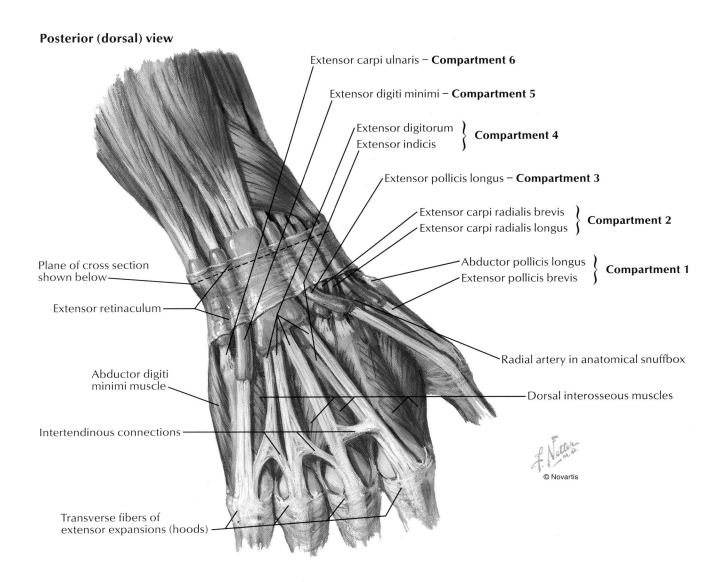

Extensor carpi ulnaris – **Compartment 6**

Extensor digiti minimi – **Compartment 5**

Extensor digitorum
Extensor indicis
} **Compartment 4**

Extensor pollicis longus – **Compartment 3**

Extensor carpi radialis brevis
Extensor carpi radialis longus
} **Compartment 2**

Abductor pollicis longus
Extensor pollicis brevis
} **Compartment 1**

Plane of cross section shown below

Extensor retinaculum

Abductor digiti minimi muscle

Intertendinous connections

Transverse fibers of extensor expansions (hoods)

Radial artery in anatomical snuffbox

Dorsal interosseous muscles

**Cross section of most distal portion of forearm**

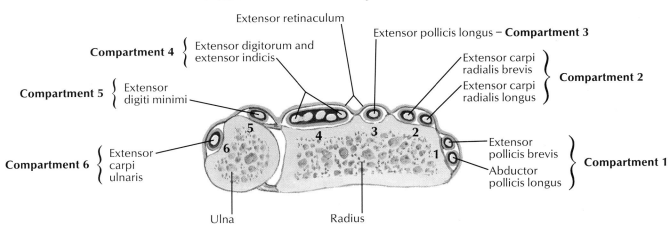

Extensor retinaculum

Extensor pollicis longus – **Compartment 3**

**Compartment 4** { Extensor digitorum and extensor indicis

**Compartment 5** { Extensor digiti minimi

**Compartment 6** { Extensor carpi ulnaris

Extensor carpi radialis brevis
Extensor carpi radialis longus
} **Compartment 2**

Extensor pollicis brevis
Abductor pollicis longus
} **Compartment 1**

Ulna

Radius

# Fingers

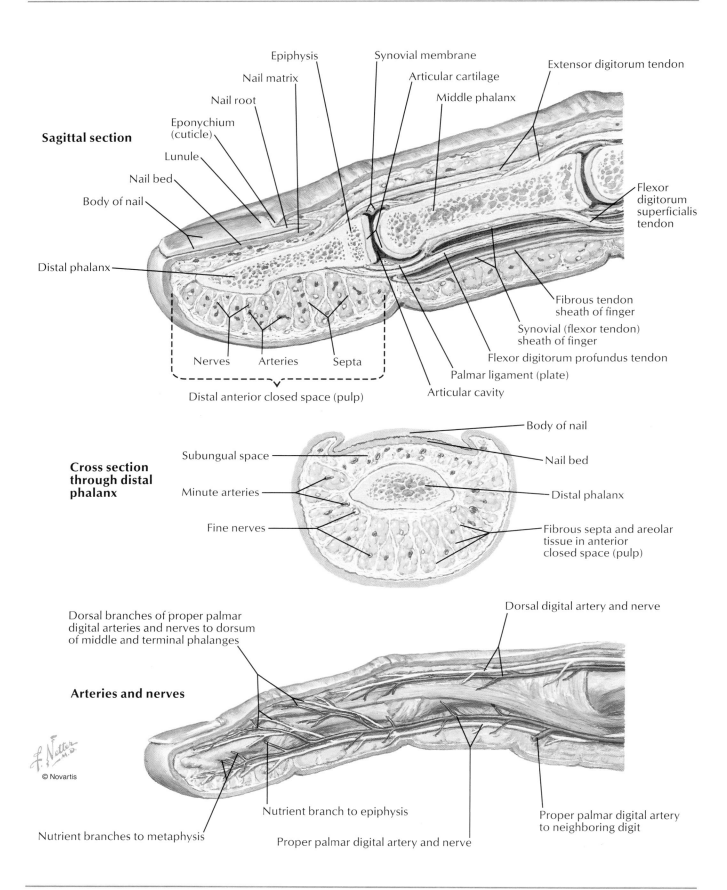

**Sagittal section**

Epiphysis

Nail matrix

Nail root

Eponychium (cuticle)

Lunule

Nail bed

Body of nail

Distal phalanx

Synovial membrane

Articular cartilage

Middle phalanx

Extensor digitorum tendon

Flexor digitorum superficialis tendon

Fibrous tendon sheath of finger

Synovial (flexor tendon) sheath of finger

Flexor digitorum profundus tendon

Palmar ligament (plate)

Articular cavity

Nerves     Arteries     Septa

Distal anterior closed space (pulp)

**Cross section through distal phalanx**

Subungual space

Minute arteries

Fine nerves

Body of nail

Nail bed

Distal phalanx

Fibrous septa and areolar tissue in anterior closed space (pulp)

**Arteries and nerves**

Dorsal branches of proper palmar digital arteries and nerves to dorsum of middle and terminal phalanges

Dorsal digital artery and nerve

Nutrient branches to metaphysis

Nutrient branch to epiphysis

Proper palmar digital artery and nerve

Proper palmar digital artery to neighboring digit

© Novartis

**PLATE 440**

**UPPER LIMB**

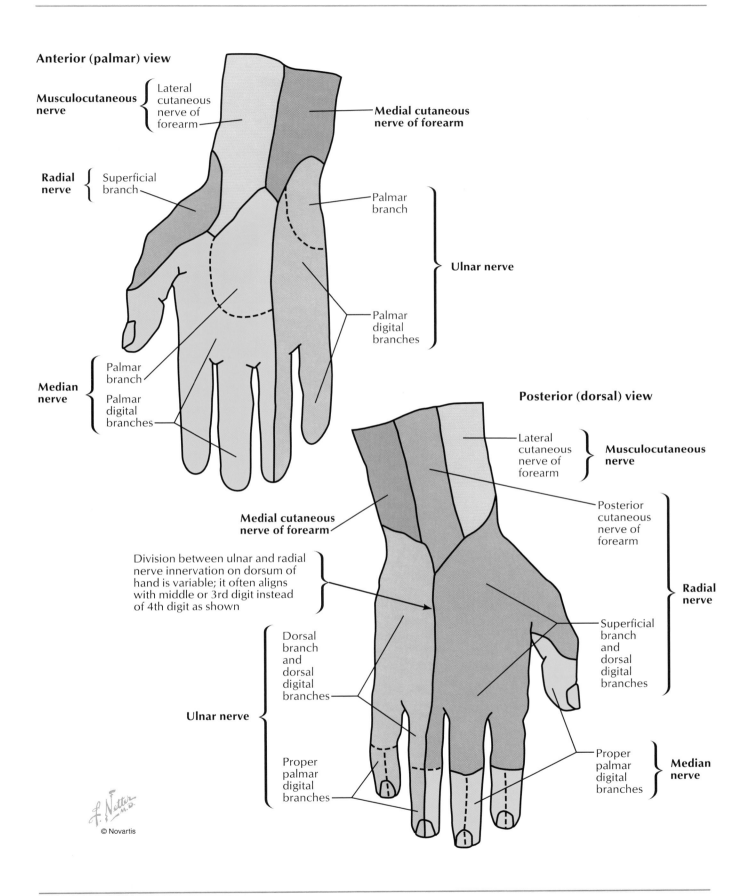

**Anterior (palmar) view**

**Musculocutaneous nerve** — Lateral cutaneous nerve of forearm

**Medial cutaneous nerve of forearm**

**Radial nerve** — Superficial branch

Palmar branch

**Ulnar nerve**

Palmar digital branches

**Median nerve** — Palmar branch

Palmar digital branches

**Posterior (dorsal) view**

Lateral cutaneous nerve of forearm — **Musculocutaneous nerve**

Posterior cutaneous nerve of forearm

**Medial cutaneous nerve of forearm**

**Radial nerve**

Division between ulnar and radial nerve innervation on dorsum of hand is variable; it often aligns with middle or 3rd digit instead of 4th digit as shown

**Ulnar nerve** — Dorsal branch and dorsal digital branches

Superficial branch and dorsal digital branches

Proper palmar digital branches

Proper palmar digital branches — **Median nerve**

© Novartis

# Arteries and Nerves of Upper Limb

**Anterior view**

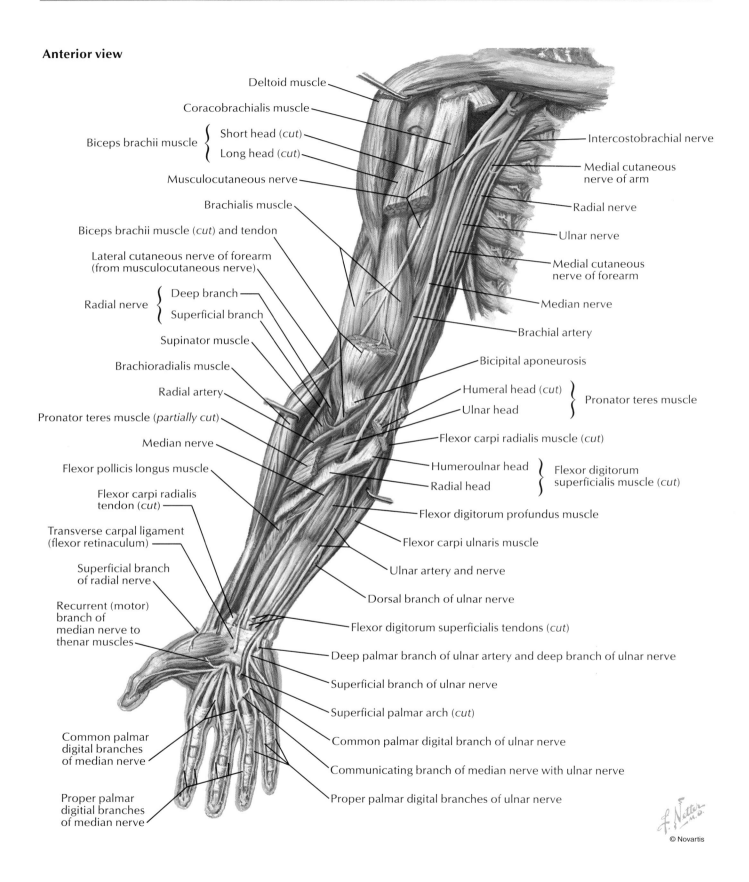

Deltoid muscle

Coracobrachialis muscle

Biceps brachii muscle { Short head (*cut*)
Long head (*cut*)

Musculocutaneous nerve

Brachialis muscle

Biceps brachii muscle (*cut*) and tendon

Lateral cutaneous nerve of forearm
(from musculocutaneous nerve)

Radial nerve { Deep branch
Superficial branch

Supinator muscle

Brachioradialis muscle

Radial artery

Pronator teres muscle (*partially cut*)

Median nerve

Flexor pollicis longus muscle

Flexor carpi radialis
tendon (*cut*)

Transverse carpal ligament
(flexor retinaculum)

Superficial branch
of radial nerve

Recurrent (motor)
branch of
median nerve to
thenar muscles

Common palmar
digital branches
of median nerve

Proper palmar
digitial branches
of median nerve

Intercostobrachial nerve

Medial cutaneous
nerve of arm

Radial nerve

Ulnar nerve

Medial cutaneous
nerve of forearm

Median nerve

Brachial artery

Bicipital aponeurosis

Humeral head (*cut*) }
Ulnar head } Pronator teres muscle

Flexor carpi radialis muscle (*cut*)

Humeroulnar head }
Radial head } Flexor digitorum superficialis muscle (*cut*)

Flexor digitorum profundus muscle

Flexor carpi ulnaris muscle

Ulnar artery and nerve

Dorsal branch of ulnar nerve

Flexor digitorum superficialis tendons (*cut*)

Deep palmar branch of ulnar artery and deep branch of ulnar nerve

Superficial branch of ulnar nerve

Superficial palmar arch (*cut*)

Common palmar digital branch of ulnar nerve

Communicating branch of median nerve with ulnar nerve

Proper palmar digital branches of ulnar nerve

© Novartis

**PLATE 442**

**UPPER LIMB**

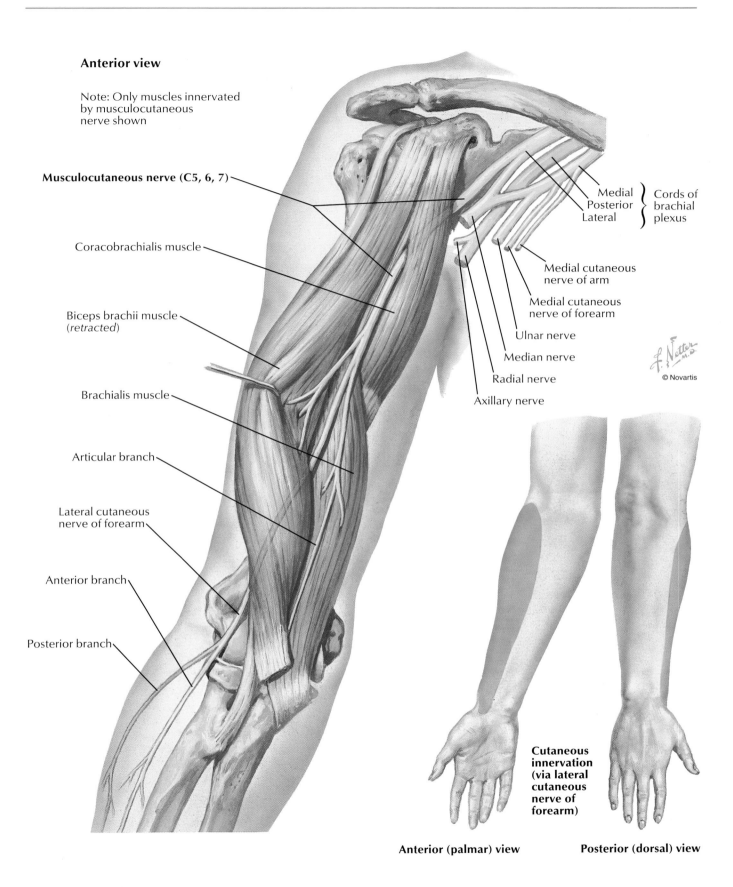

**Anterior view**

Note: Only muscles innervated by musculocutaneous nerve shown

**Musculocutaneous nerve (C5, 6, 7)**

Coracobrachialis muscle

Biceps brachii muscle (*retracted*)

Brachialis muscle

Articular branch

Lateral cutaneous nerve of forearm

Anterior branch

Posterior branch

Medial  
Posterior  } Cords of  
Lateral    } brachial plexus

Medial cutaneous nerve of arm

Medial cutaneous nerve of forearm

Ulnar nerve

Median nerve

Radial nerve

Axillary nerve

**Cutaneous innervation (via lateral cutaneous nerve of forearm)**

Anterior (palmar) view

Posterior (dorsal) view

**Anterior view**

Note: Only muscles innervated by median nerve shown

Musculocutaneous nerve

**Median nerve (C5, 6, 7, 8, T1)**

**Inconstant contribution**

Pronator teres muscle (humeral head)

Articular branch

Flexor carpi radialis muscle

Palmaris longus muscle

Pronator teres muscle (ulnar head)

Flexor digitorum superficialis muscle
(*turned up*)

Flexor digitorum profundus muscle
(lateral part supplied by median
[anterior interosseous] nerve;
medial part supplied by ulnar nerve)

Anterior interosseous nerve

Flexor pollicis longus muscle

Pronator quadratus muscle

Palmar branch of median nerve

Thenar
muscles
{
Abductor pollicis brevis
Opponens pollicis
Superficial head of
flexor pollicis brevis
(deep head
supplied by
ulnar nerve)

1st and 2nd
lumbrical muscles

Dorsal branches to
dorsum of middle and
distal phalanges

Medial
Posterior
Lateral
} Cords of
brachial
plexus

Medial cutaneous
nerve of arm

Medial cutaneous
nerve of forearm

Axillary nerve

Radial nerve

Ulnar nerve

*f. Netter*
*M.D.*
© Novartis

Communicating branch
of median nerve with
ulnar nerve

Common palmar
digital nerves

Proper palmar
digital nerves

**Cutaneous
innervation**

**Palmar view**

**Posterior (dorsal) view**

*PLATE 444*

**UPPER LIMB**

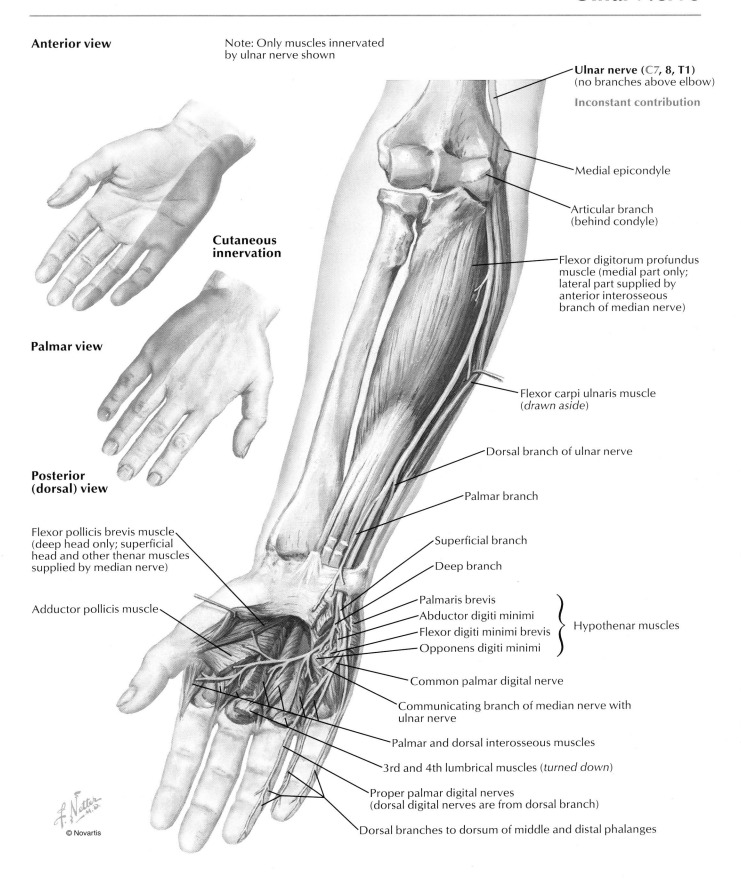

**Anterior view**

Note: Only muscles innervated
by ulnar nerve shown

**Ulnar nerve (C7, 8, T1)**
(no branches above elbow)

Inconstant contribution

Medial epicondyle

Articular branch
(behind condyle)

Flexor digitorum profundus
muscle (medial part only;
lateral part supplied by
anterior interosseous
branch of median nerve)

Flexor carpi ulnaris muscle
(*drawn aside*)

Dorsal branch of ulnar nerve

Palmar branch

Superficial branch

Deep branch

Palmaris brevis
Abductor digiti minimi
Flexor digiti minimi brevis
Opponens digiti minimi
} Hypothenar muscles

Common palmar digital nerve

Communicating branch of median nerve with
ulnar nerve

Palmar and dorsal interosseous muscles

3rd and 4th lumbrical muscles (*turned down*)

Proper palmar digital nerves
(dorsal digital nerves are from dorsal branch)

Dorsal branches to dorsum of middle and distal phalanges

**Cutaneous
innervation**

**Palmar view**

**Posterior
(dorsal) view**

Flexor pollicis brevis muscle
(deep head only; superficial
head and other thenar muscles
supplied by median nerve)

Adductor pollicis muscle

© Novartis

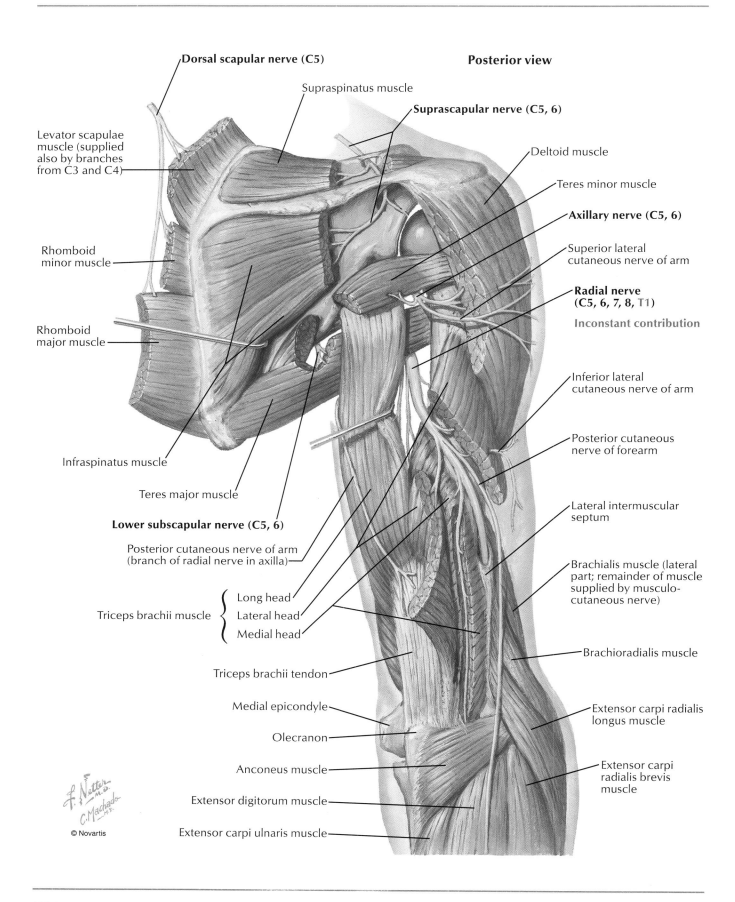

**Posterior view**

Dorsal scapular nerve (C5)

Supraspinatus muscle

**Suprascapular nerve (C5, 6)**

Levator scapulae muscle (supplied also by branches from C3 and C4)

Deltoid muscle

Teres minor muscle

**Axillary nerve (C5, 6)**

Superior lateral cutaneous nerve of arm

Rhomboid minor muscle

**Radial nerve (C5, 6, 7, 8, T1)**

Inconstant contribution

Rhomboid major muscle

Inferior lateral cutaneous nerve of arm

Posterior cutaneous nerve of forearm

Infraspinatus muscle

Teres major muscle

**Lower subscapular nerve (C5, 6)**

Lateral intermuscular septum

Posterior cutaneous nerve of arm (branch of radial nerve in axilla)

Brachialis muscle (lateral part; remainder of muscle supplied by musculocutaneous nerve)

Long head

Lateral head

Medial head

Triceps brachii muscle

Brachioradialis muscle

Triceps brachii tendon

Medial epicondyle

Extensor carpi radialis longus muscle

Olecranon

Anconeus muscle

Extensor carpi radialis brevis muscle

Extensor digitorum muscle

Extensor carpi ulnaris muscle

F. Netter M.D.
C. Machado M.D.

© Novartis

**PLATE 446**

**UPPER LIMB**

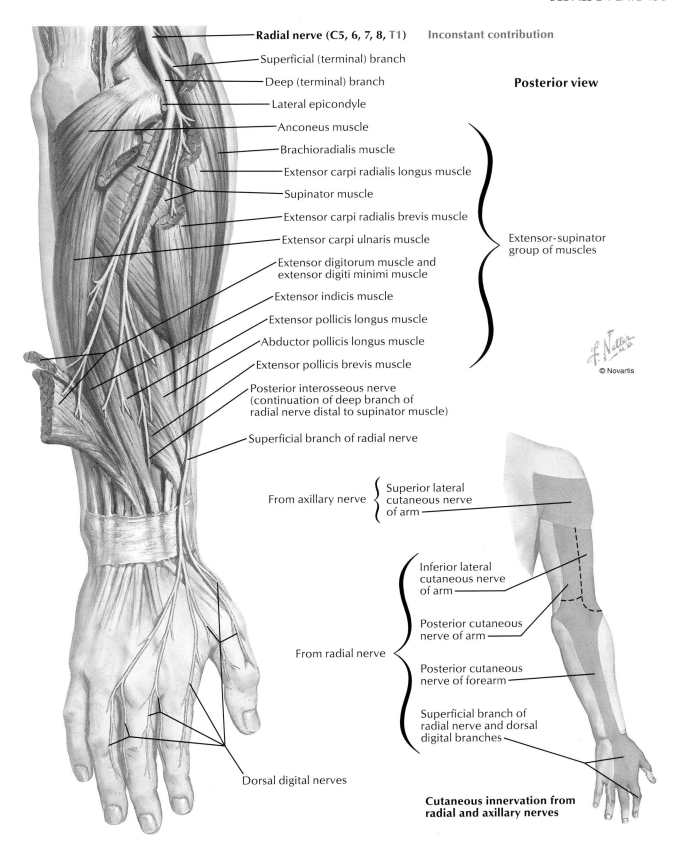

**Radial nerve (C5, 6, 7, 8, T1)**   Inconstant contribution

Superficial (terminal) branch

Deep (terminal) branch

**Posterior view**

Lateral epicondyle

Anconeus muscle

Brachioradialis muscle

Extensor carpi radialis longus muscle

Supinator muscle

Extensor carpi radialis brevis muscle

Extensor carpi ulnaris muscle

Extensor-supinator group of muscles

Extensor digitorum muscle and extensor digiti minimi muscle

Extensor indicis muscle

Extensor pollicis longus muscle

Abductor pollicis longus muscle

Extensor pollicis brevis muscle

Posterior interosseous nerve (continuation of deep branch of radial nerve distal to supinator muscle)

Superficial branch of radial nerve

From axillary nerve { Superior lateral cutaneous nerve of arm

Inferior lateral cutaneous nerve of arm

Posterior cutaneous nerve of arm

From radial nerve

Posterior cutaneous nerve of forearm

Superficial branch of radial nerve and dorsal digital branches

Dorsal digital nerves

**Cutaneous innervation from radial and axillary nerves**

© Novartis

# Cutaneous Nerves and Superficial Veins of Shoulder and Arm

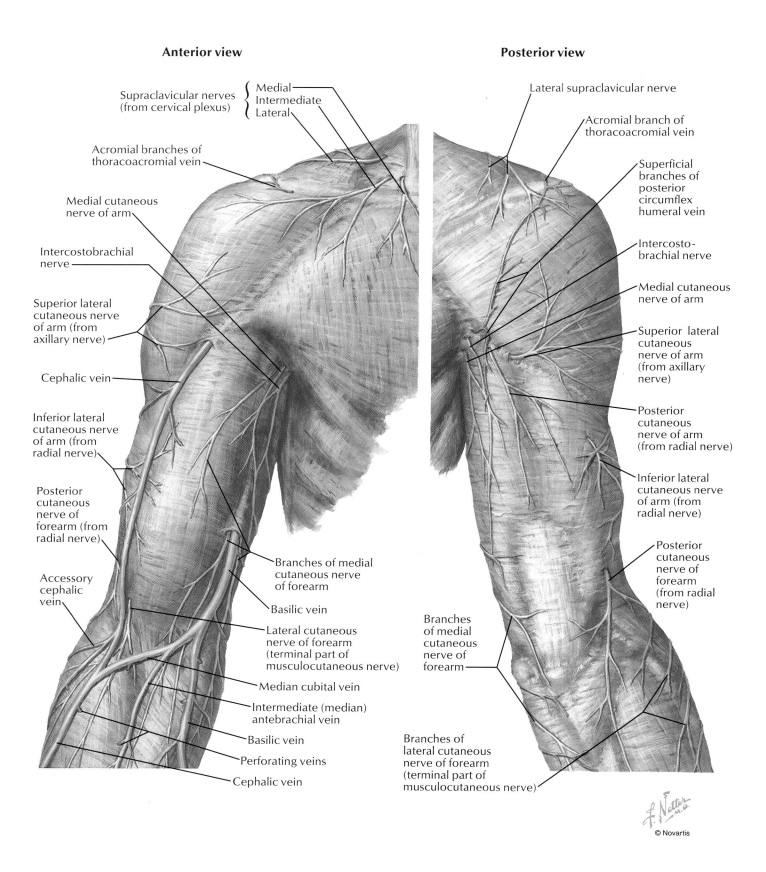

**Anterior view**

Supraclavicular nerves (from cervical plexus)
{ Medial / Intermediate / Lateral }

Acromial branches of thoracoacromial vein

Medial cutaneous nerve of arm

Intercostobrachial nerve

Superior lateral cutaneous nerve of arm (from axillary nerve)

Cephalic vein

Inferior lateral cutaneous nerve of arm (from radial nerve)

Posterior cutaneous nerve of forearm (from radial nerve)

Accessory cephalic vein

Branches of medial cutaneous nerve of forearm

Basilic vein

Lateral cutaneous nerve of forearm (terminal part of musculocutaneous nerve)

Median cubital vein

Intermediate (median) antebrachial vein

Basilic vein

Perforating veins

Cephalic vein

**Posterior view**

Lateral supraclavicular nerve

Acromial branch of thoracoacromial vein

Superficial branches of posterior circumflex humeral vein

Intercosto-brachial nerve

Medial cutaneous nerve of arm

Superior lateral cutaneous nerve of arm (from axillary nerve)

Posterior cutaneous nerve of arm (from radial nerve)

Inferior lateral cutaneous nerve of arm (from radial nerve)

Posterior cutaneous nerve of forearm (from radial nerve)

Branches of medial cutaneous nerve of forearm

Branches of lateral cutaneous nerve of forearm (terminal part of musculocutaneous nerve)

© Novartis

*PLATE 448*

**UPPER LIMB**

**Anterior (palmar) view**

**Posterior (dorsal) view**

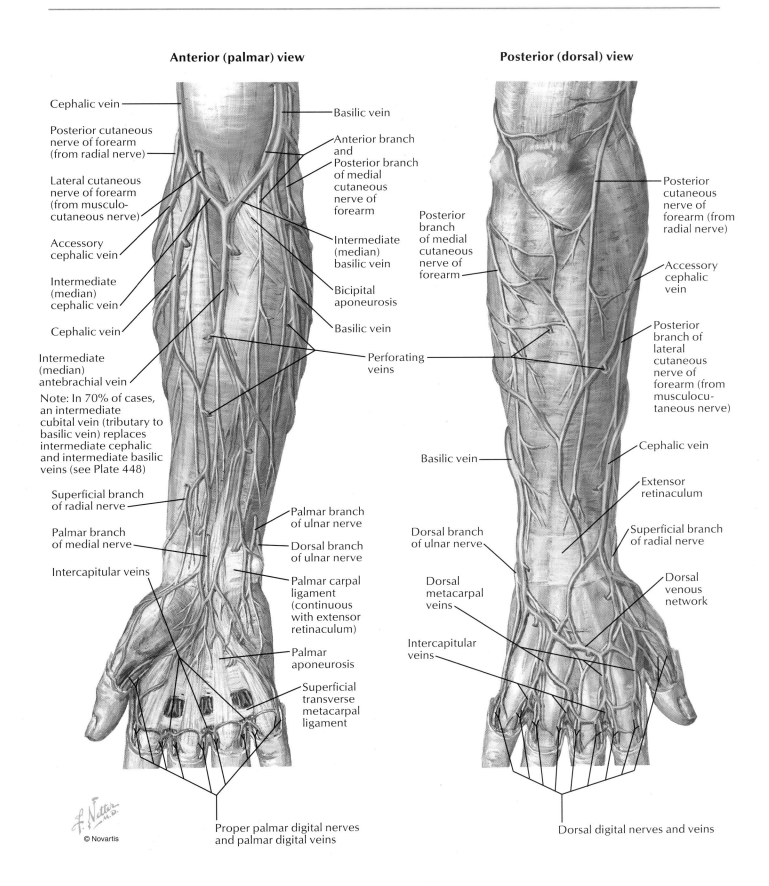

Cephalic vein

Posterior cutaneous
nerve of forearm
(from radial nerve)

Lateral cutaneous
nerve of forearm
(from musculo-
cutaneous nerve)

Accessory
cephalic vein

Intermediate
(median)
cephalic vein

Cephalic vein

Intermediate
(median)
antebrachial vein

Note: In 70% of cases,
an intermediate
cubital vein (tributary to
basilic vein) replaces
intermediate cephalic
and intermediate basilic
veins (see Plate 448)

Superficial branch
of radial nerve

Palmar branch
of medial nerve

Intercapitular veins

Basilic vein

Anterior branch
and
Posterior branch
of medial
cutaneous
nerve of
forearm

Intermediate
(median)
basilic vein

Bicipital
aponeurosis

Basilic vein

Perforating
veins

Palmar branch
of ulnar nerve

Dorsal branch
of ulnar nerve

Palmar carpal
ligament
(continuous
with extensor
retinaculum)

Palmar
aponeurosis

Superficial
transverse
metacarpal
ligament

Proper palmar digital nerves
and palmar digital veins

Posterior
branch
of medial
cutaneous
nerve of
forearm

Basilic vein

Dorsal branch
of ulnar nerve

Dorsal
metacarpal
veins

Intercapitular
veins

Posterior
cutaneous
nerve of
forearm (from
radial nerve)

Accessory
cephalic
vein

Posterior
branch of
lateral
cutaneous
nerve of
forearm (from
musculocu-
taneous nerve)

Cephalic vein

Extensor
retinaculum

Superficial branch
of radial nerve

Dorsal
venous
network

Dorsal digital nerves and veins

© Novartis

**NEUROVASCULATURE**

**PLATE 449**

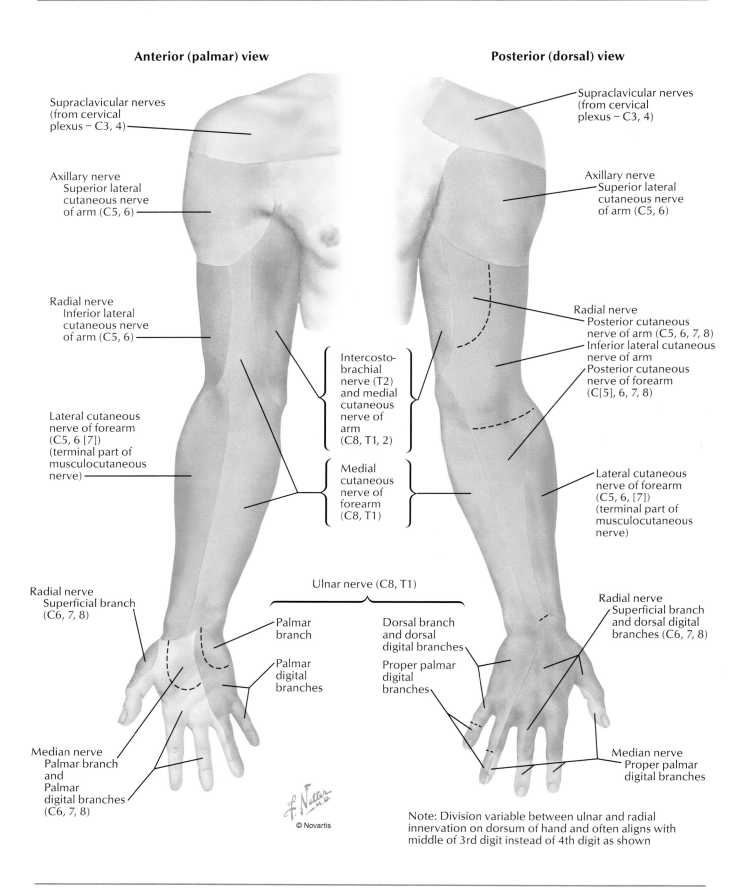

**Anterior (palmar) view**

**Posterior (dorsal) view**

Supraclavicular nerves
(from cervical
plexus – C3, 4)

Axillary nerve
Superior lateral
cutaneous nerve
of arm (C5, 6)

Radial nerve
Inferior lateral
cutaneous nerve
of arm (C5, 6)

Lateral cutaneous
nerve of forearm
(C5, 6 [7])
(terminal part of
musculocutaneous
nerve)

Radial nerve
Superficial branch
(C6, 7, 8)

Median nerve
Palmar branch
and
Palmar
digital branches
(C6, 7, 8)

Intercosto-
brachial
nerve (T2)
and medial
cutaneous
nerve of
arm
(C8, T1, 2)

Medial
cutaneous
nerve of
forearm
(C8, T1)

Ulnar nerve (C8, T1)

Palmar
branch

Palmar
digital
branches

Supraclavicular nerves
(from cervical
plexus – C3, 4)

Axillary nerve
Superior lateral
cutaneous nerve
of arm (C5, 6)

Radial nerve
Posterior cutaneous
nerve of arm (C5, 6, 7, 8)
Inferior lateral cutaneous
nerve of arm
Posterior cutaneous
nerve of forearm
(C[5], 6, 7, 8)

Lateral cutaneous
nerve of forearm
(C5, 6, [7])
(terminal part of
musculocutaneous
nerve)

Dorsal branch
and dorsal
digital branches

Proper palmar
digital
branches

Radial nerve
Superficial branch
and dorsal digital
branches (C6, 7, 8)

Median nerve
Proper palmar
digital branches

Note: Division variable between ulnar and radial
innervation on dorsum of hand and often aligns with
middle of 3rd digit instead of 4th digit as shown

© Novartis

**PLATE 450**

**UPPER LIMB**

Note: Schematic demarcation of dermatomes shown as distinct segments. There is actually considerable overlap between adjacent dermatomes

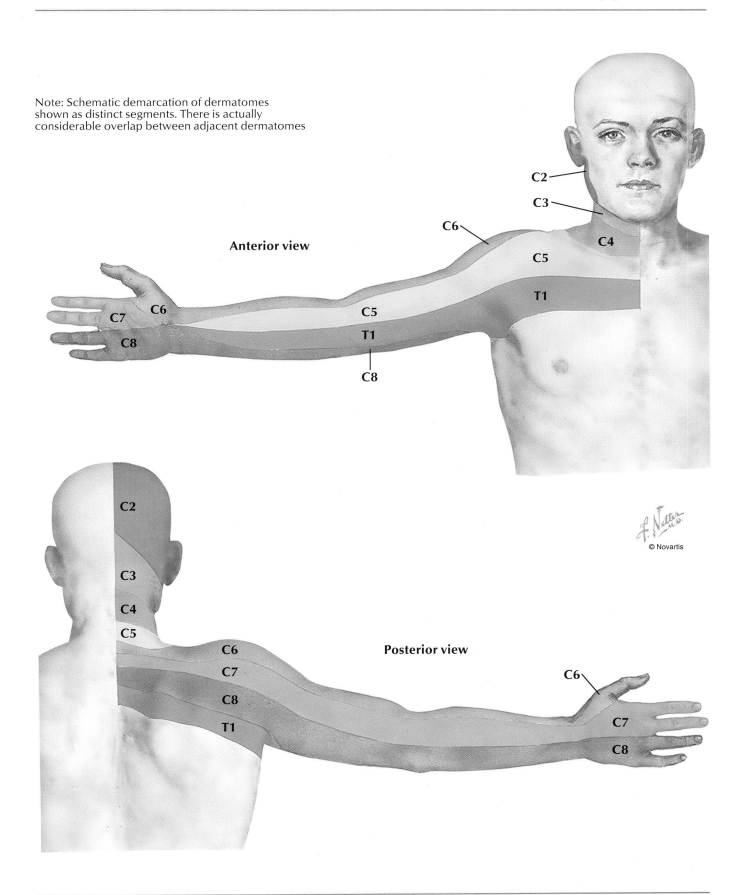

**Anterior view**

C2
C3
C6
C4
C5
T1
C5
C7 C6
C8 T1
C8

C2
C3
C4
C5
C6
C7
**Posterior view**
C8
T1
C6
C7
C8

© Novartis

SEE ALSO PLATES 169, 437

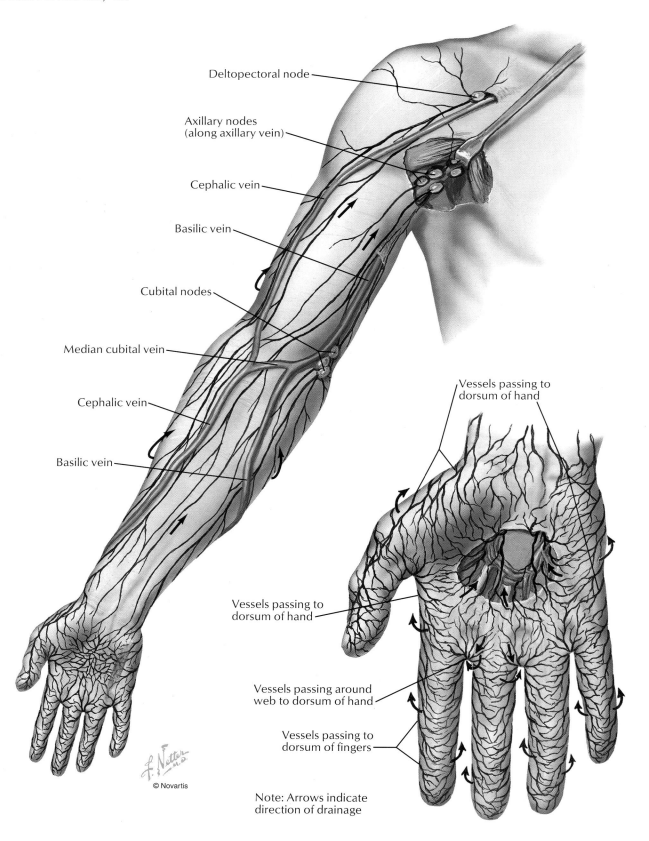

Deltopectoral node

Axillary nodes
(along axillary vein)

Cephalic vein

Basilic vein

Cubital nodes

Median cubital vein

Cephalic vein

Basilic vein

Vessels passing to
dorsum of hand

Vessels passing to
dorsum of hand

Vessels passing around
web to dorsum of hand

Vessels passing to
dorsum of fingers

Note: Arrows indicate
direction of drainage

© Novartis

**PLATE 452**

**UPPER LIMB**

**HIP AND THIGH**
*Plates 453 – 471*

453. Hip (Coxal) Bone
454. Hip Joint
455. Femur
456. Bony Attachments of Muscles of Hip and Thigh: Anterior View
457. Bony Attachments of Muscles of Hip and Thigh: Posterior View
458. Muscles of Thigh: Anterior Views
459. Muscles of Thigh: Anterior Views (*continued*)
460. Muscles of Hip and Thigh: Lateral View
461. Muscles of Hip and Thigh: Posterior Views
462. Psoas and Iliacus Muscles
463. Lumbosacral and Coccygeal Plexuses
464. Lumbar Plexus

465. Sacral and Coccygeal Plexuses
466. Arteries and Nerves of Thigh: Anterior Views
467. Arteries and Nerves of Thigh: Anterior Views (*continued*)
468. Arteries and Nerves of Thigh: Posterior View
469. Nerves of Hip and Buttock
470. Arteries of Femoral Head and Neck
471. Thigh: Serial Cross Sections

**KNEE**
*Plates 472 – 477*

472. Knee: Lateral and Medial Views
473. Knee: Anterior Views
474. Knee: Interior
475. Knee: Cruciate and Collateral Ligaments
476. Knee: Posterior and Sagittal Views
477. Arteries of Thigh and Knee: Schema

**LEG**
*Plates 478 – 487*

478. Tibia and Fibula
479. Tibia and Fibula (*continued*)
480. Attachments of Muscles of Leg
481. Muscles of Leg (Superficial Dissection): Posterior View
482. Muscles of Leg (Intermediate Dissection): Posterior View
483. Muscles of Leg (Deep Dissection): Posterior View
484. Muscles of Leg (Superficial Dissection): Anterior View
485. Muscles of Leg (Deep Dissection): Anterior View
486. Muscles of Leg: Lateral View
487. Leg: Cross Sections and Fascial Compartments

**ANKLE AND FOOT**
*Plates 488 – 501*

488. Bones of Foot
489. Bones of Foot (*continued*)
490. Calcaneus
491. Ligaments and Tendons of Ankle
492. Ligaments and Tendons of Foot: Plantar View
493. Tendon Sheaths of Ankle

494. Muscles of Dorsum of Foot: Superficial Dissection
495. Dorsum of Foot: Deep Dissection
496. Sole of Foot: Superficial Dissection
497. Muscles of Sole of Foot: First Layer
498. Muscles of Sole of Foot: Second Layer
499. Muscles of Sole of Foot: Third Layer
500. Interosseous Muscles and Deep Arteries of Foot
501. Interosseous Muscles of Foot

**NEUROVASCULATURE**
*Plates 502 – 510*

502. Femoral Nerve and Lateral Cutaneous Nerve of Thigh
503. Obturator Nerve
504. Sciatic Nerve and Posterior Cutaneous Nerve of Thigh
505. Tibial Nerve
506. Common Fibular (Peroneal) Nerve
507. Dermatomes of Lower Limb
508. Superficial Nerves and Veins of Lower Limb: Anterior View
509. Superficial Nerves and Veins of Lower Limb: Posterior View
510. Lymph Vessels and Nodes of Lower Limb

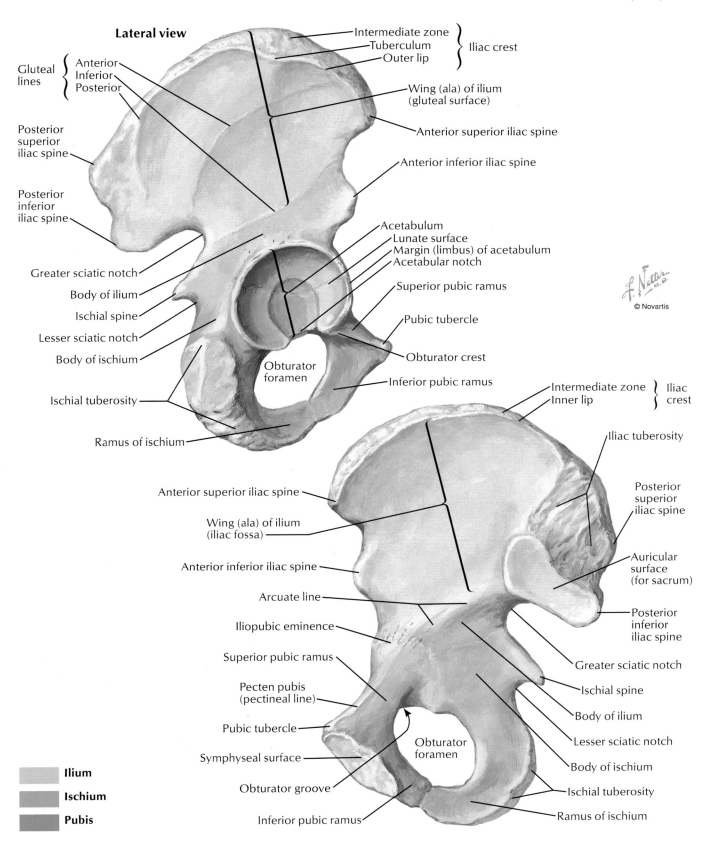

**Lateral view**

Intermediate zone
Tuberculum  } Iliac crest
Outer lip

Gluteal lines { Anterior, Inferior, Posterior

Wing (ala) of ilium (gluteal surface)

Anterior superior iliac spine

Posterior superior iliac spine

Anterior inferior iliac spine

Posterior inferior iliac spine

Acetabulum
Lunate surface
Margin (limbus) of acetabulum
Acetabular notch

Greater sciatic notch

Body of ilium

Ischial spine

Lesser sciatic notch

Body of ischium

Ischial tuberosity

Ramus of ischium

Superior pubic ramus

Pubic tubercle

Obturator crest

Obturator foramen

Inferior pubic ramus

Intermediate zone
Inner lip  } Iliac crest

Iliac tuberosity

Posterior superior iliac spine

Anterior superior iliac spine

Wing (ala) of ilium (iliac fossa)

Anterior inferior iliac spine

Arcuate line

Iliopubic eminence

Superior pubic ramus

Pecten pubis (pectineal line)

Pubic tubercle

Symphyseal surface

Obturator groove

Inferior pubic ramus

Obturator foramen

Auricular surface (for sacrum)

Posterior inferior iliac spine

Greater sciatic notch

Ischial spine

Body of ilium

Lesser sciatic notch

Body of ischium

Ischial tuberosity

Ramus of ischium

**Ilium**

**Ischium**

**Pubis**

© Novartis

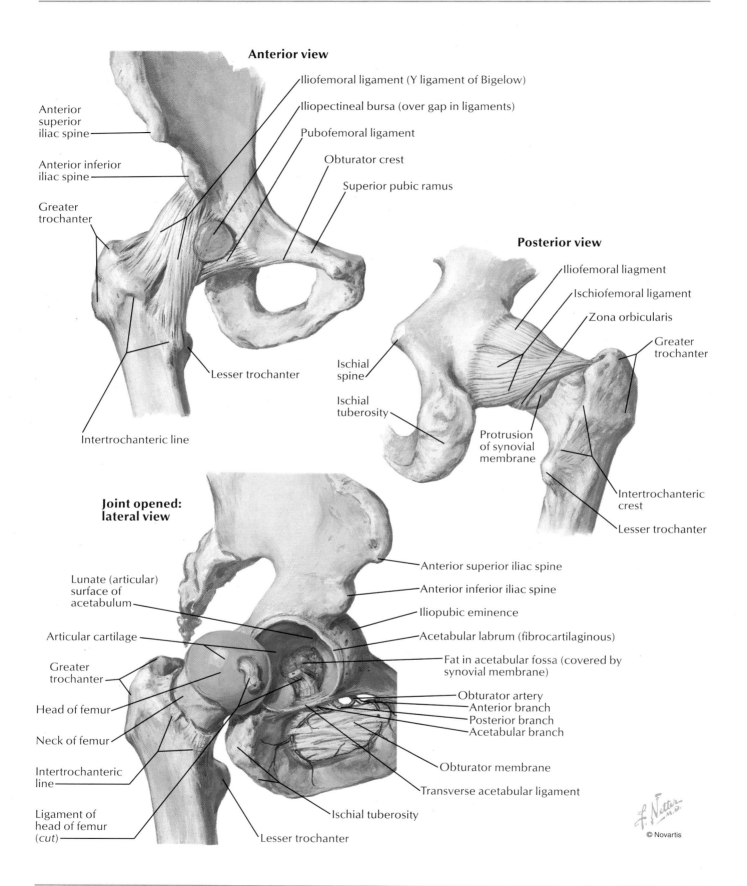

**Anterior view**

Iliofemoral ligament (Y ligament of Bigelow)

Iliopectineal bursa (over gap in ligaments)

Pubofemoral ligament

Obturator crest

Superior pubic ramus

Anterior superior iliac spine

Anterior inferior iliac spine

Greater trochanter

Lesser trochanter

Intertrochanteric line

**Posterior view**

Iliofemoral liagment

Ischiofemoral ligament

Zona orbicularis

Greater trochanter

Ischial spine

Ischial tuberosity

Protrusion of synovial membrane

Intertrochanteric crest

Lesser trochanter

**Joint opened: lateral view**

Lunate (articular) surface of acetabulum

Articular cartilage

Greater trochanter

Head of femur

Neck of femur

Intertrochanteric line

Ligament of head of femur (*cut*)

Lesser trochanter

Ischial tuberosity

Anterior superior iliac spine

Anterior inferior iliac spine

Iliopubic eminence

Acetabular labrum (fibrocartilaginous)

Fat in acetabular fossa (covered by synovial membrane)

Obturator artery
Anterior branch
Posterior branch
Acetabular branch

Obturator membrane

Transverse acetabular ligament

© Novartis

**PLATE 454**

**LOWER LIMB**

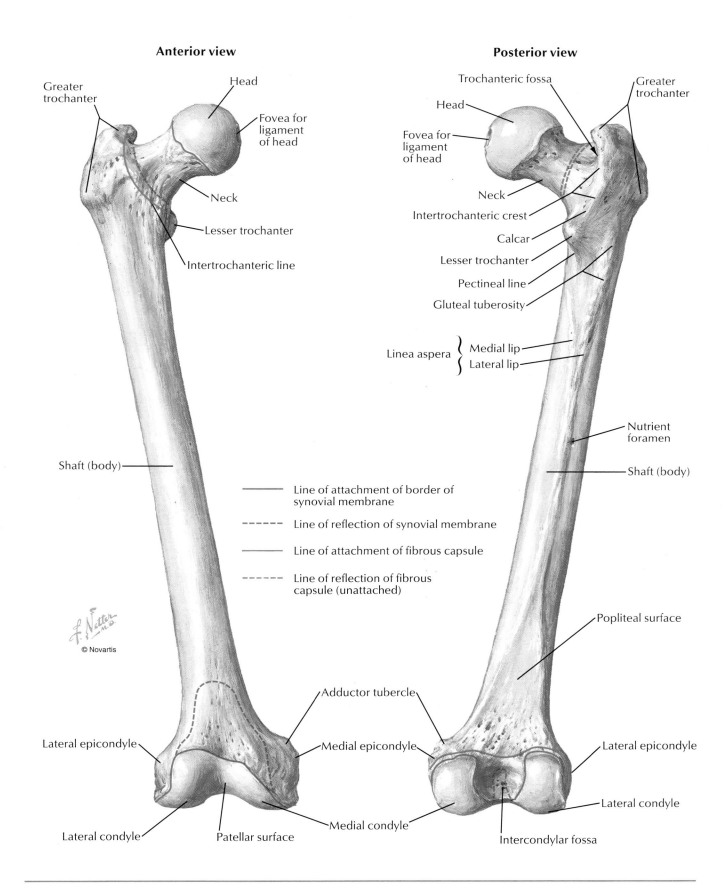

**Anterior view**

Greater trochanter

Head

Fovea for ligament of head

Neck

Lesser trochanter

Intertrochanteric line

Shaft (body)

Line of attachment of border of synovial membrane

Line of reflection of synovial membrane

Line of attachment of fibrous capsule

Line of reflection of fibrous capsule (unattached)

Lateral epicondyle

Adductor tubercle

Medial epicondyle

Lateral condyle

Patellar surface

Medial condyle

**Posterior view**

Trochanteric fossa

Head

Fovea for ligament of head

Neck

Greater trochanter

Intertrochanteric crest

Calcar

Lesser trochanter

Pectineal line

Gluteal tuberosity

Linea aspera { Medial lip
Lateral lip

Nutrient foramen

Shaft (body)

Popliteal surface

Medial epicondyle

Lateral epicondyle

Lateral condyle

Intercondylar fossa

# Bony Attachments of Muscles of Hip and Thigh: Anterior View

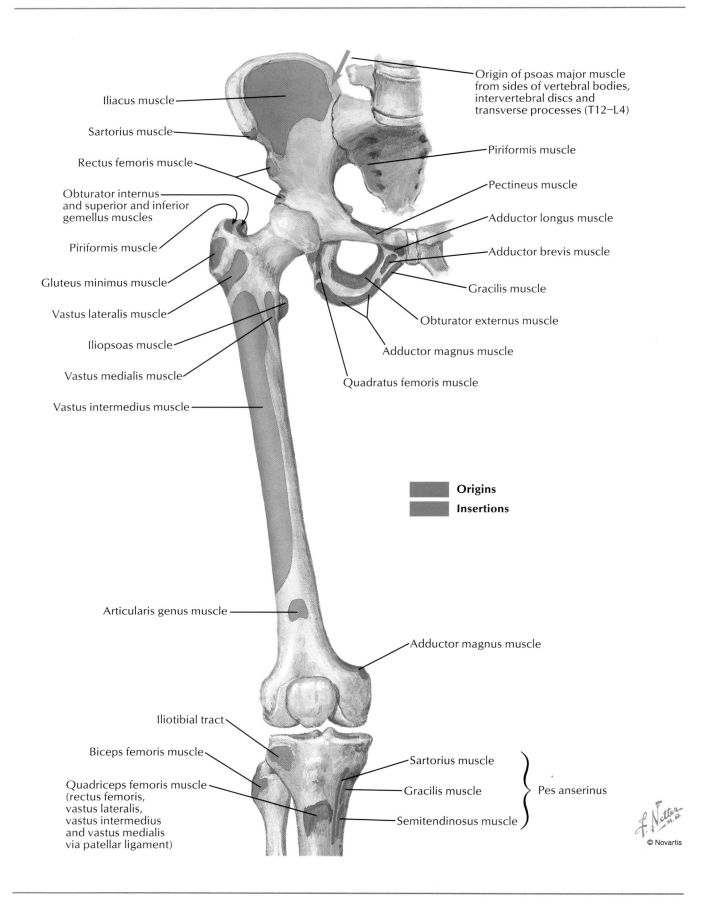

Iliacus muscle

Sartorius muscle

Rectus femoris muscle

Obturator internus and superior and inferior gemellus muscles

Piriformis muscle

Gluteus minimus muscle

Vastus lateralis muscle

Iliopsoas muscle

Vastus medialis muscle

Vastus intermedius muscle

Origin of psoas major muscle from sides of vertebral bodies, intervertebral discs and transverse processes (T12–L4)

Piriformis muscle

Pectineus muscle

Adductor longus muscle

Adductor brevis muscle

Gracilis muscle

Obturator externus muscle

Adductor magnus muscle

Quadratus femoris muscle

Origins
Insertions

Articularis genus muscle

Adductor magnus muscle

Iliotibial tract

Biceps femoris muscle

Quadriceps femoris muscle (rectus femoris, vastus lateralis, vastus intermedius and vastus medialis via patellar ligament)

Sartorius muscle

Gracilis muscle

Semitendinosus muscle

Pes anserinus

© Novartis

**PLATE 456**

**LOWER LIMB**

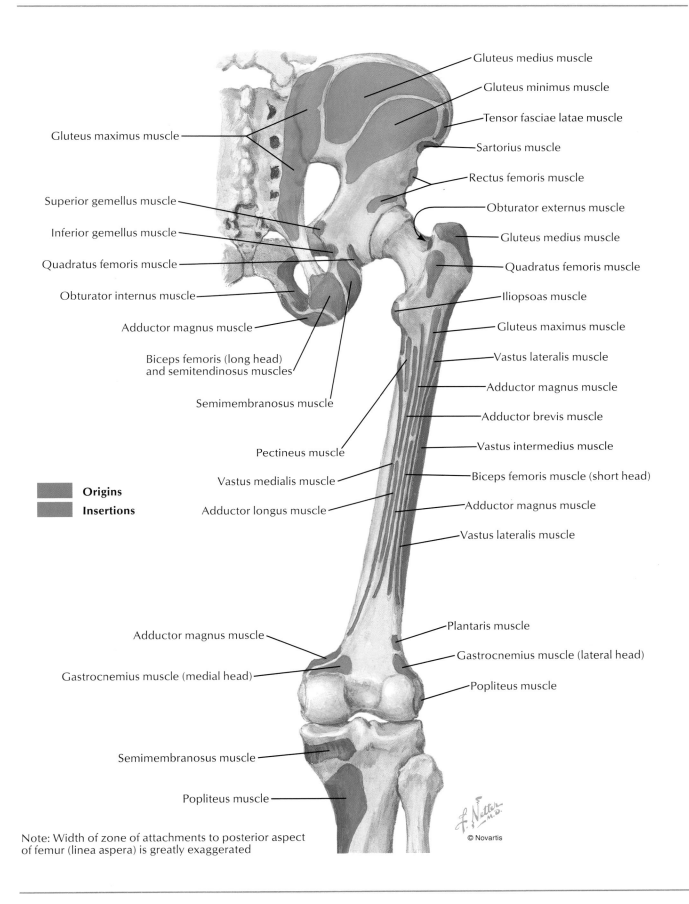

Gluteus medius muscle

Gluteus minimus muscle

Tensor fasciae latae muscle

Gluteus maximus muscle

Sartorius muscle

Rectus femoris muscle

Superior gemellus muscle

Obturator externus muscle

Inferior gemellus muscle

Gluteus medius muscle

Quadratus femoris muscle

Quadratus femoris muscle

Obturator internus muscle

Iliopsoas muscle

Adductor magnus muscle

Gluteus maximus muscle

Biceps femoris (long head) and semitendinosus muscles

Vastus lateralis muscle

Adductor magnus muscle

Semimembranosus muscle

Adductor brevis muscle

Vastus intermedius muscle

Pectineus muscle

Biceps femoris muscle (short head)

Vastus medialis muscle

Adductor magnus muscle

Adductor longus muscle

Vastus lateralis muscle

**Origins**

**Insertions**

Plantaris muscle

Gastrocnemius muscle (lateral head)

Adductor magnus muscle

Gastrocnemius muscle (medial head)

Popliteus muscle

Semimembranosus muscle

Popliteus muscle

Note: Width of zone of attachments to posterior aspect of femur (linea aspera) is greatly exaggerated

© Novartis

# Muscles of Thigh: Anterior Views

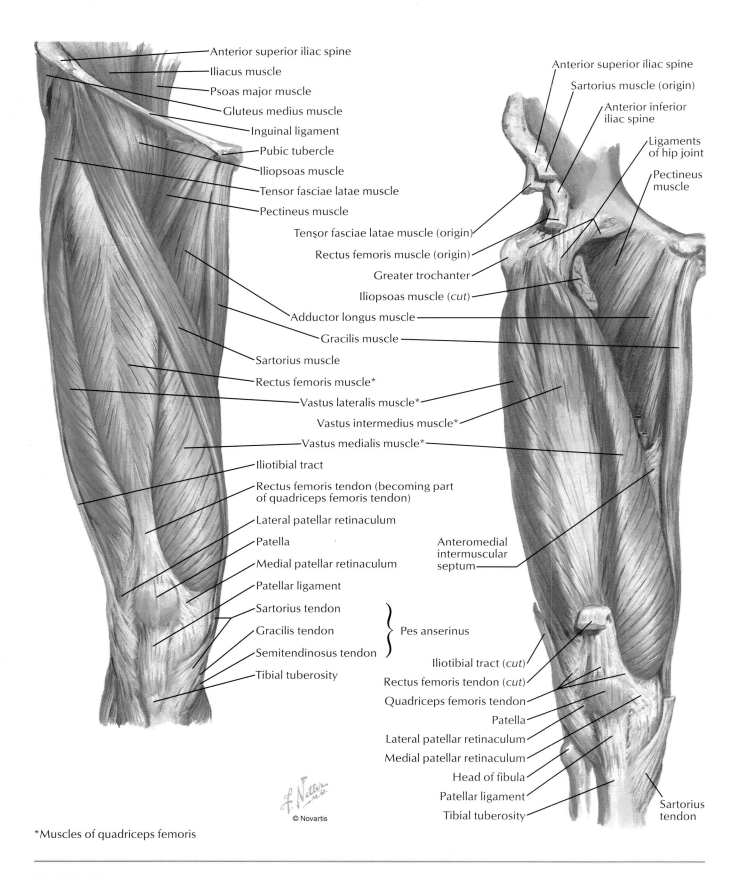

Anterior superior iliac spine
Iliacus muscle
Psoas major muscle
Gluteus medius muscle
Inguinal ligament
Pubic tubercle
Iliopsoas muscle
Tensor fasciae latae muscle
Pectineus muscle
Tensor fasciae latae muscle (origin)
Rectus femoris muscle (origin)
Greater trochanter
Iliopsoas muscle (cut)
Adductor longus muscle
Gracilis muscle
Sartorius muscle
Rectus femoris muscle*
Vastus lateralis muscle*
Vastus intermedius muscle*
Vastus medialis muscle*
Iliotibial tract
Rectus femoris tendon (becoming part of quadriceps femoris tendon)
Lateral patellar retinaculum
Patella
Medial patellar retinaculum
Patellar ligament
Sartorius tendon
Gracilis tendon
Semitendinosus tendon
Tibial tuberosity

} Pes anserinus

Anterior superior iliac spine
Sartorius muscle (origin)
Anterior inferior iliac spine
Ligaments of hip joint
Pectineus muscle

Anteromedial intermuscular septum

Iliotibial tract (cut)
Rectus femoris tendon (cut)
Quadriceps femoris tendon
Patella
Lateral patellar retinaculum
Medial patellar retinaculum
Head of fibula
Patellar ligament
Tibial tuberosity
Sartorius tendon

*Muscles of quadriceps femoris

F. Netter
© Novartis

**PLATE 458**

**LOWER LIMB**

**Deep dissection**

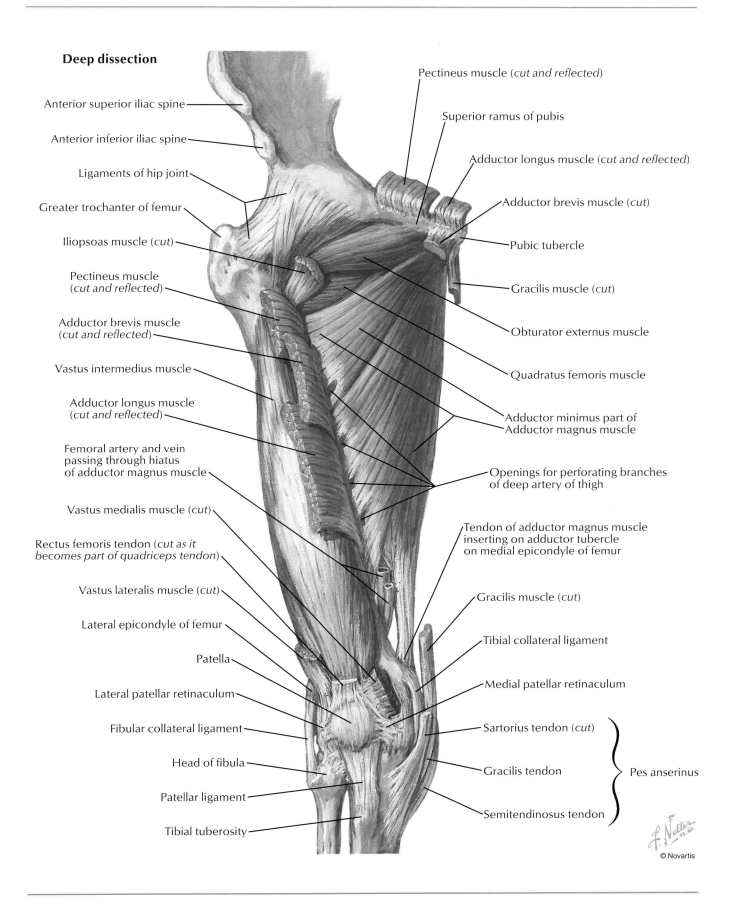

Anterior superior iliac spine

Anterior inferior iliac spine

Ligaments of hip joint

Greater trochanter of femur

Iliopsoas muscle (*cut*)

Pectineus muscle
(*cut and reflected*)

Adductor brevis muscle
(*cut and reflected*)

Vastus intermedius muscle

Adductor longus muscle
(*cut and reflected*)

Femoral artery and vein
passing through hiatus
of adductor magnus muscle

Vastus medialis muscle (*cut*)

Rectus femoris tendon (*cut as it
becomes part of quadriceps tendon*)

Vastus lateralis muscle (*cut*)

Lateral epicondyle of femur

Patella

Lateral patellar retinaculum

Fibular collateral ligament

Head of fibula

Patellar ligament

Tibial tuberosity

Pectineus muscle (*cut and reflected*)

Superior ramus of pubis

Adductor longus muscle (*cut and reflected*)

Adductor brevis muscle (*cut*)

Pubic tubercle

Gracilis muscle (*cut*)

Obturator externus muscle

Quadratus femoris muscle

Adductor minimus part of
Adductor magnus muscle

Openings for perforating branches
of deep artery of thigh

Tendon of adductor magnus muscle
inserting on adductor tubercle
on medial epicondyle of femur

Gracilis muscle (*cut*)

Tibial collateral ligament

Medial patellar retinaculum

Sartorius tendon (*cut*)

Gracilis tendon

Semitendinosus tendon

Pes anserinus

© Novartis

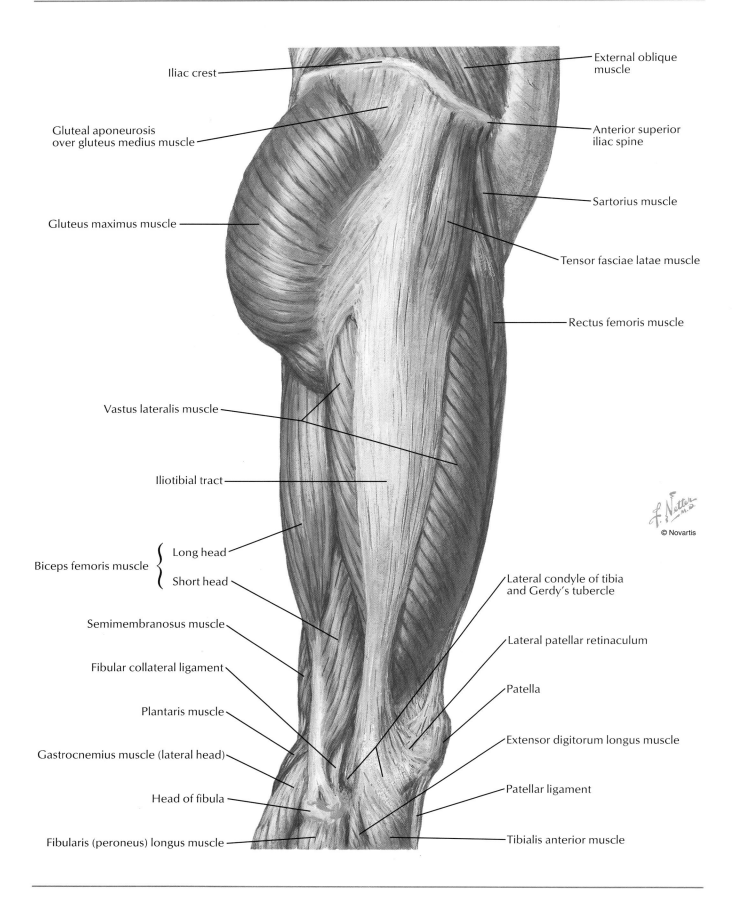

Iliac crest

External oblique muscle

Gluteal aponeurosis over gluteus medius muscle

Anterior superior iliac spine

Sartorius muscle

Gluteus maximus muscle

Tensor fasciae latae muscle

Rectus femoris muscle

Vastus lateralis muscle

Iliotibial tract

Biceps femoris muscle { Long head

Short head

Lateral condyle of tibia and Gerdy's tubercle

Semimembranosus muscle

Lateral patellar retinaculum

Fibular collateral ligament

Patella

Plantaris muscle

Extensor digitorum longus muscle

Gastrocnemius muscle (lateral head)

Head of fibula

Patellar ligament

Fibularis (peroneus) longus muscle

Tibialis anterior muscle

**PLATE 460**

**LOWER LIMB**

*FOR PIRIFORMIS AND OBTURATOR INTERNUS SEE ALSO PLATES 333, 334; FOR OBTURATOR EXTERNUS SEE PLATE 459*

**Superficial dissection**

**Deeper dissection**

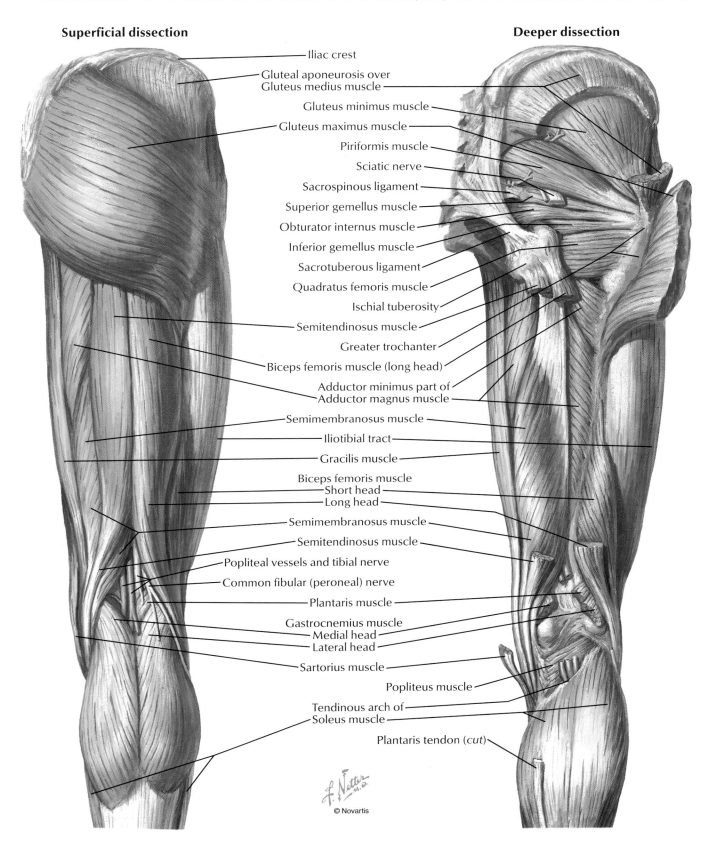

Iliac crest

Gluteal aponeurosis over
Gluteus medius muscle

Gluteus minimus muscle

Gluteus maximus muscle

Piriformis muscle

Sciatic nerve

Sacrospinous ligament

Superior gemellus muscle

Obturator internus muscle

Inferior gemellus muscle

Sacrotuberous ligament

Quadratus femoris muscle

Ischial tuberosity

Semitendinosus muscle

Greater trochanter

Biceps femoris muscle (long head)

Adductor minimus part of
Adductor magnus muscle

Semimembranosus muscle

Iliotibial tract

Gracilis muscle

Biceps femoris muscle
Short head
Long head

Semimembranosus muscle

Semitendinosus muscle

Popliteal vessels and tibial nerve

Common fibular (peroneal) nerve

Plantaris muscle

Gastrocnemius muscle
Medial head
Lateral head

Sartorius muscle

Popliteus muscle

Tendinous arch of
Soleus muscle

Plantaris tendon (*cut*)

*f. Netter*
© Novartis

**HIP AND THIGH**

*PLATE 461*

*SEE ALSO PLATE 246*

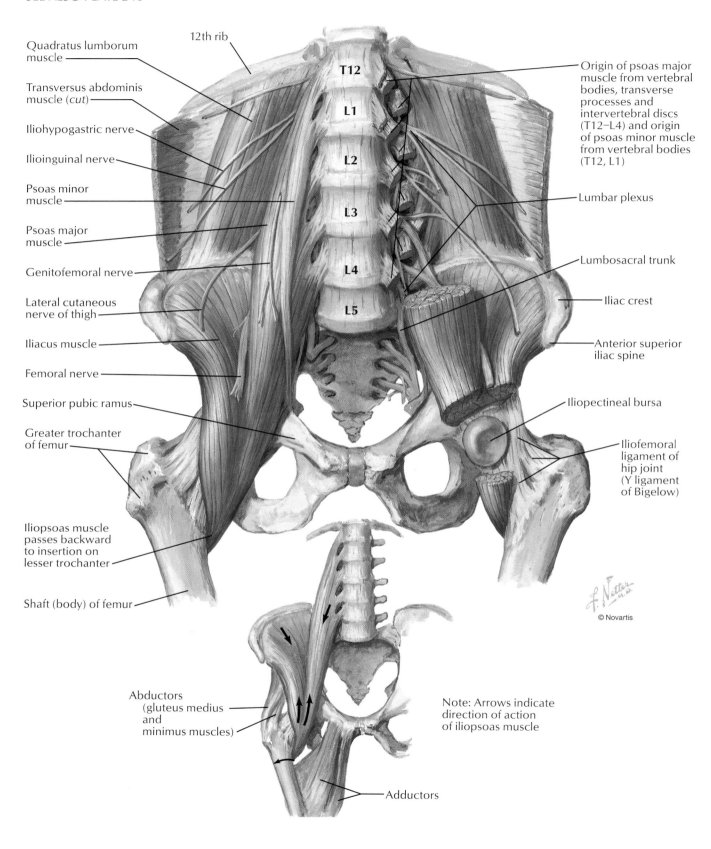

Quadratus lumborum muscle

12th rib

Transversus abdominis muscle (*cut*)

Iliohypogastric nerve

Ilioinguinal nerve

Psoas minor muscle

Psoas major muscle

Genitofemoral nerve

Lateral cutaneous nerve of thigh

Iliacus muscle

Femoral nerve

Superior pubic ramus

Greater trochanter of femur

Iliopsoas muscle passes backward to insertion on lesser trochanter

Shaft (body) of femur

T12

L1

L2

L3

L4

L5

Origin of psoas major muscle from vertebral bodies, transverse processes and intervertebral discs (T12–L4) and origin of psoas minor muscle from vertebral bodies (T12, L1)

Lumbar plexus

Lumbosacral trunk

Iliac crest

Anterior superior iliac spine

Iliopectineal bursa

Iliofemoral ligament of hip joint (Y ligament of Bigelow)

*f. Netter M.D.*

© Novartis

Abductors (gluteus medius and minimus muscles)

Note: Arrows indicate direction of action of iliopsoas muscle

Adductors

**PLATE 462**

**LOWER LIMB**

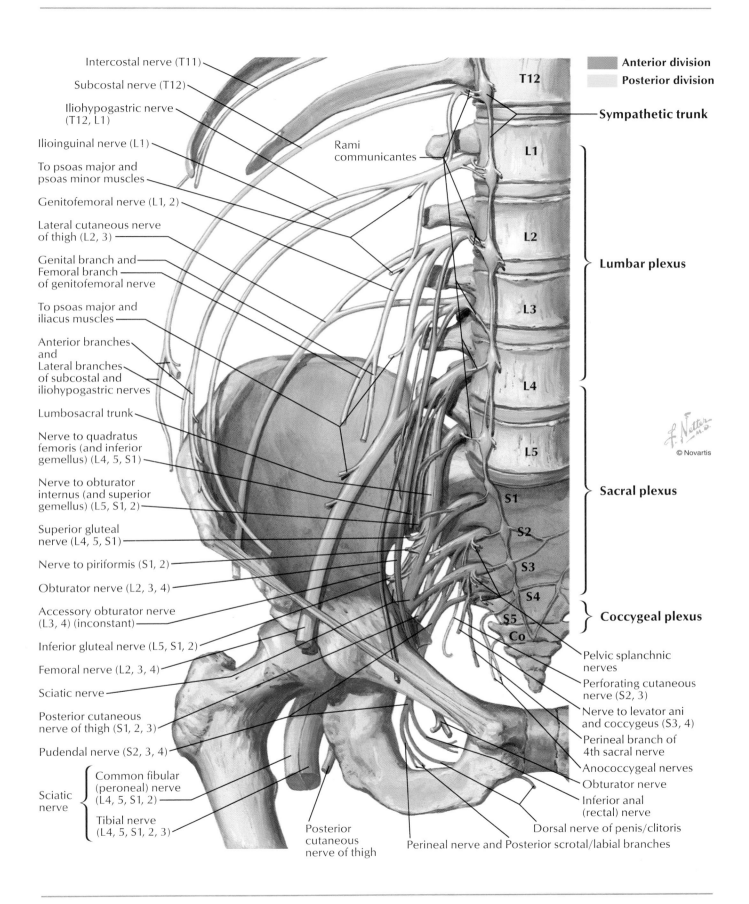

Intercostal nerve (T11)

Subcostal nerve (T12)

Iliohypogastric nerve (T12, L1)

Ilioinguinal nerve (L1)

To psoas major and psoas minor muscles

Genitofemoral nerve (L1, 2)

Lateral cutaneous nerve of thigh (L2, 3)

Genital branch and Femoral branch of genitofemoral nerve

To psoas major and iliacus muscles

Anterior branches and Lateral branches of subcostal and iliohypogastric nerves

Lumbosacral trunk

Nerve to quadratus femoris (and inferior gemellus) (L4, 5, S1)

Nerve to obturator internus (and superior gemellus) (L5, S1, 2)

Superior gluteal nerve (L4, 5, S1)

Nerve to piriformis (S1, 2)

Obturator nerve (L2, 3, 4)

Accessory obturator nerve (L3, 4) (inconstant)

Inferior gluteal nerve (L5, S1, 2)

Femoral nerve (L2, 3, 4)

Sciatic nerve

Posterior cutaneous nerve of thigh (S1, 2, 3)

Pudendal nerve (S2, 3, 4)

Sciatic nerve { Common fibular (peroneal) nerve (L4, 5, S1, 2)

Tibial nerve (L4, 5, S1, 2, 3)

Rami communicantes

Posterior cutaneous nerve of thigh

**Anterior division**
**Posterior division**

T12

**Sympathetic trunk**

L1

**Lumbar plexus**

L2

L3

L4

L5

**Sacral plexus**

S1

S2

S3

S4

S5
Co

**Coccygeal plexus**

Pelvic splanchnic nerves

Perforating cutaneous nerve (S2, 3)

Nerve to levator ani and coccygeus (S3, 4)

Perineal branch of 4th sacral nerve

Anococcygeal nerves

Obturator nerve

Inferior anal (rectal) nerve

Dorsal nerve of penis/clitoris

Perineal nerve and Posterior scrotal/labial branches

# *Lumbar Plexus*

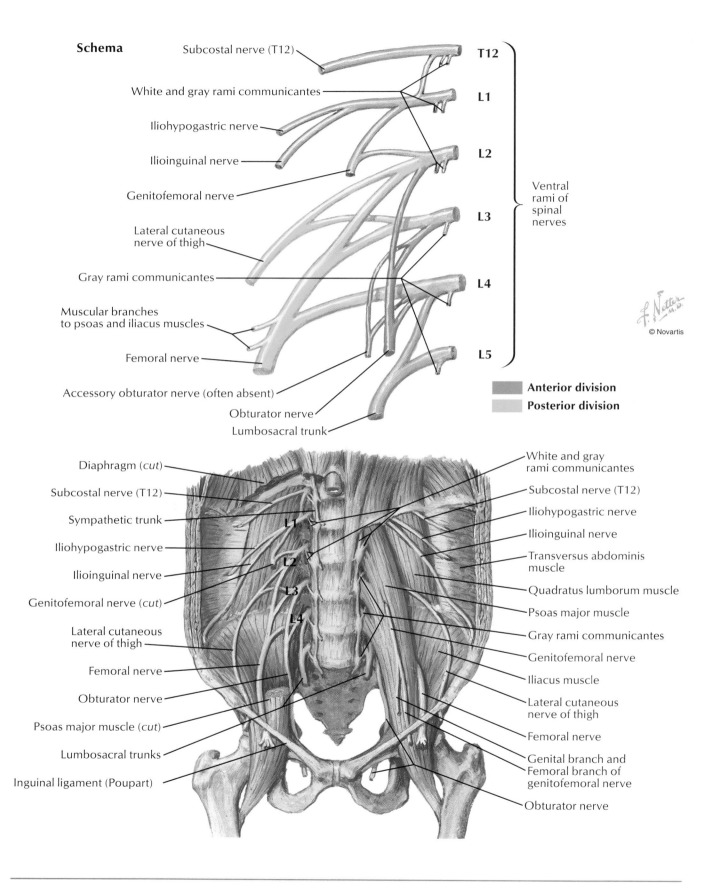

**Schema**

Subcostal nerve (T12)

White and gray rami communicantes

Iliohypogastric nerve

Ilioinguinal nerve

Genitofemoral nerve

Lateral cutaneous nerve of thigh

Gray rami communicantes

Muscular branches to psoas and iliacus muscles

Femoral nerve

Accessory obturator nerve (often absent)

Obturator nerve

Lumbosacral trunk

T12

L1

L2

L3

L4

L5

Ventral rami of spinal nerves

**Anterior division**
**Posterior division**

Diaphragm (*cut*)

Subcostal nerve (T12)

Sympathetic trunk

Iliohypogastric nerve

Ilioinguinal nerve

Genitofemoral nerve (*cut*)

Lateral cutaneous nerve of thigh

Femoral nerve

Obturator nerve

Psoas major muscle (*cut*)

Lumbosacral trunks

Inguinal ligament (Poupart)

White and gray rami communicantes

Subcostal nerve (T12)

Iliohypogastric nerve

Ilioinguinal nerve

Transversus abdominis muscle

Quadratus lumborum muscle

Psoas major muscle

Gray rami communicantes

Genitofemoral nerve

Iliacus muscle

Lateral cutaneous nerve of thigh

Femoral nerve

Genital branch and Femoral branch of genitofemoral nerve

Obturator nerve

*PLATE 464*

**LOWER LIMB**

### Schema

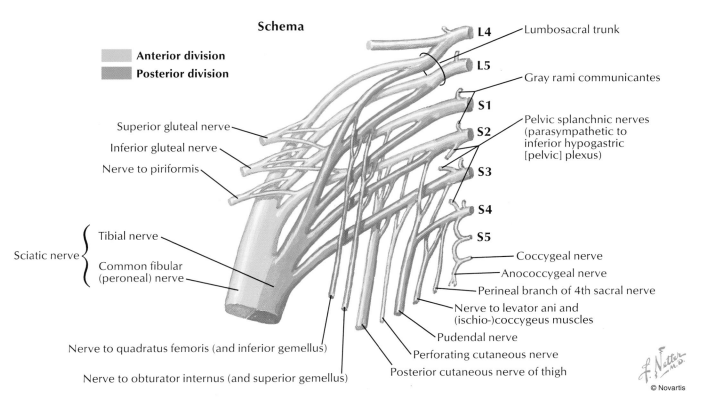

Anterior division
Posterior division

L4 — Lumbosacral trunk
L5 — Gray rami communicantes
S1
S2 — Pelvic splanchnic nerves (parasympathetic to inferior hypogastric [pelvic] plexus)
S3
S4
S5

Superior gluteal nerve
Inferior gluteal nerve
Nerve to piriformis

Sciatic nerve {
Tibial nerve
Common fibular (peroneal) nerve
}

Coccygeal nerve
Anococcygeal nerve
Perineal branch of 4th sacral nerve
Nerve to levator ani and (ischio-)coccygeus muscles
Pudendal nerve
Perforating cutaneous nerve
Posterior cutaneous nerve of thigh

Nerve to quadratus femoris (and inferior gemellus)
Nerve to obturator internus (and superior gemellus)

© Novartis

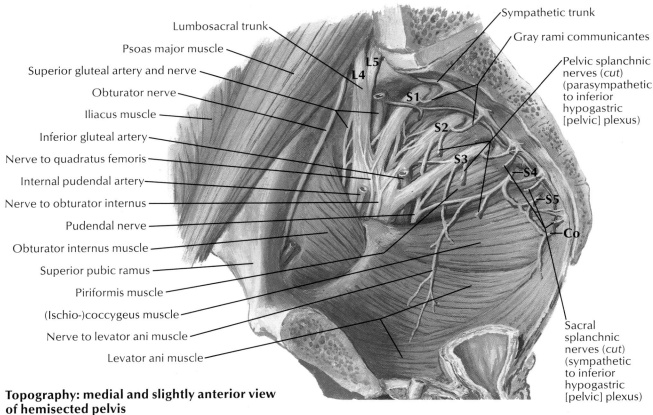

Lumbosacral trunk
Psoas major muscle
Superior gluteal artery and nerve
Obturator nerve
Iliacus muscle
Inferior gluteal artery
Nerve to quadratus femoris
Internal pudendal artery
Nerve to obturator internus
Pudendal nerve
Obturator internus muscle
Superior pubic ramus
Piriformis muscle
(Ischio-)coccygeus muscle
Nerve to levator ani muscle
Levator ani muscle

Sympathetic trunk
Gray rami communicantes
Pelvic splanchnic nerves (cut) (parasympathetic to inferior hypogastric [pelvic] plexus)

L5
L4
S1
S2
S3
S4
S5
Co

Sacral splanchnic nerves (cut) (sympathetic to inferior hypogastric [pelvic] plexus)

**Topography: medial and slightly anterior view of hemisected pelvis**

**Superficial dissections**

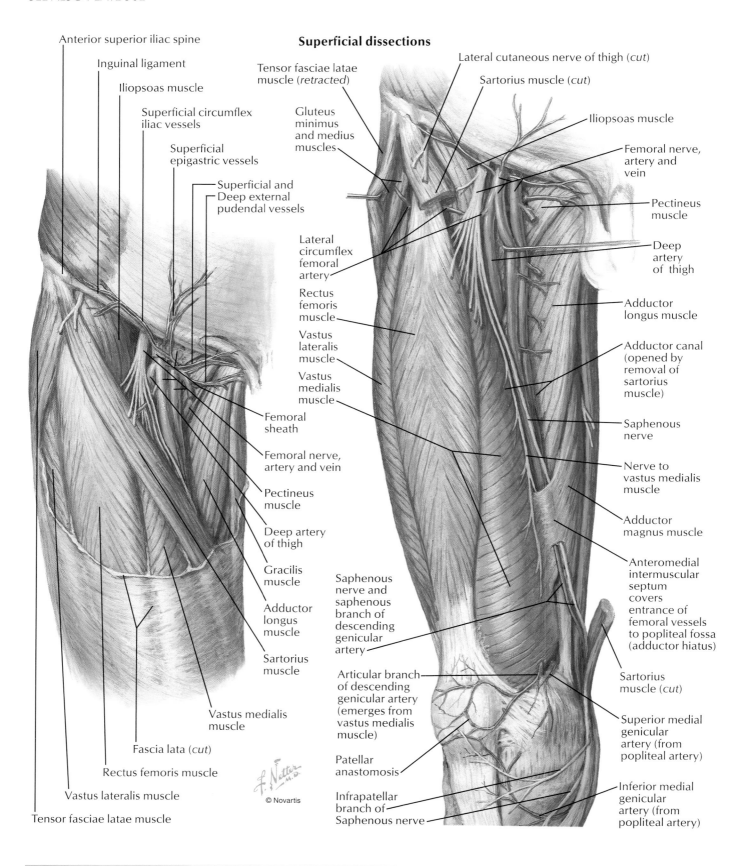

Anterior superior iliac spine

Inguinal ligament

Iliopsoas muscle

Superficial circumflex iliac vessels

Superficial epigastric vessels

Superficial and Deep external pudendal vessels

Tensor fasciae latae muscle (*retracted*)

Gluteus minimus and medius muscles

Lateral circumflex femoral artery

Rectus femoris muscle

Vastus lateralis muscle

Vastus medialis muscle

Femoral sheath

Femoral nerve, artery and vein

Pectineus muscle

Deep artery of thigh

Gracilis muscle

Adductor longus muscle

Sartorius muscle

Vastus medialis muscle

Fascia lata (*cut*)

Rectus femoris muscle

Vastus lateralis muscle

Tensor fasciae latae muscle

Lateral cutaneous nerve of thigh (*cut*)

Sartorius muscle (*cut*)

Iliopsoas muscle

Femoral nerve, artery and vein

Pectineus muscle

Deep artery of thigh

Adductor longus muscle

Adductor canal (opened by removal of sartorius muscle)

Saphenous nerve

Nerve to vastus medialis muscle

Adductor magnus muscle

Anteromedial intermuscular septum covers entrance of femoral vessels to popliteal fossa (adductor hiatus)

Sartorius muscle (*cut*)

Superior medial genicular artery (from popliteal artery)

Inferior medial genicular artery (from popliteal artery)

Saphenous nerve and saphenous branch of descending genicular artery

Articular branch of descending genicular artery (emerges from vastus medialis muscle)

Patellar anastomosis

Infrapatellar branch of Saphenous nerve

*F. Netter M.D.*

© Novartis

**PLATE 466**

**LOWER LIMB**

# Arteries and Nerves of Thigh: Anterior Views (continued)

**Deep dissection**

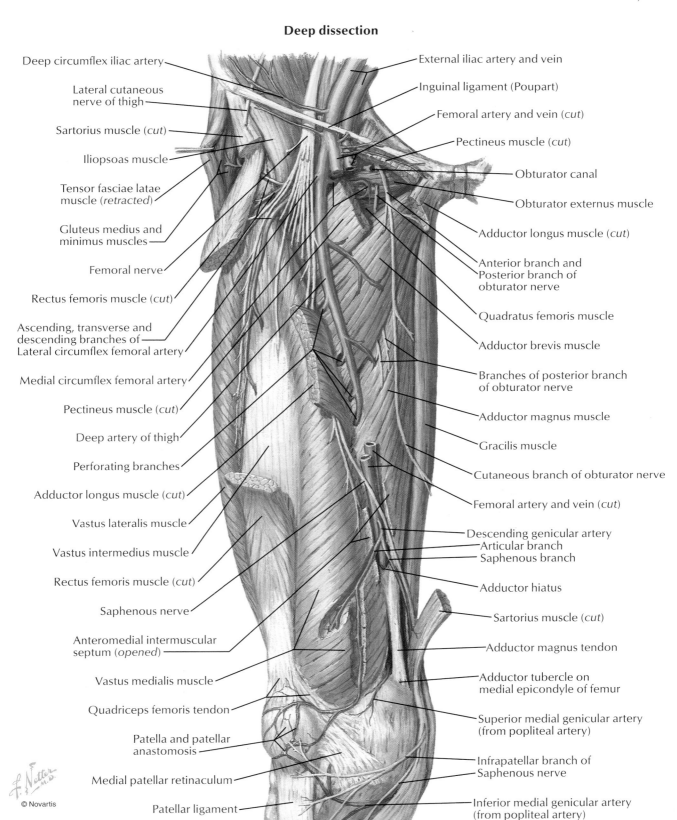

Deep circumflex iliac artery

Lateral cutaneous nerve of thigh

Sartorius muscle (*cut*)

Iliopsoas muscle

Tensor fasciae latae muscle (*retracted*)

Gluteus medius and minimus muscles

Femoral nerve

Rectus femoris muscle (*cut*)

Ascending, transverse and descending branches of Lateral circumflex femoral artery

Medial circumflex femoral artery

Pectineus muscle (*cut*)

Deep artery of thigh

Perforating branches

Adductor longus muscle (*cut*)

Vastus lateralis muscle

Vastus intermedius muscle

Rectus femoris muscle (*cut*)

Saphenous nerve

Anteromedial intermuscular septum (*opened*)

Vastus medialis muscle

Quadriceps femoris tendon

Patella and patellar anastomosis

Medial patellar retinaculum

Patellar ligament

External iliac artery and vein

Inguinal ligament (Poupart)

Femoral artery and vein (*cut*)

Pectineus muscle (*cut*)

Obturator canal

Obturator externus muscle

Adductor longus muscle (*cut*)

Anterior branch and Posterior branch of obturator nerve

Quadratus femoris muscle

Adductor brevis muscle

Branches of posterior branch of obturator nerve

Adductor magnus muscle

Gracilis muscle

Cutaneous branch of obturator nerve

Femoral artery and vein (*cut*)

Descending genicular artery
Articular branch
Saphenous branch

Adductor hiatus

Sartorius muscle (*cut*)

Adductor magnus tendon

Adductor tubercle on medial epicondyle of femur

Superior medial genicular artery (from popliteal artery)

Infrapatellar branch of Saphenous nerve

Inferior medial genicular artery (from popliteal artery)

*f. Netter*
© Novartis

**HIP AND THIGH**

*PLATE 467*

**Deep dissection**

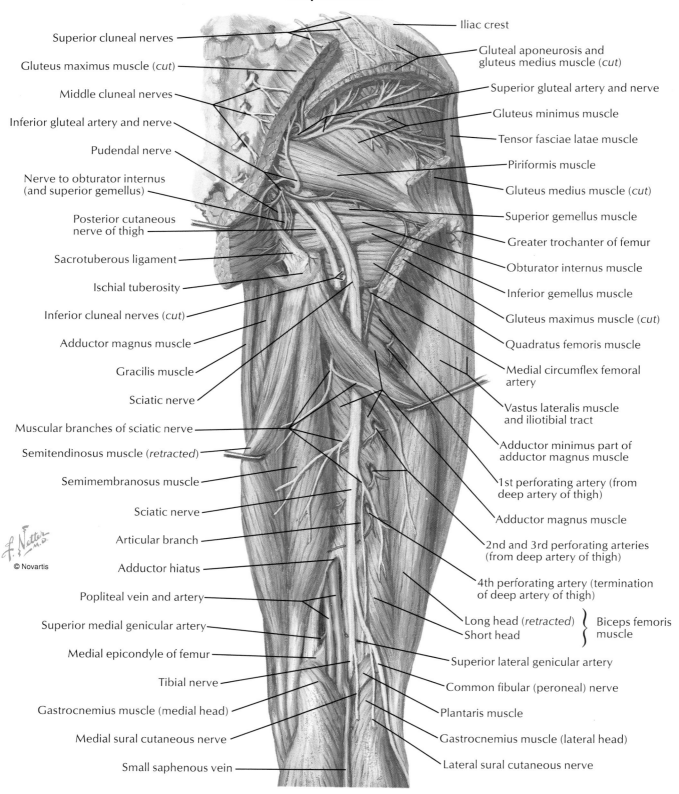

Superior cluneal nerves

Gluteus maximus muscle (*cut*)

Middle cluneal nerves

Inferior gluteal artery and nerve

Pudendal nerve

Nerve to obturator internus (and superior gemellus)

Posterior cutaneous nerve of thigh

Sacrotuberous ligament

Ischial tuberosity

Inferior cluneal nerves (*cut*)

Adductor magnus muscle

Gracilis muscle

Sciatic nerve

Muscular branches of sciatic nerve

Semitendinosus muscle (*retracted*)

Semimembranosus muscle

Sciatic nerve

Articular branch

Adductor hiatus

Popliteal vein and artery

Superior medial genicular artery

Medial epicondyle of femur

Tibial nerve

Gastrocnemius muscle (medial head)

Medial sural cutaneous nerve

Small saphenous vein

Iliac crest

Gluteal aponeurosis and gluteus medius muscle (*cut*)

Superior gluteal artery and nerve

Gluteus minimus muscle

Tensor fasciae latae muscle

Piriformis muscle

Gluteus medius muscle (*cut*)

Superior gemellus muscle

Greater trochanter of femur

Obturator internus muscle

Inferior gemellus muscle

Gluteus maximus muscle (*cut*)

Quadratus femoris muscle

Medial circumflex femoral artery

Vastus lateralis muscle and iliotibial tract

Adductor minimus part of adductor magnus muscle

1st perforating artery (from deep artery of thigh)

Adductor magnus muscle

2nd and 3rd perforating arteries (from deep artery of thigh)

4th perforating artery (termination of deep artery of thigh)

Long head (*retracted*)
Short head
} Biceps femoris muscle

Superior lateral genicular artery

Common fibular (peroneal) nerve

Plantaris muscle

Gastrocnemius muscle (lateral head)

Lateral sural cutaneous nerve

© Novartis

**PLATE 468**

**LOWER LIMB**

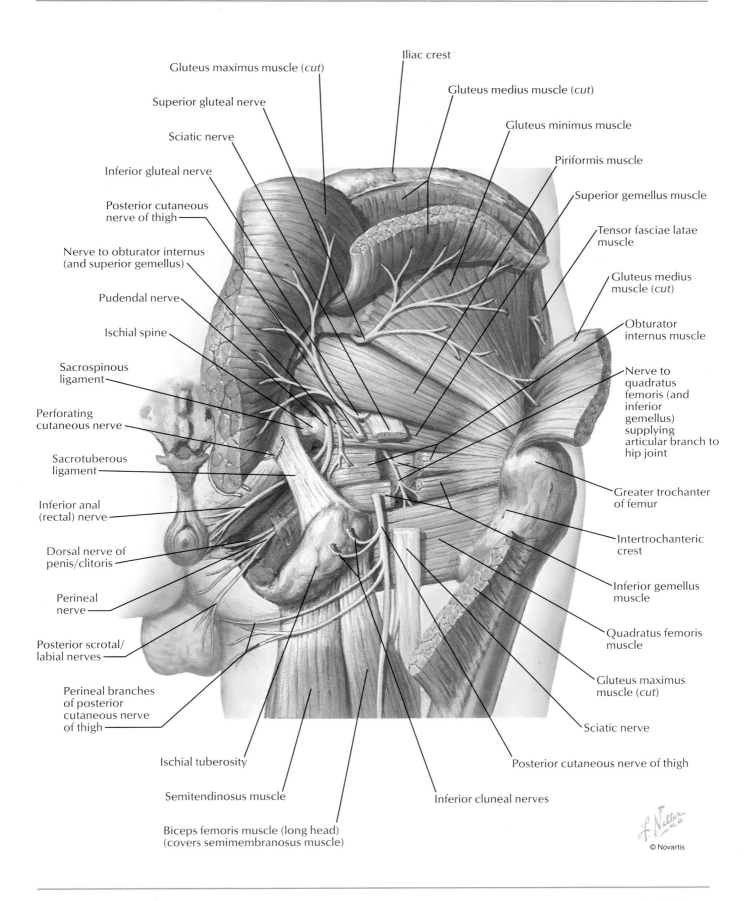

Gluteus maximus muscle (*cut*)

Superior gluteal nerve

Sciatic nerve

Inferior gluteal nerve

Posterior cutaneous nerve of thigh

Nerve to obturator internus (and superior gemellus)

Pudendal nerve

Ischial spine

Sacrospinous ligament

Perforating cutaneous nerve

Sacrotuberous ligament

Inferior anal (rectal) nerve

Dorsal nerve of penis/clitoris

Perineal nerve

Posterior scrotal/labial nerves

Perineal branches of posterior cutaneous nerve of thigh

Ischial tuberosity

Semitendinosus muscle

Biceps femoris muscle (long head) (covers semimembranosus muscle)

Iliac crest

Gluteus medius muscle (*cut*)

Gluteus minimus muscle

Piriformis muscle

Superior gemellus muscle

Tensor fasciae latae muscle

Gluteus medius muscle (*cut*)

Obturator internus muscle

Nerve to quadratus femoris (and inferior gemellus) supplying articular branch to hip joint

Greater trochanter of femur

Intertrochanteric crest

Inferior gemellus muscle

Quadratus femoris muscle

Gluteus maximus muscle (*cut*)

Sciatic nerve

Posterior cutaneous nerve of thigh

Inferior cluneal nerves

© Novartis

# *Arteries of Femoral Head and Neck*

SEE ALSO PLATE 477

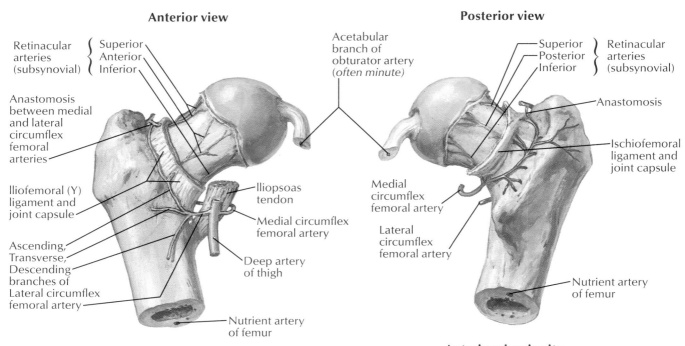

### Anterior view

Retinacular arteries (subsynovial) { Superior, Anterior, Inferior

Anastomosis between medial and lateral circumflex femoral arteries

Iliofemoral (Y) ligament and joint capsule

Ascending, Transverse, Descending branches of Lateral circumflex femoral artery

Acetabular branch of obturator artery (*often minute*)

Iliopsoas tendon

Medial circumflex femoral artery

Deep artery of thigh

Nutrient artery of femur

### Posterior view

Superior, Posterior, Inferior } Retinacular arteries (subsynovial)

Anastomosis

Ischiofemoral ligament and joint capsule

Medial circumflex femoral artery

Lateral circumflex femoral artery

Nutrient artery of femur

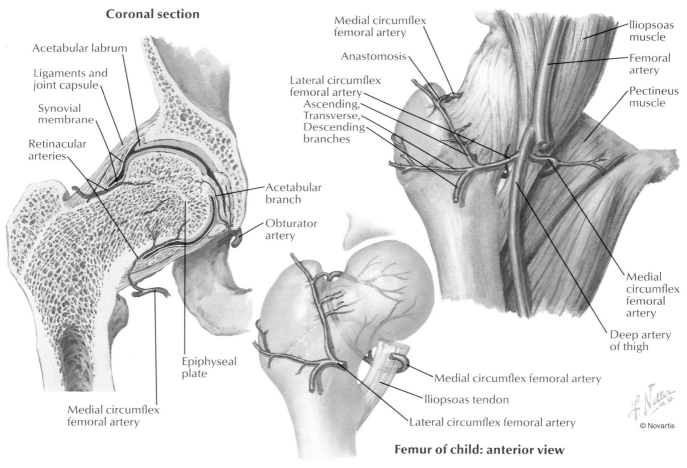

### Coronal section

Acetabular labrum

Ligaments and joint capsule

Synovial membrane

Retinacular arteries

Medial circumflex femoral artery

Acetabular branch

Obturator artery

Epiphyseal plate

### Anterior view in situ

Medial circumflex femoral artery

Anastomosis

Lateral circumflex femoral artery Ascending, Transverse, Descending branches

Iliopsoas muscle

Femoral artery

Pectineus muscle

Medial circumflex femoral artery

Deep artery of thigh

Medial circumflex femoral artery

Iliopsoas tendon

Lateral circumflex femoral artery

**Femur of child: anterior view**

© Novartis

**PLATE 470**

**LOWER LIMB**

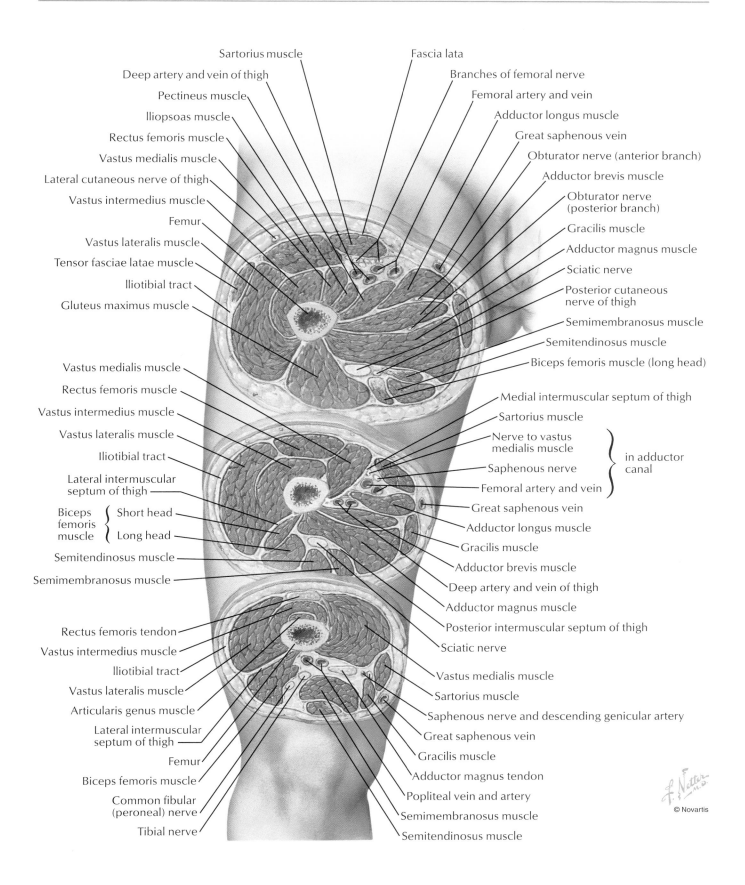

Sartorius muscle
Deep artery and vein of thigh
Pectineus muscle
Iliopsoas muscle
Rectus femoris muscle
Vastus medialis muscle
Lateral cutaneous nerve of thigh
Vastus intermedius muscle
Femur
Vastus lateralis muscle
Tensor fasciae latae muscle
Iliotibial tract
Gluteus maximus muscle

Fascia lata
Branches of femoral nerve
Femoral artery and vein
Adductor longus muscle
Great saphenous vein
Obturator nerve (anterior branch)
Adductor brevis muscle
Obturator nerve (posterior branch)
Gracilis muscle
Adductor magnus muscle
Sciatic nerve
Posterior cutaneous nerve of thigh
Semimembranosus muscle
Semitendinosus muscle
Biceps femoris muscle (long head)

Vastus medialis muscle
Rectus femoris muscle
Vastus intermedius muscle
Vastus lateralis muscle
Iliotibial tract
Lateral intermuscular septum of thigh
Biceps femoris muscle { Short head / Long head }
Semitendinosus muscle
Semimembranosus muscle

Medial intermuscular septum of thigh
Sartorius muscle
Nerve to vastus medialis muscle
Saphenous nerve
Femoral artery and vein
} in adductor canal
Great saphenous vein
Adductor longus muscle
Gracilis muscle
Adductor brevis muscle
Deep artery and vein of thigh
Adductor magnus muscle
Posterior intermuscular septum of thigh
Sciatic nerve

Rectus femoris tendon
Vastus intermedius muscle
Iliotibial tract
Vastus lateralis muscle
Articularis genus muscle
Lateral intermuscular septum of thigh
Femur
Biceps femoris muscle
Common fibular (peroneal) nerve
Tibial nerve

Vastus medialis muscle
Sartorius muscle
Saphenous nerve and descending genicular artery
Great saphenous vein
Gracilis muscle
Adductor magnus tendon
Popliteal vein and artery
Semimembranosus muscle
Semitendinosus muscle

© Novartis

# Knee: Lateral and Medial Views

## Lateral view

Iliotibial tract

Biceps femoris muscle { Long head — Short head

Bursa deep to iliotibial tract

Fibular collateral ligament and bursa deep to it

Plantaris muscle

Biceps femoris tendon and its inferior subtendinous bursa

Common fibular (peroneal) nerve

Head of fibula

Gastrocnemius muscle

Soleus muscle

Fibularis (peroneus) longus muscle

Vastus lateralis muscle

Quadriceps femoris tendon

Patella

Lateral patellar retinaculum

Joint capsule of knee

Patellar ligament

Tibial tuberosity

Tibialis anterior muscle

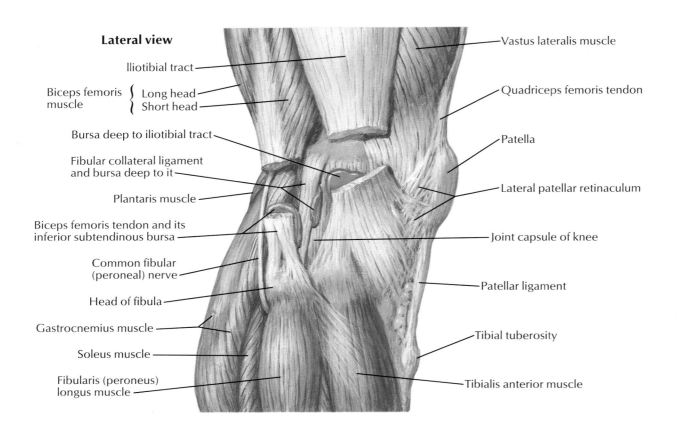

## Medial view

Vastus medialis muscle

Quadriceps femoris tendon

Medial epicondyle of femur

Patella

Medial patellar retinaculum

Joint capsule

Patellar ligament

Tibial tuberosity

Sartorius muscle

Gracilis muscle

Tendon of semitendinosus muscle

Semimembranosus muscle and tendon

Adductor magnus tendon

Parallel fibers } Tibial collateral ligament
Oblique fibers }

Semimembranosus bursa

Anserine bursa deep to Semitendinosus, Gracilis and Sartorius tendons } Pes anserinus

Gastrocnemius muscle

Soleus muscle

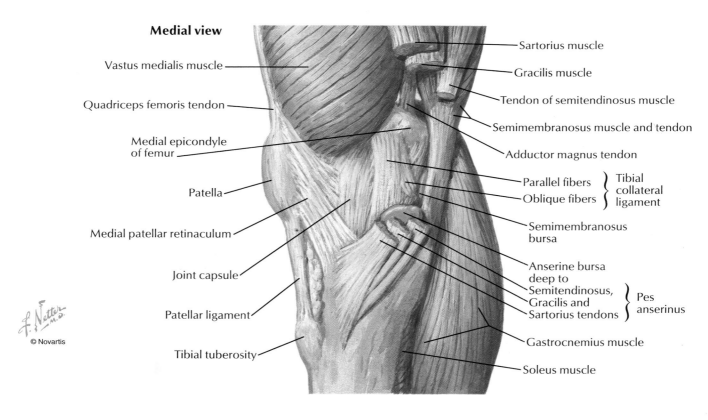

F. Netter
M.D.

© Novartis

**PLATE 472**

**LOWER LIMB**

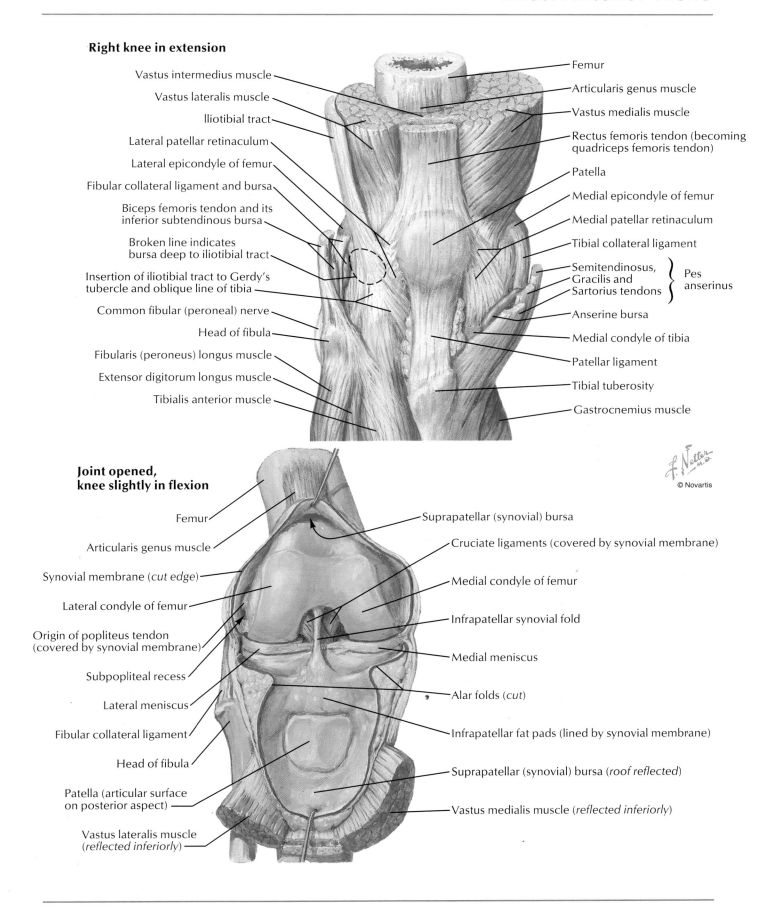

**Right knee in extension**

Vastus intermedius muscle

Vastus lateralis muscle

Iliotibial tract

Lateral patellar retinaculum

Lateral epicondyle of femur

Fibular collateral ligament and bursa

Biceps femoris tendon and its inferior subtendinous bursa

Broken line indicates bursa deep to iliotibial tract

Insertion of iliotibial tract to Gerdy's tubercle and oblique line of tibia

Common fibular (peroneal) nerve

Head of fibula

Fibularis (peroneus) longus muscle

Extensor digitorum longus muscle

Tibialis anterior muscle

Femur

Articularis genus muscle

Vastus medialis muscle

Rectus femoris tendon (becoming quadriceps femoris tendon)

Patella

Medial epicondyle of femur

Medial patellar retinaculum

Tibial collateral ligament

Semitendinosus, Gracilis and Sartorius tendons } Pes anserinus

Anserine bursa

Medial condyle of tibia

Patellar ligament

Tibial tuberosity

Gastrocnemius muscle

**Joint opened, knee slightly in flexion**

Femur

Articularis genus muscle

Synovial membrane (*cut edge*)

Lateral condyle of femur

Origin of popliteus tendon (covered by synovial membrane)

Subpopliteal recess

Lateral meniscus

Fibular collateral ligament

Head of fibula

Patella (articular surface on posterior aspect)

Vastus lateralis muscle (*reflected inferiorly*)

Suprapatellar (synovial) bursa

Cruciate ligaments (covered by synovial membrane)

Medial condyle of femur

Infrapatellar synovial fold

Medial meniscus

Alar folds (*cut*)

Infrapatellar fat pads (lined by synovial membrane)

Suprapatellar (synovial) bursa (*roof reflected*)

Vastus medialis muscle (*reflected inferiorly*)

© Novartis

## Inferior view

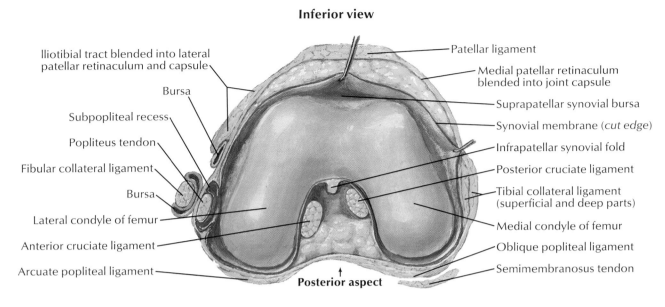

Iliotibial tract blended into lateral patellar retinaculum and capsule

Bursa

Subpopliteal recess

Popliteus tendon

Fibular collateral ligament

Bursa

Lateral condyle of femur

Anterior cruciate ligament

Arcuate popliteal ligament

Patellar ligament

Medial patellar retinaculum blended into joint capsule

Suprapatellar synovial bursa

Synovial membrane (cut edge)

Infrapatellar synovial fold

Posterior cruciate ligament

Tibial collateral ligament (superficial and deep parts)

Medial condyle of femur

Oblique popliteal ligament

Semimembranosus tendon

**Posterior aspect** ↑

## Superior view

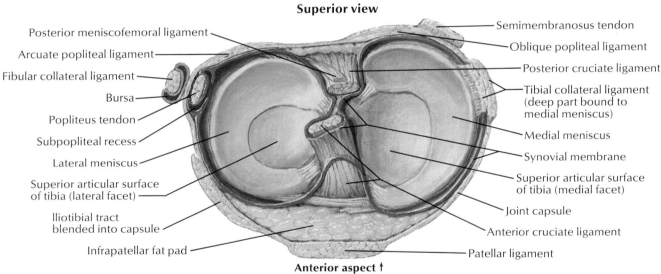

Posterior meniscofemoral ligament

Arcuate popliteal ligament

Fibular collateral ligament

Bursa

Popliteus tendon

Subpopliteal recess

Lateral meniscus

Superior articular surface of tibia (lateral facet)

Iliotibial tract blended into capsule

Infrapatellar fat pad

Semimembranosus tendon

Oblique popliteal ligament

Posterior cruciate ligament

Tibial collateral ligament (deep part bound to medial meniscus)

Medial meniscus

Synovial membrane

Superior articular surface of tibia (medial facet)

Joint capsule

Anterior cruciate ligament

Patellar ligament

**Anterior aspect** ↑

## Superior view: ligaments and cartilage removed

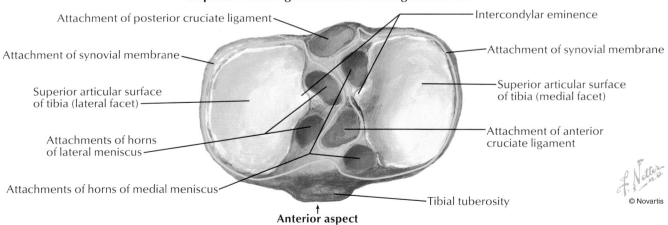

Attachment of posterior cruciate ligament

Attachment of synovial membrane

Superior articular surface of tibia (lateral facet)

Attachments of horns of lateral meniscus

Attachments of horns of medial meniscus

Intercondylar eminence

Attachment of synovial membrane

Superior articular surface of tibia (medial facet)

Attachment of anterior cruciate ligament

Tibial tuberosity

**Anterior aspect** ↑

© Novartis

**PLATE 474**　　　　　　　　　　　　　　　　　　　**LOWER LIMB**

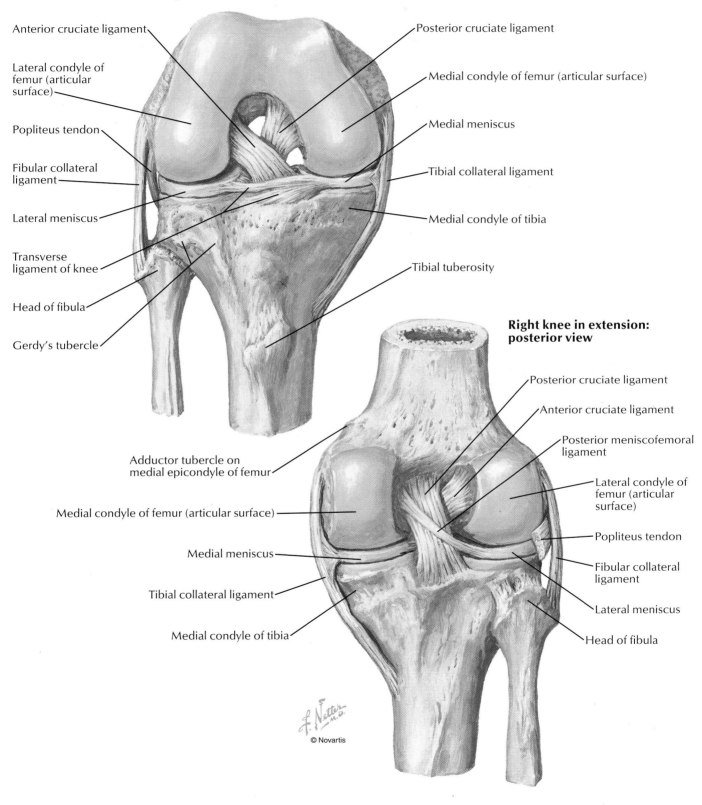

**Right knee in flexion: anterior view**

Anterior cruciate ligament

Lateral condyle of femur (articular surface)

Popliteus tendon

Fibular collateral ligament

Lateral meniscus

Transverse ligament of knee

Head of fibula

Gerdy's tubercle

Posterior cruciate ligament

Medial condyle of femur (articular surface)

Medial meniscus

Tibial collateral ligament

Medial condyle of tibia

Tibial tuberosity

**Right knee in extension: posterior view**

Adductor tubercle on medial epicondyle of femur

Medial condyle of femur (articular surface)

Medial meniscus

Tibial collateral ligament

Medial condyle of tibia

Posterior cruciate ligament

Anterior cruciate ligament

Posterior meniscofemoral ligament

Lateral condyle of femur (articular surface)

Popliteus tendon

Fibular collateral ligament

Lateral meniscus

Head of fibula

© Novartis

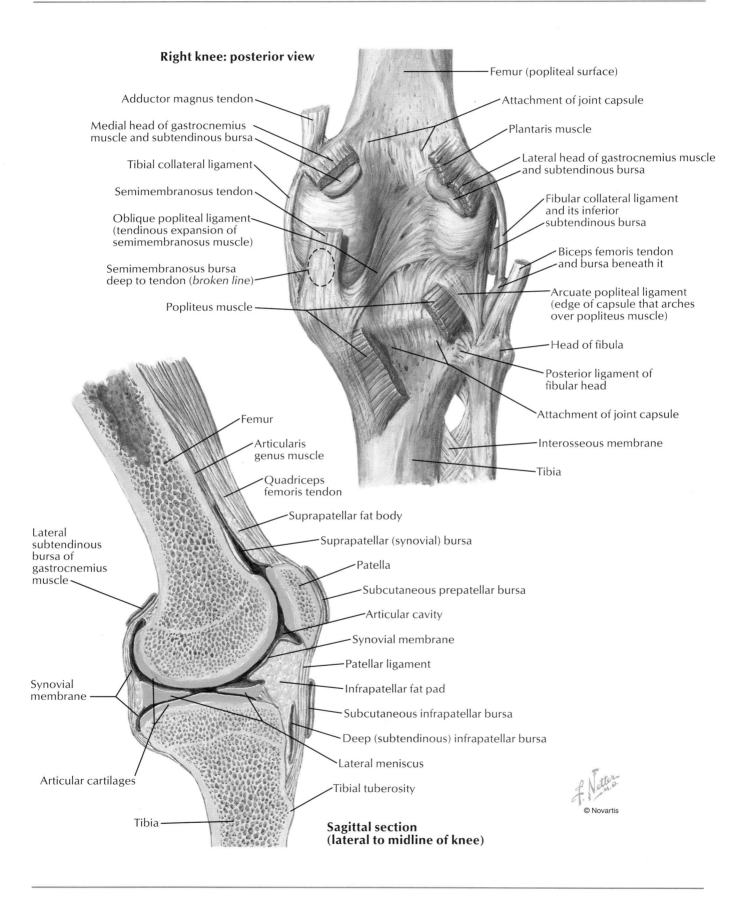

**Right knee: posterior view**

Adductor magnus tendon

Medial head of gastrocnemius muscle and subtendinous bursa

Tibial collateral ligament

Semimembranosus tendon

Oblique popliteal ligament (tendinous expansion of semimembranosus muscle)

Semimembranosus bursa deep to tendon (*broken line*)

Popliteus muscle

Femur (popliteal surface)

Attachment of joint capsule

Plantaris muscle

Lateral head of gastrocnemius muscle and subtendinous bursa

Fibular collateral ligament and its inferior subtendinous bursa

Biceps femoris tendon and bursa beneath it

Arcuate popliteal ligament (edge of capsule that arches over popliteus muscle)

Head of fibula

Posterior ligament of fibular head

Attachment of joint capsule

Interosseous membrane

Tibia

Femur

Articularis genus muscle

Quadriceps femoris tendon

Suprapatellar fat body

Suprapatellar (synovial) bursa

Patella

Subcutaneous prepatellar bursa

Articular cavity

Synovial membrane

Patellar ligament

Infrapatellar fat pad

Subcutaneous infrapatellar bursa

Deep (subtendinous) infrapatellar bursa

Lateral meniscus

Tibial tuberosity

Lateral subtendinous bursa of gastrocnemius muscle

Synovial membrane

Articular cartilages

Tibia

**Sagittal section (lateral to midline of knee)**

© Novartis

**PLATE 476**　　　　　　　　　　　　　　　　　　　**LOWER LIMB**

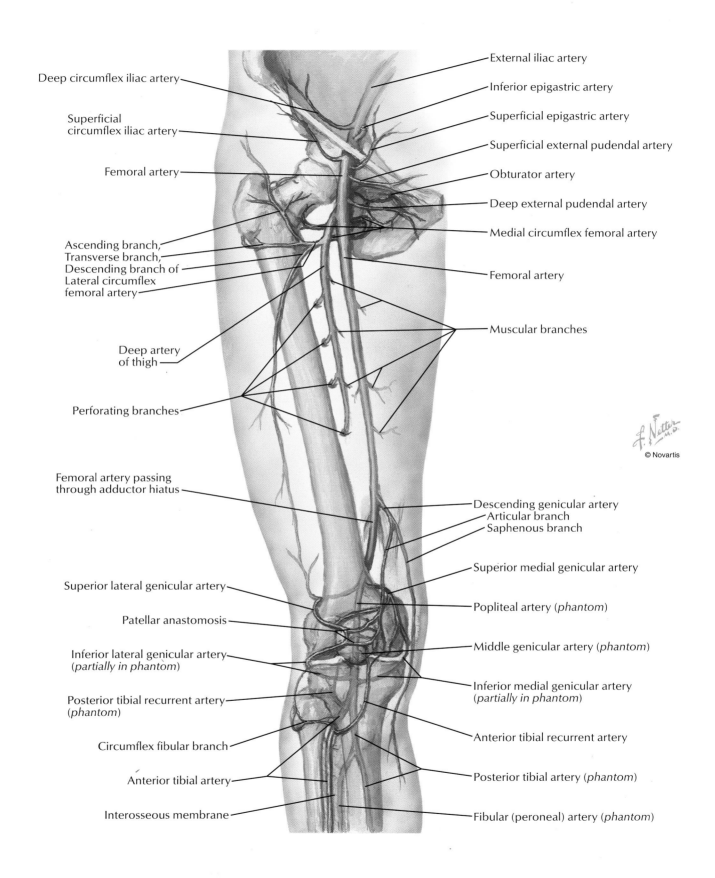

Deep circumflex iliac artery

Superficial circumflex iliac artery

Femoral artery

Ascending branch,
Transverse branch,
Descending branch of
Lateral circumflex
femoral artery

Deep artery of thigh

Perforating branches

Femoral artery passing through adductor hiatus

Superior lateral genicular artery

Patellar anastomosis

Inferior lateral genicular artery (*partially in phantom*)

Posterior tibial recurrent artery (*phantom*)

Circumflex fibular branch

Anterior tibial artery

Interosseous membrane

External iliac artery

Inferior epigastric artery

Superficial epigastric artery

Superficial external pudendal artery

Obturator artery

Deep external pudendal artery

Medial circumflex femoral artery

Femoral artery

Muscular branches

Descending genicular artery
Articular branch
Saphenous branch

Superior medial genicular artery

Popliteal artery (*phantom*)

Middle genicular artery (*phantom*)

Inferior medial genicular artery (*partially in phantom*)

Anterior tibial recurrent artery

Posterior tibial artery (*phantom*)

Fibular (peroneal) artery (*phantom*)

F. Netter M.D.
© Novartis

# Tibia and Fibula

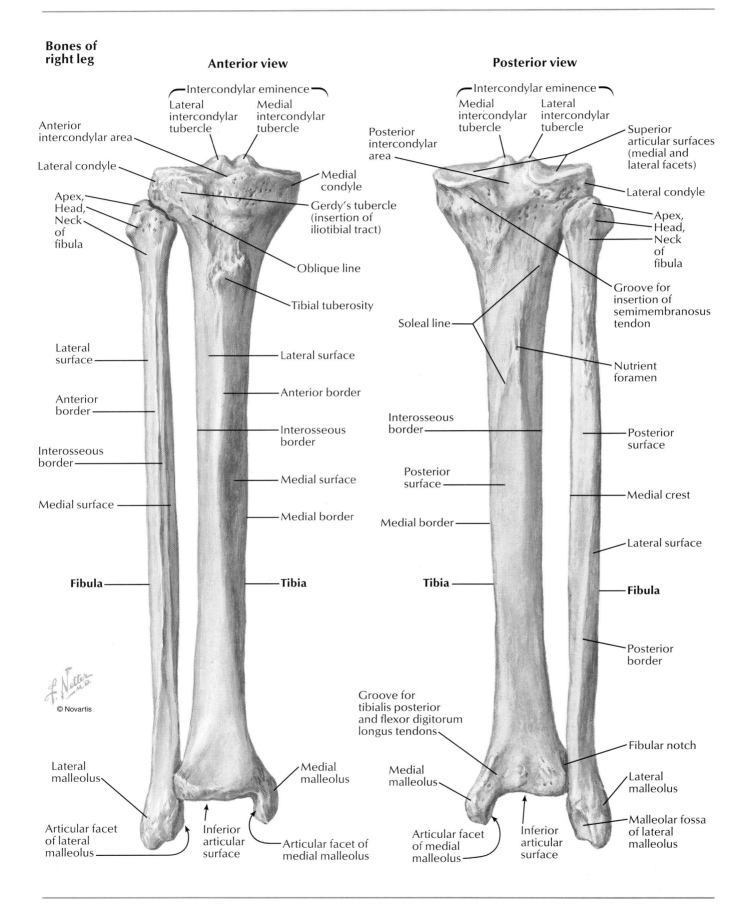

**Bones of right leg**

**Anterior view**

Intercondylar eminence
Lateral intercondylar tubercle
Medial intercondylar tubercle
Anterior intercondylar area
Lateral condyle
Apex, Head, Neck of fibula
Medial condyle
Gerdy's tubercle (insertion of iliotibial tract)
Oblique line
Tibial tuberosity
Lateral surface
Lateral surface
Anterior border
Anterior border
Interosseous border
Interosseous border
Medial surface
Medial surface
Medial border
**Fibula**
**Tibia**
Lateral malleolus
Medial malleolus
Articular facet of lateral malleolus
Inferior articular surface
Articular facet of medial malleolus

**Posterior view**

Intercondylar eminence
Medial intercondylar tubercle
Lateral intercondylar tubercle
Posterior intercondylar area
Superior articular surfaces (medial and lateral facets)
Lateral condyle
Apex, Head, Neck of fibula
Groove for insertion of semimembranosus tendon
Soleal line
Nutrient foramen
Interosseous border
Posterior surface
Posterior surface
Medial crest
Medial border
Lateral surface
**Tibia**
**Fibula**
Posterior border
Groove for tibialis posterior and flexor digitorum longus tendons
Medial malleolus
Fibular notch
Lateral malleolus
Malleolar fossa of lateral malleolus
Articular facet of medial malleolus
Inferior articular surface

© Novartis

*PLATE 478*

**LOWER LIMB**

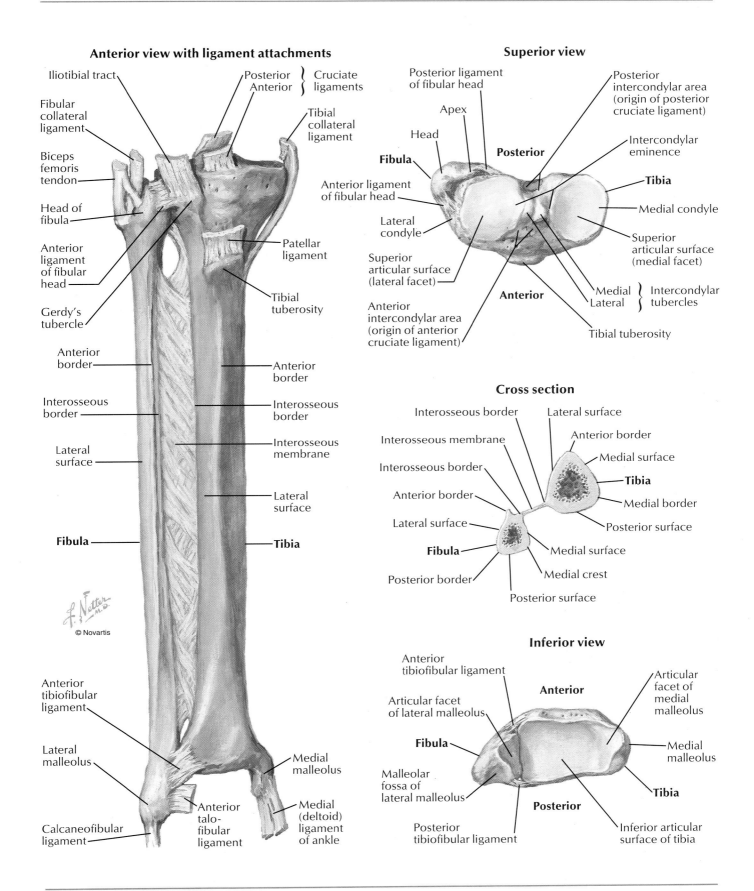

**Anterior view with ligament attachments**

Iliotibial tract
Posterior
Anterior } Cruciate ligaments
Fibular collateral ligament
Tibial collateral ligament
Biceps femoris tendon
Head of fibula
Anterior ligament of fibular head
Patellar ligament
Gerdy's tubercle
Tibial tuberosity
Anterior border
Anterior border
Interosseous border
Interosseous border
Interosseous membrane
Lateral surface
Lateral surface
**Fibula**
**Tibia**
Anterior tibiofibular ligament
Lateral malleolus
Medial malleolus
Anterior talofibular ligament
Medial (deltoid) ligament of ankle
Calcaneofibular ligament

**Superior view**

Posterior ligament of fibular head
Posterior intercondylar area (origin of posterior cruciate ligament)
Apex
Head
Intercondylar eminence
**Fibula**
**Posterior**
**Tibia**
Anterior ligament of fibular head
Medial condyle
Lateral condyle
Superior articular surface (medial facet)
Superior articular surface (lateral facet)
Medial
Lateral } Intercondylar tubercles
**Anterior**
Anterior intercondylar area (origin of anterior cruciate ligament)
Tibial tuberosity

**Cross section**

Interosseous border
Lateral surface
Interosseous membrane
Anterior border
Interosseous border
Medial surface
Anterior border
**Tibia**
Lateral surface
Medial border
**Fibula**
Posterior surface
Medial surface
Posterior border
Medial crest
Posterior surface

**Inferior view**

Anterior tibiofibular ligament
Articular facet of medial malleolus
**Anterior**
Articular facet of lateral malleolus
**Fibula**
Medial malleolus
Malleolar fossa of lateral malleolus
**Tibia**
**Posterior**
Posterior tibiofibular ligament
Inferior articular surface of tibia

© Novartis

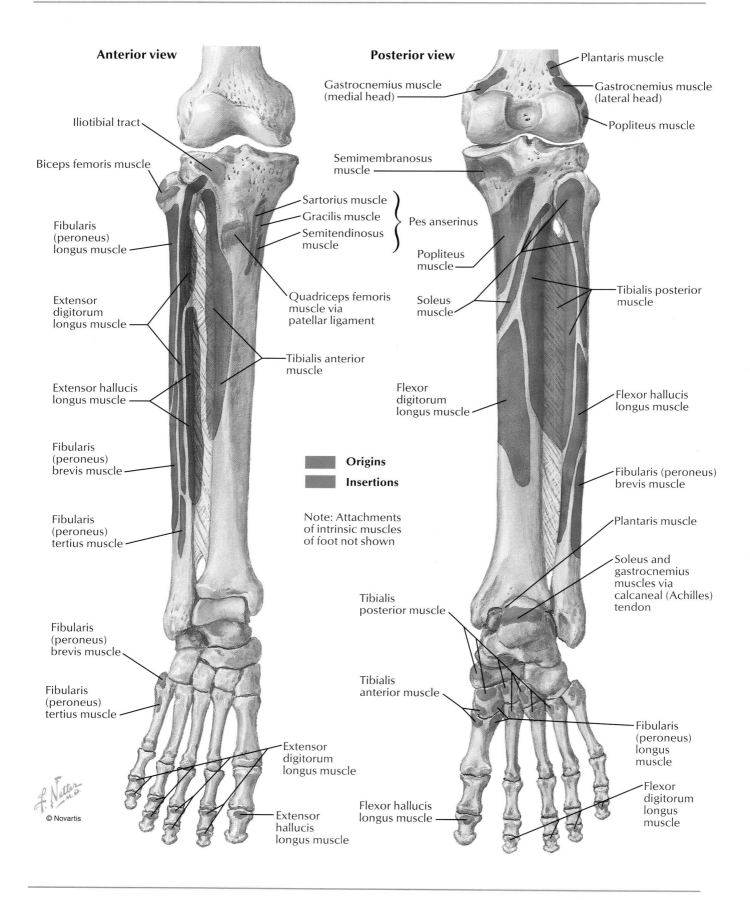

**Anterior view**

**Posterior view**

Iliotibial tract

Biceps femoris muscle

Fibularis (peroneus) longus muscle

Extensor digitorum longus muscle

Extensor hallucis longus muscle

Fibularis (peroneus) brevis muscle

Fibularis (peroneus) tertius muscle

Fibularis (peroneus) brevis muscle

Fibularis (peroneus) tertius muscle

Sartorius muscle
Gracilis muscle
Semitendinosus muscle

} Pes anserinus

Quadriceps femoris muscle via patellar ligament

Tibialis anterior muscle

Extensor digitorum longus muscle

Extensor hallucis longus muscle

Gastrocnemius muscle (medial head)

Semimembranosus muscle

Popliteus muscle

Soleus muscle

Flexor digitorum longus muscle

Tibialis posterior muscle

Tibialis anterior muscle

Flexor hallucis longus muscle

Plantaris muscle

Gastrocnemius muscle (lateral head)

Popliteus muscle

Tibialis posterior muscle

Flexor hallucis longus muscle

Fibularis (peroneus) brevis muscle

Plantaris muscle

Soleus and gastrocnemius muscles via calcaneal (Achilles) tendon

Fibularis (peroneus) longus muscle

Flexor digitorum longus muscle

**Origins**

**Insertions**

Note: Attachments of intrinsic muscles of foot not shown

*f. Netter*
M.D.

© Novartis

*PLATE 480*

**LOWER LIMB**

# Muscles of Leg (Superficial Dissection): Posterior View

SEE ALSO PLATE 504

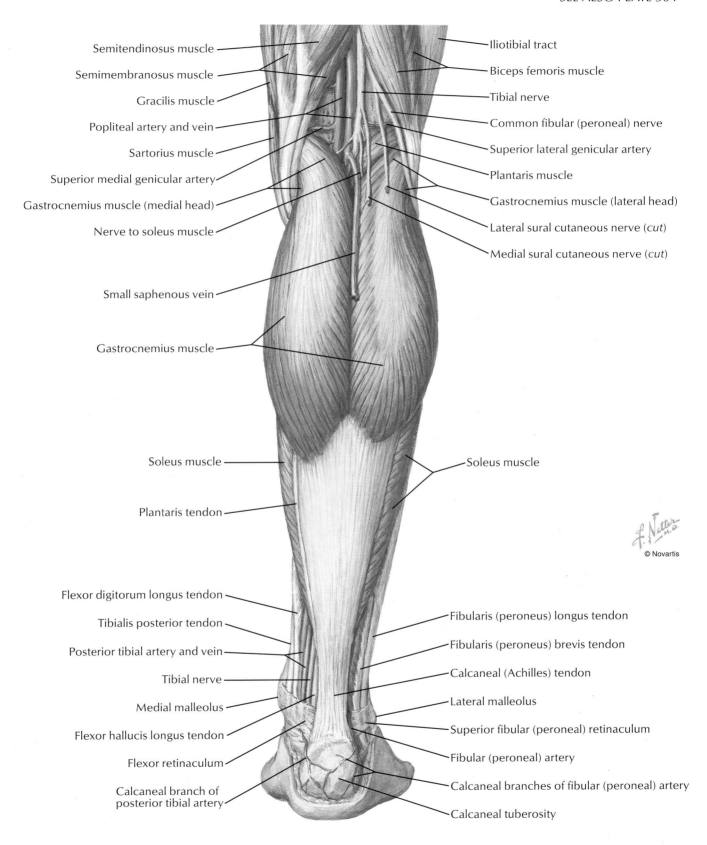

Semitendinosus muscle

Semimembranosus muscle

Gracilis muscle

Popliteal artery and vein

Sartorius muscle

Superior medial genicular artery

Gastrocnemius muscle (medial head)

Nerve to soleus muscle

Small saphenous vein

Gastrocnemius muscle

Soleus muscle

Plantaris tendon

Flexor digitorum longus tendon

Tibialis posterior tendon

Posterior tibial artery and vein

Tibial nerve

Medial malleolus

Flexor hallucis longus tendon

Flexor retinaculum

Calcaneal branch of
posterior tibial artery

Iliotibial tract

Biceps femoris muscle

Tibial nerve

Common fibular (peroneal) nerve

Superior lateral genicular artery

Plantaris muscle

Gastrocnemius muscle (lateral head)

Lateral sural cutaneous nerve (cut)

Medial sural cutaneous nerve (cut)

Soleus muscle

Fibularis (peroneus) longus tendon

Fibularis (peroneus) brevis tendon

Calcaneal (Achilles) tendon

Lateral malleolus

Superior fibular (peroneal) retinaculum

Fibular (peroneal) artery

Calcaneal branches of fibular (peroneal) artery

Calcaneal tuberosity

© Novartis

SEE ALSO PLATE 505

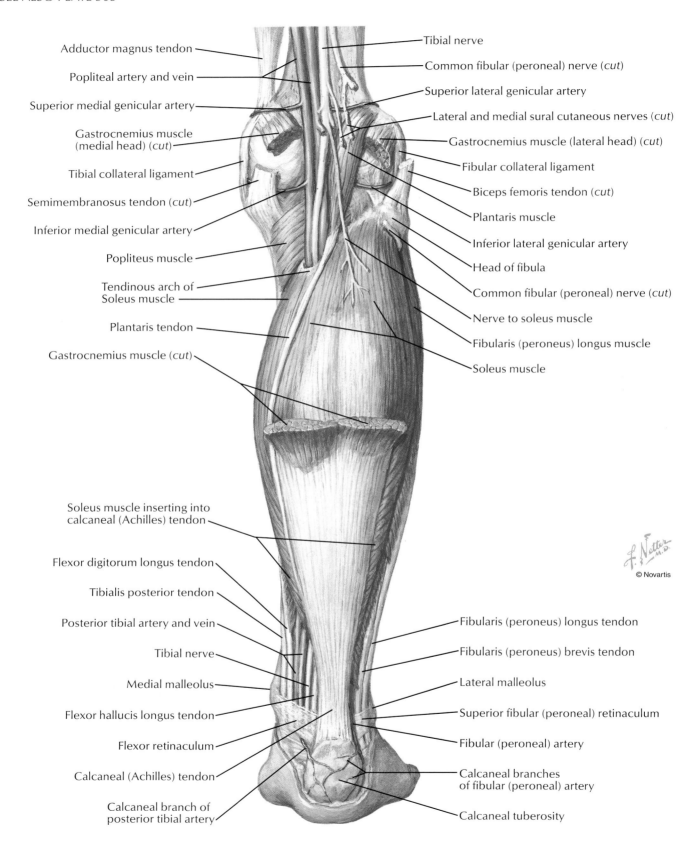

Adductor magnus tendon

Popliteal artery and vein

Superior medial genicular artery

Gastrocnemius muscle (medial head) (*cut*)

Tibial collateral ligament

Semimembranosus tendon (*cut*)

Inferior medial genicular artery

Popliteus muscle

Tendinous arch of Soleus muscle

Plantaris tendon

Gastrocnemius muscle (*cut*)

Soleus muscle inserting into calcaneal (Achilles) tendon

Flexor digitorum longus tendon

Tibialis posterior tendon

Posterior tibial artery and vein

Tibial nerve

Medial malleolus

Flexor hallucis longus tendon

Flexor retinaculum

Calcaneal (Achilles) tendon

Calcaneal branch of posterior tibial artery

Tibial nerve

Common fibular (peroneal) nerve (*cut*)

Superior lateral genicular artery

Lateral and medial sural cutaneous nerves (*cut*)

Gastrocnemius muscle (lateral head) (*cut*)

Fibular collateral ligament

Biceps femoris tendon (*cut*)

Plantaris muscle

Inferior lateral genicular artery

Head of fibula

Common fibular (peroneal) nerve (*cut*)

Nerve to soleus muscle

Fibularis (peroneus) longus muscle

Soleus muscle

Fibularis (peroneus) longus tendon

Fibularis (peroneus) brevis tendon

Lateral malleolus

Superior fibular (peroneal) retinaculum

Fibular (peroneal) artery

Calcaneal branches of fibular (peroneal) artery

Calcaneal tuberosity

F. Netter M.D.

© Novartis

**PLATE 482**

**LOWER LIMB**

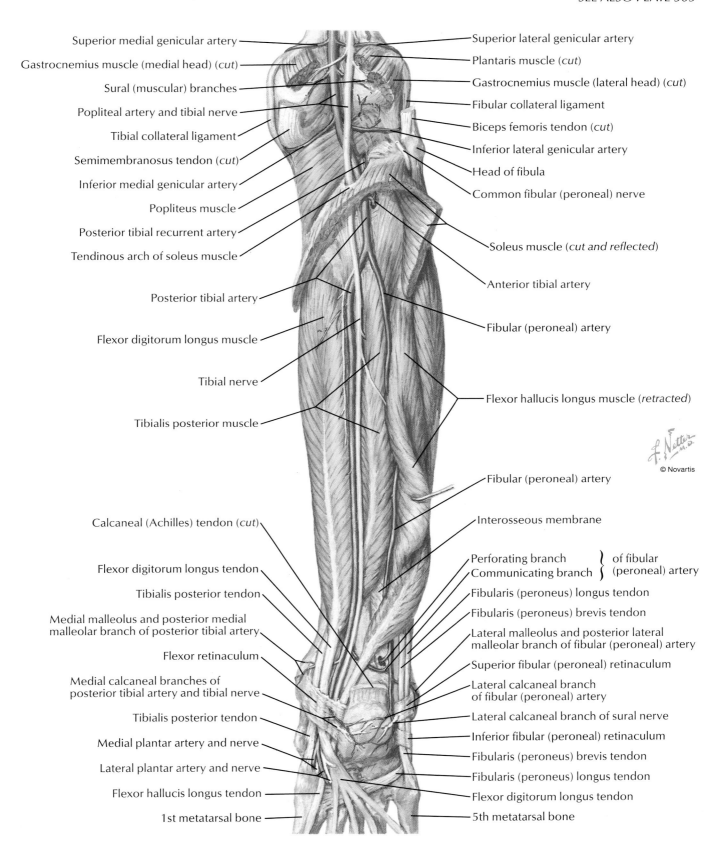

Superior medial genicular artery

Gastrocnemius muscle (medial head) (*cut*)

Sural (muscular) branches

Popliteal artery and tibial nerve

Tibial collateral ligament

Semimembranosus tendon (*cut*)

Inferior medial genicular artery

Popliteus muscle

Posterior tibial recurrent artery

Tendinous arch of soleus muscle

Posterior tibial artery

Flexor digitorum longus muscle

Tibial nerve

Tibialis posterior muscle

Calcaneal (Achilles) tendon (*cut*)

Flexor digitorum longus tendon

Tibialis posterior tendon

Medial malleolus and posterior medial malleolar branch of posterior tibial artery

Flexor retinaculum

Medial calcaneal branches of posterior tibial artery and tibial nerve

Tibialis posterior tendon

Medial plantar artery and nerve

Lateral plantar artery and nerve

Flexor hallucis longus tendon

1st metatarsal bone

Superior lateral genicular artery

Plantaris muscle (*cut*)

Gastrocnemius muscle (lateral head) (*cut*)

Fibular collateral ligament

Biceps femoris tendon (*cut*)

Inferior lateral genicular artery

Head of fibula

Common fibular (peroneal) nerve

Soleus muscle (*cut and reflected*)

Anterior tibial artery

Fibular (peroneal) artery

Flexor hallucis longus muscle (*retracted*)

Fibular (peroneal) artery

Interosseous membrane

Perforating branch } of fibular
Communicating branch } (peroneal) artery

Fibularis (peroneus) longus tendon

Fibularis (peroneus) brevis tendon

Lateral malleolus and posterior lateral malleolar branch of fibular (peroneal) artery

Superior fibular (peroneal) retinaculum

Lateral calcaneal branch of fibular (peroneal) artery

Lateral calcaneal branch of sural nerve

Inferior fibular (peroneal) retinaculum

Fibularis (peroneus) brevis tendon

Fibularis (peroneus) longus tendon

Flexor digitorum longus tendon

5th metatarsal bone

*SEE ALSO PLATE 506*

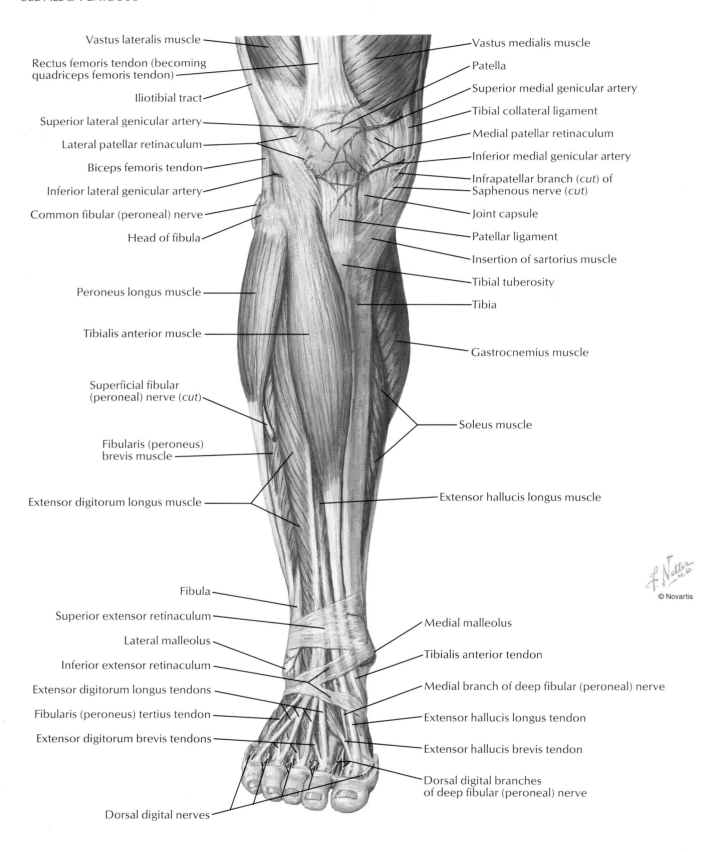

Vastus lateralis muscle

Rectus femoris tendon (becoming quadriceps femoris tendon)

Iliotibial tract

Superior lateral genicular artery

Lateral patellar retinaculum

Biceps femoris tendon

Inferior lateral genicular artery

Common fibular (peroneal) nerve

Head of fibula

Peroneus longus muscle

Tibialis anterior muscle

Superficial fibular (peroneal) nerve (*cut*)

Fibularis (peroneus) brevis muscle

Extensor digitorum longus muscle

Fibula

Superior extensor retinaculum

Lateral malleolus

Inferior extensor retinaculum

Extensor digitorum longus tendons

Fibularis (peroneus) tertius tendon

Extensor digitorum brevis tendons

Dorsal digital nerves

Vastus medialis muscle

Patella

Superior medial genicular artery

Tibial collateral ligament

Medial patellar retinaculum

Inferior medial genicular artery

Infrapatellar branch (*cut*) of Saphenous nerve (*cut*)

Joint capsule

Patellar ligament

Insertion of sartorius muscle

Tibial tuberosity

Tibia

Gastrocnemius muscle

Soleus muscle

Extensor hallucis longus muscle

Medial malleolus

Tibialis anterior tendon

Medial branch of deep fibular (peroneal) nerve

Extensor hallucis longus tendon

Extensor hallucis brevis tendon

Dorsal digital branches of deep fibular (peroneal) nerve

© Novartis

**PLATE 484**

**LOWER LIMB**

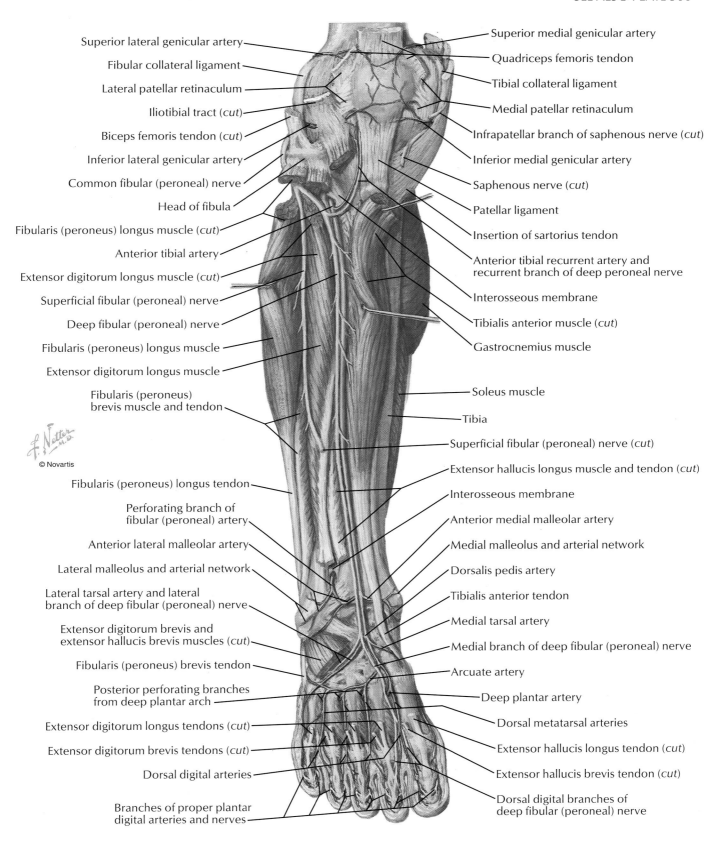

Superior lateral genicular artery

Fibular collateral ligament

Lateral patellar retinaculum

Iliotibial tract (*cut*)

Biceps femoris tendon (*cut*)

Inferior lateral genicular artery

Common fibular (peroneal) nerve

Head of fibula

Fibularis (peroneus) longus muscle (*cut*)

Anterior tibial artery

Extensor digitorum longus muscle (*cut*)

Superficial fibular (peroneal) nerve

Deep fibular (peroneal) nerve

Fibularis (peroneus) longus muscle

Extensor digitorum longus muscle

Fibularis (peroneus) brevis muscle and tendon

Fibularis (peroneus) longus tendon

Perforating branch of fibular (peroneal) artery

Anterior lateral malleolar artery

Lateral malleolus and arterial network

Lateral tarsal artery and lateral branch of deep fibular (peroneal) nerve

Extensor digitorum brevis and extensor hallucis brevis muscles (*cut*)

Fibularis (peroneus) brevis tendon

Posterior perforating branches from deep plantar arch

Extensor digitorum longus tendons (*cut*)

Extensor digitorum brevis tendons (*cut*)

Dorsal digital arteries

Branches of proper plantar digital arteries and nerves

Superior medial genicular artery

Quadriceps femoris tendon

Tibial collateral ligament

Medial patellar retinaculum

Infrapatellar branch of saphenous nerve (*cut*)

Inferior medial genicular artery

Saphenous nerve (*cut*)

Patellar ligament

Insertion of sartorius tendon

Anterior tibial recurrent artery and recurrent branch of deep peroneal nerve

Interosseous membrane

Tibialis anterior muscle (*cut*)

Gastrocnemius muscle

Soleus muscle

Tibia

Superficial fibular (peroneal) nerve (*cut*)

Extensor hallucis longus muscle and tendon (*cut*)

Interosseous membrane

Anterior medial malleolar artery

Medial malleolus and arterial network

Dorsalis pedis artery

Tibialis anterior tendon

Medial tarsal artery

Medial branch of deep fibular (peroneal) nerve

Arcuate artery

Deep plantar artery

Dorsal metatarsal arteries

Extensor hallucis longus tendon (*cut*)

Extensor hallucis brevis tendon (*cut*)

Dorsal digital branches of deep fibular (peroneal) nerve

*F. Netter M.D.*

© Novartis

*SEE ALSO PLATE 506*

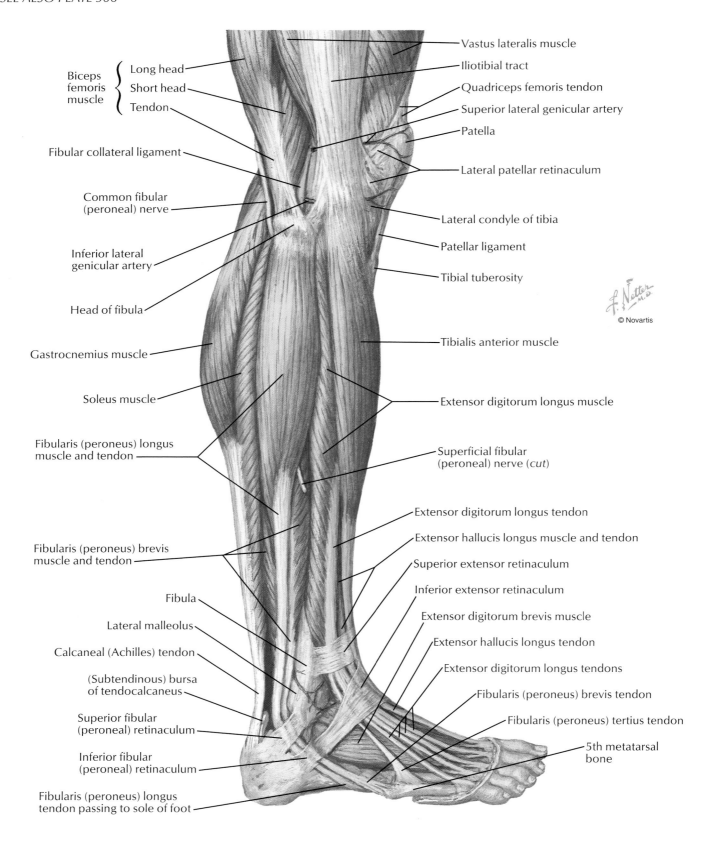

Biceps femoris muscle { Long head / Short head / Tendon

Vastus lateralis muscle

Iliotibial tract

Quadriceps femoris tendon

Superior lateral genicular artery

Patella

Fibular collateral ligament

Lateral patellar retinaculum

Common fibular (peroneal) nerve

Lateral condyle of tibia

Inferior lateral genicular artery

Patellar ligament

Tibial tuberosity

Head of fibula

© Novartis

Gastrocnemius muscle

Tibialis anterior muscle

Soleus muscle

Extensor digitorum longus muscle

Fibularis (peroneus) longus muscle and tendon

Superficial fibular (peroneal) nerve (*cut*)

Extensor digitorum longus tendon

Extensor hallucis longus muscle and tendon

Fibularis (peroneus) brevis muscle and tendon

Superior extensor retinaculum

Inferior extensor retinaculum

Extensor digitorum brevis muscle

Fibula

Lateral malleolus

Extensor hallucis longus tendon

Calcaneal (Achilles) tendon

Extensor digitorum longus tendons

(Subtendinous) bursa of tendocalcaneus

Fibularis (peroneus) brevis tendon

Superior fibular (peroneal) retinaculum

Fibularis (peroneus) tertius tendon

5th metatarsal bone

Inferior fibular (peroneal) retinaculum

Fibularis (peroneus) longus tendon passing to sole of foot

**PLATE 486**

**LOWER LIMB**

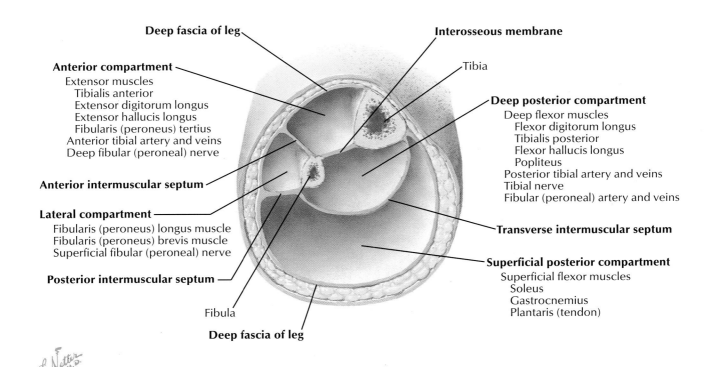

**Deep fascia of leg**

**Interosseous membrane**

Tibia

**Anterior compartment**
Extensor muscles
Tibialis anterior
Extensor digitorum longus
Extensor hallucis longus
Fibularis (peroneus) tertius
Anterior tibial artery and veins
Deep fibular (peroneal) nerve

**Anterior intermuscular septum**

**Lateral compartment**
Fibularis (peroneus) longus muscle
Fibularis (peroneus) brevis muscle
Superficial fibular (peroneal) nerve

**Posterior intermuscular septum**

Fibula

**Deep fascia of leg**

**Deep posterior compartment**
Deep flexor muscles
Flexor digitorum longus
Tibialis posterior
Flexor hallucis longus
Popliteus
Posterior tibial artery and veins
Tibial nerve
Fibular (peroneal) artery and veins

**Transverse intermuscular septum**

**Superficial posterior compartment**
Superficial flexor muscles
Soleus
Gastrocnemius
Plantaris (tendon)

© Novartis

**Cross section just above middle of leg**

Tibialis anterior muscle

Extensor hallucis longus muscle

Extensor digitorum longus muscle

Superficial fibular (peroneal) nerve

Anterior intermuscular septum

Deep fascia of leg

Fibularis (peroneus) longus muscle

Fibularis (peroneus) brevis muscle

Posterior intermuscular septum

Fibula

Lateral sural cutaneous nerve

Transverse intermuscular septum

Soleus muscle

Gastrocnemius muscle (lateral head)

Sural communicating branch of lateral sural cutaneous nerve

Anterior tibial artery and veins and deep fibular (peroneal) nerve

Tibia

Interosseous membrane

Great saphenous vein and saphenous nerve

Tibialis posterior muscle

Flexor digitorum longus muscle

Fibular (peroneal) artery and veins

Posterior tibial artery and veins and tibial nerve

Flexor hallucis longus muscle

Deep fascia of leg

Plantaris tendon

Gastrocnemius muscle (medial head)

Medial sural cutaneous nerve

Small saphenous vein

# Bones of Foot

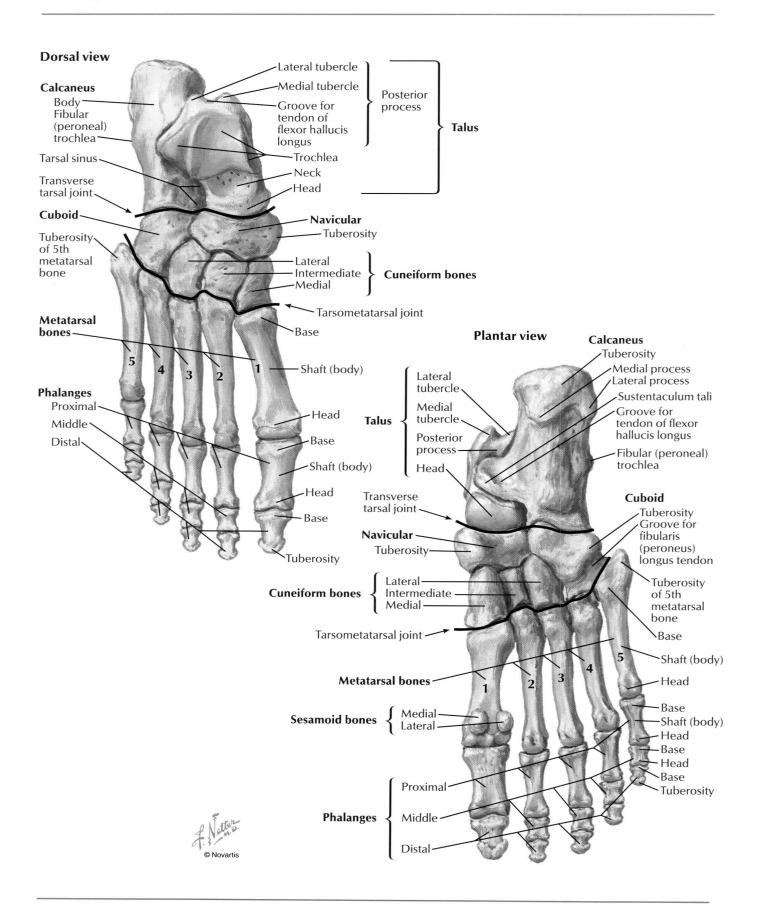

**Dorsal view**

**Calcaneus**
Body
Fibular (peroneal) trochlea
Tarsal sinus
Transverse tarsal joint
**Cuboid**
Tuberosity of 5th metatarsal bone
**Metatarsal bones**
**Phalanges**
Proximal
Middle
Distal

Lateral tubercle
Medial tubercle
Groove for tendon of flexor hallucis longus
Trochlea
Neck
Head

Posterior process

**Talus**

**Navicular**
Tuberosity
Lateral
Intermediate
Medial
Tarsometatarsal joint
Base
Shaft (body)

**Cuneiform bones**

5  4  3  2  1

Head
Base
Shaft (body)
Head
Base
Tuberosity

**Plantar view**

Lateral tubercle
Medial tubercle
Posterior process
Head

**Talus**

Transverse tarsal joint
**Navicular**
Tuberosity

**Cuneiform bones**
Lateral
Intermediate
Medial
Tarsometatarsal joint

**Metatarsal bones**

**Sesamoid bones**
Medial
Lateral

**Phalanges**
Proximal
Middle
Distal

**Calcaneus**
Tuberosity
Medial process
Lateral process
Sustentaculum tali
Groove for tendon of flexor hallucis longus
Fibular (peroneal) trochlea

**Cuboid**
Tuberosity
Groove for fibularis (peroneus) longus tendon
Tuberosity of 5th metatarsal bone
Base
Shaft (body)
Head
Base
Shaft (body)
Head
Base
Head
Base
Tuberosity

1  2  3  4  5

F. Netter M.D.
© Novartis

*PLATE 488*

**LOWER LIMB**

**Lateral view**

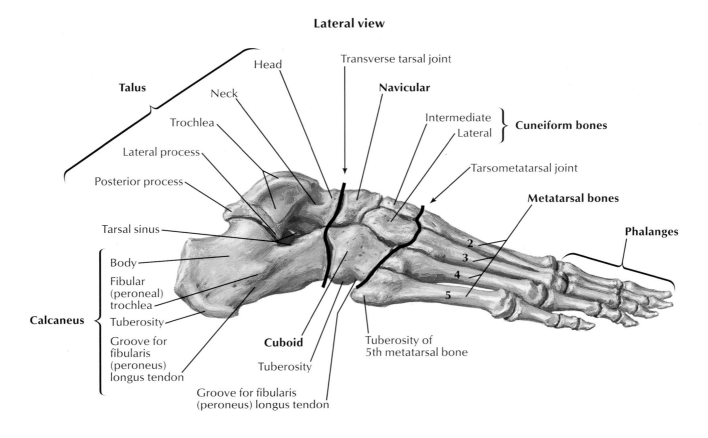

Transverse tarsal joint

Head

Neck

**Talus**

Trochlea

Lateral process

Posterior process

Tarsal sinus

**Navicular**

Intermediate
Lateral } **Cuneiform bones**

Tarsometatarsal joint

**Metatarsal bones**

**Phalanges**

**Calcaneus** {
Body
Fibular (peroneal) trochlea
Tuberosity
Groove for fibularis (peroneus) longus tendon

2
3
4
5

**Cuboid**

Tuberosity

Groove for fibularis (peroneus) longus tendon

Tuberosity of 5th metatarsal bone

**Medial view**

f. Netter
© Novartis

Transverse tarsal joint

**Navicular**
Tuberosity

Neck

**Talus**

Head

Trochlea

Posterior process

**Cuneiform bones** {
Intermediate
Medial

Tarsometatarsal joint

**Metatarsal bones**

**Phalanges**

2
1

Tuberosity of 1st metatarsal bone

**Sesamoid bone**

Tuberosity

Groove for tendon of flexor hallucis longus

Sustentaculum tali

**Calcaneus**

# *Calcaneus*

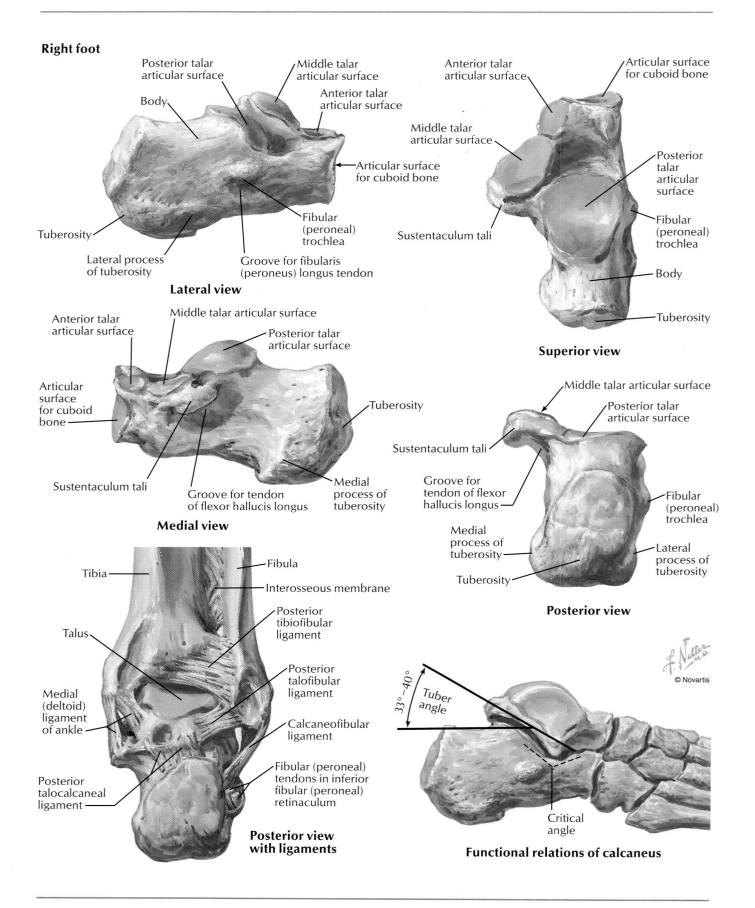

Posterior talar articular surface

Middle talar articular surface

Body

Anterior talar articular surface

Articular surface for cuboid bone

Tuberosity

Fibular (peroneal) trochlea

Lateral process of tuberosity

Groove for fibularis (peroneus) longus tendon

**Lateral view**

Anterior talar articular surface

Middle talar articular surface

Posterior talar articular surface

Articular surface for cuboid bone

Tuberosity

Sustentaculum tali

Groove for tendon of flexor hallucis longus

Medial process of tuberosity

**Medial view**

Anterior talar articular surface

Middle talar articular surface

Articular surface for cuboid bone

Posterior talar articular surface

Sustentaculum tali

Fibular (peroneal) trochlea

Body

Tuberosity

**Superior view**

Middle talar articular surface

Posterior talar articular surface

Sustentaculum tali

Groove for tendon of flexor hallucis longus

Medial process of tuberosity

Tuberosity

Fibular (peroneal) trochlea

Lateral process of tuberosity

**Posterior view**

Tibia

Fibula

Interosseous membrane

Talus

Posterior tibiofibular ligament

Posterior talofibular ligament

Medial (deltoid) ligament of ankle

Calcaneofibular ligament

Posterior talocalcaneal ligament

Fibular (peroneal) tendons in inferior fibular (peroneal) retinaculum

**Posterior view with ligaments**

33°–40°

Tuber angle

Critical angle

**Functional relations of calcaneus**

© Novartis

**PLATE 490**

**LOWER LIMB**

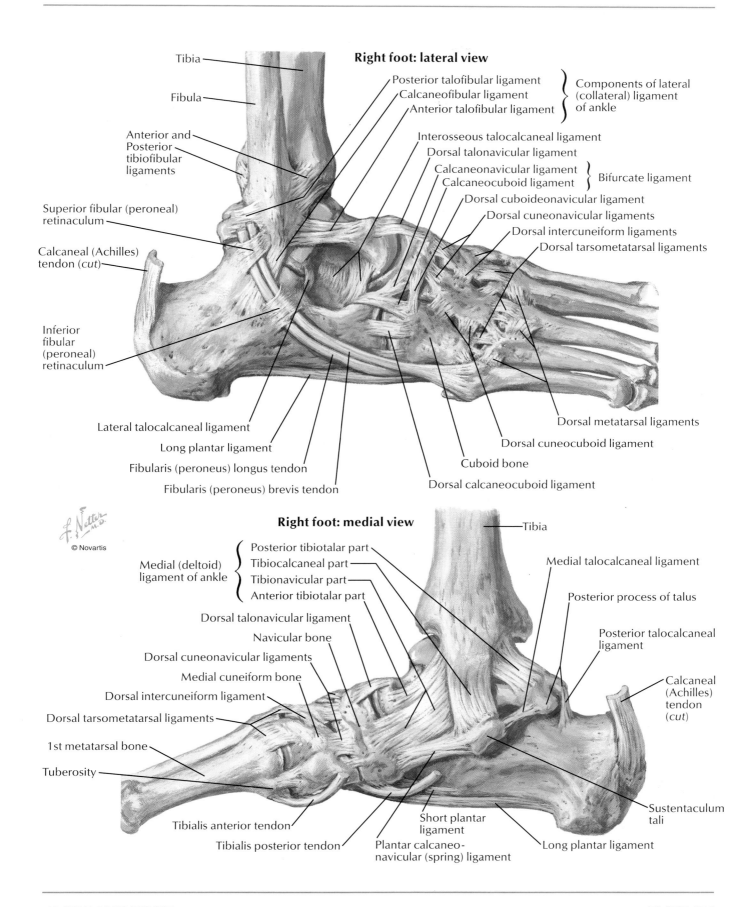

**Right foot: lateral view**

Tibia

Fibula

Anterior and Posterior tibiofibular ligaments

Superior fibular (peroneal) retinaculum

Calcaneal (Achilles) tendon (*cut*)

Inferior fibular (peroneal) retinaculum

Posterior talofibular ligament
Calcaneofibular ligament
Anterior talofibular ligament

Components of lateral (collateral) ligament of ankle

Interosseous talocalcaneal ligament
Dorsal talonavicular ligament
Calcaneonavicular ligament
Calcaneocuboid ligament

Bifurcate ligament

Dorsal cuboideonavicular ligament
Dorsal cuneonavicular ligaments
Dorsal intercuneiform ligaments
Dorsal tarsometatarsal ligaments

Dorsal metatarsal ligaments

Dorsal cuneocuboid ligament

Cuboid bone

Dorsal calcaneocuboid ligament

Lateral talocalcaneal ligament
Long plantar ligament
Fibularis (peroneus) longus tendon
Fibularis (peroneus) brevis tendon

**Right foot: medial view**

Tibia

Medial (deltoid) ligament of ankle

Posterior tibiotalar part
Tibiocalcaneal part
Tibionavicular part
Anterior tibiotalar part

Dorsal talonavicular ligament
Navicular bone
Dorsal cuneonavicular ligaments
Medial cuneiform bone
Dorsal intercuneiform ligament
Dorsal tarsometatarsal ligaments
1st metatarsal bone
Tuberosity

Medial talocalcaneal ligament

Posterior process of talus

Posterior talocalcaneal ligament

Calcaneal (Achilles) tendon (*cut*)

Sustentaculum tali

Tibialis anterior tendon
Tibialis posterior tendon
Plantar calcaneo-navicular (spring) ligament
Short plantar ligament
Long plantar ligament

© Novartis

ℱ. Netter M.D.

# Ligaments and Tendons of Foot: Plantar View

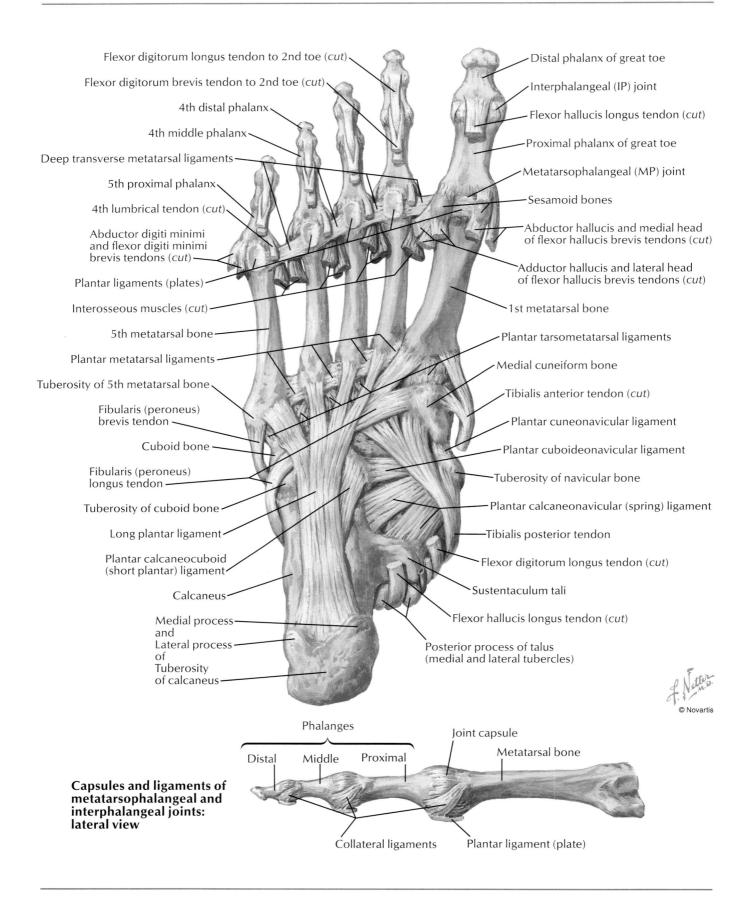

Flexor digitorum longus tendon to 2nd toe (*cut*)

Flexor digitorum brevis tendon to 2nd toe (*cut*)

4th distal phalanx

4th middle phalanx

Deep transverse metatarsal ligaments

5th proximal phalanx

4th lumbrical tendon (*cut*)

Abductor digiti minimi and flexor digiti minimi brevis tendons (*cut*)

Plantar ligaments (plates)

Interosseous muscles (*cut*)

5th metatarsal bone

Plantar metatarsal ligaments

Tuberosity of 5th metatarsal bone

Fibularis (peroneus) brevis tendon

Cuboid bone

Fibularis (peroneus) longus tendon

Tuberosity of cuboid bone

Long plantar ligament

Plantar calcaneocuboid (short plantar) ligament

Calcaneus

Medial process and Lateral process of Tuberosity of calcaneus

Distal phalanx of great toe

Interphalangeal (IP) joint

Flexor hallucis longus tendon (*cut*)

Proximal phalanx of great toe

Metatarsophalangeal (MP) joint

Sesamoid bones

Abductor hallucis and medial head of flexor hallucis brevis tendons (*cut*)

Adductor hallucis and lateral head of flexor hallucis brevis tendons (*cut*)

1st metatarsal bone

Plantar tarsometatarsal ligaments

Medial cuneiform bone

Tibialis anterior tendon (*cut*)

Plantar cuneonavicular ligament

Plantar cuboideonavicular ligament

Tuberosity of navicular bone

Plantar calcaneonavicular (spring) ligament

Tibialis posterior tendon

Flexor digitorum longus tendon (*cut*)

Sustentaculum tali

Flexor hallucis longus tendon (*cut*)

Posterior process of talus (medial and lateral tubercles)

Phalanges

Distal   Middle   Proximal

Joint capsule

Metatarsal bone

**Capsules and ligaments of metatarsophalangeal and interphalangeal joints: lateral view**

Collateral ligaments

Plantar ligament (plate)

© Novartis

**PLATE 492**   **LOWER LIMB**

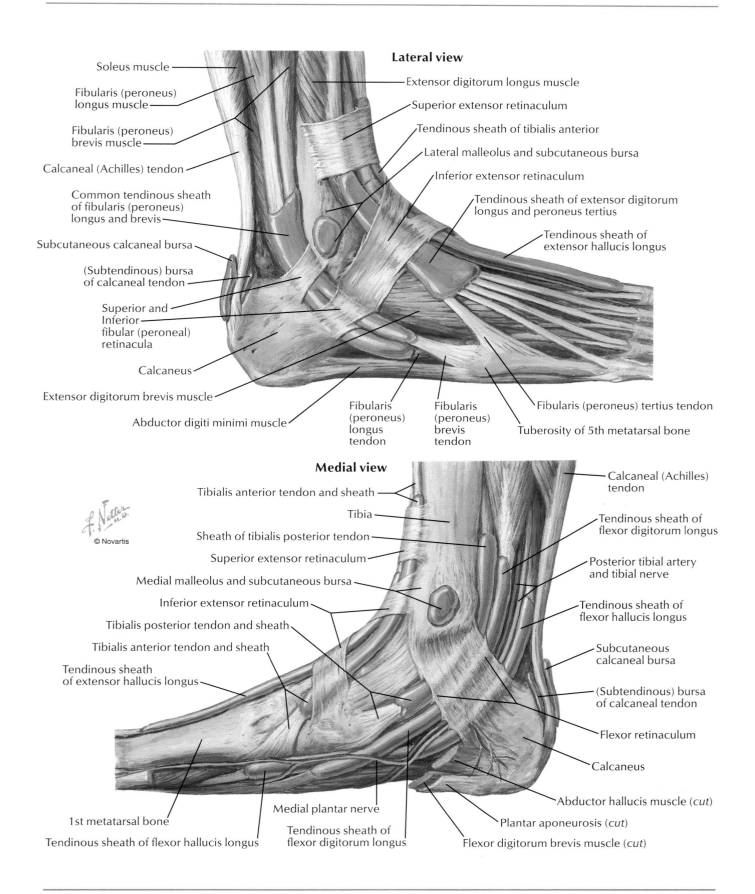

**Lateral view**

Soleus muscle

Fibularis (peroneus) longus muscle

Fibularis (peroneus) brevis muscle

Calcaneal (Achilles) tendon

Common tendinous sheath of fibularis (peroneus) longus and brevis

Subcutaneous calcaneal bursa

(Subtendinous) bursa of calcaneal tendon

Superior and Inferior fibular (peroneal) retinacula

Calcaneus

Extensor digitorum brevis muscle

Abductor digiti minimi muscle

Extensor digitorum longus muscle

Superior extensor retinaculum

Tendinous sheath of tibialis anterior

Lateral malleolus and subcutaneous bursa

Inferior extensor retinaculum

Tendinous sheath of extensor digitorum longus and peroneus tertius

Tendinous sheath of extensor hallucis longus

Fibularis (peroneus) longus tendon

Fibularis (peroneus) brevis tendon

Fibularis (peroneus) tertius tendon

Tuberosity of 5th metatarsal bone

**Medial view**

Tibialis anterior tendon and sheath

Tibia

Sheath of tibialis posterior tendon

Superior extensor retinaculum

Medial malleolus and subcutaneous bursa

Inferior extensor retinaculum

Tibialis posterior tendon and sheath

Tibialis anterior tendon and sheath

Tendinous sheath of extensor hallucis longus

1st metatarsal bone

Tendinous sheath of flexor hallucis longus

Medial plantar nerve

Tendinous sheath of flexor digitorum longus

Calcaneal (Achilles) tendon

Tendinous sheath of flexor digitorum longus

Posterior tibial artery and tibial nerve

Tendinous sheath of flexor hallucis longus

Subcutaneous calcaneal bursa

(Subtendinous) bursa of calcaneal tendon

Flexor retinaculum

Calcaneus

Abductor hallucis muscle (cut)

Plantar aponeurosis (cut)

Flexor digitorum brevis muscle (cut)

F. Netter M.D.
© Novartis

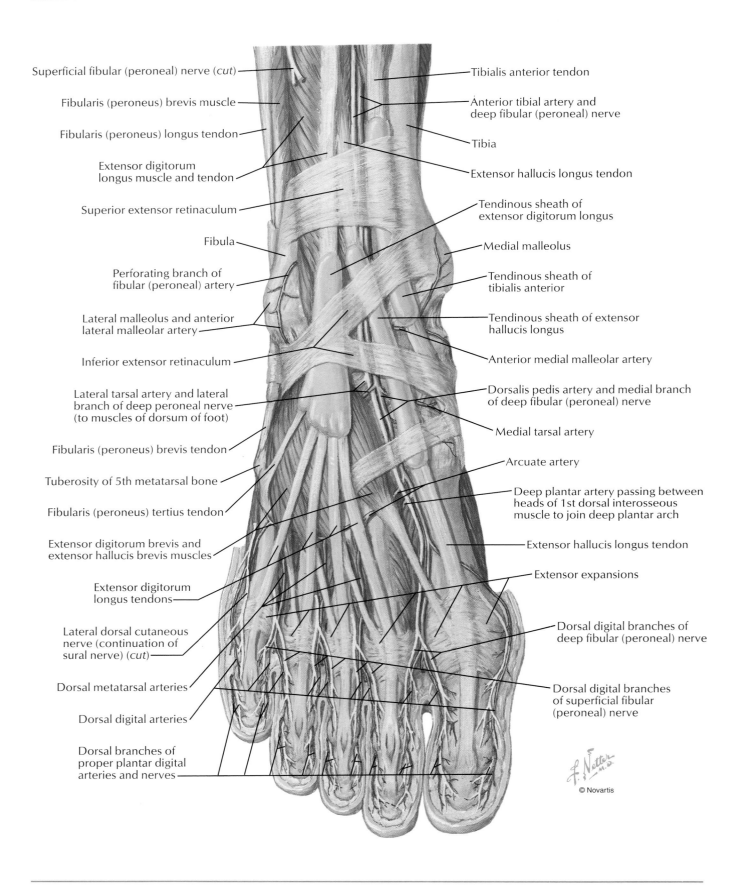

Superficial fibular (peroneal) nerve (*cut*)

Fibularis (peroneus) brevis muscle

Fibularis (peroneus) longus tendon

Extensor digitorum longus muscle and tendon

Superior extensor retinaculum

Fibula

Perforating branch of fibular (peroneal) artery

Lateral malleolus and anterior lateral malleolar artery

Inferior extensor retinaculum

Lateral tarsal artery and lateral branch of deep peroneal nerve (to muscles of dorsum of foot)

Fibularis (peroneus) brevis tendon

Tuberosity of 5th metatarsal bone

Fibularis (peroneus) tertius tendon

Extensor digitorum brevis and extensor hallucis brevis muscles

Extensor digitorum longus tendons

Lateral dorsal cutaneous nerve (continuation of sural nerve) (*cut*)

Dorsal metatarsal arteries

Dorsal digital arteries

Dorsal branches of proper plantar digital arteries and nerves

Tibialis anterior tendon

Anterior tibial artery and deep fibular (peroneal) nerve

Tibia

Extensor hallucis longus tendon

Tendinous sheath of extensor digitorum longus

Medial malleolus

Tendinous sheath of tibialis anterior

Tendinous sheath of extensor hallucis longus

Anterior medial malleolar artery

Dorsalis pedis artery and medial branch of deep fibular (peroneal) nerve

Medial tarsal artery

Arcuate artery

Deep plantar artery passing between heads of 1st dorsal interosseous muscle to join deep plantar arch

Extensor hallucis longus tendon

Extensor expansions

Dorsal digital branches of deep fibular (peroneal) nerve

Dorsal digital branches of superficial fibular (peroneal) nerve

© Novartis

**PLATE 494**

**LOWER LIMB**

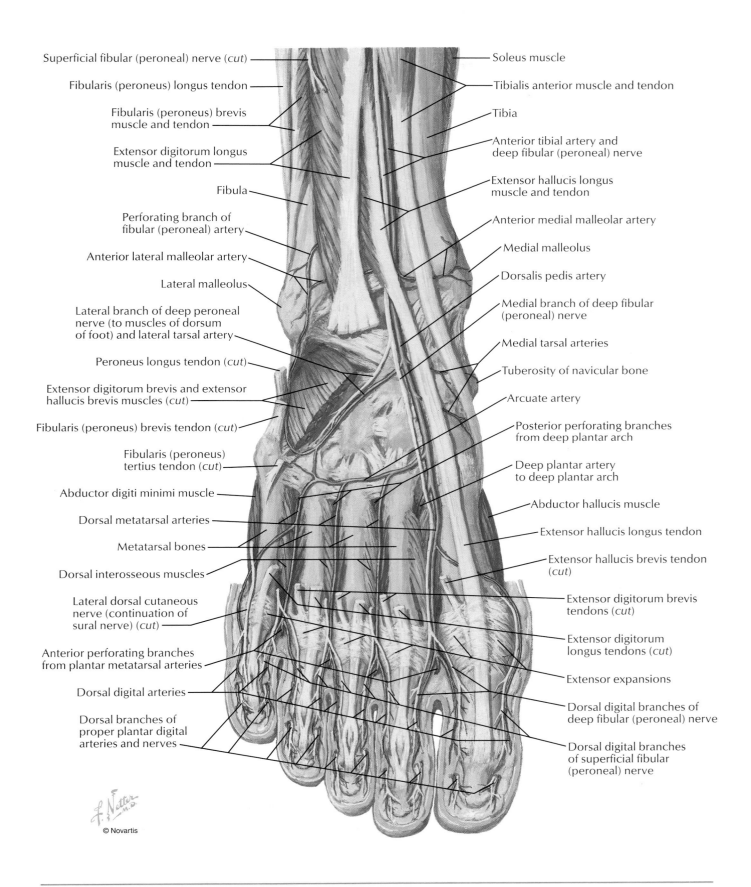

Superficial fibular (peroneal) nerve (*cut*)

Fibularis (peroneus) longus tendon

Fibularis (peroneus) brevis muscle and tendon

Extensor digitorum longus muscle and tendon

Fibula

Perforating branch of fibular (peroneal) artery

Anterior lateral malleolar artery

Lateral malleolus

Lateral branch of deep peroneal nerve (to muscles of dorsum of foot) and lateral tarsal artery

Peroneus longus tendon (*cut*)

Extensor digitorum brevis and extensor hallucis brevis muscles (*cut*)

Fibularis (peroneus) brevis tendon (*cut*)

Fibularis (peroneus) tertius tendon (*cut*)

Abductor digiti minimi muscle

Dorsal metatarsal arteries

Metatarsal bones

Dorsal interosseous muscles

Lateral dorsal cutaneous nerve (continuation of sural nerve) (*cut*)

Anterior perforating branches from plantar metatarsal arteries

Dorsal digital arteries

Dorsal branches of proper plantar digital arteries and nerves

Soleus muscle

Tibialis anterior muscle and tendon

Tibia

Anterior tibial artery and deep fibular (peroneal) nerve

Extensor hallucis longus muscle and tendon

Anterior medial malleolar artery

Medial malleolus

Dorsalis pedis artery

Medial branch of deep fibular (peroneal) nerve

Medial tarsal arteries

Tuberosity of navicular bone

Arcuate artery

Posterior perforating branches from deep plantar arch

Deep plantar artery to deep plantar arch

Abductor hallucis muscle

Extensor hallucis longus tendon

Extensor hallucis brevis tendon (*cut*)

Extensor digitorum brevis tendons (*cut*)

Extensor digitorum longus tendons (*cut*)

Extensor expansions

Dorsal digital branches of deep fibular (peroneal) nerve

Dorsal digital branches of superficial fibular (peroneal) nerve

F. Netter
M.D.
© Novartis

Superficial transverse
metatarsal ligaments

Proper plantar digital
arteries and nerves

Superficial branch of
medial plantar artery

Transverse fasciculi

Digital slips of
plantar aponeurosis

Medial plantar fascia

Lateral plantar fascia

Cutaneous branches of medial
plantar artery and nerve

Cutaneous branches
of lateral plantar
artery and nerve

Plantar aponeurosis

Lateral band of plantar aponeurosis
(calcaneometatarsal ligament)

Medial calcaneal branches of tibial
nerve and posterior tibial artery

Tuberosity of calcaneus
with overlying fat
pad (partially cut away)

© Novartis

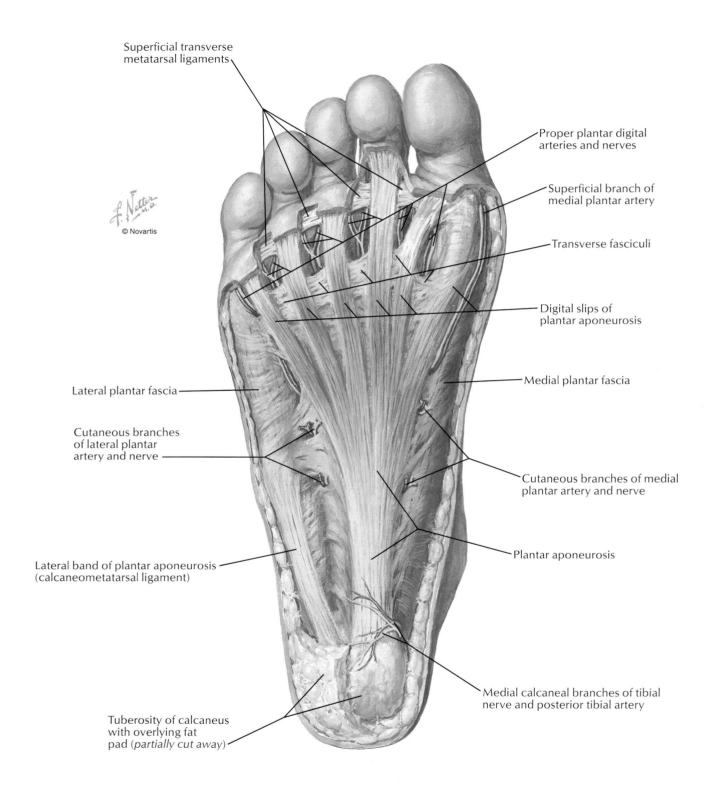

**PLATE 496**

**LOWER LIMB**

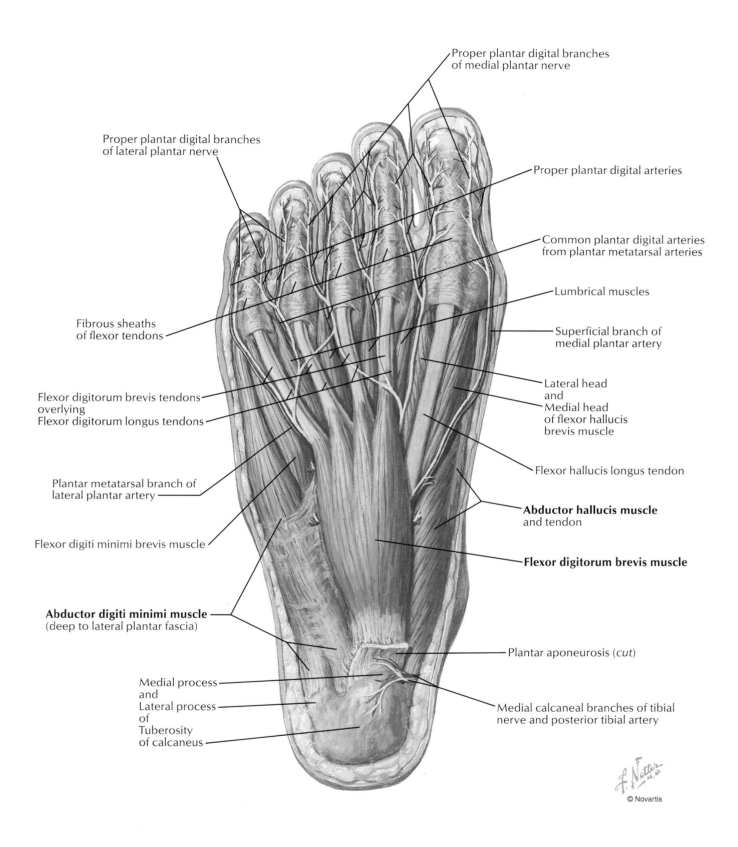

Proper plantar digital branches
of medial plantar nerve

Proper plantar digital branches
of lateral plantar nerve

Proper plantar digital arteries

Common plantar digital arteries
from plantar metatarsal arteries

Lumbrical muscles

Fibrous sheaths
of flexor tendons

Superficial branch of
medial plantar artery

Flexor digitorum brevis tendons
overlying
Flexor digitorum longus tendons

Lateral head
and
Medial head
of flexor hallucis
brevis muscle

Flexor hallucis longus tendon

Plantar metatarsal branch of
lateral plantar artery

**Abductor hallucis muscle**
and tendon

Flexor digiti minimi brevis muscle

**Flexor digitorum brevis muscle**

**Abductor digiti minimi muscle**
(deep to lateral plantar fascia)

Plantar aponeurosis (cut)

Medial process
and
Lateral process
of
Tuberosity
of calcaneus

Medial calcaneal branches of tibial
nerve and posterior tibial artery

© Novartis

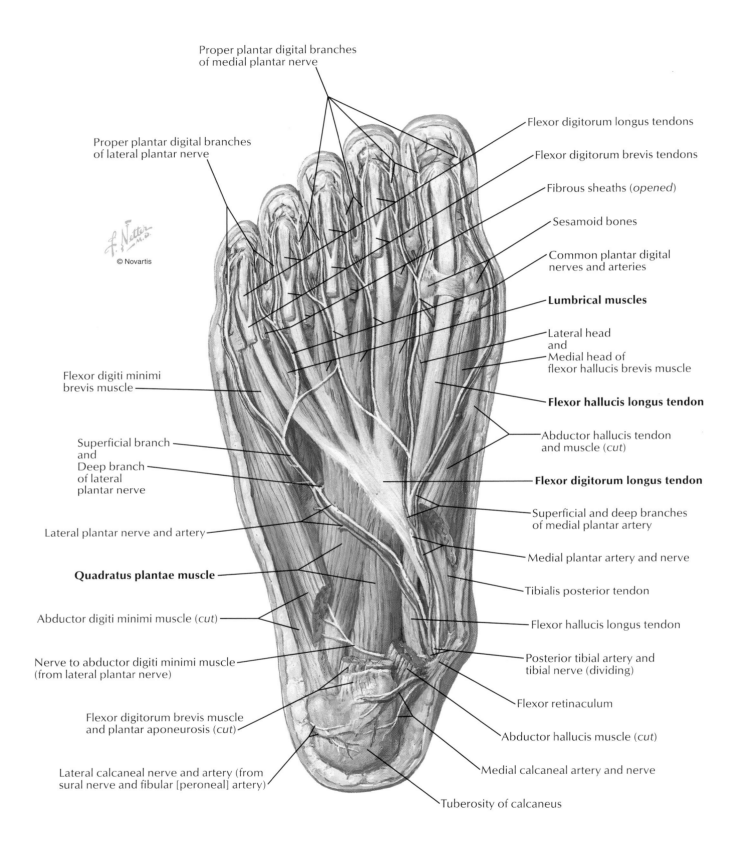

Proper plantar digital branches
of medial plantar nerve

Proper plantar digital branches
of lateral plantar nerve

Flexor digitorum longus tendons

Flexor digitorum brevis tendons

Fibrous sheaths (opened)

Sesamoid bones

Common plantar digital
nerves and arteries

**Lumbrical muscles**

Lateral head
and
Medial head of
flexor hallucis brevis muscle

**Flexor hallucis longus tendon**

Abductor hallucis tendon
and muscle (cut)

**Flexor digitorum longus tendon**

Superficial and deep branches
of medial plantar artery

Medial plantar artery and nerve

Tibialis posterior tendon

Flexor hallucis longus tendon

Posterior tibial artery and
tibial nerve (dividing)

Flexor retinaculum

Abductor hallucis muscle (cut)

Medial calcaneal artery and nerve

Tuberosity of calcaneus

Flexor digiti minimi
brevis muscle

Superficial branch
and
Deep branch
of lateral
plantar nerve

Lateral plantar nerve and artery

**Quadratus plantae muscle**

Abductor digiti minimi muscle (cut)

Nerve to abductor digiti minimi muscle
(from lateral plantar nerve)

Flexor digitorum brevis muscle
and plantar aponeurosis (cut)

Lateral calcaneal nerve and artery (from
sural nerve and fibular [peroneal] artery)

© Novartis

**PLATE 498**     **LOWER LIMB**

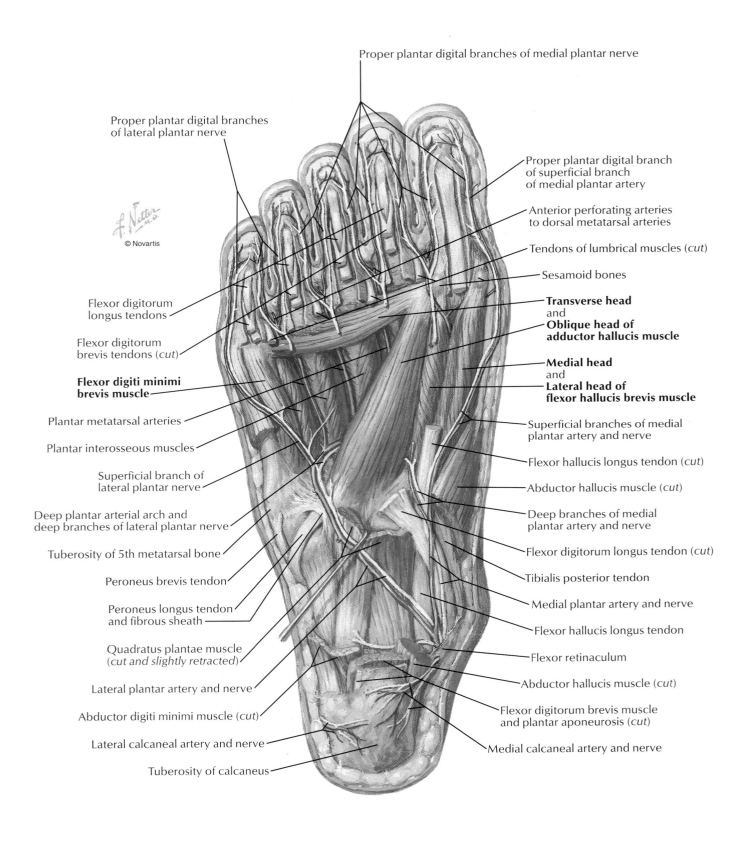

Proper plantar digital branches of medial plantar nerve

Proper plantar digital branches of lateral plantar nerve

Proper plantar digital branch of superficial branch of medial plantar artery

Anterior perforating arteries to dorsal metatarsal arteries

Tendons of lumbrical muscles (*cut*)

Sesamoid bones

**Transverse head** and **Oblique head of adductor hallucis muscle**

**Medial head** and **Lateral head of flexor hallucis brevis muscle**

Flexor digitorum longus tendons

Flexor digitorum brevis tendons (*cut*)

**Flexor digiti minimi brevis muscle**

Plantar metatarsal arteries

Plantar interosseous muscles

Superficial branch of lateral plantar nerve

Deep plantar arterial arch and deep branches of lateral plantar nerve

Tuberosity of 5th metatarsal bone

Peroneus brevis tendon

Peroneus longus tendon and fibrous sheath

Quadratus plantae muscle (*cut and slightly retracted*)

Lateral plantar artery and nerve

Abductor digiti minimi muscle (*cut*)

Lateral calcaneal artery and nerve

Tuberosity of calcaneus

Superficial branches of medial plantar artery and nerve

Flexor hallucis longus tendon (*cut*)

Abductor hallucis muscle (*cut*)

Deep branches of medial plantar artery and nerve

Flexor digitorum longus tendon (*cut*)

Tibialis posterior tendon

Medial plantar artery and nerve

Flexor hallucis longus tendon

Flexor retinaculum

Abductor hallucis muscle (*cut*)

Flexor digitorum brevis muscle and plantar aponeurosis (*cut*)

Medial calcaneal artery and nerve

© Novartis

# Interosseous Muscles and Deep Arteries of Foot

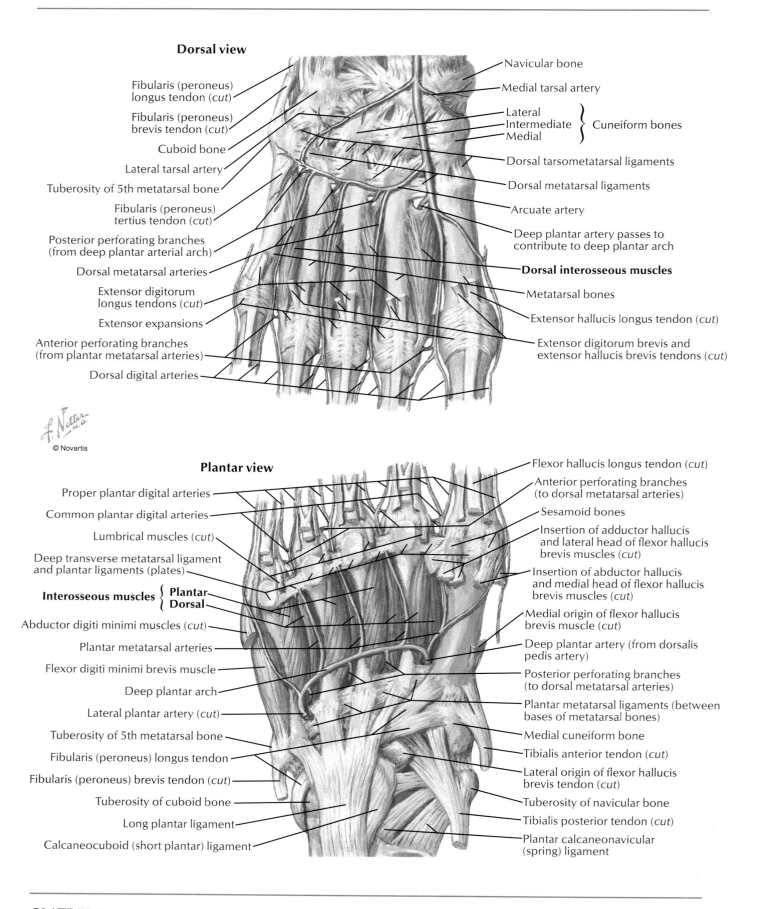

**Dorsal view**

Fibularis (peroneus) longus tendon (*cut*)

Fibularis (peroneus) brevis tendon (*cut*)

Cuboid bone

Lateral tarsal artery

Tuberosity of 5th metatarsal bone

Fibularis (peroneus) tertius tendon (*cut*)

Posterior perforating branches (from deep plantar arterial arch)

Dorsal metatarsal arteries

Extensor digitorum longus tendons (*cut*)

Extensor expansions

Anterior perforating branches (from plantar metatarsal arteries)

Dorsal digital arteries

Navicular bone

Medial tarsal artery

Lateral
Intermediate } Cuneiform bones
Medial

Dorsal tarsometatarsal ligaments

Dorsal metatarsal ligaments

Arcuate artery

Deep plantar artery passes to contribute to deep plantar arch

**Dorsal interosseous muscles**

Metatarsal bones

Extensor hallucis longus tendon (*cut*)

Extensor digitorum brevis and extensor hallucis brevis tendons (*cut*)

© Novartis

**Plantar view**

Proper plantar digital arteries

Common plantar digital arteries

Lumbrical muscles (*cut*)

Deep transverse metatarsal ligament and plantar ligaments (plates)

**Interosseous muscles** { Plantar
Dorsal

Abductor digiti minimi muscles (*cut*)

Plantar metatarsal arteries

Flexor digiti minimi brevis muscle

Deep plantar arch

Lateral plantar artery (*cut*)

Tuberosity of 5th metatarsal bone

Fibularis (peroneus) longus tendon

Fibularis (peroneus) brevis tendon (*cut*)

Tuberosity of cuboid bone

Long plantar ligament

Calcaneocuboid (short plantar) ligament

Flexor hallucis longus tendon (*cut*)

Anterior perforating branches (to dorsal metatarsal arteries)

Sesamoid bones

Insertion of adductor hallucis and lateral head of flexor hallucis brevis muscles (*cut*)

Insertion of abductor hallucis and medial head of flexor hallucis brevis muscles (*cut*)

Medial origin of flexor hallucis brevis muscle (*cut*)

Deep plantar artery (from dorsalis pedis artery)

Posterior perforating branches (to dorsal metatarsal arteries)

Plantar metatarsal ligaments (between bases of metatarsal bones)

Medial cuneiform bone

Tibialis anterior tendon (*cut*)

Lateral origin of flexor hallucis brevis tendon (*cut*)

Tuberosity of navicular bone

Tibialis posterior tendon (*cut*)

Plantar calcaneonavicular (spring) ligament

**PLATE 500**

**LOWER LIMB**

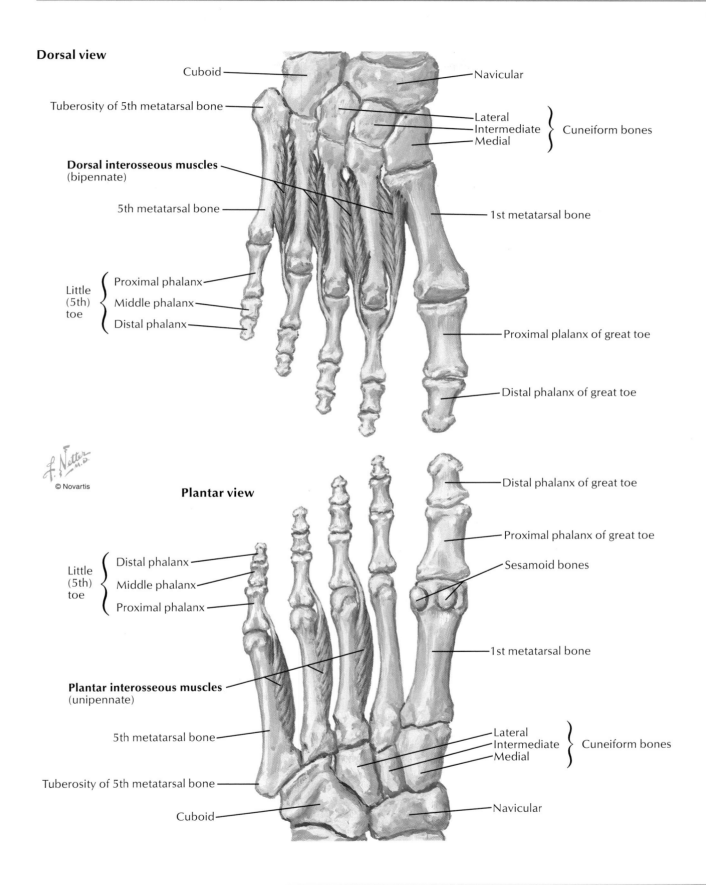

**Dorsal view**

Cuboid

Tuberosity of 5th metatarsal bone

Navicular

Lateral

Intermediate — Cuneiform bones

Medial

**Dorsal interosseous muscles**
(bipennate)

5th metatarsal bone

1st metatarsal bone

Little
(5th)
toe
— Proximal phalanx

Middle phalanx

Distal phalanx

Proximal plalanx of great toe

Distal phalanx of great toe

**Plantar view**

Distal phalanx of great toe

Proximal phalanx of great toe

Little
(5th)
toe
— Distal phalanx

Middle phalanx

Proximal phalanx

Sesamoid bones

1st metatarsal bone

**Plantar interosseous muscles**
(unipennate)

5th metatarsal bone

Lateral

Intermediate — Cuneiform bones

Medial

Tuberosity of 5th metatarsal bone

Cuboid

Navicular

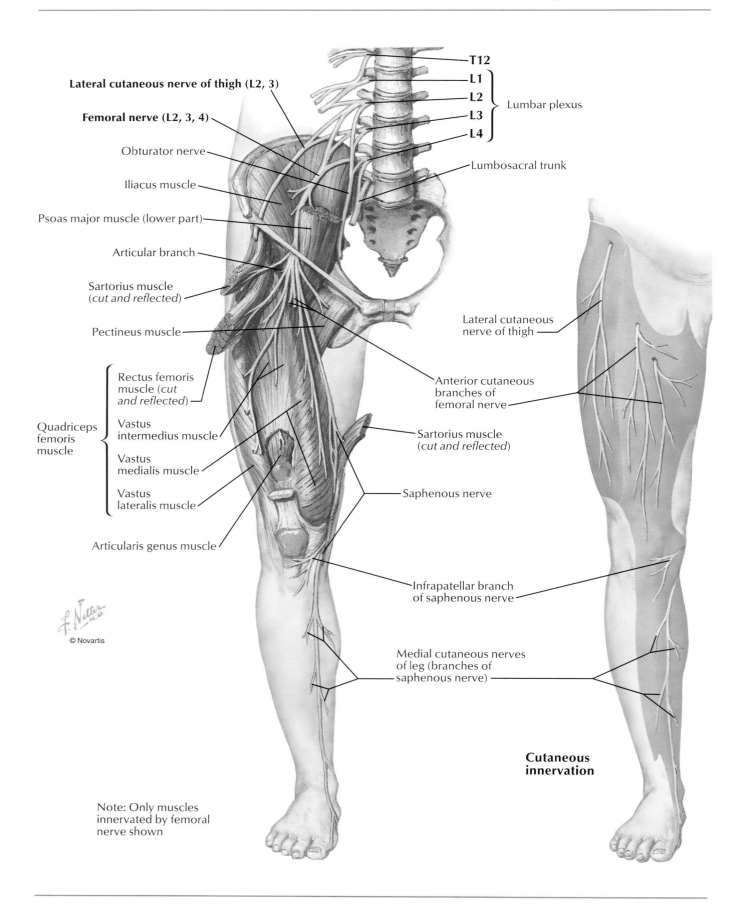

**Lateral cutaneous nerve of thigh (L2, 3)**

**Femoral nerve (L2, 3, 4)**

Obturator nerve

Iliacus muscle

Psoas major muscle (lower part)

Articular branch

Sartorius muscle
(*cut and reflected*)

Pectineus muscle

Rectus femoris
muscle (*cut
and reflected*)

Quadriceps
femoris
muscle

Vastus
intermedius muscle

Vastus
medialis muscle

Vastus
lateralis muscle

Articularis genus muscle

T12

L1

L2

L3

L4

Lumbar plexus

Lumbosacral trunk

Lateral cutaneous
nerve of thigh

Anterior cutaneous
branches of
femoral nerve

Sartorius muscle
(*cut and reflected*)

Saphenous nerve

Infrapatellar branch
of saphenous nerve

Medial cutaneous nerves
of leg (branches of
saphenous nerve)

**Cutaneous
innervation**

*f. Netter*
*M.D.*

© Novartis

Note: Only muscles
innervated by femoral
nerve shown

*PLATE 502*                                                                                **LOWER LIMB**

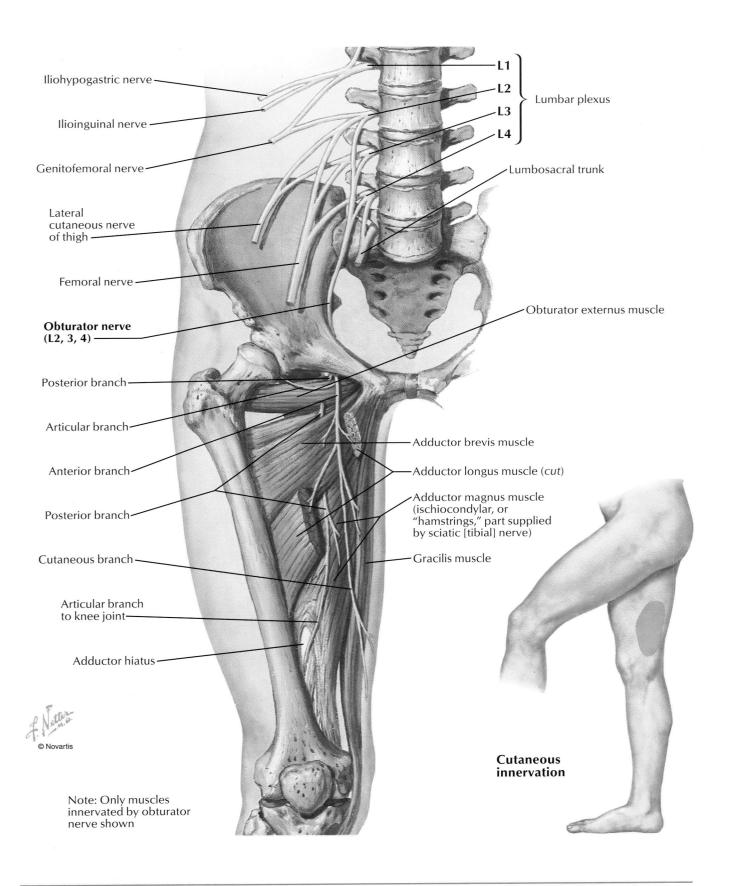

Iliohypogastric nerve

Ilioinguinal nerve

Genitofemoral nerve

Lateral cutaneous nerve of thigh

Femoral nerve

**Obturator nerve (L2, 3, 4)**

Posterior branch

Articular branch

Anterior branch

Posterior branch

Cutaneous branch

Articular branch to knee joint

Adductor hiatus

L1
L2
L3
L4

Lumbar plexus

Lumbosacral trunk

Obturator externus muscle

Adductor brevis muscle

Adductor longus muscle (*cut*)

Adductor magnus muscle (ischiocondylar, or "hamstrings," part supplied by sciatic [tibial] nerve)

Gracilis muscle

**Cutaneous innervation**

Note: Only muscles innervated by obturator nerve shown

© Novartis

# *Sciatic Nerve and Posterior Cutaneous Nerve of Thigh*

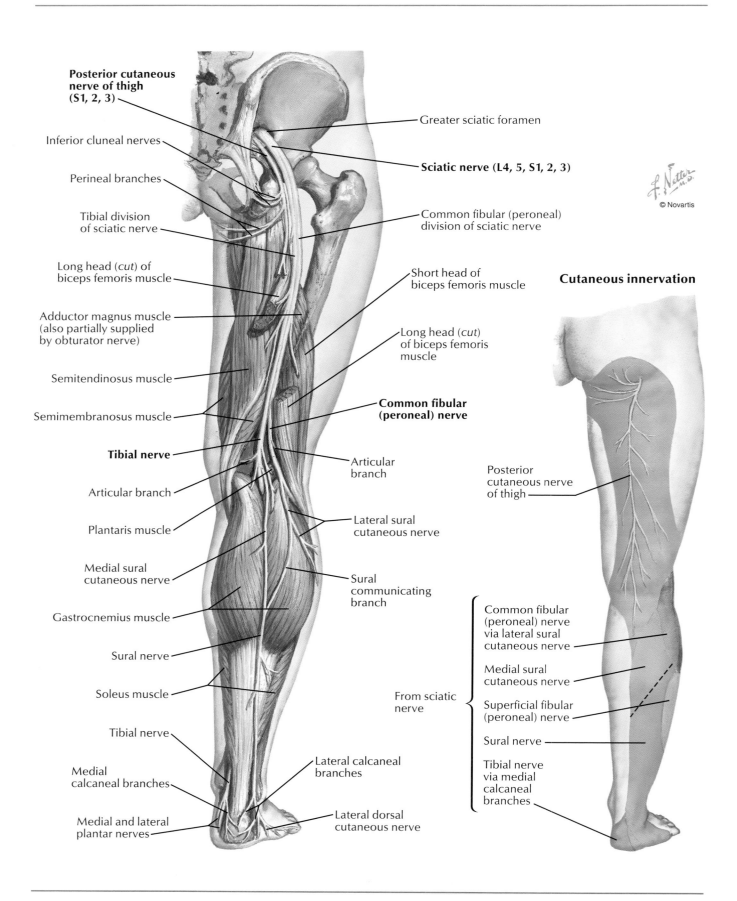

**Posterior cutaneous nerve of thigh (S1, 2, 3)**

Inferior cluneal nerves

Perineal branches

Tibial division of sciatic nerve

Long head (*cut*) of biceps femoris muscle

Adductor magnus muscle (also partially supplied by obturator nerve)

Semitendinosus muscle

Semimembranosus muscle

**Tibial nerve**

Articular branch

Plantaris muscle

Medial sural cutaneous nerve

Gastrocnemius muscle

Sural nerve

Soleus muscle

Tibial nerve

Medial calcaneal branches

Medial and lateral plantar nerves

Greater sciatic foramen

**Sciatic nerve (L4, 5, S1, 2, 3)**

Common fibular (peroneal) division of sciatic nerve

Short head of biceps femoris muscle

Long head (*cut*) of biceps femoris muscle

**Common fibular (peroneal) nerve**

Articular branch

Lateral sural cutaneous nerve

Sural communicating branch

Lateral calcaneal branches

Lateral dorsal cutaneous nerve

**Cutaneous innervation**

Posterior cutaneous nerve of thigh

Common fibular (peroneal) nerve via lateral sural cutaneous nerve

Medial sural cutaneous nerve

Superficial fibular (peroneal) nerve

Sural nerve

Tibial nerve via medial calcaneal branches

From sciatic nerve

*F. Netter M.D.*
© Novartis

*PLATE 504*

**LOWER LIMB**

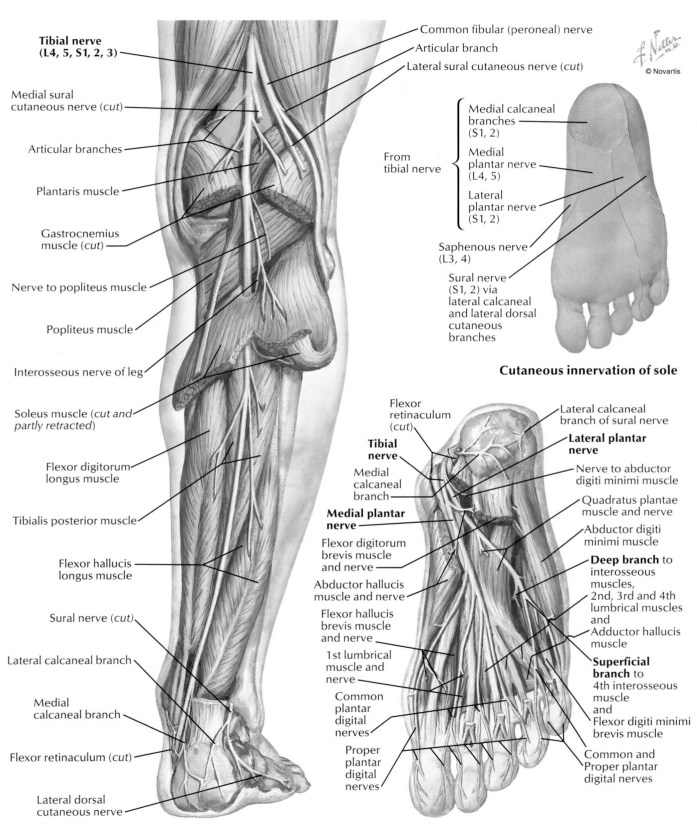

**Tibial nerve**
**(L4, 5, S1, 2, 3)**

Medial sural cutaneous nerve (*cut*)

Articular branches

Plantaris muscle

Gastrocnemius muscle (*cut*)

Nerve to popliteus muscle

Popliteus muscle

Interosseous nerve of leg

Soleus muscle (*cut and partly retracted*)

Flexor digitorum longus muscle

Tibialis posterior muscle

Flexor hallucis longus muscle

Sural nerve (*cut*)

Lateral calcaneal branch

Medial calcaneal branch

Flexor retinaculum (*cut*)

Lateral dorsal cutaneous nerve

Common fibular (peroneal) nerve
Articular branch
Lateral sural cutaneous nerve (*cut*)

© Novartis

From tibial nerve {
Medial calcaneal branches (S1, 2)
Medial plantar nerve (L4, 5)
Lateral plantar nerve (S1, 2)
}

Saphenous nerve (L3, 4)

Sural nerve (S1, 2) via lateral calcaneal and lateral dorsal cutaneous branches

**Cutaneous innervation of sole**

Flexor retinaculum (*cut*)

**Tibial nerve**

Medial calcaneal branch

**Medial plantar nerve**

Flexor digitorum brevis muscle and nerve

Abductor hallucis muscle and nerve

Flexor hallucis brevis muscle and nerve

1st lumbrical muscle and nerve

Common plantar digital nerves

Proper plantar digital nerves

Lateral calcaneal branch of sural nerve

**Lateral plantar nerve**

Nerve to abductor digiti minimi muscle

Quadratus plantae muscle and nerve

Abductor digiti minimi muscle

**Deep branch** to interosseous muscles, 2nd, 3rd and 4th lumbrical muscles and Adductor hallucis muscle

**Superficial branch** to 4th interosseous muscle and Flexor digiti minimi brevis muscle

Common and Proper plantar digital nerves

Note: Articular branches not shown

# *Common Fibular (Peroneal) Nerve*

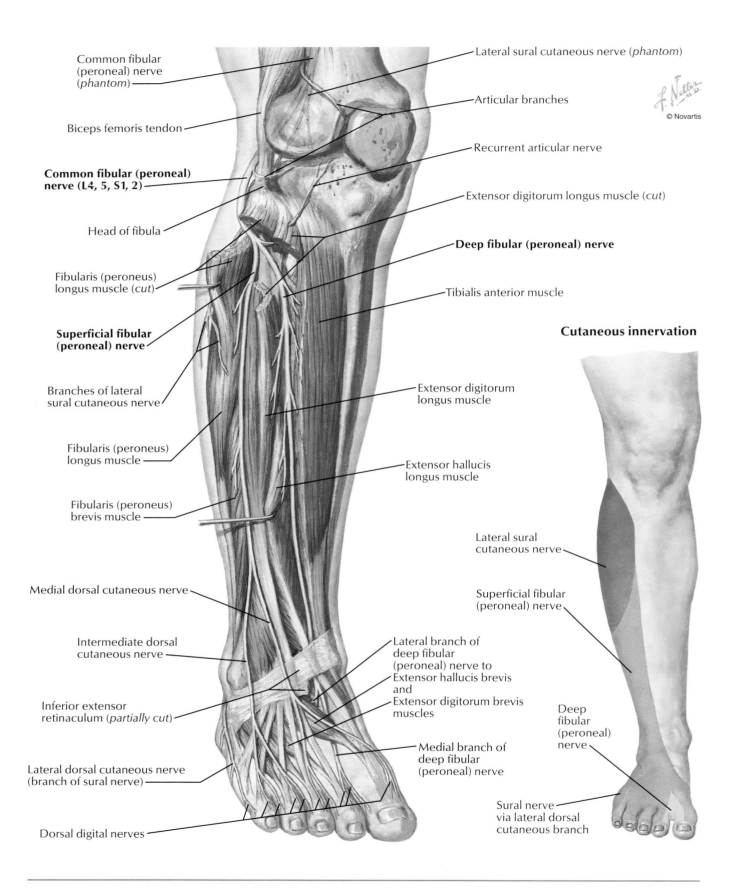

Common fibular (peroneal) nerve (*phantom*)

Biceps femoris tendon

**Common fibular (peroneal) nerve (L4, 5, S1, 2)**

Head of fibula

Fibularis (peroneus) longus muscle (*cut*)

**Superficial fibular (peroneal) nerve**

Branches of lateral sural cutaneous nerve

Fibularis (peroneus) longus muscle

Fibularis (peroneus) brevis muscle

Medial dorsal cutaneous nerve

Intermediate dorsal cutaneous nerve

Inferior extensor retinaculum (*partially cut*)

Lateral dorsal cutaneous nerve (branch of sural nerve)

Dorsal digital nerves

Lateral sural cutaneous nerve (*phantom*)

Articular branches

Recurrent articular nerve

Extensor digitorum longus muscle (*cut*)

**Deep fibular (peroneal) nerve**

Tibialis anterior muscle

Extensor digitorum longus muscle

Extensor hallucis longus muscle

Lateral branch of deep fibular (peroneal) nerve to Extensor hallucis brevis and Extensor digitorum brevis muscles

Medial branch of deep fibular (peroneal) nerve

**Cutaneous innervation**

Lateral sural cutaneous nerve

Superficial fibular (peroneal) nerve

Deep fibular (peroneal) nerve

Sural nerve via lateral dorsal cutaneous branch

**PLATE 506**

**LOWER LIMB**

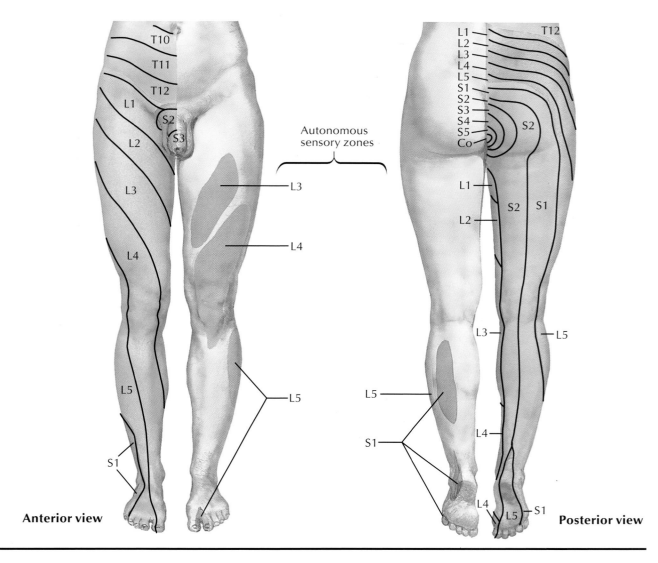

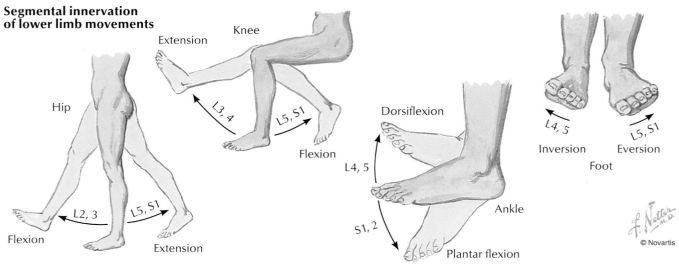

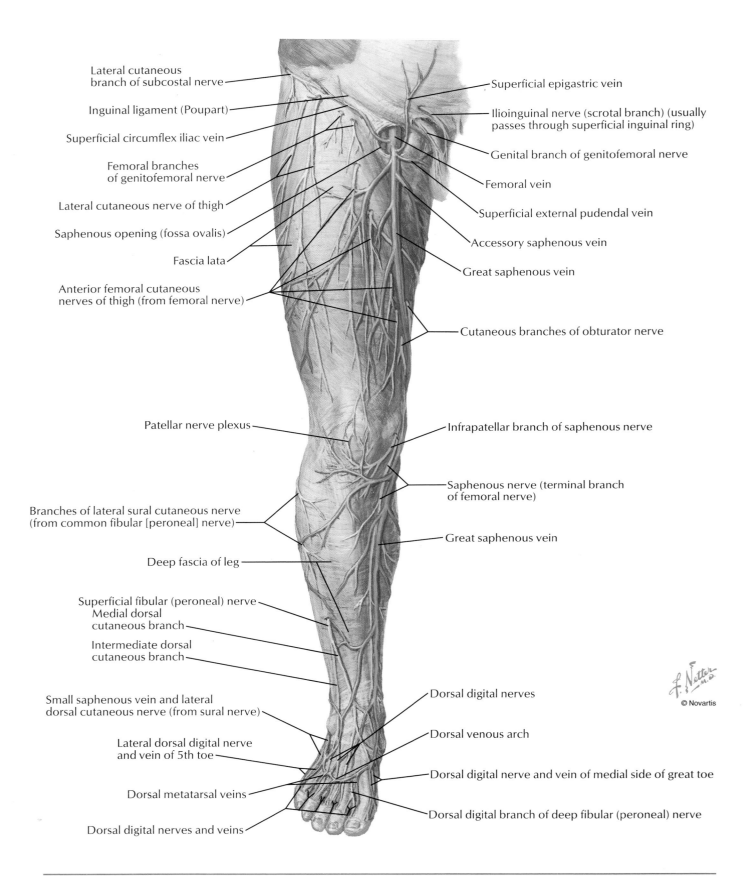

Lateral cutaneous branch of subcostal nerve

Inguinal ligament (Poupart)

Superficial circumflex iliac vein

Femoral branches of genitofemoral nerve

Lateral cutaneous nerve of thigh

Saphenous opening (fossa ovalis)

Fascia lata

Anterior femoral cutaneous nerves of thigh (from femoral nerve)

Patellar nerve plexus

Branches of lateral sural cutaneous nerve (from common fibular [peroneal] nerve)

Deep fascia of leg

Superficial fibular (peroneal) nerve
Medial dorsal cutaneous branch

Intermediate dorsal cutaneous branch

Small saphenous vein and lateral dorsal cutaneous nerve (from sural nerve)

Lateral dorsal digital nerve and vein of 5th toe

Dorsal metatarsal veins

Dorsal digital nerves and veins

Superficial epigastric vein

Ilioinguinal nerve (scrotal branch) (usually passes through superficial inguinal ring)

Genital branch of genitofemoral nerve

Femoral vein

Superficial external pudendal vein

Accessory saphenous vein

Great saphenous vein

Cutaneous branches of obturator nerve

Infrapatellar branch of saphenous nerve

Saphenous nerve (terminal branch of femoral nerve)

Great saphenous vein

Dorsal digital nerves

Dorsal venous arch

Dorsal digital nerve and vein of medial side of great toe

Dorsal digital branch of deep fibular (peroneal) nerve

© Novartis

**PLATE 508**　　　　　　　　　　　　　　　　**LOWER LIMB**

# Superficial Nerves and Veins of Lower Limb: Posterior View

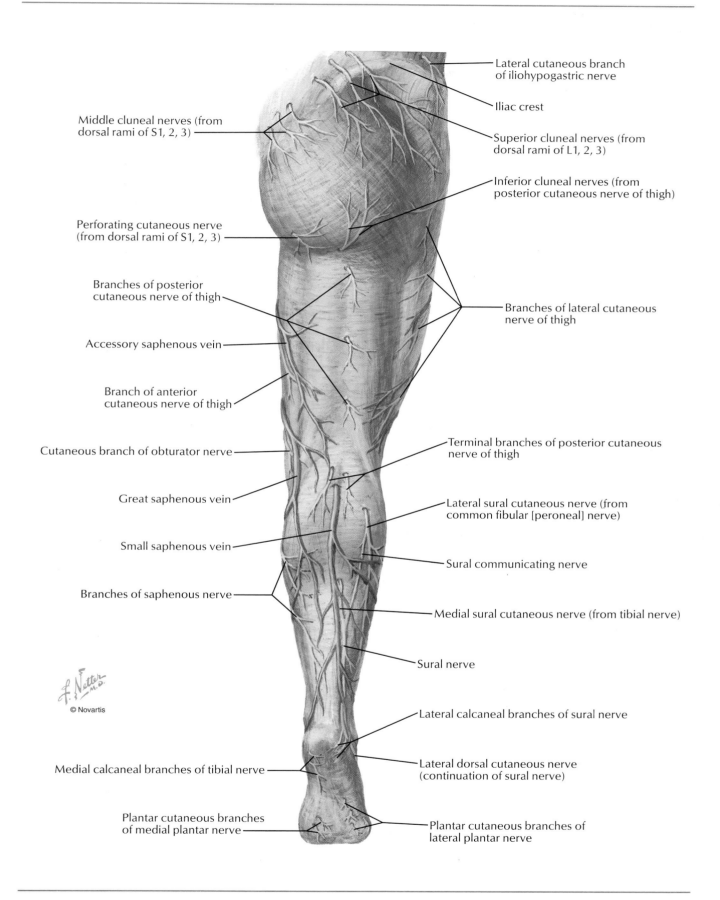

Lateral cutaneous branch of iliohypogastric nerve

Iliac crest

Middle cluneal nerves (from dorsal rami of S1, 2, 3)

Superior cluneal nerves (from dorsal rami of L1, 2, 3)

Inferior cluneal nerves (from posterior cutaneous nerve of thigh)

Perforating cutaneous nerve (from dorsal rami of S1, 2, 3)

Branches of posterior cutaneous nerve of thigh

Branches of lateral cutaneous nerve of thigh

Accessory saphenous vein

Branch of anterior cutaneous nerve of thigh

Terminal branches of posterior cutaneous nerve of thigh

Cutaneous branch of obturator nerve

Great saphenous vein

Lateral sural cutaneous nerve (from common fibular [peroneal] nerve)

Small saphenous vein

Sural communicating nerve

Branches of saphenous nerve

Medial sural cutaneous nerve (from tibial nerve)

Sural nerve

Lateral calcaneal branches of sural nerve

Medial calcaneal branches of tibial nerve

Lateral dorsal cutaneous nerve (continuation of sural nerve)

Plantar cutaneous branches of medial plantar nerve

Plantar cutaneous branches of lateral plantar nerve

© Novartis

**NEUROVASCULATURE**

*PLATE 509*

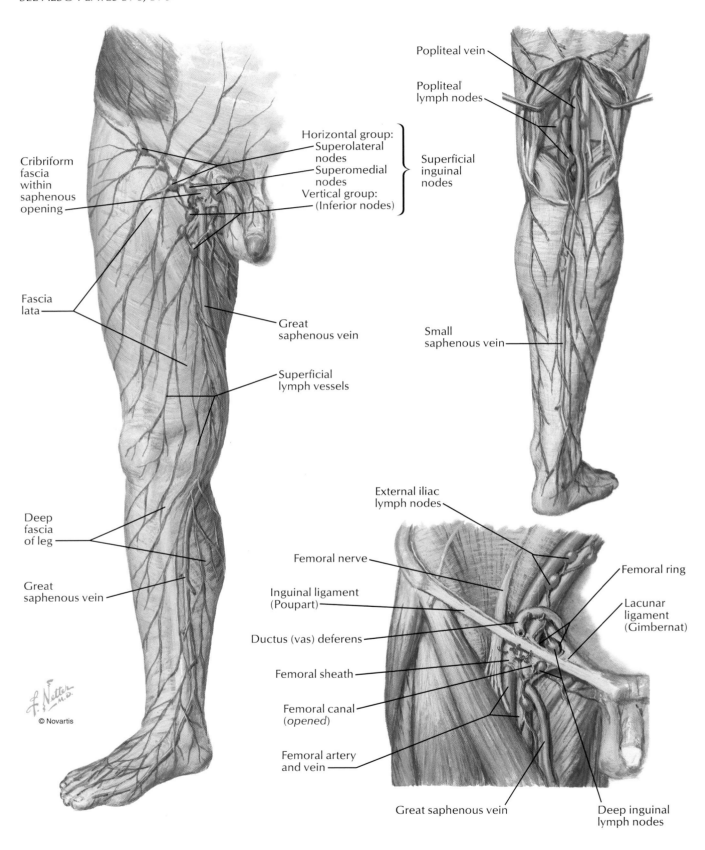

Popliteal vein

Popliteal lymph nodes

Superficial inguinal nodes

Small saphenous vein

Horizontal group:
Superolateral nodes
Superomedial nodes
Vertical group:
(Inferior nodes)

Cribriform fascia within saphenous opening

Fascia lata

Great saphenous vein

Superficial lymph vessels

Deep fascia of leg

Great saphenous vein

External iliac lymph nodes

Femoral nerve

Femoral ring

Inguinal ligament (Poupart)

Lacunar ligament (Gimbernat)

Ductus (vas) deferens

Femoral sheath

Femoral canal (*opened*)

Femoral artery and vein

Great saphenous vein

Deep inguinal lymph nodes

*f. Netter M.D.*

© Novartis

**PLATE 510**

**LOWER LIMB**

# Section VIII
# CROSS-SECTIONAL ANATOMY

**SKIN**
*Plate 511*
511. Skin: Cross-Sectional View

**CROSS-SECTION OVERVIEW**
*Plate 512*
512. Key Figure for Cross Sections

**THORAX**
*Plates 513 – 516*
513. Thorax: Brachiocephalic Vessels
514. Thorax: Aortic and Azygos Arches
515. Thorax: Pulmonary Trunk
516. Thorax: Four Chambers of Heart

**ABDOMEN**
*Plates 517 – 522*
517. Abdomen: Esophagogastric Junction

518. Abdomen: Pylorus and Body of
     Pancreas
519. Abdomen: Origins of Celiac Artery
     and Portal Vein
520. Abdomen: Renal Hilum and Vessels
521. Abdomen: Ileocecal Junction
522. Abdomen: Sacral Promontory

**MALE PELVIS**
*Plate 523*
523. Male Pelvis: Bladder-Prostate
     Junction

**THORAX**
*Plates 524 – 525*
524. Thorax: Heart, Ascending Aorta
525. Thorax: Tracheal Bifurcation,
     Left Atrium

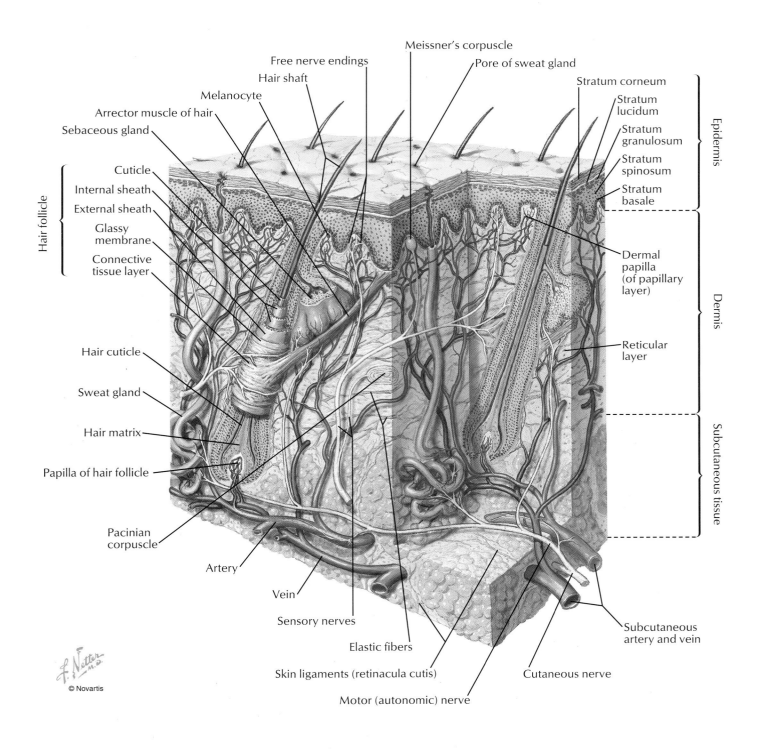

Meissner's corpuscle

Free nerve endings

Hair shaft

Pore of sweat gland

Melanocyte

Stratum corneum

Arrector muscle of hair

Stratum lucidum

Sebaceous gland

Stratum granulosum

Cuticle

Stratum spinosum

Internal sheath

Stratum basale

External sheath

Epidermis

Glassy membrane

Connective tissue layer

Hair follicle

Dermal papilla (of papillary layer)

Hair cuticle

Dermis

Reticular layer

Sweat gland

Hair matrix

Papilla of hair follicle

Subcutaneous tissue

Pacinian corpuscle

Artery

Vein

Sensory nerves

Subcutaneous artery and vein

Elastic fibers

Skin ligaments (retinacula cutis)

Cutaneous nerve

Motor (autonomic) nerve

*f. Netter*
*M.D.*

© Novartis

# Key Figure for Cross Sections

513
514
515

516

517

518
519
520

521

522

523

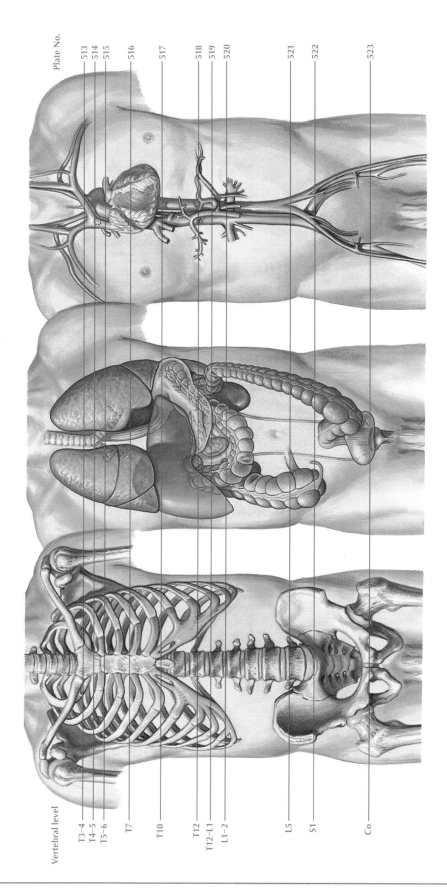

© Novartis

Vertebral level

T3–4
T4–5
T5–6

T7

T10

T12
T12–L1
L1–2

L5

S1

Co

**Transverse Section: Upper Level of T4, Sternoclavicular Joint**

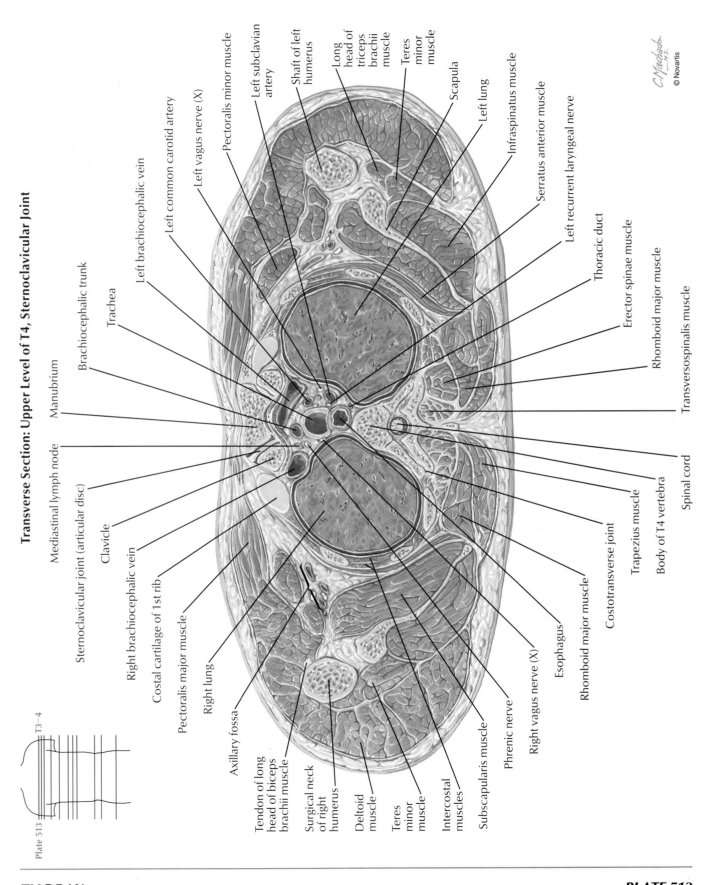

Pectoralis minor muscle

Left subclavian artery

Shaft of left humerus

Long head of triceps brachii muscle

Teres minor muscle

Scapula

Left lung

Infraspinatus muscle

Serratus anterior muscle

Left recurrent laryngeal nerve

Thoracic duct

Erector spinae muscle

Rhomboid major muscle

Transversospinalis muscle

Left vagus nerve (X)

Left common carotid artery

Left brachiocephalic vein

Trachea

Brachiocephalic trunk

Manubrium

Mediastinal lymph node

Sternoclavicular joint (articular disc)

Clavicle

Right brachiocephalic vein

Costal cartilage of 1st rib

Pectoralis major muscle

Right lung

Axillary fossa

Tendon of long head of biceps brachii muscle

Surgical neck of right humerus

Deltoid muscle

Teres minor muscle

Intercostal muscles

Subscapularis muscle

Phrenic nerve

Right vagus nerve (X)

Rhomboid major muscle

Esophagus

Costotransverse joint

Trapezius muscle

Body of T4 vertebra

Spinal cord

Plate 513

T3–4

**THORAX**

*PLATE 513*

**Transverse Section: T4–5 Intervertebral Disc, Manubrium**

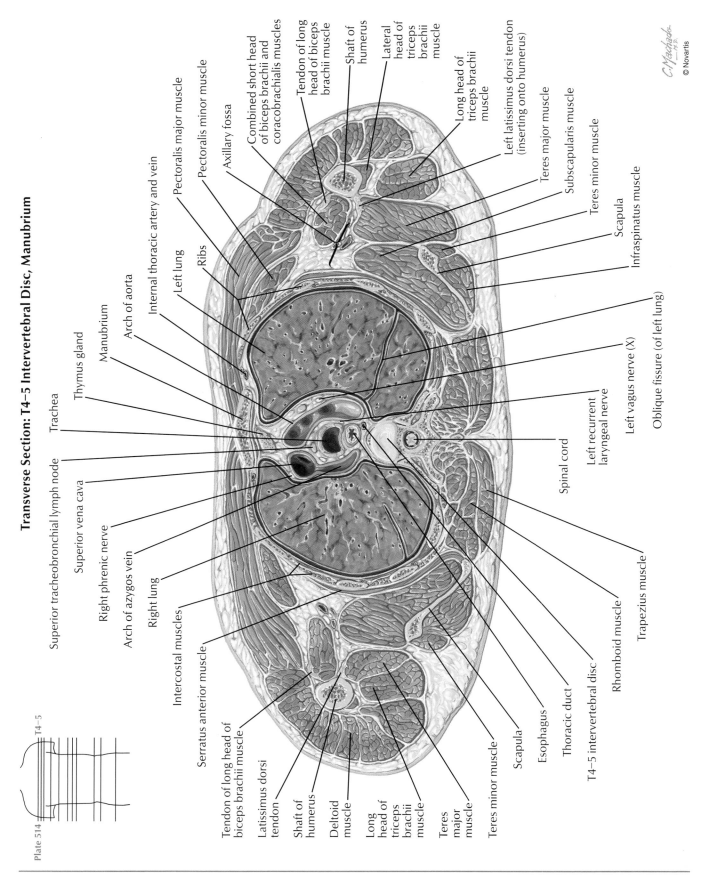

Superior tracheobronchial lymph node

Trachea

Thymus gland

Manubrium

Arch of aorta

Internal thoracic artery and vein

Left lung

Ribs

Axillary fossa

Pectoralis minor muscle

Pectoralis major muscle

Combined short head of biceps brachii and coracobrachialis muscles

Tendon of long head of biceps brachii muscle

Shaft of humerus

Lateral head of triceps brachii muscle

Long head of triceps brachii muscle

Left latissimus dorsi tendon (inserting onto humerus)

Teres major muscle

Subscapularis muscle

Teres minor muscle

Scapula

Infraspinatus muscle

Oblique fissure (of left lung)

Left vagus nerve (X)

Left recurrent laryngeal nerve

Spinal cord

Trapezius muscle

Rhomboid muscle

T4–5 intervertebral disc

Thoracic duct

Esophagus

Scapula

Teres minor muscle

Teres major muscle

Long head of triceps brachii muscle

Deltoid muscle

Shaft of humerus

Latissimus dorsi tendon

Tendon of long head of biceps brachii muscle

Serratus anterior muscle

Intercostal muscles

Right lung

Arch of azygos vein

Right phrenic nerve

Superior vena cava

Right phrenic nerve

Plate 514

T4–5

**PLATE 514**

**CROSS-SECTIONAL ANATOMY**

**Transverse Section: T5–6 Intervertebral Disc, Sternal Angle**

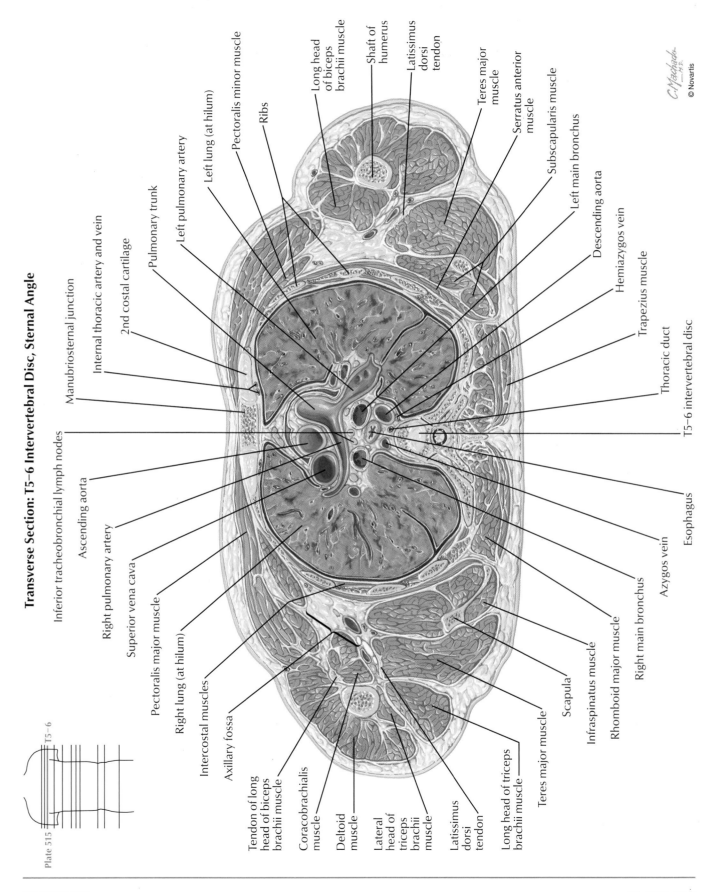

Inferior tracheobronchial lymph nodes

Manubriosternal junction

Internal thoracic artery and vein

2nd costal cartilage

Pulmonary trunk

Left pulmonary artery

Left lung (at hilum)

Pectoralis minor muscle

Ribs

Long head of biceps brachii muscle

Shaft of humerus

Latissimus dorsi tendon

Teres major muscle

Serratus anterior muscle

Subscapularis muscle

Left main bronchus

Descending aorta

Hemiazygos vein

Trapezius muscle

Thoracic duct

T5–6 intervertebral disc

Esophagus

Azygos vein

Right main bronchus

Rhomboid major muscle

Infraspinatus muscle

Scapula

Teres major muscle

Long head of triceps brachii muscle

Latissimus dorsi tendon

Lateral head of triceps brachii muscle

Deltoid muscle

Coracobrachialis muscle

Tendon of long head of biceps brachii muscle

Axillary fossa

Intercostal muscles

Right lung (at hilum)

Pectoralis major muscle

Superior vena cava

Right pulmonary artery

Ascending aorta

Plate 515

T5–6

C. Machado
—M.D.
© Novartis

**Transverse Section: Level of T7, 3rd Interchondral Space**

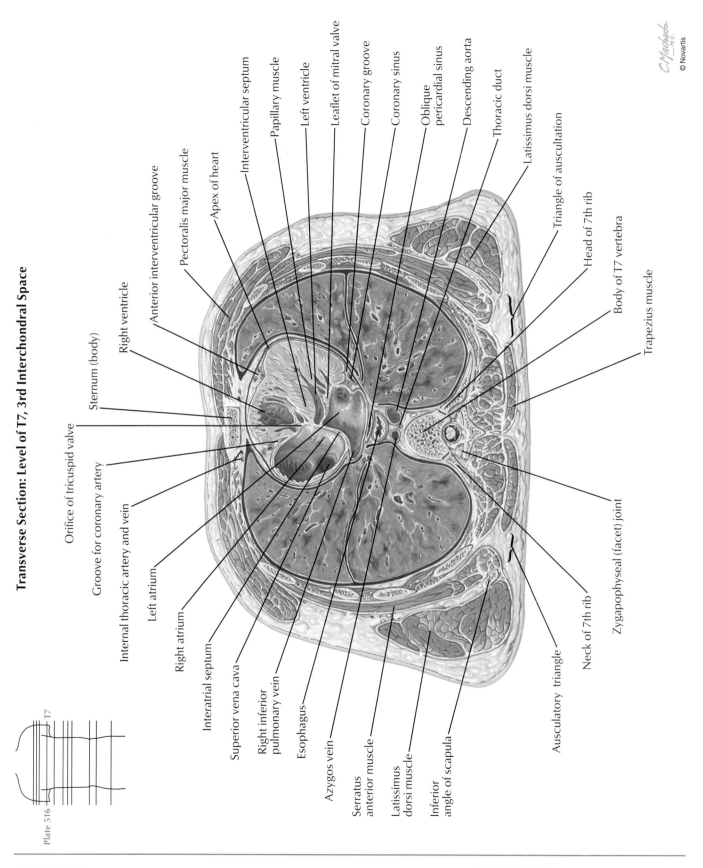

Orifice of tricuspid valve

Groove for coronary artery

Internal thoracic artery and vein

Left atrium

Right atrium

Interatrial septum

Superior vena cava

Right inferior pulmonary vein

Esophagus

Azygos vein

Serratus anterior muscle

Latissimus dorsi muscle

Inferior angle of scapula

Sternum (body)

Right ventricle

Anterior interventricular groove

Pectoralis major muscle

Apex of heart

Interventricular septum

Papillary muscle

Left ventricle

Leaflet of mitral valve

Coronary groove

Coronary sinus

Oblique pericardial sinus

Descending aorta

Thoracic duct

Latissimus dorsi muscle

Triangle of auscultation

Head of 7th rib

Body of T7 vertebra

Trapezius muscle

Zygapophyseal (facet) joint

Neck of 7th rib

Auscultatory triangle

C. Machado M.D.
© Novartis

Plate 516

T7

**PLATE 516**

**CROSS-SECTIONAL ANATOMY**

**Transverse Section: Level of T10, Xiphisternal Junction**

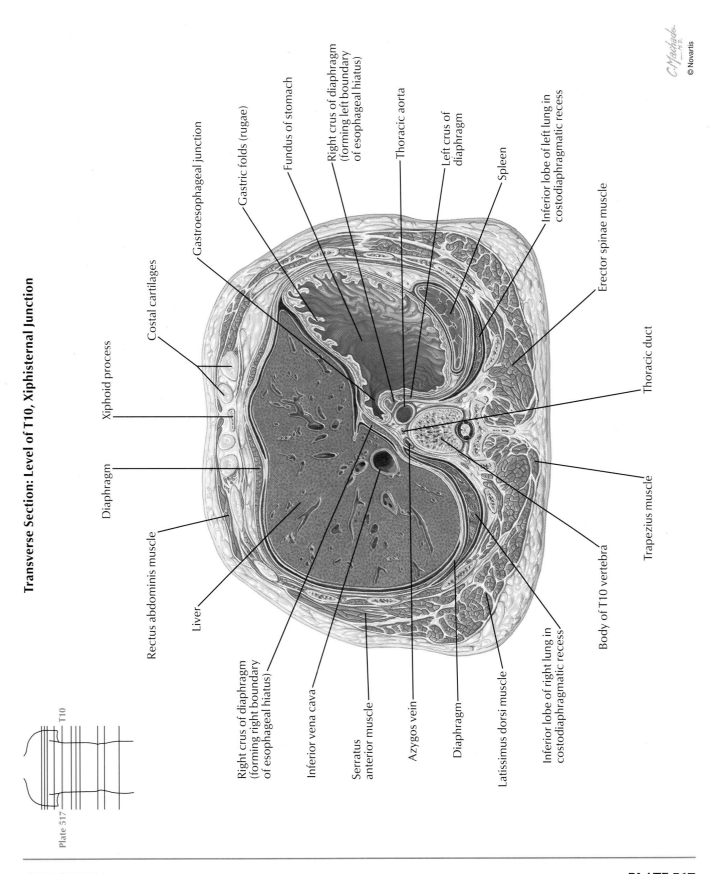

Gastroesophageal junction

Gastric folds (rugae)

Fundus of stomach

Right crus of diaphragm (forming right boundary of esophageal hiatus)

Thoracic aorta

Left crus of diaphragm

Spleen

Inferior lobe of left lung in costodiaphragmatic recess

Erector spinae muscle

Costal cartilages

Xiphoid process

Thoracic duct

Diaphragm

Rectus abdominis muscle

Liver

Trapezius muscle

Body of T10 vertebra

Right crus of diaphragm (forming right boundary of esophageal hiatus)

Inferior vena cava

Serratus anterior muscle

Azygos vein

Diaphragm

Latissimus dorsi muscle

Inferior lobe of right lung in costodiaphragmatic recess

T10

Plate 517

© Novartis

**Transverse Section: Level of T12, Inferior to Xiphoid**

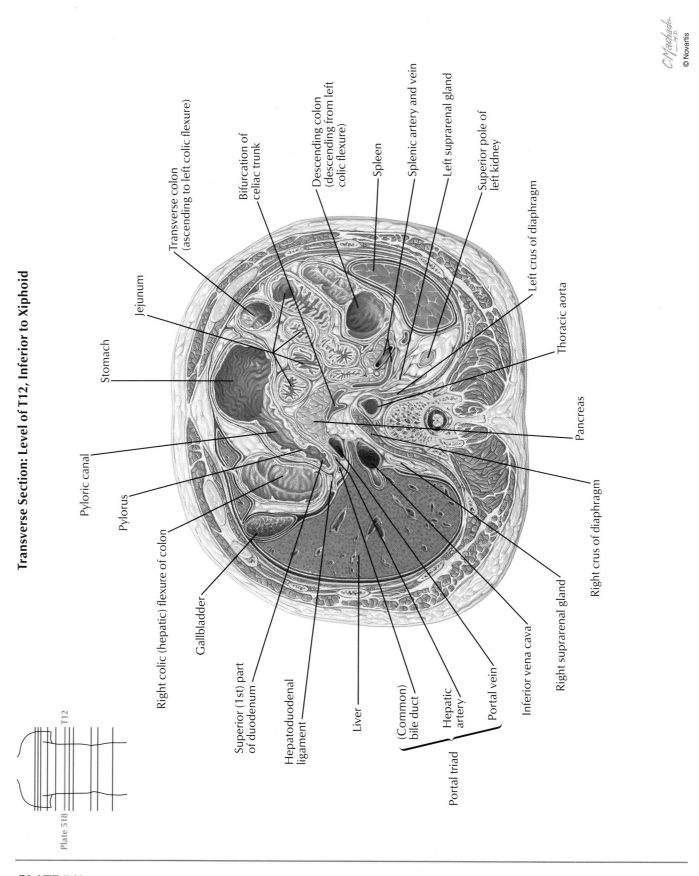

Transverse colon (ascending to left colic flexure)

Bifurcation of celiac trunk

Descending colon (descending from left colic flexure)

Spleen

Splenic artery and vein

Left suprarenal gland

Superior pole of left kidney

Left crus of diaphragm

Thoracic aorta

Pancreas

Right crus of diaphragm

Right suprarenal gland

Inferior vena cava

Portal vein

Hepatic artery

(Common) bile duct

Portal triad

Liver

Hepatoduodenal ligament

Superior (1st) part of duodenum

Gallbladder

Right colic (hepatic) flexure of colon

Pylorus

Pyloric canal

Stomach

Jejunum

C. Machado M.D.
© Novartis

Plate 518

**PLATE 518**

**CROSS-SECTIONAL ANATOMY**

**Transverse Section: Level of T12–L1 Intervertebral Disc**

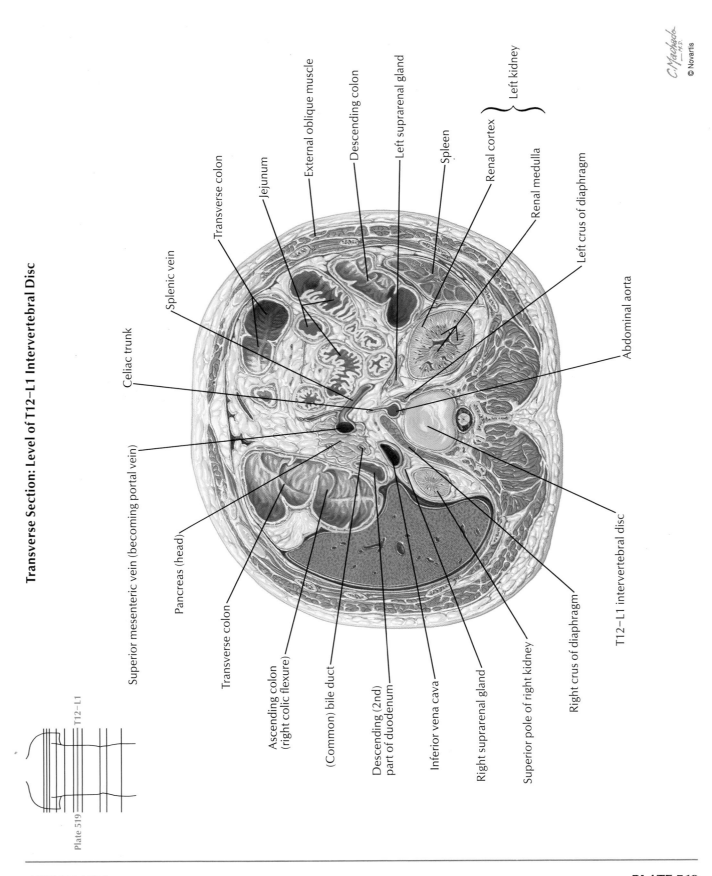

Transverse colon

Jejunum

External oblique muscle

Descending colon

Left suprarenal gland

Spleen

Renal cortex

Left kidney

Renal medulla

Left crus of diaphragm

Abdominal aorta

Splenic vein

Celiac trunk

Superior mesenteric vein (becoming portal vein)

Pancreas (head)

Transverse colon

Ascending colon (right colic flexure)

(Common) bile duct

Descending (2nd) part of duodenum

Inferior vena cava

Right suprarenal gland

Superior pole of right kidney

Right crus of diaphragm

T12–L1 intervertebral disc

T12–L1

Plate 519

**Transverse Section: Level of L1–2 Intervertebral Disc**

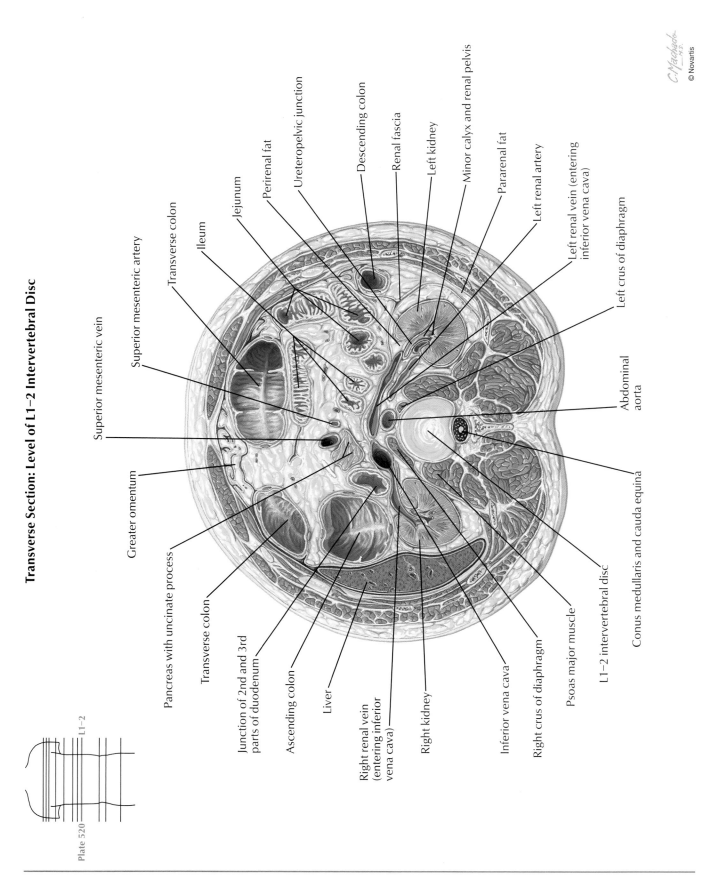

Perirenal fat

Ureteropelvic junction

Descending colon

Renal fascia

Left kidney

Minor calyx and renal pelvis

Pararenal fat

Left renal artery

Left renal vein (entering inferior vena cava)

Left crus of diaphragm

Jejunum

Transverse colon

Ileum

Superior mesenteric artery

Superior mesenteric vein

Abdominal aorta

Conus medullaris and cauda equina

Greater omentum

Pancreas with uncinate process

Transverse colon

Ascending colon

Liver

Junction of 2nd and 3rd parts of duodenum

Right renal vein (entering inferior vena cava)

Right kidney

Inferior vena cava

Right crus of diaphragm

Psoas major muscle

L1–2 intervertebral disc

L1–2

Plate 520

C Machado MD.
© Novartis

**PLATE 520**

**CROSS-SECTIONAL ANATOMY**

**Transverse Section: Level of L5, Near Transtubercular Plane**

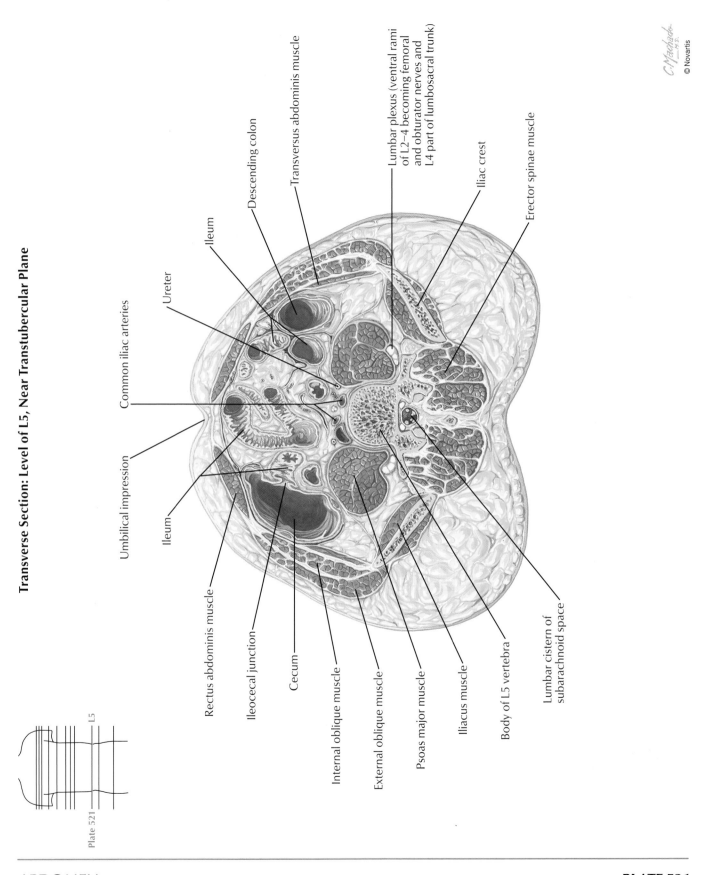

Descending colon

Transversus abdominis muscle

Lumbar plexus (ventral rami of L2–4 becoming femoral and obturator nerves and L4 part of lumbosacral trunk)

Iliac crest

Erector spinae muscle

Ileum

Ureter

Common iliac arteries

Umbilical impression

Ileum

Rectus abdominis muscle

Ileocecal junction

Cecum

Internal oblique muscle

External oblique muscle

Psoas major muscle

Iliacus muscle

Body of L5 vertebra

Lumbar cistern of subarachnoid space

L5

Plate 521

**ABDOMEN**

*PLATE 521*

© Novartis

**Transverse Section: Level of S1, Anterior Superior Iliac Spines**

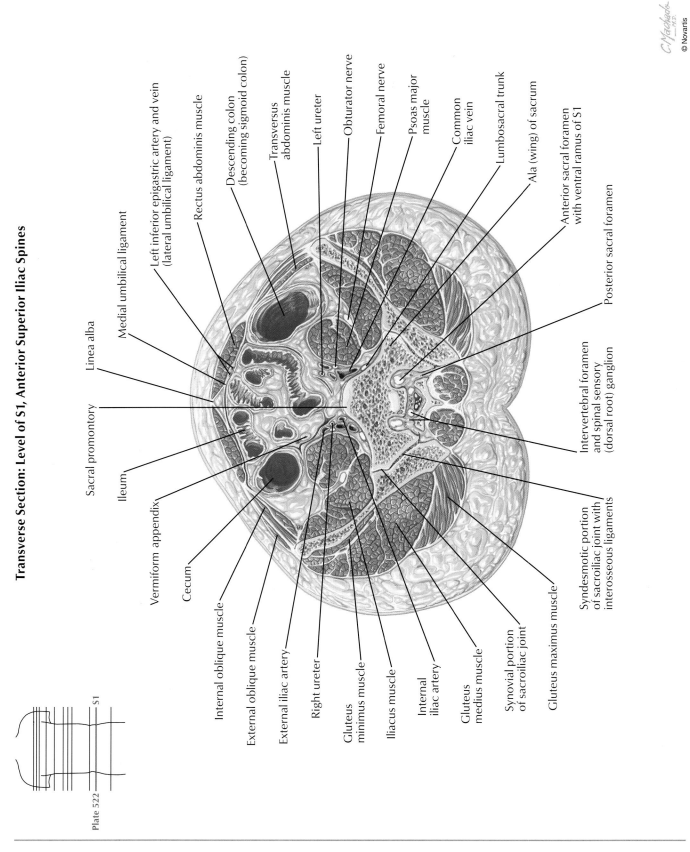

Left inferior epigastric artery and vein (lateral umbilical ligament)

Rectus abdominis muscle

Descending colon (becoming sigmoid colon)

Transversus abdominis muscle

Left ureter

Obturator nerve

Femoral nerve

Psoas major muscle

Common iliac vein

Lumbosacral trunk

Ala (wing) of sacrum

Anterior sacral foramen with ventral ramus of S1

Posterior sacral foramen

Intervertebral foramen and spinal sensory (dorsal root) ganglion

Medial umbilical ligament

Linea alba

Sacral promontory

Ileum

Vermiform appendix

Cecum

Internal oblique muscle

External oblique muscle

External iliac artery

Right ureter

Gluteus minimus muscle

Iliacus muscle

Internal iliac artery

Gluteus medius muscle

Synovial portion of sacroiliac joint

Gluteus maximus muscle

Syndesmotic portion of sacroiliac joint with interosseous ligaments

S1

Plate 522

**PLATE 522**

**CROSS-SECTIONAL ANATOMY**

© Novartis

**Transverse Section: Pubic Crest, Femoral Heads, Coccyx**

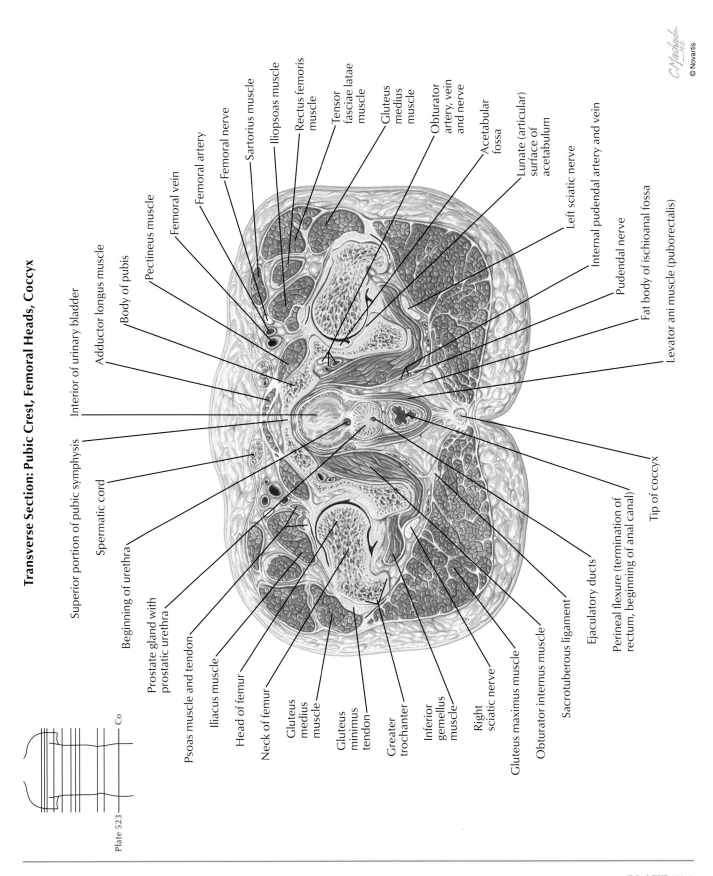

Femoral vein

Femoral artery

Femoral nerve

Sartorius muscle

Iliopsoas muscle

Rectus femoris muscle

Tensor fasciae latae muscle

Gluteus medius muscle

Obturator artery, vein and nerve

Acetabular fossa

Lunate (articular) surface of acetabulum

Left sciatic nerve

Internal pudendal artery and vein

Pudendal nerve

Fat body of ischioanal fossa

Levator ani muscle (puborectalis)

Pectineus muscle

Body of pubis

Adductor longus muscle

Interior of urinary bladder

Superior portion of pubic symphysis

Spermatic cord

Beginning of urethra

Prostate gland with prostatic urethra

Psoas muscle and tendon

Iliacus muscle

Head of femur

Neck of femur

Gluteus medius muscle

Gluteus minimus tendon

Greater trochanter

Inferior gemellus muscle

Right sciatic nerve

Gluteus maximus muscle

Obturator internus muscle

Sacrotuberous ligament

Ejaculatory ducts

Perineal flexure (termination of rectum, beginning of anal canal)

Tip of coccyx

Co

Plate 523

**Coronal Section: Anterior Axillary Line**

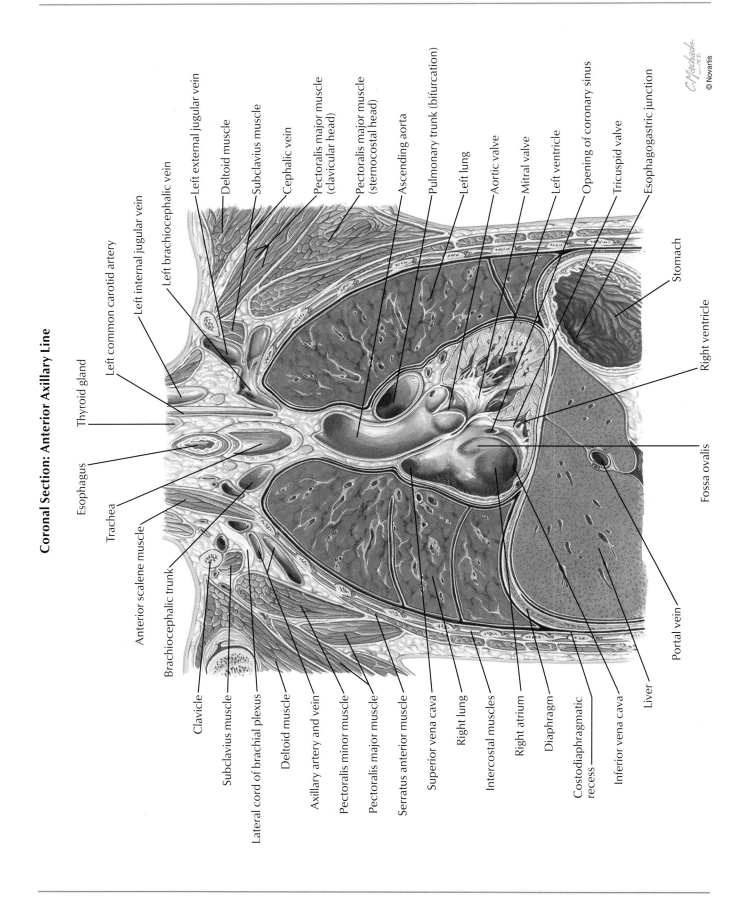

Left external jugular vein

Deltoid muscle

Subclavius muscle

Cephalic vein

Pectoralis major muscle (clavicular head)

Pectoralis major muscle (sternocostal head)

Ascending aorta

Pulmonary trunk (bifurcation)

Left lung

Aortic valve

Mitral valve

Left ventricle

Opening of coronary sinus

Tricuspid valve

Esophagogastric junction

Left internal jugular vein

Left brachiocephalic vein

Left common carotid artery

Thyroid gland

Esophagus

Trachea

Anterior scalene muscle

Brachiocephalic trunk

Clavicle

Subclavius muscle

Lateral cord of brachial plexus

Deltoid muscle

Axillary artery and vein

Pectoralis minor muscle

Pectoralis major muscle

Serratus anterior muscle

Superior vena cava

Right lung

Intercostal muscles

Right atrium

Diaphragm

Costodiaphragmatic recess

Inferior vena cava

Liver

Portal vein

Fossa ovalis

Right ventricle

Stomach

C. Machado M.D.

© Novartis

**PLATE 524**

**CROSS-SECTIONAL ANATOMY**

**Coronal Section: Midaxillary Line**

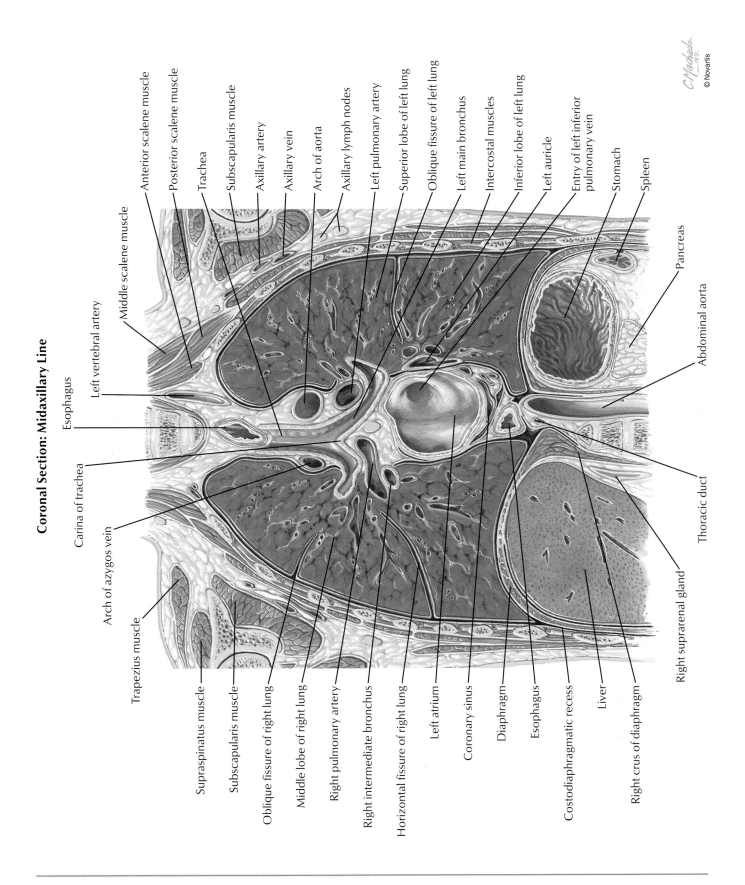

Anterior scalene muscle
Posterior scalene muscle
Trachea
Subscapularis muscle
Axillary artery
Axillary vein
Arch of aorta
Axillary lymph nodes
Left pulmonary artery
Superior lobe of left lung
Oblique fissure of left lung
Left main bronchus
Intercostal muscles
Inferior lobe of left lung
Left auricle
Entry of left inferior pulmonary vein
Stomach
Spleen

Middle scalene muscle

Left vertebral artery

Esophagus

Pancreas

Abdominal aorta

Carina of trachea

Thoracic duct

Arch of azygos vein

Right suprarenal gland

Trapezius muscle

Supraspinatus muscle
Subscapularis muscle
Oblique fissure of right lung
Middle lobe of right lung
Right pulmonary artery
Right intermediate bronchus
Horizontal fissure of right lung
Left atrium
Coronary sinus
Diaphragm
Esophagus
Costodiaphragmatic recess
Liver
Right crus of diaphragm

# REFERENCES

*Plate 52*

Braus H. Anatomie des Menschen. Berlin, Verlag von Julius Springer, 1924

*Plate 85*

Nishida S. The Structure of the Eye. New York, Elsevier North-Holland, 1982

*Plate 150*

Keegan JJ. J Neurosurg 1947;4:115

*Plate 158*

Turnbull IM. Blood supply of the spinal cord. In Vinken PJ, Bruyn GW (eds). Handbook of Clinical Neurology, XII. Amsterdam, North-Holland, 1972, pp 478-491

*Plate 188, 189*

Jackson CL, Huber JF. Correlated applied anatomy of the bronchial tree and lungs with a system of nomenclature. Dis Chest 1943;9:319–326

*Plate 191*

Ikeda S, Ono Y, Miyazawa S, et al. Flexible broncho-fiberscope. Otolaryngology (Tokyo) 1970;42:855–861

*Plates 236, 343, 345, 353 & 357*

Myers RP, King BF, Cahill DR. Deep perineal "space" as defined by magnetic resonance imaging. Presented at 14th Annual Scientific Session of the American Association of Clinical Anatomists, Honolulu, HI, 1997. (Abstract:Clin Anat 1998;11)

*Plate 265*

DiDio LJA. Anatomo-Fisiologia do Piloro ileo-ceco-colica no homen, Actas das Primeiras Jornadas Inter-universitarías Argentinas de Gastroenterologia, Rosario, 1954

———. Dados anatomicos sobre o "piloro" ileo-ceco-colico. (Com observacao direta in vivo de "papila" ileo-ceco-colica.) (English summary). Thesis, Fac Med, Univ de São Paulo, 1952

*Plate 273*

Healey JE Jr, Schroy. Anatomy of the biliary duct within the human liver; analysis of the prevailing pattern of branchings and the major variations of the biliary ducts. Arch Surg 1953;66:599

———, Sörensen. The intrahepatic distribution of the hepatic artery in man. J Int Coll Surg 1953;20:133

*Plates 274, 275*

Elias H. Liver morphology. Biol Rev 1955;30:263

———. Origin and early development of the liver in various vertebrates. Act Hepat 1955;3:1

———. Morphology of the liver. In "Liver Injury," Trans 11th Conference. New York, Macy Foundation, 1953

———. A re-examination of the structure of the mammalian liver; the hepatic lobule and its relation to the vascular and biliary system. Am J Anat 1949;85:379

———. A re-examination of the structure of the mammalian liver; parenchymal architecture. Am J Anat 1949;84:311

*Plates 288, 289*

Michels NA. Blood Supply and Anatomy of the Upper Abdominal Organs, With a Descriptive Atlas. Philadelphia, JB Lippincott, 1955

*Plate 312*

Thomas MD. In The Ciba Collection of Medical Illustrations, Vol 3, Part II. Summit NJ, CIBA, p 78

*Plates 329, 338, 358, 368, 385*

Stormont TJ, Cahill DR, King BF, Myers RP. Fascias of the male external genitalia and perineum. Clin Anat 1994;7:115

*Plates 333, 337, 342, 345, 351, 352*

Oelrich TM. The striated urogenital sphincter muscle in the female. Anat Rec 1983;205:223

*Plates 336, 338*

Myers RP, Goellner JR, Cahill DR. Prostate shape, external striated urethral sphincter and radical prostatectomy: the apical dissection. J Urol 1987;138:543

*Plates 336, 338, 357, 358*

Oelrich TM. The urethral sphincter muscle in the male. Am J Anat 1980;158:229

*Plate 378*

Flocks RH, Kerr HD, Elkins HB, et al. Treatment of carcinoma of the prostate by interstitial radiation with radio-active gold (Au198):A preliminary report. J Urol 1952;68(2):510–522

*Plate 455*

Keegan JJ, Garrett FD. The segmental distribution of the cutaneous nerves in the limbs of man. Anat Rec 1948;102:409–437

*Plate 511*

Keegan JJ. J Bone Joint Surg 1944;26:238

Last RJ. Innervation of the limbs. J Bone Joint Surg 1949;31(B):452

# INDEX

References are to plate numbers; numbers in bold refer to primary sources. In most cases, structures are listed under singular nouns.

## A

**Abdomen**
arteries of 238, 247–see also arteries of individual organs
bony framework of 231
cross sections of 517–522
lymph vessels and nodes of 249, 295–297, 321–see also lymph nodes of individual organs
muscles of 232–237, 246
nerves of 240, 241, 250–see also nerves of individual organs
autonomic 300
planes of 251
quadrants of 251
regions of 251
veins of 239, 248–see also veins of individual organs
viscera of 252, 258–268–see also individual organs
**Acetabulum** 334, 453
Achilles–see Tendon, calcaneal (Achilles)
**Acinus** 192
**Acromion** 22, 170, 174, 178, **392**–398, 400, 402, 403
**Action** of
extrinsic eye muscles 79
infrahyoid muscles 24
intrinsic laryngeal muscles 73
jaws 11
suprahyoid muscles 24
wrist 423
Adam's apple–see Prominence, laryngeal
Adamkiewicz–see Artery, segmental medullary, major anterior
**Adenohypophysis** 133, 140
Adenoid–see Tonsil, pharyngeal
**Adhesion,** interthalamic 100, 102, 105, 109, 139
**Aditus** of larynx 57, 60, 223
**Adnexa**
of orbit–see Apparatus, lacrimal; Eyelids
of uterus 346
**Adrenergic** 154
synapsis–see Synapsis, adrenergic
terminal–see Terminal, adrenergic
**Agger nasi** 32, 33
Air cell–see Cell (air)
**Airway,** intrapulmonary 192
**Ala** (wing)
of central cerebellar lobule–see Wing, of central (cerebellar) lobule
ilium 231, 330, 335, 453
sacrum 145, 522
vomer 5

**Ala** cont.
Albini–see Nodule, Albini's
ALS–see System, anterolateral
**Alveolus** of
lung 192, 193
pancreas 279
**Alveus** of hippocampus 106
**Ampulla**
of ductus deferens 359
of duodenum 262, 276
hepatopancreatic 278
of inner ear 87
labyrinthine 90, 118
of lactiferous duct 167
of semicircular duct 90, 118
of uterine tube 346
of Vater–see Ampulla, hepatopancreatic
of vestibule 91
**Anastomosis**
around
elbow 405
eye/orbit 80
knee 477
scapula 398
between
angular and dorsal nasal arteries 35, 80
carotid and vertebral arteries 131
cervical and occipital arteries 28
circumflex femoral arteries 470
external and internal carotid arteries 80, 131
inferior phrenic and left gastric arteries 288
intercostal and lumbar arteries 218, 238
lacrimal and middle meningeal arteries 95
median and ulnar nerves 462, 444, 445
pancreatic arteries 284–286
posterior septal branch of sphenopalatine artery and greater palatine artery 36
pubic branches of obturator and inferior epigastric arteries 243, 340, 341
right and left carotid arteries 131
right and left hepatic arteries 288
subclavian and carotid arteries 131
subclavian and vertebral arteries 131
superior and inferior mesenteric arteries (arc of Riolan) 289
paravertebral 158
portacaval 293
prevertebral 158
scapular 398
Anesthesia, perineal 384
Angiogram, coronary–see Arteriogram of coronary arteries
**Angle**
anterior chamber, of eye–see Angle, iridocorneal
iridocorneal 82, 83, 86
of Louis–see Angle, sternal
of mandible 9, 10, 60
of mastoid 6

**Angle** cont.
of rib 170, 171
of scapula 392, 393, 516
sternal 170
subpubic 332
tuber 490
**Ankle**
bones of 378, 479, 488–490
ligaments of 491
lymph nodes of 510
tendinous sheaths of 493
tendons of 491
**Anulus** fibrosus
of heart–see Ring, fibrous, of heart
of intervertebral disc 144
**Anoderm** 365
**Anomaly** of
cervical ribs 173
right inferior laryngeal nerve 74
right subclavian artery 74
**Ansa**
cervicalis 26, **27,** 29, 65, 68, 122, 123
subclavia 124, 198, 214, 215, 228
**Anteflexion** of uterus 348
**Antihelix** of external ear 88
**Antitragus** of external ear 88
**Antrum**
mastoid 89
pyloric 258
tympanic 89
**Anus** 337, 350, 354, 356, 367, 369, 389
**Aorta**
abdominal 165, 181, 217, 220, 246, **247,** 253, 256, 257, 261, 279, 282, 284, 290, 306, 309, 311, 312, 314, 320, 324, 325, 327–329, 339, 340, 344, 369, 371–374, 383, 519–520, 525
ureteric branches 320
arch of 30, 68, 69, 74, 131, 184, 195, 196, 199–203, 208, 209, 213, 217, 219, **220,** 221, 225, 514, 525
ascending 131, 194, 203, 208, 211, 212, 515, 524
descending 131, 180, 194, 196, 219, 220, 225, 230, 515, 516
thoracic 156, 158, 179, 217, 219, 221, **225,** 517, 518
esophageal branches 225
ureteric branch 320
**Aperture**–see also Opening
lateral, of 4th ventricle (Luschka) 102, 103, 139
median, of 4th ventricle (Magendie) 102, 103, 109, 139
**Apex** of
bladder 338
fibula 478, 479
heart 201, 202, 516
lung 184, 185, 187
sacrum 145
tongue 52

**Aponeurosis**
  bicipital 402, 404, 416, 442, 449
  epicranial (galea aponeurotica) 17, 20, 21, 96, 164
  external abdominal oblique 232–235, 240, 242, 244, 327, 328
  gluteal 312, 460, 461, 468
  internal abdominal oblique 234, 235, 240, 328
  palatine 46, 59
  palmar 412, 416, 417, 424, 428, 429, 431, 449
  pharyngeal 59, 61, 223
  plantar 493, 496–499
  of scalp–see Aponeurosis, epicranial
  transversus abdominis 161, 162, 165, 235, 237, 238, 312, 324, 329
**Apparatus**
  lacrimal 77
Appendage, atrial–see Auricle, of left antrium; of right antrium
**Appendix**
  epididymidis 361, 390
  epiploic–see Appendix, omental
  fibrous, of liver 270
  omental (epiploic) 254, 267, 328
  of testis 365, 394
  vermiform 120, 254, 265, **266,** 267, 339, 340, 522
  vesicular 346, 390
**Aqueduct**
  cerebral 100, 102, 103, 109, 139
  cochlear 91
  of Sylvius (midbrain aqueduct) 100, 102, 103, 109
  vestibular 90–92
**Arachnoid**
  granulation 94–96, 103
  mater 94, 96, 103, 155, 156
Arantius, nodules of–see Nodule, of semilunar valve
**Arc**
  omental (epiploic) arterial 288
  of Riolan–see Anastomosis, between superior and inferior mesenteric arteries
**Arch**
  anterior, of atlas 12, 57
  lumbocostal, of diaphragm 181, 246–see also Ligament, arcuate, of diaphragm
  of obturator fascia–see Arch, tendinous, of levator ani muscle
  palatoglossal 45, 52, 54, 58
  palatopharyngeal 45, 52, 54, 58, 60
  of pelvic diaphragm–see Arch, tendinous, of levator animuscle
  of pelvic fascia–see Arch, tendinous, of pelvic fascia
  pharyngopalatine–see Arch, palatopharyngeal
  posterior, of atlas 12, 164

**Arch** *cont.*
  pubic 231, 332
  of soleus muscle–see Arch, tendinous, of soleus muscle
  tendinous
    of levator ani muscle 236, 246, 333–**336,** 341–343, 345, 352, 364
    of pelvic fascia 45, 343
    of soleus 482, 483
  zygomatic 2, 9, 48
**Arch** (arterial)
  of aorta 68, 69, 74, 131, 195, 199–**202,** 203, 209, 219, 220, 225, 514, 525
  deep
    palmar 434, 435
    plantar 485, 495, 500
  dorsal carpal 438
  palmar carpal 434
  palpebral 80
  superficial palmar 429, 430, 435, 442
**Arch** (venous)
  of azygos vein 514, 525
  dorsal
    of foot 508
    of hand 441, 449
  superficial palmar 429
**Area**
  bare
    of diaphragm 257, 270, 311
    of liver 270, 311, 324, 329
    of pericardium 184
  cribriform, of kidney 321
  intercondylar, of tibia 478, 479
  of Laimer 69, 222, 223
  of liver–see Segment, of liver
  parolfactory 100, 113
  of referred pain
    biliary 309
    pancreatic 310
  pontine taste 129
  septal (pellucidum) 113
  subcallosal 100, 113
  vestibular, of 4th ventricle 109
**Arm**
  arteries of 404, 405, 442
  bones of 392, 393
  cross sections of 406
  fascia/fascial compartments 406, 448
  lymph nodes and vessels of 452
  muscles of 402, 403
  nerves of 442, 443, 446, 448
Arteria recta–see Artery, straight
**Arteriogram** of coronary arteries 206, 207
**Arteriole**
  of kidney
    afferent 317, 318
    aglomerular 318
    cortical radiate 315, 318
    efferent 317, 318
    interlobular–see Arteriole, of kidney cortical radiale
  of liver
    intralobular 274

**Arteriole** *cont.*
  periportal 274
  portal 274
  macular (of retina) 86
  nasal (of retina) 86
  temporal (of retina) 86
**Artery**
  of abdominal wall 238, 247
  accessory
    left gastric 288
    hepatic 288, 289
    meningeal 35, 95
    middle colic 291
    renal 316
  acetabular–see Artery, obturator, acetabular branch
  acoustic, internal–see Artery, labyrinthine
  acromial–see Acromial branch under Artery, suprascapular; thoracoacromial
  of Adamkiewicz–see Artery, segmental medullary, major anterior
  alveolar
    anterior superior 35
    inferior 35, 47, 54, 63, 64
      lingual branch 63
      mental branch 35, 63
      mylohyoid branch 35, 63
    middle superior 35
    posterior superior 35, 63
  of anal canal 369
  angular (of face) 17, 31, 35, 63, 80, 131–see also Artery, cerebral, middle, branch to angular gyrus
  anomalous right subclavian 74
  anterolateral central (lentriculostriate) 132–134, 136
  anteromedial central (perforating) 133
  aortic intercostal–see Artery, intercostal, posterior
  appendicular 264, 286, 287, 293, 304
  arcuate
    of foot 485, 494, 495, 500
    of kidney 315, 318
    of arm 404, 405, 442
  ascending
    branch–see under Artery, iliac, circumflex, deep; femoral circumflex, lateral; humeral, circumflex, posterior
    cervical–see Artery, cervical, ascending
    frontal–see Artery, prefrontal
    palatine–see Artery, palatine, ascending
    pharyngeal–see Artery, pharyngeal, ascending
  atrial, anterior right–see under Artery, coronary, right
  atrioventricular–see under Artery, coronary, left, circumflex branch
  of atrioventricular node–see Artery, coronary, right, atrioventricular (AV) nodal branch

**Artery** *cont.*

auricular
anterior–see Artery, temporal, superficial,
anterior auricular branches
deep 35
posterior 17, 29, 35, 63, 95, 130, 131,
164
axillary 168, 175, 186, 238, **398**–400,
404, 524, 525
basilar 130–134, 136, 157
brachial 168, 398, 400, 402, **404**–406,
416–418, 442
deep–see Artery, deep, of arm
muscular branches of 404
brachiocephalic–see Trunk (arterial),
brachiocephalic
of brain 130–136, 141
bronchial 187, 193, **196,** 218, 219, 225
esophageal branches 225
variations in 196
buccal 35, 63
of bulb
of penis 376
of vestibule 345, 375
calcaneal 481, 482
lateral–see Artery, fibular (peroneal),
calcaneal branch
medial–see Artery, tibial, posterior,
calcaneal branch
calcarine–see Artery, cerebral, posterior,
calcarine branch
callosomarginal 134, 135
medial frontal branches 134, 135
candelabra–see Artery, prefrontal
capsular
of kidney 318
of liver 288
caroticotympanic 131
carotid 29
common 17, 25–**29,** 63–65, 68–70, 74,
119, 122, 124, 125, 127, 128, **130,**
131, 176, 182, 186, 195, 199, 200,
202, 220, 225, 513, 525
external 17, 23, 24, 26–**29,** 35, 36,
53–55, 63–65, 68–70, 95, 119, 124,
125, 127, 128, **130,** 131
internal 17, 27–**29,** 30, 39, 54, 63, 65,
68–70, 80, 81, 89, 93, 95, 98, 115,
117, 119, 122, 124–128, **130,**
131–136
cavernous branch of 95
meningeal branch of 95
meningohypophyseal trunk of 95
tentorial branch of 95, 98
carpal–see Carpal branches under Artery,
radial; ulnar
of cauda equina 157
of cavernous sinus–see Artery, carotid,
internal, cavernous branch
cecal 264, 286, 287, 293, 305
celiac–see Trunk (arterial), celiac
central
anterolateral (lenticulostriate) 132, 134, 136

**Artery** *cont.*

anteromedial (perforating) 133
of retina–see Artery, retinal, central
posteromedial (perforating) 133
sulcal (rolandic), of brain–see Artery,
sulcal, central (rolandic)
cerebellar
anterior inferior 130–134, 136, 157
posterior inferior 130–132, 134, 136,
157
cerebellar tonsillar branch 136
choroidal branch to 4th ventricle 136
superior 130–134, 136, 157
superior vermian branch 136
cerebral
anterior 130–136
terminal branches 135
middle 130, 132–136
branch to angular gyrus 134, 135
temporal branches 135
terminal branches (trunks) 135
posterior 130–136
calcarine branch 135, 136
dorsal branch to corpus callosum 135,
136
parietooccipital branch 135, 136
temporal branches 135
terminal branches 135
cervical
ascending 28, 63, 65, 68–70, 130, 131,
157
deep 28, 130, 131, 157
transverse 27, 28, 63, 68–70, 131, 163,
398, 400
choroidal
anterior 132–134, 136
posterior
lateral 132, 136
medial 132, 136
to 4th ventricle–see Artery, cerebellar,
posterior inferior, choroidal branch
to 4th ventricle
ciliary
anterior 86
posterior 80, 86
cingular 135
of Circle of Willis 133
circumflex
coronary–see Artery, coronary, left,
circumflex branch
femoral–see Artery, femoral, circumflex
fibular–see Artery, tibial, posterior,
circumflex fibular branch
humeral–see Artery, humeral, circumflex
iliac–see Artery, iliac, circumflex
scapular–see Artery, scapular, circumflex
clavicular–see Artery, thoracoacromial,
clavicular branch
of clitoris
deep 375
dorsal 375
colic 289

**Artery** *cont.*

branch of ileocolic–see Artery, ileocolic,
colic branch
left 247, 287, 289, 300, 305, 306, 319,
369
large branch replacing middle colic
289
middle 279, 283, 284, 286, 287, 289,
304, 305, 329
common trunk with right colic 289
right 286, 287, 289, 304, 305, 319, 328
common trunk
with ileocolic 289
with middle colic 289
variations in 289
collateral
of gallbladder 288
of liver 288
medial 403, 405, 405, 415
radial 403, 405, 406
ulnar
inferior 404, 405, 415
superior 404–406, 415
communicating
anterior 130–135
posterior 98, 130–136
coronary (in general) 204, 205
left 204, 205, 207
anterior descending (LAD)–see Artery,
coronary, left, anterior
interventricular branch of
anterior interventricular branch of 201,
204, 205, 207
interventricular septal branch 204
circumflex branch of 204, 205, 207
atrioventricular branch of 207
lateral branch of 207
posterolateral branch of 207
marginal–see Artery, coronary, right, right
marginal branch
posterior descending–see Artery,
coronary, right, posterior
interventricular branch
right 201, 202, 204–206
anterior right atrial branch 204
conus branch 206
posterior interventricular branch 202,
204, 206
atrioventricular (AV) nodal branch
206, 210
interventricular septal branch 204
right marginal branch 204, 206
sinuatrial (SA) nodal branch 204, 206
right marginal–see Artery, coronary, right,
right marginal branch
of conjunctiva 86
of conus arteriosus–see Artery, coronary,
right, conus branch
cortical radiate (interlobular) of kidney
315, 318
costocervical–see Trunk (arterial),
costocervical
of cranial fossa, posterior 136

**Artery** *cont.*

cremasteric 234, 236, 238, 244, 245, 247, 372

cricothyroid–see Artery, thryoid, superior, cricothyroid branch

cystic 276, 282, 284, 288

deep

of arm (deep brachial) 397, 400, 403, 406

of clitoris 375

of penis 355, 357, 359, 376

of thigh (deep femoral) 466, 467, 468, 470, 471, 477

muscular branches 477

perforating branches 468, 477

deferential–see Artery, of ductus deferens

deltoid–see Artery, thoracoacromial, deltoid branch

descending

branch of

lateral femoral circumflex–see under Artery, femoral, circumflex, lateral

posterior humeral circumflex–see under Artery, humeral, circumflex, posterior

coronary–see Artery, coronary, left, anterior interventricular branch; right, posterior interventricular branch

genicular–see Artery, genicular, descending

palatine–see Artery, palatine, descending

digital (hand)

common palmar 428, 429, 431, 434, 435

dorsal 438, 440

proper palmar 428, 429, 431, 435, 440

digital (foot)

common plantar 497, 498, 500

dorsal 485, 494, 495, 500

proper plantar 485, 494–497, 500

dorsal

of clitoris 375

branch to corpus callosum–see Artery, cerebral, posterior, branch to corpus callosum

of foot 485, 494, 495, 500

of penis 238, 355, 357, 372, 374

scapular–see Artery, scapular, dorsal

dorsalis pedis–see Artery, dorsal, of foot

to ductus deferens 238, 247, 319, 361, 369, 372, 374

branch from inferior vesicle artery 247, 319, 369, 372

of duodenum 279–281

of Drummond–see Artery, marginal (Drummond)

of elbow 405, 442

epigastric

inferior 234, 236, 238, 243, **244,** 247, 257, 320, 328, 339–341, 369, 371, 372, 374, 477

cremasteric branch–see Artery, cremasteric

pubic branch 234, 236, 244, 247, 340, 341

superficial 232, 234, 238, 242, 247, 466, 477

superior 174–176, 179, 200, 234, 238, 327

episcleral 86

esophageal branch from

aorta–see Aorta, thoracic, esophageal branch

bronchial–see Artery, bronchial, esophageal branch

inferior phrenic–see Artery, phrenic, inferior, esophageal branch

inferior thyroid–see Artery, thyroid, inferior, esophageal branch

left gastric–see Artery, gastric, left, esophageal branch

ethmoidal

anterior 36, 80, 95

anterior meningeal branch 80, 95

nasal (external and anterior lateral) branch 36

anterior septal branch 36

posterior 80, 95

lateral nasal branch 36

septal branch 36

of eye 86–see also Artery, ophthalmic

of eyelids 80

facial **17,** 26, 27, 29, 31, 35, 54, 55, 63, 64, 69, 80, 125, 127, 130, 131

lateral nasal branch 36

alar branch 36

inferior labial branch 63

superior labial branch 63

nasal septal branch 36

tonsillar branch (tonsillar artery) 35, 58, 63

transverse 17, 29, 31, 55, 63, 80

femoral 234, 238, 244, 245, 247, 354, 372, 378, 459, 466, 467, 470, 471, **477,** 510 523

circumflex

lateral 466, 467, 470, 477

ascending branch 470, 477

descending branch 470, 477

tranverse branch 470, 477

medial 467, 468, 470, 477

deep–see Artery, deep, of thigh

muscular branch 477

of proximal femur 470

fibular (peroneal) 477, 481–483, 487, 494

(lateral) calcaneal branch 481–483, 498, 499

communicating branch 483

perforating branch 483, 484

posterior lateral malleolar branch 483

of foot 495, 497–500

of forearm 442

foveolar–see Artery, obturator, acetabular branch

frontal

ascending (middle cerebral)–see Artery, prefrontal

branch of middle meningeal–see Artery, meningeal, middle, frontal branch

branch of superficial temporal–see Artery, temporal, superficial, frontal branch

medial frontal branch–see Artery, callosomarginal, medial frontal branch

polar (frontopolar) 134, 135

frontobasal (orbitofrontal) 132, 134, 135

frontopolar–see Artery, frontal, polar

gastric

accessory left 288

left 225, 247, 255, 257, 282, **283,** 284, 286, 288, 300–305, 327, 329, 381

esophageal branch 225, 228, 282, 283

right 262, 276, 282–284, 286, 288, 301–304

short 257, 281–284, 286, 288, 327

gastroduodenal 262, 276, 283–286, 288, 290, 302–304, 309

gastroepiploic–see Artery, gastro-omental

gastro-omental (gastroepiploic)

left 255, 281–284, 286, 288; 301–303

right 255, 257, 282–284, 286, 288, 301–303

genicular

descending 466, 467, 471, 477

articular branch 466, 467, 477

saphenous branch 466, 467, 477

lateral

inferior 477, 481–486

superior 468, 477, 481–486

medial

inferior 466, 467, 477, 482–485

superior 466–468, 481–485

middle 477

gluteal

inferior 247, 320, 369, 373, 374, 465, 468

superior 247, 320, 369, 373, 374, 465, 468

of hand 435, 438, 442

of head of femur 470

of heart 204–207

hemorrhoidal–see Artery, rectal

hepatic

accessory 288

common 247, 255, 262, 276, **282–**288, 300, 303, 309, 327, 518

intermediate 284

left 276, 284, 288

accessory/replaced 288

proper 257, 261, 262, 270–273, 276, 279, 282–**284,** 285, 288, 299, 303, 327, 329

replaced 288

**Artery** *cont.*
right 276, 284, 288
accessory/replaced 288
of Heubner–see Artery, striate, medial
of hip 470, 477
humeral
circumflex
anterior 398, 400, 402, 404, 405
posterior 398, 400, 403–405
ascending and descending branches 398
hypogastric–see Artery, iliac, internal
hypophyseal 133, 141
hypothalamic 133, 141
ileal 264, 286, 287, 291
branch from ileocolic–see under Artery, ileocolic
ileocolic **264,** 286, 287, 289, 304, 305, 319
colic branch 264, 286, 287
ileal branch 264, 286, 287
of ileum 286
iliac
circumflex
ascending branch–see under Artery, iliac, circumflex, deep
deep 236, 238, 244, 247, 341, 374, 467, 477
ascending branch 238, 247
superficial 232, 234, 238, 242, 247, 466, 477
common 247, 254, 257, 300, 311, 319, 320, **369,** 371–374, 383, 521
ureteric branch 320
external 236, 243–**245,** 247, 254, 257, 264, 292, 300, 311, 319, 337–341, 344, 364, 369, 371–374, 383, 467, 477, 522
internal 247, 287, 300, 305, 311, 319, 321, 341, 345, 369, 371–**373, 374,** 383, 522
iliolumbar 247, 373, 374
infraorbital 17, 31, 35, 63, 76, 80
of infratemporal fossa 35
innominate–see Trunk (arterial), brachiocephalic
intercostal 158, 174, 175, 177, 179, 196, 218, 225, 238, 288, 331
anterior 176, 179, 238
highest–see Artery, intercostal, supreme
lateral cutaneous branch of 174, 175, 177, 196
posterior 157, 158, 168, 174, 175, 177, 179, 196, 218, 219, 225, 238
dorsal branch of 158, 179
supreme 28, 130, 131
interlobar, of kidney 315, 318
interlobular, of kidney–see Artery, cortical radiate
internal acoustic–see Artery, labyrinthine
internal mammary–see Artery, thoracic,

**Artery** *cont.*
internal
internal spermatic–see Artery, testicular
interosseous (forearm)
anterior 405, 415, 417–419
common 405, 417–419
posterior 405, 415, 418, 419
recurrent 405, 415
interventricular–see Artery, coronary, left, anterior interventricular branch; right, posterior interventricular branch
intestinal–see Artery, ileal, jejunal, of small intestine
intrahepatic 274, 275
intrapulmonary 193
intrarenal–see Interlobar, interlobular, and segmental arteries under Artery, of kidney
of iris 83, 86
greater arterial circle 83, 86
lesser arterial circle 83, 86
jejunal 286–288, 291, 301
juxtacolic–see Artery, marginal
of kidney 315, 318–see also Artery, renal, segmental, renal
arcuate 315, 318
cortical radiate 315, 318
interlobar 315, 318
interlobular–see Artery, of kidney, cortical radiate
segmental 315
of knee 477
labial branches–see Labial branches under Artery, facial, perineal
labyrinthine (internal acoustic) 130, 132–134, 136
lacrimal 80, 131
anastomotic branch with middle meningeal 95
zygomatic branches 80
laryngeal, superior 29, 63, 68–70, 130, 223
of larynx 68, 70
of leg 481–485
lenticulostriate–see Artery, anterolateral central
of ligament of femoral head–see Artery, obturatory, acetabular branch
lingual 17, 27, 29, 35, 53, 54, 63, 69, 127, 130, 131
deep 45, 53
dorsal 53
tonsillar branch 58
suprahyoid branch 53, 63
of liver 282–284–see also Artery, hepatic
lumbar 157, 238, 247
of lung 194, 195–see also Artery, pulmonary
macular–see Arteriole, macular (of retina)
malleolar–see also Malleolar branch under

**Artery** *cont.*
Artery, fibular, tibial, posterior
anterior
lateral 485, 494, 495
medial 485, 494, 495
mammary 168–see Mammary branch under Artery, thoracic, internal; lateral internal–see Artery, thoracic, internal
of mammary gland 168
marginal
branch of right coronary–see Artery, coronary, right, right marginal branch
(juxtacolic, of Drummond) 287, 292, 305
masseteric 35, 48, 49, 63
mastoid–see Artery, occipital, mastoid branch
maxillary 11, 29, **35,** 36, 41, 48, 49, 63, 65, 95, 125, 127, 128, 130, 131
pterygoid branch 35
medullary
segmental 131, 157, 158, 179
major anterior (Adamkiewicz) 157
meningeal
accessory 35, 95
branch–see under Artery, carotid, internal; ethmoidal, anterior; occipital; pharyngeal, ascending; vertebral
branch of lacrimal–see Artery, lacrimal, anastomotic branch with middle meningeal
middle 11, 35, 41, 49, 63, 65, 94–96, 98, 125, 130, 131
frontal branch 95
parietal branch 95
mental–see Artery, alveolar, inferior; mental branch
mesenteric
inferior 152, 247, 253, 261, 287, 289, 300, 305, 306, 311, 314, 319, 320, 328, 329, 369, 371, 372, 381
superior 152, 165, 217, 247, 253, 257, 261, 262, 264, 279, 283–289, 291, 299, 301, 303, 304, 306, 310, 311, 314, 319, 320, 324, 328, 329, 381, 520
ileal branch 286, 287, 291
jejunal branch 286, 287, 291
metacarpal
dorsal 438
palmar 434, 435
metatarsal
dorsal 485, 494, 495, 500
plantar 497, 499, 500
anterior perforating branches of, to dorsal metatarsal arteries 495, 499, 500
of mouth 63
musculophrenic 175, 176, 186, 200, 238
mylohyoid–see Artery, alveolar, inferior, mylohyoid branch

**Artery** *cont.*
nasal
dorsal 17, 31, 35, 63, 76, 80, 131
external—see External nasal branch under
Artery, ethmoidal, anterior
lateral—see Lateral nasal branch under
Artery, ethmoidal, facial,
sphenopalatine
septal—see Nasal septal branch under
Artery, ethmoidal (anterior and
posterior); facial, superior labial
branch; posterior; sphenopalatine
of nasal cavity 35, 36
of neck 28, 29, 63
of femur 470
obliterated umbilical—see Artery, umbilical,
occluded part
obturator 236, 243, 247, 287, 319, 320,
341, 344, 369, 371, **373,** 374, 381,
454, 470, 477, 523
acetabular branch (to ligament of
femoral head) 454, 470
pubic branch (anastomiosis with inferior
epigastric pubic branch) 243, 340,
341
occipital 17, 29, 64, 95, 130, 131, 164
descending branch 28
mastoid branch 95, 130
medial 135
meningeal branch 17
sternocleidomastoid branch 29, 63
omental (epiploic) 288
ophthalmic 35, 78, 80, 126, 130, 131,
133, 136
of orbit 80
orbitofrontal—see Artery, frontobasal
ovarian 247, 292, 300, 311, 314, 319,
320, 322, 328, 339, 341, 344, 346,
349, **371,** 374, 383, 386
branch from uterine—see Artery, uterine,
ovarian branch
tubal branch 375
ureteric branch 320
palatine
ascending 35, 58, 63
tonsillar branch 35, 58
descending 35, 63
greater 35, 36, 46
lesser 35, 36, 46, 58
tonsillar branch 58
palmar
branch of median nerve—see Artery,
median, palmar branch
carpal—see Palmar carpal branch under
Artery, radial, ulnar; see also Arch
(arterial), palmar carpal
deep—see Artery, ulnar, deep palmar
branches; see also Arch (arterial),
deep, palmar
digital 435
common—see Artery, digital, common
palmar
proper—see Artery, digital, proper
palmar

**Artery** *cont.*
metacarpal—see Artery, metacarpal,
palmar
superficial—see Arch (arterial), superficial
palmar
palpebral 80
pancreatic 283–285, 288
caudal 283, 284
dorsal (superior) 282–286, 288, 292
great 283–285
inferior 283–286, 288
superior—see Artery, pancreatic, dorsal
transverse 283–286
pancreaticoduodenal
common inferior 286, 287
inferior 283–285, 288, 301, 304, 305
anterior branch 283–288, 301–303
posterior branch 282–287, 302, 303
superior
anterior 255, 282–286, 288, 301–303
posterior 282–286, 288, 302, 303
paracentral 134, 135
cingular branch 135
paramedian—see Artery, posteromedial
central
of parathyroid glands 70
parietal 134, 135
branch of middle meningeal—see Artery,
meningeal, middle, parietal branch
branch of superficial temporal—see
Artery, temporal, superficial, parietal
branch
parietooccipital 135, 136
pectoral—see Artery, thoracoacromial,
pectoral branch
of pelvic viscera 371, 373–376
of penis 238, 355, 372, 374, 376
of bulb—see Artery, of bulb, of penis
deep—see Artery, deep, of penis
dorsal—see Artery, dorsal, of penis
perforating—see also Artery, posteromedial
central
of Circle of Willis 133
branch—see Perforating branch under
Artery, deep, of thigh; fibular
(peroneal); metatarsal, plantar;
thoracic, internal
pericallosal 134, 135
posterior—see Artery, cerebral,
posterior, dorsal branch to corpus
callosum
pericardiacophrenic 176, 180, 182, 195,
200, 201, 203, 218, 219, 230, 238
perineal 345, 357, 374–376
posterior labial branch 375
posterior scrotal branch 374, 376
transverse 375, 376
of perineum 372; 375–376
peroneal—see Artery, fibular (peroneal)
pharyngeal, ascending 29, 35, 63, 130,
131

**Artery** *cont.*
meningeal branch 95, 130
tonsillar branch 35, 58
of pharyngeal region 63
phrenic, inferior **181,** 220, 225, 228, 247,
255, 257, 282–284, 286, 288,
300–302, 304, 305, 314, 316, 325,
326, 381
recurrent esophageal branch 181, 225,
247, 282, 283, 304
plantar
deep 485, 494, 495, 500
digital—see Artery, digital (foot), common
plantar; proper plantar
lateral 483, 498–500
medial 483, 496–498
metatarsal—see Artery, metatarsal, plantar
polar frontal 134, 135
pontine 132–134, 136
popliteal 461, 468, 471, 477, 481–483
sural (muscular) branch 483
postcentral sulcal—see Artery, sulcal,
postcentral
precentral sulcal—see Artery, sulcal,
precentral
precuneal 135
prefrontal 132, 134, 135
pre-rolandic—see Artery, sulcal, precentral
princeps pollicis 435
profunda
brachii—see Artery, deep, of arm
femoris—see Artery, deep, of thigh
prostatic 374
pterygoid—see Artery, maxillary, pterygoid
branches
of pterygoid canal 35
pubic
branch of inferior epigastric—see under
Artery, epigastric, inferior
branch of obturator 243—see also
Anastomosis, between pubic branch
of obturator and inferior epigastric
arteries
pudendal
external
deep 238, 247, 372, 466, 477
superficial 232, 234, 238, 247, 372,
466, 477
internal 247, 287, 320, 357, 369, 370,
373–376, 465, 523
pulmonary 187, 193, **194,** 195, 201, 202,
208, 209, 217–219
radial 404, 405, 415–**417,** 418, 419, 424,
429, 430, 434–436, 439, 442
dorsal carpal branch 436
palmar carpal branch 418, 434, 435
superficial palmar branch of 417, 418,
424, 429, 434, 435
radialis indicis 435
radicular 157, 158, 179
rectal
inferior 287, 369, 373–376
middle 247, 287, 305, 319, 320, 341,
369, 371, 373, 374

**Artery** *cont.*
   superior 247, 257, 287, 300, 305, 306,
     319, 341, 369, 371, 381
  rectosigmoid 287, 305, 369
  recurrent
    branch of inferior phrenic–see Artery,
     phrenic, inferior, recurrent
     esophageal branch
    esophageal branch–see Artery, phrenic,
     inferior, recurrent esophageal
     branch
    of Heubner–see Artery, striate, medial
    interosseous–see Artery, interosseous,
     recurrent
    meningeal branch of lacrimal–see Artery,
     lacrimal, anastomotic branch with
     middle meningeal
    radial 404, 405, 417, 418
    tibial
     anterior 477, 485
     posterior 477, 483
    ulnar
     anterior 405, 417, 418
     posterior 404, 414, 415, 418
  renal 247, 300, 303, 305, 311, 313,
    **314**–316, 320, 323–325, 329, 371,
    372, 381, 388, 520
    accessory 316
    pelvic branch 315
    segmental–see Artery, segmental (renal)
    ureteric branch 314, 315, 320
    variations 316
  retinal
    central 80, 82, 86
    macular–see Arteriole, macular
    nasal–see Arteriole, nasal
    temporal–see Arteriole, temporal
  retinacular (to femoral neck/head) 470
  retroesophageal right subclavian 74
  of round ligament
    of femur–see Artery, obturator, acetabular
     branch
    of uterus–see Artery, uterine, branch to
     round ligament
  rolandic–see Artery, central sulcal
  sacral
    lateral 157, 247, 369, 373, 374
    middle 157, 247, 287, 341, 344, 369,
     371, 373, 374
  saphenous–see Artery, genicular,
    descending, saphenous branch
  scapular
    circumflex 397, 398, 400, 402, 405
    dorsal 27, 28, 398, 400
  scrotal, posterior–see Artery, perineal,
    posterior scrotal branch
  segmental
    medullary–see Artery, medullary,
     segmental

**Artery** *cont.*
  septal, nasal–see Septal branch under
    Artery, ethmoidal (anterior and
    posterior); facial, superior labial
    branch; sphenopalatine
  of shoulder 28
  sigmoid 247, 257, 287, 305, 319, 328, 369
  sinuatrial–see Artery, coronary, right,
    sinuatrial (SA) nodal branch
  of small intestine 286
  sphenopalatine 35, 36, 63
    posterior lateral nasal branch 35, 36
    posterior septal branch 35, 36
  spermatic, internal–see Artery, testicular
  spinal
    anterior 131, 132, 134, 136, 157, 158
    posterior 132, 134, 136, 157, 158
  splenic 225, 247, 257, 261, 279, 281, 282,
    **283**–286, 288, 300–303, 309, 310,
    327, 329, 518
    splenic branch 282
  sternocleidomastoid–see Artery, occipital,
    sternocleidomastoid branch
  of stomach 282, 283
  straight (arteria recta) of small intestine
    263, 286, 287, 308
  striate, medial (recurrent artery of Heubner)
    132–135
  subclavian 25, 27, **28**, 63–65, 68–70, 74,
    120, 124, 130, 131, 157, 168, 173,
    175–177, 182, 186, 195, 200–202,
    218–220, 225, 238, 398, 400, 513
    retroesophageal right 74
  subcostal 238, 247
  sublingual 53, 55
  submental 35, 63
  subscapular 238, 397, 398, 400, 405
  sulcal
    central (rolandic) 134, 135
    precentral (pre-rolandic) 134, 135
    postcentral 135
    of spinal cord 158
  superior vena cava–see Artery, coronary,
    right, sinuatrial (SA) branch
  supraduodenal 282–286
  suprahyoid–see Artery, lingual, suprahyoid
    branch
  supraorbital 17, 31, 35, 63, 76, 80, 131
  suprarenal
    inferior 247, 314, 315, 320, 325
    middle 247, 314, 325
    superior 181, 247, 314, 325
  suprascapular 27, 28, 63,
    68–70, 131, 397, 398, 400
    infraspinous branch 398
  supratrochlear 17, 31, 35, 63, 76, 80, 131
  of tail of pancreas–see Artery, pan-
    creatic, caudal
  tarsal
    lateral 485, 494, 495, 500
    medial 485, 494, 495, 500
  of teeth 35

**Artery** *cont.*
  temporal
    branch of
     middle cerebral–see Artery, cerebral,
      middle, temporal branch
     posterior cerebral–see Artery, cerebral,
      posterior, temporal branch
    deep 35, 63, 94
    superficial 17, 29, 35, 55, 63–65, 80,
     94, 95, 128, 130, 131
     anterior auricular branch 17
     frontal branch 17, 80, 94
     parietal branch 17, 94
  tentorial–see Artery, carotid, internal,
    tentorial branch; Trunk (arterial),
    meningohypophyseal, tentorial branch
  terminal–see Terminal branch under Artery,
    cerebral, anterior, middle; posterior
  testicular 238, 243–245, 247, 257, 292,
    300, 311, 314, 319, 320, 322, 328,
    340, 361, **372,** 374, 380, 387
  thalamogeniculate 136
  thalamoperforating 133, 136
  thalamotuberal 133
  of thigh 470–472, 481
  thoracic
    internal 28, 69, 130, 131, **168,** 174–**176,**
     179, 180, 182, 186, 195, 200, 201,
     218–220, 225, 230, 238, 288,
     514–516
     medial mammary branch 168
     perforating branch 168, 176, 177, 179
    lateral 168, 174, 175, 177, 238, 398,
     400, 405
     lateral mammary branch 168
    superior 175, 177, 398, 400, 405
  thoracoacromial 174, 175, 398–400, 405
    acromial branch 398, 400, 405
    clavicular branch 398, 400, 405
    deltoid branch 395, 398, 400, 405
    pectoral branch 398, 400, 405
  thoracodorsal 238, 397, 398, 400, 405
  thyrocervical–see Trunk (arterial),
    thyrocervical
  thyroid
    inferior 27, 28, 63, 68–70, 130, 131,
     176, 214, 225, 398
     esophageal branch 225
    superior 26, 27, 29, 63, 68–70, 130, 131
     cricothyroid branch 63
  of thyroid gland 68, 70
  tibial
    anterior 477, 483, 485, 487, 494, 495
    posterior 477, 481–483, 487, 493,
     497–499
     calcaneal branch 481–483, 496–499
     circumflex fibular branch 477
     medial malleolar branch 483
  of tongue 53–see also Artery, lingual
  tonsillar–see Tonsillar branch under Artery,
    facial; lingual, dorsal; palatine,
    (ascending and lesser); pharyngeal,
    ascending–see also Cerebellar tonsillar

**Artery** cont.
branch under Artery, cerebellar, posterior inferior
tubal–see Tubal branch under Artery, ovarian, uterine
tympanic, anterior 35, 131
ulnar 404, 405, 414–**418,** 419, 424, 428–430, 434, 435, 442
deep palmar branch of 417, 418, 424, 428, 429, 434, 435, 442
dorsal carpal branch of 438
palmar carpal branch 418, 434, 425
umbilical 217
occluded part 234, 236, 244, 245, 257, 319, 339–341, 371, 373, 374
patent part 236, 247, 369, 371, 373, 374
ureteric–see Ureteric branch under Aorta, abdominal; and under Artery, iliac, common; vesical (inferior and superior); ovarian; renal
urethral 357, 374, 376
of urinary bladder 320
uterine 319, 320, 341, 344–346, 371, 373, **375**
ovarian branch 375
branch to round ligament 375
tubal branch 375
vaginal branch 375
vaginal 319, 320, 341, 342, 345, 371, 373, 375
vermian–see Artery, cerebellar, superior, superior vermian branch
vertebral 14, 16, 27, 28, 63, 65, 69, 70, 95, 124, **130–**134, 136, 157, 164, 176, 214, 225, 525
meningeal branch 95, 130, 136
vesical
inferior 247, 287, 319, 320, 341, 342, 369, 371, 373, 374
ureteric branch 320
superior 236, 247, 287, 319, 320, 341, 369, 371, 373, 374
ureteric branch 324
of bulb of vestibule 345, 375
of wrist 442
zygomatic branch from lacrimal–see Artery, lacrimal, zygomatic branch
zygomaticofacial 17, 80
zygomaticoorbital 17
zygomaticotemporal 17
Articulation–see Joint
Arytenoid–see Cartilage, arytenoid
**Atlas (C2)** 9, **12,** 14–16, 32, 57, 142
**Atrium**
left 194, 202, 203, 208, **209,** 211, 212, 230, 516, 525
right 194, 201–203, **208,** 211, 212, 218, 230, 516, 524
**Attachment** of
ascending colon 257
cecum 264
descending colon 257
greater omentum 257

**Attachment** cont.
lesser omentum 257
muscles–see also origins and insertions of individual muscles
sigmoid mesocolon 257
transverse mesocolon 257, 279
Auerbach–see Plexus (nerve), myenteric
**Auricle**
of ear 87, 88
of left atrium 201–203, 209, 212, 213, 525
of right atrium 201, 202, 208, 212
**Autonomic** nervous system–see System, nervous, autonomic (ANS)
**Axilla** 402–405–see also Fossa, axillary
cross sections of 399, 513–**515,** 524, 525
**Axis (C2)** 9, **12,** 15, 54
of lens 85
celiac–see Trunk (arterial), celiac

# B

**Back**
bones of 142–145
cross section (of lumbar region) 165
joints of 146–147
ligaments of 146–147
muscles of 160–162, 164
nerves of 163
**Band**–see also Fiber
central, of extensor (digitorum) tendon
lateral
of extensor (digitorum) tendon 421, 433
of plantar aponeurosis 500
longitudinal, of cruciate ligament 15, 16
moderator 208, 212, 213
parietal, of supraventricular crest–see Limb, parietal, of supraventricular crest
septal 208, 211, 212
Bartholin–see Duct, sublingual; Gland, vestibular, greater
**Base**
cranial 5–7
bones of 6
foramina of 7
of heart 202
of metacarpal bones 426
of metatarsal bones 488
of phalanges (hand) 426
of phalanges (foot) 488
of renal pyramid 313
of sacrum 145
of skull–see Base, cranial
Basiocciput–see Part, basilar, of occipital bone
**Bed**
of liver 270
of nail 439
of parotid gland 29, 54
of sublingual gland 54
of submandibular gland 54
Bertin–see Column, renal

Bigelow–see Ligament, iliofemoral
**Bladder,** urinary 154, 236, 245, 252, 305, 311, 319, 329, 337–**343,** 344, 351, 353, 357, 358, 360, 363, 371, 388, 523
Blood supply–see Artery; Vein
Blood vessels, innervation of 216
**Body**
adipose–see Fat, pararenal
amygdaloid 104, 106, 113
anococcygeal 351, 352
of Arantius–see Nodule, of semilunar valve
of axis 12
of bladder 338, 343
of caudate nucleus 102, 104
carotid 29, 65, 119, 124, 130, 199
cell, of presynaptic sympathetic neurons 126–128
ciliary 82, 83, 85, 86
of clitoris 337, 389
of epididymis 362
fat
infrapatellar 476
of ischioanal fossa 351, 354, 364, 523
of orbit 42, 78
of femur 455, 462
of fibula 478, 479
of fornix 100, 102, 106
of gallbladder 276
gastric–see Body, of stomach
geniculate
lateral 101, 104, 105, **108–**110, 114, 126, 132, 136–138
medial 105, 105, 108, 109, 132, 136–138
of hyoid bone 9, 47
of ilium 334, 453
of ischium 453
mammillary 100, 101, 106, 108, 140
of mandible 1, 2, 9, 10, 22
of metacarpal bones 426
of metatarsal bones 488
of pancreas 279
of penis 393
perineal 338, 342, 350–352, 356–358, 363, 367, 376
of phalanges
hand 426
foot 488
pineal 100, 104, 105, 108, 109
of pubis 523
of rib 170
of scapula 399
of sphenoid bone 3, 34, 36, 44
of sternum 170, 174, 176, 231, 516
of stomach 258, 259
of tibia 478, 479
of tongue 42, 52
of uterus 337, 344, 346
vertebral 13, 143, 144, 146, 147, 156, 165, 513, 516, 517, 521
vitreous, of eye 82
**Bone**
of abdomen 231

**Bone** *cont.*
  of ankle 478, 479, 488–490
  of arm 392, 393
  auditory–see Ossicles, auditory
  of back 142–145
  breast–see Sternum
  calcaneal–see Calcaneous
  capitate–see Capitate
  carpal 422–426
  clavicle–see Clavicle
  conchal–see Concha, nasal
  coxal–see Bone, hip (coxal)
  of cranial base 6
  cuboid–see Cuboid
  cuneiform–see Cuneiform
  of ear–see Ossicles, auditory
  of elbow 411
  ethmoid 1–3, 6–8, 32–34, 38, 44
  femur–see Femur
  fibula–see Fibula
  of foot 488–490
  of forearm 409
  frontal 1–6, 8, 31, 33, 34, 76, 77
  "funny"–see Nerve, ulnar
  hamate–see Hamate
  of hand 430
  hip (coxal) 330–332 453, 454–457
  hyoid **9,** 22–24, 26, 29, 47, 53–55, 57, 59,
      61, 62, 68, 70, 71
  ilial–see Ilium
  ischial–see Ischium
  lacrimal 1–3, 8, 33, 44
  of leg 478, 479
  lunate–see Lunate
  mandibular–see Mandible
  maxillary–see Maxilla
  metacarpal 420–427, 430, 433, 436
  metatarsal 483, 486, 488, 489, 491–493,
      495, 500, 501
  nasal 1–3, 8, 31, 33, 34, 44
  of nasal cavity 33, 44
  navicular–see Navicular
  of neck 9–13
  occipital 2–6, 8, 14, 25, 32–34, 57–61
    basilar part–see Part, basilar, of occipital
        bone
  palatine 1, 3, 5, 8, 9, 33, 44
  parietal 1–6, 8
  of pelvis 330–331–see also Pelvis, bony
  pisiform–see Pisiform
  pubic–see Pubis
  scaphoid–see Scaphoid
  sesamoid 426, 488, 489, 494, 498–501
  of shoulder 391–393
  sphenoid 1–3, 5, 6, 8, 9, 33, 34
  sternum–see Sternum
  talus–see Talus
  tarsal–see Bone(s), of foot
  temporal 1–3, 5, 6, 8, 9
  of thigh 471, 454
  of thorax 170, 171
  tibia–see Tibia
  trapezium–see Trapezium

**Bone** *cont.*
  trapezoid–see Trapezoid
  triquetrum–see Triquetrum
  vertebra–see Vertebra
  vomer–see Vomer
  of wrist 422, 423, 426
  zygomatic 1, 2, 5, 8, 76
**Bony framework**–see Framework, bony
**Border**
  anterior
    of fibula 478, 479
    of radius 409
    of tibia 478, 479
    of ulna 409
  of fibula–see Border, anterior; interosseous,
      posterior; of fibula
  of heart–see Border, inferior; left, right, of
      heart
  inferior
    of heart 201
    of liver 269, 270
    of lung 184, 185
  interosseous
    of fibula 478, 479
    of radius 409
    of tibia 478, 479
    of ulna 409
  lateral, of scapula 392, 393
  left, of heart 184, 201
  of liver–see Border, inferior, of liver
  of lung–see Border, inferior, of lung
  medial, of scapula 394, 393
  posterior
    of fibula 478, 479
    of radius 409
    of ulna 409
  of radius–see Border, anterior; interosseous;
      posterior; of radius
  right, of heart 184
  of scapula–see Border, lateral; medial;
      superior; of scapula
  superior, of scapula 394, 393
  of tibia–see Border, anterior; interosseous;
      medial; of tibia
  of ulna–see Border, anterior; interosseous;
      posterior; of ulna
**Bowel**–see Colon; Intestine, large; small
**Bowman**–see Capsule, glomerular
**Boyden**–see Sphincter, of common bile
    duct
**Brachium**–see also Arm
  of inferior colliculus 105, 108
  of superior colliculus 105, 108
**Brain** 96, 99–109
  arteries of 130–135
    schema 131
  meninges of 94–96
  veins of
    deep 138
    subependymal 139
    superficial 96
  venous sinuses 97–98

**Brainstem  108,** 110, 111
**Branch**
  bundle, of conducting system of heart–see
      Bundle, left; right, of conductive fibers
      of heart
  subendocardial, of conductive system of
      heart 213
**Branch** (of artery)–see under parent artery
  acetabular–see under Artery, obturator
  acromial–see under Artery, suprascapular,
      thoracoacromial
  alar–see under Artery, facial, lateral nasal
      branch
  anastomotic, of lacrimal with middle
      meningeal artery  95
  angular–see Branch to angular gyrus under
      Artery, cerebral, middle
  to angular gyrus–see under Artery, cerebral,
      middle
  articular–see under Artery, genicular,
      descending
  ascending–see under Artery, iliac,
      circumflex, deep; femoral, circumflex,
      lateral
  atrial–see under Artery, coronary, right
  atrioventricular–see under Artery, coronary,
      left, circumflex branch of
  atrioventricular (AV) nodal–see under
      Artery, coronary, right, posterior
      interventricular branch of
  auricular–see under Artery, temporal,
      superficial
  calcaneal
    lateral–see under Artery, fibular
        (peroneal)
    medial–see under Artery, tibial, posterior
  calcarine–see under Artery, cerebral,
      posterior
  carpal–see under Artery, radial, ulnar
  cavernous–see under Artery, carotid,
      internal
  cerebellar tonsillar–see under Artery,
      cerebellar, posterior inferior
  choroidal–see under Artery, cerebellar,
      posterior inferior
  circumflex–see under Artery, coronary, left;
      fibular (peroneal); tibial, posterior
      (circumflex fibular branch)
  clavicular–see under Artery,
      thoracoacromial
  colic–see under Artery, ileocolic
  communicating–see under Artery, fibular
      (peroneal)
  conus–see under Artery, coronary, right
  to corpus callosum (dorsal)–see under
      Artery, cerebral, posterior
  cremasteric–see Artery, cremasteric
  cricothyroid–see under Artery, thyroid,
      superior
  deferential–see under Artery, of ductus
      deferens
  deltoid–see under Artery, thoracoacromial

**Branch** *cont.*

descending–see under Artery, coronary,
    left; right; Artery, femoral, circumflex,
    lateral; occipital
esophageal–see under Aorta, thoracic;
    Artery, bronchial; gastric, left; phrenic,
    inferior, left; thyroid, inferior
frontal–see under Artery, meningeal,
    middle; temporal, superficial
medial–see under Artery, callosomarginal
genicular–see Artery, genicular
ileal–see under Artery, ileocolic
infraspinous–see under Artery,
    suprascapular
interventricular, posterior–see under Artery,
    coronary, right
labial
    inferior and superior–see under Artery,
        facial
    posterior–see under Artery, perineal
lateral–see under Artery, coronary, left,
    circumflex branch of
malleolar–see under Artery, fibular
    (peroneal); tibial, posterior–see also
    Artery, malleolar, anterior
mammary–see under Artery, thoracic,
    internal and lateral
marginal–see under Artery, coronary, right
mastoid–see under Artery, occipital
meningeal–see under Artery, carotid,
    internal; ethmoidal (anterior and
    posterior); occipital; pharyngeal,
    ascending; vertebral
mental–see under Artery, alveolar, inferior
muscular–see under Artery, brachial;
    femoral
mylohyoid–see under Artery, alveolar,
    inferior;
nasal, lateral–see under Artery, ethmoidal
    (anterior and posterior); facial;
    sphenopalatine
nodal–see Artery, coronary, right
    atrioventricular (AV) nodal branch;
    sinuatrial (SA) nodal branch
palmar, deep–see under Artery, ulnar
parietal–see under Artery, meningeal,
    middle; temporal, superficial
parietooccipital–see under Artery, cerebral,
    posterior
pectoral–see under Artery, thoracoacromial
pelvic–see under Artery, renal
perforating–see under Artery, deep, of
    thigh; fibular (peroneal); metatarsal,
    plantar; thoracic, internal
posterolateral–see under Artery, coronary,
    left, circumflex branch of
pterygoid–see under Artery, maxillary
pubic–see under Artery, epigastric, inferior;
    obturator
to round ligament–see under Artery, uterine
saphenous–see under Artery, genicular,

**Branch** *cont.*

descending
scrotal, posterior–see under Artery, perineal
septal
    interventricular–see under Artery,
        coronary, left, anterior
        interventricular branch; coronary,
        right, posterior interventricular
        branch
    nasal–see under Artery, ethmoidal
        (anterior and posterior); facial;
        superior labial branch;
        sphenopalatine
sinuatrial (SA) nodal–see under Artery,
    coronary, right
splenic–see under Artery, splenic
sternocleidomastoid–see under Artery,
    occipital
suprahyoid–see under Artery, lingual
sural (muscular)–see under Artery, popliteal
emporal–see under Artery, cerebral,
    middle; posterior
tentorial–see under Artery, carotid, internal
terminal–see under Artery, cerebral,
    anterior; middle; posterior
tonsillar–see under Artery, facial; lingual,
    dorsal; palatine (ascending and lesser);
    pharyngeal, ascending–see also Artery,
    tonsillar and Cerebellar tonsillar
    branch under Artery, cerebellar,
    posterior inferior
transverse–see under Artery, femoral,
    circumflex, lateral
tubal–see under Artery, ovarian
ureteric–see under Aorta, abdominal; and
    Artery, iliac, common; vesical (inferior
    and superior); ovarian; renal
vermian–see under Artery, cerebellar,
    superior
zygomatic–see under Artery, lacrimal,
**Branch** (of nerve)–see under parent nerve
anterior–see under Nerve, obturator
anterior cutaneous–see under Nerve,
    femoral
articular–see under Nerve, auriculo-
    temporal; fibular (peroneal), common;
    median; obturator; tibial; ulnar
auricular–see under Nerve, mandibular;
    vagus
buccal–see under Nerve, facial–see also
    Nerve, buccal (of mandibular nerve)
calcaneal–see under Nerve, sural; tibial
carotid (to carotid sinus and body)–see
    under Nerve, glossopharyngeal
celiac–see under Nerve, vagus
cervical–see under Nerve, facial
communicating
    of cervical plexus
        to brachial plexus 123
        to vagus 27

**Branch** *cont.*

of glossopharyngeal nerve
    with auricular branch of vagus 119
    with chorda tympani of facial 119
of intercostal with intercostal 241
of median nerve with ulnar nerve 444
between nasopalatine and greater
    palatine 37
of vagus with glossopharyngeal nerve
    120
of zygomatic to lacrimal 40, 116, 127
cutaneous–see under Nerve, femoral;
    iliohypogastric; intercostal; plantar
    (lateral and medial); subcostal
deep–see under Nerve, plantar, lateral;
    radial; ulnar
dental–see under Nerve, maxillary
dorsal–see under Nerve, digital, proper,
    (palmar and plantar); radial; ulnar
external–see under Nerve, accessory;
    laryngeal, superior
femoral–see under Nerve, genitofemoral
ganglionic–see Nerve, maxillary, branches
    to pterygopalatine ganglion
gastric–see under Nerve, vagus
genital–see under Nerve, genitofemoral
gingival–see under Nerve, maxillary
hepatic–see under Nerve, vagus
infrapatellar–see under Nerve, saphenous
internal–see under Nerve, accessory;
    laryngeal, superior
intestinal–see under Nerve, vagus
labial–see under Nerve, ilioinguinal;
    perineal
laryngopharyngeal–see under Ganglion,
    cervical, superior
lingual–see under Nerve, glossopharyngeal
marginal mandibular–see under Nerve,
    facial
meningeal–see under Nerve,
    glossopharyngeal; hypoglossal;
    mandibular; maxillary; spinal;
    vagus–see also Nerve, ophthalmic,
    tentorial (meningeal) branch
motor, to thenar muscles–see under Nerve,
    median
nasal–see under Ganglion, pterygopalatine;
    and under Nerve, alveolar, superior;
    ethmoidal, anterior; palatine, greater;
    infraorbital; maxillary
occipital–see under Nerve, auricular,
    posterior
palmar–see under Nerve, median; ulnar
palpebral–see under Nerve, lacrimal
parotid–see under Nerve, auriculotemporal
pericardial–see under Nerve, phrenic
perineal–see under Nerve, cutaneous,
    posterior, of thigh; spinal, sacral
pharyngeal–see under Ganglion,
    pterygopalatine; and under Nerve,

**Branch** *cont.*
  glossopharyngeal; vagus
  posterior–see under Nerve, obturator
  pterygopalatine–see Nerve, maxillary,
      ganglionic branch to pterygopalatine
      ganglion
  pyloric–see under Nerve, vagus, hepatic
      branch
  recurrent–see under Nerve, fibular
      (peroneal), deep; mandibular–see also
      Nerve, spinal, (recurrent) meningeal
      branch
  scrotal
    anterior–see under Nerve, ilioinguinal;
        genitofemoral
    posterior–see under Nerve, perineal
  stylohyoid–see under Nerve, facial
  stylopharyngeal–see under Nerve,
      glossopharyngeal
  superficial–see under Nerve, plantar,
      lateral; radial; ulnar
  temporal–see under Nerve, facial
  tentorial–see under Nerve, ophthalmic
  tonsillar–see under Nerve,
      glossopharyngeal
  zygomatic–see under Nerve, facial–see also
      Nerve, zygomatic
  zygomaticofacial–see under Nerve,
      zygomatic
  zygomaticotemporal–see under Nerve,
      zygomatic
**Breast** 167–169
  artery of 168
  cross section of 167
  mammary gland 167
  lymph vessels and nodes 169
**Bregma** 4
**Brim**, pelvic 145, 345–see also Linea,
    terminalis of pelvis
**Bronchiole** 192, 193
**Bronchus**
  arteries of 196
  cardiac (left lung) 191
  eparterial 187, 190, 191, 194, 195, 220
  extrapulmonary 190
  innervation of 199
  intermediate 191, 195
  intrapulmonary 190, 192
  lingular 190, 191
  lobar
    inferior 187, 190, 191, 194
    lower–see Bronchus, lobar, inferior
    middle 190, 191, 194
    superior
      left 190, 191, 194
      right (eparterial) 187, 190–191, 194,
          195
    upper–see Bronchus, lobar superior
  main 187, **190,** 191, 194–196, 198,
      218–222, 230, 515, 525
  nomenclature of 191
  2nd order–see Bronchus, lobar
  3rd order–see Bronchus,
      segmental

**Bronchus** *cont.*
  4th order–see Bronchus, subsegmental
  primary–see Bronchus, main
  segmental 191, 192
  subsegmental 191, 192
  superior division 190, 191
  veins of 196
Brunner–see Gland, duodenal
Buck–see Fascia, deep, of penis (Buck's)
**Bulb**–see also Eyeball
  of corpus spongiosum 356
  duodenal 259, 262
  of penis 356, 357
  olfactory 38, 101, 113
  urethral–see Urethra, spongy, bulbous
      portion
  of vestibule 343, 345, 351–353, 375
**Bulla**, ethmoidal 32, 33
**Bundle**
  atrioventricular (His) 213
  left, of conductive fibers of heart 213
  of His–see Bundle, atrioventricular
  oval–see Fasciculus, septomarginal
  right, of conductive fibers of heart 213
Burns–see Space, suprasternal (Burns)
**Bursa**
  anserine 472, 473
  of biceps femoris tendon–see Bursa,
      subtendinous, inferior, of biceps
      femoris
  of fibular collateral ligament 472–474,
      476
  of gastrocnemius muscle–see Bursa,
      subtendinous, inferior, of biceps
      femoris
  iliopectineal 454, 462
  of iliotibial tract 472–474
  olecranon–see Bursa, subcutaneous,
      olecranon
  omental 255, 256, 327, 329
    cross section of 256
    inferior recess of 329
    superior recess of 255, 257, 270, 329
  radial–see Sheath, tendinous, of flexor
      pollicis longus
  semimembranosus 472, 476
  subcutaneous
    calcaneal 493
    infrapatellar 476
    lateral malleolar 493
    medial malleolar 493
    olecranon 408
    prepatellar 476
  subdeltoid 398, 402
  subscapular–see Bursa, subtendinous, of
      subscapularis
  subtendinous
    calcaneal 486, 493
    inferior, of biceps femoris 472, 473, 476
    infrapatellar 476
    of gastrocnemius muscle 476
    of subscapularis 394
  suprapatellar 473, 474, 476

**Bursa** *cont.*
  ulnar–see Sheath, flexor, common
**Buttock**, nerves of 468, 469, 509


# C

**Calcaneus** 488–**490,** 492, 493
**Calcar** avis 105, 106
Calot–see Lymph node, of Calot; Triangle,
    cystic
**Calvaria** 4, 96
**Calyx** of kidney 313, 520
Camera–see Chamber
Camper–see Tissue, subcutaneous, fatty layer,
    of abdomen
**Canal**
  adductor 466, 467, 471
  Alcock's–see Canal, pudendal
  anal 337, 364, 365–see also Rectum/anal
      canal
  carotid 5, 93
  central, of spinal cord 102, 103, 109
  cervical, of uterus 346
  condylar 5, 7
  dental root 51
  facial 118
  femoral 244, 510
  gastric 259
  of Hering–see Ductule, bile, periportal
  Hunter–see Canal, adductor
  hyaloid, of eye 82
  hypoglossal 3, 5, 7, 16, 122
  incisive 3, 32–37, 38
  infraorbital 40
  inguinal 244
  mandibular 54
  nasofrontal 33
  nasolacrimal 33
  obturator 236, 330, 333, 335, 341, 342,
      344, 373
  optic 1, 3, 7, 78
  pudendal 287, 296, 364, 369, 370, 373,
      375, 376, 382, 384
  pyloric 258
  sacral 145, 335
  Schlemm's–see Sinus venous of sclera
  semicircular 90–92
  spinal–see Canal, vertebral
  vertebral 13, 143, 144
**Canaliculus**
  bile 275
  lacrimal 77
  mastoid 5
  tympanic 5
**Cap** of duodenum 259, 262
**Capillary**
  intrapulmonary 193
  subpleural 193
**Capitate** 422, 426
**Capitulum** of humerus 392, 407
**Capsule**–see also Ligament; Joint
  atlantoaxial–see Capsule, joint, atlantoaxial

**Capsule** *cont.*
  atlantooccipital–see Capsule, joint,
      atlantooccipital
  of basal nuclei
      external 104
      internal 102, 104, 134
  Bowman's–see Capsule, glomerular
  fat, perirenal–see Fat, perirenal
  fibrous, of thyroid gland 70
  glomerular 317
  joint
      atlantoaxial 14, 15
      atlantooccipital 14, 15
      temporomandibular 11
      zygapophyseal 14, 15, 146
  of kidney 313, 317, 318, 324
  lens 82, 83, 85
  of liver 273
  of suprarenal gland 325
  temporomandibular–see Capsule, joint,
      temporomandibular
  Tenon's–see sheath, fascial, of eyeball
  of vertebral joint, lateral–see Capsule, joint,
      zygapophyseal
  zygapophyseal–see Capsule, joint,
      zygapophyseal
**Caput** of mandible–see Head, of mandible
Carina, of trachea 525
Carpal–see Bone, carpal
**Cartilage**
  alar 31, 33, 34
  arytenoid 59, 71, 72
  of auditory tube 46, 49, 59, 61, 93
  corniculate 59, 71
  costal 170, 171, 180, 184, 231, 241, 513,
      514, 517
  cricoid 9, 23, 24, 57, 59, 62, 68, 71, 72,
      184, 190, 195, 221–223
  laryngeal 71
  nasal
      lateral 31, 33, 34
      septal 31, 34
  thyroid 9, 23, 24, 26, 57, 59, 62, 68, 71,
      72, 184, 190, 195, 221–223
  tracheal 190
**Caruncle**
  hymenal 345, 350
  lacrimal 76, 77
  sublingual 45, 55
**Cauda** equina 148, 149, 156, 165, 520
**Cavity**
  of concha 88
  glenoid, of scapula 170, 392, 394
  nasal 32–44, 77, 78
      arteries of 36
      autonomic innervation of 39
      nerves of 37–38
      paranasal sinuses 42–44
  oral 42, 45–see also Mouth
      inspection of 45
  pericardial 230
  peritoneal 251–257
  pleural 230
  tympanic 39, 41, 87, **89,** 91, 118, 119

**Cavum** conchae–see Cavity, of concha
**Cecum** 120, 252, 254, 267, 339, 340,
      521–522
**Cell**
  amacrine, of retina 114
  argentaffine, of stomach 259
  bipolar, of retina 114
  body–see Body, cell
  epithelial, of stomach 259
  ethmoidal (air) 42–44, 78
  ganglion, of retina 114
  granule, of olfactory bulb 113
  hair, of spiral organ 91
  horizontal, of retina 114
  mastoid (air) 89
  melanocyte 511
  mitral, of olfactory bulb 113
  mucous, of stomach 259
  olfactory 113
  parietal, of stomach 259
  periglomerular, of olfactory bulb 113
  pigment, of retina 114
  pillar, of spiral organ 91
  of retina 114
  rod, of spiral organ 91
  of spiral organ 91
  of stomach 259
  of taste bud, sustentacular 52
  tufted, of olfactory bulb 113
  tympanic (air) 89
  zymogenic, of stomach 259
**Cementum** 51
**Cerebellum** 92, 100, 105, **107, 109,** 137,
      139
**Cerebrospinal fluid** (CSF) 103
**Cerebrum** 96, 99–104
**Cervix** of uterus 337, 341, 344–346, 386
**Chamber** of eye
  anterior 76, 82, 83, 85, 86
  posterior 76, 82, 83, 85, 86
  vitreous 86
**Chiasm,** optic 98, 100, 101, 108, 114, 133,
      134, 138–140
**Choana** 5, 9, 34, 46, 49, 60, 61, 93
**Cholangiole** 274, 275
**Cholinergic**
  synapses 154
  terminals 199
Chorda tympani–see Nerve, chorda
      tympani
**Chordae** tendineae 208, 209, 211
**Choroid** 82, 85, 86, 114
**Cilia** of eyelid–see Eyelash
**Circle,** arterial
  cerebral (Willis) 132, 133
  major, of iris 83
  minor, of iris 83
  of Willis–see Circle, arterial, cerebral
      (Willis)
**Circulation**
  of cerebrospinal fluid (CSF) 103
  intrapulmonary (schema) 193
  prenatal 217
  postnatal 217

**Cistern**
  cerebellomedullary (posterior) 103
  chiasmatic 103
  of corpus callosum 103
  chyle–see Cisterna chyli
  of great cerebral vein–see Cistern,
      quadrigeminal
  interpeduncular 103
  lumbar 521
  prepontine 103
  quadrigeminal 103
**Cisterna**
  chyli 249, 296, 300
  magna–see Cistern, cerebello-
      medullary (posterior)
**Claustrum** 104
**Clavicle** 22–24, 26, 170, 171, 174–176,
      184–186, 218, 219, **391–**396, 398–400,
      513, 524
**Clitoris** 347, 350, 352, 367, 389
**Clivus** 6, 15
Cloquet–see Lymph node, highest deep
      inguinal
**Coccyx** 142, 145, 147–149, 231, 330–336,
      352, 354, 356, 363, 367, 523
**Cochlea** 87, 89–92
**Collar** of Helvetius 224, 260
Colles–see Fascia, perineal, superficial
**Colliculus**
  facial, of 4th ventricle 109
  inferior 100, 105, 108, 109, 137
  seminal 343, 358
  superior 100, 101, 105, 108–110, 126,
      136, 137
**Colon**–see also Intestine, large
  ascending 120, 252, **254,** 261, 267, 312,
      328, 339, 340, 519, 520
  descending 252, **254,** 261, 267, 324, 328,
      339, 340, 518–521
  flexure of–see Flexure, colic
  sigmoid 252, 254, 267, **268,** 339, 340,
      344, 363–366, 383, 520
  transverse 252–**254,** 256, 261, 267, 270,
      276, 279, 281, 295, 328, 329,
      518–520
**Column**
  anal 365
  of Bertin–see Column, renal
  of fornix 100, 104–106, 138
  of Morgagni–see Column, anal
  rectal–see Column, anal
  renal 313, 318
  spinal–see Column, vertebral
  vertebral 142
      arteries of 158
      relationship to spinal cord/nerves 148,
          149
      veins of 159
**Commissure**
  cerebral
      anterior 100, 109, 113, 139, 140
      posterior 100, 105, 109
  of fornix 106
  of gray matter 151

**Commissure** *cont.*
habenular 100, 105, 109
labial 350
white, of spinal cord 151
**Compartment**
of extensor tendons at wrist 414, 415, 439
fascial, of
arm 406
forearm 419
leg 487
thigh 471
perineal, superficial–see Space, perineal, superficial
Compressor urethrae 333, 345, 352, 375
**Concha**
of external ear 88
nasal
inferior 1, 3, 32, 33, 42–44, 77
middle 1, 3, 32, 33, 42–44, 77
superior 3, 32, 33, 44
sphenoidal 44
Conduction fiber–see Bundle, atrioventricular; left; right; and Fiber, subendocardial
Conductive system, see System, conductive
**Condyle**
of femur 455, 473–475
of humerus 392, 407
occipital 3, 5, 6, 25, 93, 122
of tibia 460, 473, 475, 478, 479, 486
**Cone**
of light 88
medullary–see Conus, medullaris
of retina 114
**Confluence** of sinuses 97, 98, 137, 138
**Conjunctiva** 76, 78, 82, 83, 86
**Constrictions** of esophagus 221
Constrictor of pupil–see Muscle, sphincter, of pupil
**Conus**
arteriosus 201, 208–210, 212
elasticus 72
medullaris 148, 149, 156, 520
Cooper–see Ligament, suspensory, of breast; pectineal
**Cord**
of brachial plexus 401, 443, 444, 524
genital 390
oblique, of radioulnar syndesmosis 408, 409
spermatic 232, 236, 238, 240, 242–245, 372, 376, 523
spinal 39, 126–128, **148,** 151, 154, 156, 199, 306, 307, 309, 310, 323, 326, 388, 513–520
arteries of 157–158
cross sections of 151
fiber tracts of 151
in situ 148, 156
relationship to vertebrae 149
veins of 159
tendinous–see Chorda tendinae

**Cord** *cont.*
vocal–see Ligament, vocal
**Cornea** 76, 78, 82, 83, 86
**Cornu**–see also Horn
coccygeal 145
sacral 145
**Corona**
of glans 356
radiata of ovarian follicle 349
**Corpus**–see also Body
albicans 350, 353
adiposum–see Body, fat
Arantii–see Nodule, of semilunar valve
callosum **100**–102, 104–106, 134, 136, 138, 139
cavernosum 338, 355–357, 359
clitoris–see Body, of clitoris
of gallbladder–see Body, of gallbladder
hemorrhagicum, of ovary 349
luteum 346, 349
of penis–see Body, of penis
spongiosum 338, 355–357, 359
of stomach–see Body, of stomach
striatum 104, 134
of uterus–see Body, of uterus
**Corpuscle**
cortical renal 317
juxtamedullary renal 317
Malpighian–see Corpuscle, renal
Meissner's 511
Pacinian 511
renal 317
**Cortex**
of kidney 313, 317, 318, 519
of lens 85
of ovary 349
of suprarenal gland 325, 326
Corti–see Organ, spiral, of Corti
**Cough** receptors 199
Cowper–see Gland, bulbourethral (Cowper)
Coxa–see Bone, hip (coxal)
**Cranium** 1–9–see also Base, cranial
neonatal 8
view
anterior 1
inferior 5
lateral 2
median section 3
superior 4
**Crest**
frontal 4, 6
of humeral tubercle 392
iliac 147, 160–163, 178, 231, 237, 311, 312, 324, 330, 331, **453,** 460–462, 468, 469, 509, 521
infratemporal 2
intertrochanteric 454, 455, 469
nasal
of maxilla 34
of palatine bone 34
obturator 330, 454
occipital

**Crest** *cont.*
external 5
internal 6
pubic 243, 335
sacral 145, 330, 334
of sphenoid bone 34
supracondylar 392, 393, 407
supraventricular 208, 212
urethral 358, 359
**Cricoid**–see Cartilage, cricoid
**Crista**
galli 3, 6, 34
terminalis 208, 213
**Cross section**
abdomen
abdominal wall, anterior (transverse) 235
abdominal wall, lateral (coronal) 236
abdominal wall and viscera (median) 329
abdominal wall and viscera at T10 (transverse) 517
abdominal wall and viscera at T12 (transverse) 327, 518
abdominal wall and viscera at T12–L1 (transverse) 519
abdominal wall and viscera at L1–2 (transverse) 520
abdominal wall and viscera at L2–3 (transverse) 328
abdominal wall and viscera at L5 (transverse) 521
abdominal wall and viscera at S1 (transverse) 522
appendix (transverse) 266
duodenum (coronal) 262
esophagogastric junction (coronal) 224
gallbladder/biliary tract (sagittal) 276
kidney (multisectional) 317
kidney with arteries (coronal) 315
omental bursa (transverse) 256
pylorus (coronal) 260
retroperitoneum at level of renal hilum (transverse) 324
retroperitoneum, kidney, suprarenal gland (sagittal) 324
stomach (coronal) 259
back
lumbar region of back (transverse) 165
lumbar vertebra/spinal cord (transverse) 156
spinal cord with arteries (transverse and median) 158
spinal cord with veins (transverse) 159
thoracic vertebra/spinal cord (transverse) 156
thoracic vertebra/spinal cord with arteries (transverse) 158
head and neck
hemisections (median sections)
hemisected cranium 3
hemisected cranium with meningeal

**Cross section** *cont.*
    arteries 95
    hemisected head and neck 57
  brain/cranial cavity
    brain with arteries (coronal) 134
    brain with arteries (median) 135
    brain with basal nuclei (transverse) 104
    cavernous/sphenoidal sinuses (coronal) 98
    cerebellum (in plane of cerebellar peduncle) 107
    cerebellum/brainstem (median) 109
    hemisected cranium with meninges/dural sinuses 97
    hemisected cranium and brain 100
    hemisected brain/brainstem/spinal cord with subarachnoid space 103
    hemisected brain minus brainstem 100
    thalamus (schema) 105
    ventricles of brain (coronal) 102
  ear
    cochlea, section through turn 91
    external, middle, internal (schema) 87
    labyrinth (bony, membranous) 91
    pharyngotympanic (auditory) tube 93
  mouth
    oral cavity/oropharynx/parotid region (transverse) 54
    tongue and floor of mouth (coronal) 54
  nasal cavity
    lateral wall (median) 32
    lateral wall (bony, median) 3, 33
    septum (median) 34
    septum (bony, median) 34
    arteries (hinged bony specimen) 36
    nerves (hinged bony specimen) 37
    paranasal sinuses (coronal) 42
    paranasal sinuses (transverse) 42
    paranasal sinuses (sagittal) 43
  orbits
    anterior orbit (sagittal) 76
    eyeball, whole (transverse) 82
      blood vessels (schema) 86
      anterior/posterior chambers 83
    left and right orbits (coronal) 42
    left and right orbits (transverse) 42
    left orbit/maxillary sinus (sagittal) 43
    middle of orbit (coronal) 78
    right orbit (transverse) 78
    right orbit (sagittal) with veins 80
  parotid region
    (transverse) 19, 54
  pharynx
    mucosa (median) 57
    muscles (median) 59
  tongue
    (coronal) 54
    (sagittal) 57

**Cross section** *cont.*
    tooth 51
    neck
      fascial layers (schematic, median) 30
      fascial layers (schematic, transverse) 30
  lower limb
    hip joint with arteries (coronal) 470
    knee (sagittal lateral to midline) 376
    leg (above middle) (transverse) 487
    thigh (serial transverse) 471
  pelvis and perineum
    ischioanal fossae (coronal) 364
    pelvic viscera and perineum: female (median) 337, 346
    pelvic viscera and perineum: male (median) 338
    pelvis wall and floor (coronal) 236
    pelvic wall and viscera at level of femoral heads, tip of coccyx 523
    perineopelvic spaces (median) 368
    perineum and urethra: male (coronal) 357
    prostate (transverse) 358
    prostate with arteries (coronal) 374
    prostatic and bulbous urethra (coronal) 358
    prostatic, seminal vesicles and penile urethra (median) 358
    rectum (coronal) 365
    scrotum and testis (coronal) 362
    testis (coronal) 362
    urethra: female (coronal) 353
    urethra: male (coronal) 359
    urinary bladder and urethra: female (coronal) 343
    urinary bladder and urethra: male (coronal) 343
    uterus: age changes (coronal) 347
    uterus and adnexa (coronal) 346
    vagina and endopelvic fascia (coronal) 245
    wall of anal canal (coronal) 366
  skin 511
  thorax
    breast (sagittal) 167
    heart: atria, ventricles and interventricular septum (oblique) 212
    mediastinum (transverse) 230
    ribs and sterncostal joints (coronal) 171
    thoracic wall/spinal nerve (transverse) 166 (schema), 241
    thoracic wall and viscera, T4 level (transverse) 513
    thoracic wall and viscera, T4 –5 level (transverse) 514
    thoracic wall and viscera, T5–6 level (transverse) 515
    thoracic wall and viscera, T7 level (transverse) 516
    thoracic wall and viscera at anterior axillary line (coronal) 524

**Cross section** *cont.*
    thoracic wall and viscera at midaxillary line (coronal) 525
    trachea (transvserse) 190
  upper limb
    arm (serial transverse) 406
    axilla (sagittal) 399
    finger, distal (sagittal) 440
    finger, distal (transverse) 440
    forearm (serial transverse) 419
    hand at midpalm (transverse) 431
    shoulder (coronal) 394
    sternoclavicular joint (coronal) 391
    wrist/carpal tunnel (transverse) 430
    wrist joints (coronal) 425
**Crown** of tooth 51
**Crus**–see also Limb
  of antihelix 88
  of clitoris 337, 343, 345, 352
  cerebral 100, 101, 107, 109, 132, 138
  of diaphragm–see under Diaphragm, thoracic
  of fornix 100, 104, 106, 136
  of helix 88
  of incus 88, 89
  of penis 343, 356, 357, 359
  of stapes 87–89
  of superficial inguinal ring 243
**Crypt**
  anal 369
  of intestinal glands (Lieberkühn) 266
  of lingual tonsil 52
  of Lieberkühn–see Crypt, of intestinal glands
**Cuboid** 488, 489, 491, 492, 500, 501
**Cuff**
  musculotendinous–see Cuff, rotator
  rotator 398, 401, 400
**Cul-de-sac** of Douglas 337, 339, 341, 344, 346, 363
**Culmen**
  of cerebellum 107, 109, 137
  of left lung 188, 189
**Cumulus** oöphorus of ovarian follicle 349
**Cuneiform** 488, 489, 491, 492, 500, 501
**Cuneus** 100, 101
**Cupula** of
  cochlea 90
  pleura 68, 184, 185, 218, 219
**Curvature**
  cervical 13
  lumbar 142
  of vertebral column 142
  sacral 142
  thoracic 142
  of stomach 258
**Cusp**
  anterior
    of mitral valve 209–212, 230
    of pulmonary valve–see Cusp, semilunar, anterior, of pulmonary valve

**Cusp** *cont.*
    of tricuspid valve 210–212, 230
    of aortic valve–see Cusp, semilunar, left;
        right; posterior; of aortic valve
    commissural, of mitral valve 210, 211
    coronary–see Cusp, semilunar, left; right; of
        aortic valve
    mitral valve–see Cusp, anterior; posterior;
        commissural; of mitral valve
    noncoronary–see Cusp, semilunar,
        posterior, of aortic valve
    posterior
        of aortic valve–see Cusp, semilunar,
            posterior, of aortic valve
        of mitral valve 209–212, 230
        of tricuspid valve 208, 210–212, 230
    of pulmonary valve–see Cusp, semilunar,
        anterior; left; right; of pulmonary valve
    semilunar
        anterior, of pulmonary valve 208, 210
        left
            of aortic valve 209–213
            of pulmonary valve 208, 213
        right
            of aortic valve 209–213
            of pulmonary valve 208, 213
        posterior (noncoronary), of aortic valve
            209–213
    septal, of tricuspid valve 208, 210–212,
        230
    of tricuspid valve–see Cusp, anterior;
        posterior; septal; of tricuspid valve
**Cuticle** of hair follicle 511
**Cymba** conchae of external ear 88


**D**

Dartos–see Fascia, superficial (dartos), of
    penis; scrotum
Darwin–see Tubercle, of external ear
**Declive** of cerebellum 107, 109, 137
**Decussation**
    of pyramids 108, 109
    of superior cerebellar peduncles 107
Denonvilliers'–see Fascia, rectovesical
    (Denonvilliers')
**Dens** (of axis) 12, 13, 15, 16, 32, 57
**Dentin** 51
**Depression** for trigeminal ganglion–see
    Impression, trigeminal
Depressor–see Muscle, depressor
**Dermis** 511
**Dermatomes**–see also Plate 18 for zones of
    head and neck
    of lower limb 150, 507
    of neck 451
    of trunk 150
    of upper limb 150, 451
Descemet–see Membrane, posterior limiting
    (of cornea)
**Descendens**
cervicalis–see Root, of ansa cervicalis,

**Descendens** *cont.*
    inferior
    hypoglossi–see Root, of ansa cervicalis,
        superior
**Descent** of testis 360
**Diameters** of pelvic inlet 332
**Diaphragm**
    pelvic **333**–338, 363, 364, 366–see also
        Muscle, levator ani
        female 333–334
        male 335–336
    thoracic 176, **180, 181, 183,** 184, 186,
        195, 198, 200, 218–221, 224–226,
        236, 238, 241, 246, 248, 255, 256,
        258, 269, 270, 281, 309, 311, 312,
        324, 327, 329, 381, 464
        arteries 181, 247
        central tendon 180, 181, 246
        crura 165, 181, 246, 253, 324, 327,
            517–520, 525
        function 183
        innervation (schema) 182
        nerves 181, 182
        surface
            abdominal 181
            projection 184
            thoracic 180
        veins 248, 318
**Diastole** 210
**Dilator** of pupil–see Muscle, dilator, of pupil
**Diploë** 4
**Disc**
    articular
        of sternoclavicular joint 171, 391, 513
        of temporomandibular joint 11, 49
        of wrist 423–425
    intervertebral 14, **144,** 146, 147, 180, 514,
        515, 519, 520
    optic 86
Disse–see Space, perisinusoidal (Disse)
**Division**
    of brachial plexus 401
    of left lung–see Culmen, of left lung;
        Lingula, left lung
    of mandibular nerve 41
    of oculomotor nerve 78, 81, 115
    of vestibular nerve 90, 118
**Dome**
    of diaphragm 184, 185
    of pleura–see Cupula, of pleura
**Dorsum**
    of foot 484, 485, 485, 494, 495
    of hand 431, 437–439, 441, 450
    sellae 6
    of tongue 52
Douglas–see Line, arcuate, of rectus sheath;
    Pouch, rectouterine
Down–see Syndrome, Down's
Drummond–see Artery, marginal, juxtacolic,
    of Drummond
**Duct**–see also Opening
    alveolar 192
    Bartholin–see Duct, sublingual

**Duct** *cont.*
    bile
        (common) 256, 257, 261, 262, 271, 276,
            278, 279, 282, 284, 285, 290, 299,
            518, 519
        intrahepatic 274, 275
    bulbourethral 361
    cochlear 87, 90–92
    cystic 270, 276, 277, 282, 284, 327
        parts of 276
        variations of 277
    ejaculatory 358, 390, 523
    endolymphatic 91, 92
    epididymal 362
    Gartner's–see Duct, longitudinal, of
        epoöphoron (Gartner)
    hepatic
        accessory 277
        common, 270, 272, 273, 276, 277, 284,
            289, 290, 327
    of labyrinth 90–92, 118
    of lacrimal gland 77
    lactiferous 167
    longitudinal, of epoöphoron (Gartner) 390
    lymph–see also Duct, thoracic; Trunk
        (lymphatic)
        right 197
    mesonephric (wolffian) 360, 390
    müllerian–see Duct, paramesonephric
        (müllerian)
    nasofrontal–see Canal, nasofrontal
    nasolacrimal 32, 44, 77–see also Canal,
        nasolacrimal
    pancreatic 276, 278
        accessory 262, 279, 280
        interlobular 279
        principal 262, 279, 280
        variations in 280
    paramesonephric (müllerian) 360, 390
    paraurethral 353
    parotid 19, 48, 49, 55, 63
    of Santorini–see Duct, pancreatic,
        accessory
    semicircular, of labyrinth 90–92, 118
    Skene's–see Duct, paraurethral
    Stenson's–see Duct, parotid
    sublingual 55
    submandibular 45, 47, 53–55
    thoracic 66, 175, 180, 186, 195, 197, 198,
        200, 219, 220, 226, **227,** 230, 246,
        249, 296, 300, 327, 513–517, 525
    Wharton's–see Duct, submandibular
    of Wirsung–see Duct, pancreatic,
        principal
    wolffian–see Duct, mesonephric (wolffian)
**Ductule**
    bile 274, 275
    of testis 362, 390
**Ductus**
    arteriosus 217
    choledochus–see Duct, bile, (common)
    deferens 236, 243–245, 247, 319, 338,

**Ductus** *cont.*
 340, 343, 358, 360–**362,** 363, 374,
 380, 381, 387, 390, 510
 reuniens 91
 venosus 217
**Duodenojejunal** flexure–see Flexure,
 duodenojejunal
**Duodenum** 120, 256, 257, **261, 262,** 279,
 285, 311, 319
 ampulla 259, 262
 arteries of 283–285
 ascending (4th) part 253
 cap of 259, 262
 cross sections 324, 329, 518, 519
 descending (2nd) part 165, 255, 258, 276,
 278, 324, 519, 520
 flexures of 262
 inferior (horizontal–3rd) part 253, 329, 520
 innervation of (schema) 303
 in situ 261
 mucosa of 262
 musculature of 262
 nerves of 301–303
 superior (1st) part 256, 258, 259, 270, 276,
 518
 veins of 290
**Dura mater** 34, 93–97, 103, 148, 149, 155,
 156, 165


**E**

**Ear** 87–89
 drum–see Membrane, tympanic
 external 88
 inner 87
 lobe–see Lobule, of auricle
 middle 87, 88–see also Cavity, tympanic
Ebner–see Gland, serous (Ebner)
Edinger-Westphal–see Nucleus, accessory
 oculomotor
**Elbow**
 arteries of 446
 bones of 407
 collateral circulation at–see Anastomoses,
 around elbow
 joint–see Joint, elbow
 ligaments of 408
**Eminence**
 collateral 105
 iliopectineal–see Eminence, iliopubic
 iliopubic 231, 330–332, 335, 453, 454
 intercondylar, of tibia 474, 478, 479
 medial, of 4th ventricle 109
 median, of tuber cinereum 140
 pyramidal, in tympanic cavity 89
**Enamel** of tooth 51
**Endometrium** 346
**Endothelium**
 of anterior chamber (cornea) 83
**Ependyma** 102

**Epicondyle**
 of femur
 lateral 455, 459
 medial 455, 459, 467, 468, 472, 475
 of humerus
 lateral 392, 393, 402, 403, 407, 408,
 410–413, 415, 418, 447
 medial 392, 393, 402–404, 407, 408,
 410–418, 445, 446
**Epidermis** 511
**Epididymis** 360–362, 387, 390
**Epiglottis** 52, 57, 58, 60, 61, 70–72, 75, 129,
 221, 223
**Epithelium**
 germinal, of ovary 349
 gingival 51
 pigment 83
 superficial, of ovary 349
 of tongue 52
**Epoöphoron** 346, 390
**Equator** of lens 85
**Eruption** of teeth 50
**Esophagus** 30, 57, 59–62, 69, 70, 75, 120,
 180, 195, 196, 218–**222,** 223–226,
 228–230, 246, 248, 253, 257, 258, 260,
 305, 311, 314, 329
 arteries of 225
 constrictions 221
 cross section 230, 513–517, 524, 525
 in situ 220
 junctions
 esophagogastric 224
 pharyngoesophageal 223
 lymph vessels and nodes 227
 mucosa/submucosa 223, 224, 229
 musculature **222,** 223, 260
 nerves 228
 intrinsic 229
 variations 229
Ethmoid–see Bone, ethmoid
Eustachian–see Tube, pharyngotympanic
 (auditory); Valve, of inferior vena cava
 (Eustachian)
**Expiration** 183
**Eye** 42, 76, 79, 82–86, 115, 153–see also
 Orbit
**Eyeball** 42, **82–86**
 arteries of 86
 chambers of 83–84
 extrinsic muscles of 79
 lens and supporting structures of 85
 veins of 86
**Eyelashes** 76
**Eyelids** 76


**F**

**Face**
 arteries of 17, 35, 63
 lymph nodes of 66, 67
 muscles of 20, 21, 48

**Face** *cont.*
 nerves of 18, 19, 65
 veins of 17, 64
 wrinkling, in skin of 20
 zones of sensory innervation 18
**Facet**
 articular–see also Surface, articular
 anterior (of dens) for atlas 12
 of atlas
 for axis–see Surface, articular, inferior
 (of atlas for axis)
 for dens 12
 for occipital condyle–see Surface,
 articular, superior (of atlas for
 occipital condyle)
 of axis
 for atlas–see Facet, articular, anterior
 (of dens for atlas); Surface,
 articular, superior (of axis for
 atlas)
 for C3 vertebra–see Facet, articular,
 inferior (of axis for C3)
 for transverse ligament–see Facet,
 articular, posterior (of dens for
 transverse ligament)
 costal
 superior (for head of rib) 13, 143, 172
 transverse (for tubercle of rib) 13, 143,
 172
 of cricoid cartilage for thyroid cartilage
 74
 of dens for transverse ligament–see
 Facet, articular, posterior (of dens for
 transverse ligament)
 inferior (of axis) for C3 12
 posterior (of dens for transverse ligament)
 12, 15
 (of rib)
 for transverse process 171
 for vertebral body 171
 (of sacrum) for vertebra 145
 (of transverse process) for rib 143, 172
 (of vertebra)
 for rib–see Facet, costal, (for head of
 rib); transverse (for tubercle of rib)
 for sacrum 144
 tropism 147
Fallopius–see Tube, uterine
False
 pelvis–see Pelvis, greater (false)
 vocal cords–see Fold, vestibular
**Falx**
 cerebelli 97, 137
 cerebri 34, 96–98, 134, 137
 inguinal (conjoint tendon) 233, 234, 236,
 242, 243
**Fascia**
 alar 30, 31, 33
 antebrachial 419, 449
 of arm–see Fascia, brachial
 axillary 399, 448
 brachial 406, 448

**Facia** *cont.*
buccopharyngeal 30, 54, 57, 59
Buck's–see Fascia, deep (Buck's), of penis
Camper's–see Tissue, subcutaneous, fatty
layer, of abdomen
cervical 21, 23, **30,** 57, 174, 395
investing layer 21, 23, 26, 30, 57
pretracheal layer 23, 30, 57
prevertebral layer 30, 54, 57, 59
superficial–see Tissue, subcutaneous, of
neck
superficial layer (of deep)–see Fascia,
cervical, investing layer
clavipectoral 174, 399
Colles'–see Fascia, perineal, superficial
(Colles')
cremasteric 233, 234, 245, 361, 362
cribriform 232, 242, 510
crural–see Fascia, deep, of leg
dartos–see Fascia, superficial (dartos), of
penis; of scrotum
deep
of arm–see Fascia, brachial
(Buck's), of penis 232–234, 238, 239,
329, 338, 354, 355, 356, 357, 359,
361, 367, 368, 372, 374, 376
of deep perineal muscles 333
of forearm–see Fascia, antebrachial
of hand–see Aponeurosis, palmar; Fascia,
dorsal, of hand
of leg 487, 508–510
deltoid 21
Denonvilliers'–see Fascia, rectovesical
(Denonvilliers')
dorsal, of hand 431, 437
diaphragmatic 224, 236, 324, 327, 329
endopelvic 341
paravesical 343
extraperitoneal 165, 234, 235, 244, 245,
383–see also Fascia, endopelvic
of eyeball–see Sheath, fascial, of eyeball
Gallaudet's–see Fascia, perineal, deep
(investing–Gallaudet's)
geniohyoid 30
gluteus medius–see Aponeurosis,
gluteal
iliac 236, 243–245, 341, 364
infradiaphragmatic 224
infraspinatus 160, 163, 178, 237, 395
intercavernous, of deep fascia of penis
(Buck's) 356
investing–see also under names of
individual muscles or regions
cervical–see Fascia, cervical, investing
layer
of perineum (Gallaudet's)–see Fascia,
perineal, deep (investing–
Gallaudet's)
lata **232–**234, 242, 345, 350, 354, 355,
378, **466,** 471, 508, 510
levator ani, superior–see Fascia, of pelvic
diaphragm, superior

**Facia** *cont.*
lumbodorsal–see Fascia,
thoracolumbar
masseteric 21
nasal fibrofatty 31, 33
of neck–see Fascia, cervical
obturator 333, 335, 341, 342, 344, 345,
352, 364, 373, 382
of orbit 78
paravesical–see under Fascia, endopelvic
parotid 21
pectineal 234, 244
pectoral 21, 167, 403
pelvic–see Fascia, endopelvic
tendinous arch of–see Arch, tendinous,
of pelvic fascia
of pelvic diaphragm
deep–see Fascia, of pelvic diaphragm,
superior
inferior 345, 351, 352, 364, 366, 368,
376
superficial–see Fascia, of pelvic
diaphragm, inferior
superior 341, 342, 344, 345, 351, 364,
366, 368
of penis
deep (Buck's)–see Fascia, deep (Buck's),
of penis
superficial (dartos)–see Fascia, superficial
(dartos), of penis
perineal
deep (investing–Gallaudet's) 338, 343,
345, 351, **352,** 353, **355–**357, 363,
368
superficial (Colles') 329, 338, 343, 345,
351–**353, 354–**357, 363, 367, 368,
375, 376, 382
pharyngobasilar 32, 46, 53, 57–59, 61, 62,
67
plantar 500
presacral 329, 341, 368
pretracheal–see Fascia, cervical,
pretracheal layer
prevertebral–see Fascia, cervical,
prevertebral layer
prostatic 338, 343, 358
psoas 165, 324
rectal 329, 341, 344, 351, 358, 363–366,
368
rectovesical (Denonvilliers') 329, 336, 338,
358, 363, 368
renal 165, **324,** 325, 520
Scarpa's–see Tissue, subcutaneous,
membranous layer, of abdomen
of scrotum–see Fascia, superficial (dartos),
of scrotum
Sibson's–see Membrane, suprapleural
spermatic
external 232–234, 243, 245, 338,
354–356, **361,** 362, 3761
internal 234, 244, 245, 361, 362

**Facia** *cont.*
subcutaneous–see Tissue, subcutaneous
of abdomen 232, 235, 329, 338, 351,
354, 355
subserous 165, 234, 235, 244, 245, 383
superficial
of abdomen–see Tissue, subcutaneous,
fatty layer; membranous layer, of
abdomen
cervical (investing)–see Fascia, cervical,
investing layer
(dartos), of penis 232–234, 329, 338,
354–356, 361
(dartos), of scrotum 232–234, 329, 338,
354, 361, 362, 367, 376
of penis–see Fascia, superficial (dartos),
of penis; deep (Buck's), of penis
supradiaphragmatic 224
temporalis 21, 41, 48
of thigh–see Fascia lata
thoracolumbar **160–**163, 165, 177, 178,
237, 312, 328
transversalis 165, 224, 234–**236,** 243–245,
247, 257, 324, 327–329, 338–342,
351
trapezius 21
umbilical prevesical 234–236, 244, 245,
329, 338, 341, 342
of urogenital diaphragm
inferior–see membrane, perineal
uterine 341
uterovaginal 344, 345, 351
vaginal 344, 363
vesical 329, 338, 341, 343, 344, 351, 363,
368
Fascicle–see Fiber
**Fasciculus**–see also Fiber
cuneate 108, 109, 151
dorsal longitudinal 140
dorsolateral 151
gracile 108, 109, 151
interfascicular 151
mammillothalamic 100
medial longitudinal 107, 109, 151
proprii 151
semilunar–see Fasciculus, interfascicular
septomarginal 151
sulcomarginal–see Fasciculus, medial
longitudinal
transverse, of
palmar aponeurosis 428
plantar aponeurosis 496
**Fat**–see also Body, fat
of anterior abdominal wall–see Tissue,
subcutaneous, fatty layer, of abdomen
of breast 167
in epidural space 156
extraperitoneal 383
hilar 322
in ischioanal fossa–see Body, fat, of
ischioanal fossa
orbital–see Body, fat, of orbit
pararenal 165, 324, 520

**Fat** *cont.*
  pericardial 218, 219
  perirenal 165, 317, 324, 520
  in prevesical space 234
  subcutaneous–see Fascia, subcutaneous
  of subhiatal ring 224
**Fauces** 58
**Femur** 231, **455,** 470, 471, 473, 476
**Fenestra**
  cochleae–see Window, round
  vestibuli–see Window, oval
**Fiber**–see also Fasciculus
  of ciliary zonule 82, 83, 85, 86
  elastic, of skin 511
  of His–see Bundle, atrioventricular
  intercrural inguinal 232, 242, 245
  of Luschka–see Muscle, levator ani,
      prerectal fibers
  nerve
    afferent (sensory) 110–113, 115–120,
        122, 123, 126, 199, 306, 307, 309,
        310, 323, 386–388
      vagal 215, 303
    antidromic conduction 153, 154, 307
    efferent (motor) 110–112, 115–117,
        119–123, 306–see also Fiber
        (nerve), somatic efferent
    mixed 110, 111
    motor–see Fiber, efferent
    olfactory 113
    parasympathetic 39, 115–117, 119, 120,
        152, 199, 306
      presynaptic/postsynaptic 126–128,
          153, 154, 303, 307, 309, 310
    proprioceptive 116, 121, 123
    sensory–see Fiber, afferent
    somatic efferent 154, 306, 388
    spinoreticular 151
    sympathetic 115–117, 152, 199, 306
      presynaptic/postsynaptic 126–128,
          153, 154, 215, 216, 303, 307,
          309, 310, 323, 326, 386, 388
  to olfactory bulb 113
  Purkinje–see Branch, subendocardial, of
      conductive system of heart
  transverse, of antebrachial fascia (palmar
      carpal ligament) 416, 417, 424,
      428–430, 435, 449
  vaginorectal fascial 341
  vesicocervical fascial 341
  zonular 85, 86–see also Fiber, of ciliary
      zonule
**Fibula 478,** 479, 484, 486, 487, 490 491,
    494, 495
**Filum** terminale, (dural and pial) 148, 149
**Fimbria**
  of hippocampus 100, 102, 104–106, 113
  of uterine tube 346
**Finger** 433, 440
**Fingernail**–see Nail (of finger)
**Fissure**–see also Sulcus
  of cerebellum 107
  cerebral

**Fissure** *cont.*
    lateral–see Sulcus, cerebral, lateral
    longitudinal 101, 136, 138
    sylvian–see Sulcus, cerebral, lateral
  for roung ligament of liver 270
  for ligamentum venosum 270
  of lung 184–187, 514, 525
  orbital
    inferior 1, 2, 78
    superior 1, 7, 78
  petrosquamous 8
  petrotympanic 5
  pterygomaxillary 2
  ventral median, of spinal cord 151
**Flexure**
  colic
    hepatic–see Flexure, colic, right
    left (splenic) 252–255, 258, 261, 267,
        271, 279, 321
    right (hepatic) 252, 254, 255, 258, 261,
        267, 271, 279, 324
    splenic–see Flexure, colic, left
  of duodenum 262
  duodenojejunal 165, 253, 261, 262, 279,
      238, 325
  hepatic–see Flexures, colic, right
  perineal (of rectum and anal canal) 523
  splenic–see Flexure, colic, left
**Flocculus** of cerebellum 107, 108
**Floor**
  of mouth 47
  of nasal cavity 32
  of urethra 363
**Fluid,** cerebrospinal 103
**Fold**–see also Ligament; Plica
  alar, of knee 477
  aryepiglottic 60, 61, 72, 75
  bloodless, of Treves–see Fold, ileocecal
  cecal 264, 339, 340
  circular
    of duodenum 262, 278
    ileum 263
    jejunum 263
  duodenal 253, 261
  duodenojejunal–see Fold, duodenal
  fimbriated, of tongue 45
  gastric 224, 259, 517
  gastropancreatic 255
  glossoepiglottic 52, 75
  ileocecal 264
  infrapatellar 477
  inguinal 390
  interureteric 343
  of iris 83
  of Kerckring–see Fold, circular, of
      duodenum; ileum; jejunum
  of left vena cava 203, 209
  mallear 89
  palatine, transverse 46
  palmate, of cervical canal 346
  pharyngoepiglottic 59, 61, 223
  pubovesical 236
  rectal–see Fold, transverse, of rectum

**Fold** *cont.*
  rectosacral–see Fold, uterosacral;
      sacrogenital
  sacrogenital 257, 340, 364–see also Fold,
      uterosacral
  salpingopharyngeal 58, 60
  semilunar
    of conjunctiva 76, 77
    of fauces 58
    of large intestine 267
  sublingual 45, 55
  transverse, of rectum 365
  triangular, of fauces 58
  umbilical
    lateral 236, 257, 339, 340, 522
    medial 235, 236, 257, 339, 340, 371
    median 235, 236, 257, 339, 341, 344
  ureteric 339, 340, 344
  urethral 389
  urogenital 389
  of uterine tube 346
  uterosacral 319, 339, 344, 364–see also
      Fold, sacrogenital
  vascular cecal 264
  ventricular, of larynx–see Fold, vestibular,
      of larynx
  vesical, transverse 236, 339, 340
  vesicosacral 340
  vestibular, of larynx 75
  vocal 57, 75
**Folium** of cerebellum 107, 109, 137
**Follicle**
  graffian–see Follicle, vesicular ovarian
  hair 153, 154, 511
  lingual–see Tonsil, lingual
  lymph
    of appendix–see Lymph nodule, of
        appendix
    of small intestine–see Lymph nodule, of
        small intestine
    of stomach–see Lymph nodule, of
        stomach
  ovarian–see Follicle, vesicular ovarian
  vesicular ovarian 346, 349
Fontana–see Space, of iridocorneal angle
**Fontanelle** 8
**Foot**
  arteries of 500
  bones of 488–490
  ligaments of 491, 492
  lymph nodes of 510
  muscles of 494–501
  nerves of 504, 505
  sole of 496–499
  tendons of 492
**Footplate** of stapes, 87, 89
**Foramen**–see also Aperture; Opening
  alveolar, of maxilla 2
  apical dental 51
  cecum of
    frontal bone 6, 7
    tongue 52, 57

**Foramen** *cont.*
of cranial base 7
cribriform 7
of emissary veins 4–see also Canal,
    condylar; Foramen, mastoid; parietal;
    sphenoidal emissary
epiploic–see Foramen, omental
ethmoidal
    anterior 1, 7, 8
    posterior 1, 7
for inferior vena cava–see Opening, caval
infraorbital 1, 2, 8, 31
interventricular (Monro) 100, 102, 103,
    105, 109, 138, 139
intervertebral 13, 144–147, 166, 522
ischiatic–see Foramen, sciatic
jugular 3, 5, 6, 97, 98, 119–121
lacerum 5, 7, 93
of Luschka–see Aperture, lateral, of 4th
    ventricle
of Magendie–see Aperture, median, of 4th
    ventricle
magnum 3, 5, 7, 16, 93, 121
mandibular 10, 41
mastoid 5, 7
mental 1, 2, 10
of Monro–see Foramen, interventricular
    (Monro)
nasolacrimal 44
nutrient, of femur 455, 478
obturator 231, 331, 453, 467
omental (epiploic) 255–258, 271, 327, 329
optic 1
ovale of
    cranium 2, 5, 7, 9, 40, 41, 93
    heart 209, 217
palatine
    greater 5, 33, 34, 36, 46, 50
    lesser 5, 33, 34, 36, 46, 50
parietal 4
rotundum 7, 39, 40
sacral
    anterior (ventral) 145, 331, 335, 522
    posterior 145, 331, 334, 522
sciatic
    greater 147, 330, 331, 334, 504
    lesser 147, 330, 331
sphenoidal emissary 7
sphenopalatine 2, 3, 9, 33, 35, 36
spinosum 5, 7, 9, 41, 93
stylomastoid 5, 19, 89, 117, 119
supraorbital 1, 2, 8
of transverse process 12, 13
vena caval–see Opening, caval
vertebral 12, 13, 143, 144
of Vesalius–see Foramen, sphenoidal
    emissary
of Winslow–see Foramen, omental
    (epiploic)
zygomaticofacial 1, 2, 8
**Forearm**
arteries of 442

**Forearm** *cont.*
bones of 409
cross sections of 419
fascia/fascial compartments of 419, 449
lymph nodes of 452
muscles of 414–418
nerves of 444, 447
    cutaneous 449
superficial veins of 448
Foreskin–see Prepuce
**Fornix**
cerebral 100, 105, **106,** 138, 140
    body of 102, 106, 109
    column of 104, 106, 138
    commissure of 106
    crus 104, 106, 136
conjunctival 76
vaginal 337, 346
**Fossa**
acetabular 330, 453, 454, 523
axillary 513–515–see also Axilla
of cochlear window–see Fossa, of round
    window
condylar, of occipital bone 5
coronoid, of humerus 392, 411
cranial 6
digastric, of mandible 10
duodenal 253, 261
glenoid–see Cavity, glenoid, of scapula
hypophyseal of sphenoid bone 6, 44
ileocecal 264
ileocolic–see Recess, ileocecal
iliac 330, 331, 339, 340, 453
incisive 5, 46, 50
infraspinous 170, 393
infratemporal 2, 9
intercondylar, of femur 455
interpeduncular 101
intersigmoid 254
ischioanal 345, 351, 352, 354–356, **364,**
    366, 368, 376
    anterior recess of 236, 343, 345
jugular 5, 89
for lacrimal sac 1, 2
mandibular 2, 5, 8, 11
mesentericoparietal 253
navicular, of urethra 338, 359
olecranon, of humerus 393, 407
of oval window 89
ovalis
    of fascia lata–see Opening, saphenous
    heart 208, 217, 524
paraduodenal–see Recess, paraduodenal
pararectal 340
parotid–see Space, parotid; Bed, of parotid
    gland
piriform 60, 75, 221
pterygoid
    of mandible–see Fovea, pterygoid, of
        mandible
    of sphenoid bone 5
pterygopalatine 2, 9, 35, 39

**Fossa** *cont.*
radial, of humerus 392, 407
retrocecal–see Recess, retrocecal
rhomboid, of 4th ventricle 108
of round window 88, 89
scaphoid,
    of external ear 88
    of sphenoid bone 5, 93
sublingual 10
submandibular 10
subscapular 170, 392
supraspinous 170, 393
supratonsillar 58
supravesical 236
temporal 2, 9
triangular, of ear 88
trochanteric, of femur 455
of vestibular window–see Fossa, of oval
    window
Fourchette–see Commissure, labial
**Fovea**
caudal–see Fovea, inferior, of 4th ventricle
centralis, in macula lutea 82, 86
of head of femur 455
inferior, of 4th ventricle 109
pterygoid, of mandible 10
superior, of 4th ventricle 109
**Foveola,** granular 4, 94, 96
**Framework,** bony
of abdomen 231
of head and neck 9
of thorax 170
**Frenulum**
of clitoris 350
of ileal orifice 265
of lip 45
of penis 356
of tongue 45, 55
**Fundus**
of gallbladder 270, 276
of stomach 221, 224, 258, 259, 517
of urinary bladder 338, 343
of uterus 337, 339, 344, 346
**Funiculus,** lateral 109


**G**

Galea aponeurotica–see Aponeurosis,
    epicranial
Galen–see Vein, cerebral, great (of Galen)
Gallaudet–see Fascia, perineal, deep
**Gallbladder** 120, 153, 184, 252, 255, 258,
    269–271, **276,** 277, 284, 327, 518
artery (cystic) of 282, 284
innervation (schema) 313
parts 276
referred pain from 313
surface projection of 269
**Ganglion**
aorticorenal 152, 153, 250, **300,**
    302–308, 322, **323,** 326, 380, 381,
    385–388

**Ganglion** *cont.*
basal–see Nucleus, basal
celiac 120, 152–154, 228, 250, **300, 301–306,** 307, 309, 310, 322, 326, 327, 380, 381, 385–388
cervical sympathetic
inferior–see Ganglion, cervicothoracic (stellate)
middle 65, 124, 152, 154, 214, 215, 228
superior 28, 39, 54, 119, 122, **124, 125–**128, 152, 154, 199, 214, 215, 228
laryngopharyngeal branch 129
cervicothoracic (stellate) 124, 152, 198, 214, 215, 228
ciliary 40, 81, 115, 116, 125, **126,** 152, 153
cochlea (spiral) 91, 118
dorsal root–see Ganglion, spinal sensory
geniculate 39, 41, 110, 117–119, 125, 129
of glossopharyngeal nerve
inferior 119, 128, 129
superior 119
inferior
of glossopharyngeal nerve 119, 128, 129
of vagus nerve 120–122, 129, 228
jugular–see Ganglion, superior, of glossopharyngeal nerve; of vagus nerve
lumbar sympathetic 156, 216, 300, 322, 323, **380, 381,** 383, 385–387
mesenteric
inferior 152–154, 300, **305,** 306, 322, 380, 381, 385–388
superior 120, 152–154, 250, 300, 302–**304, 305–**307, 310, 322, 323, 326, 380, 381, 385–388
nodose–see Ganglion, inferior, of vagus nerve
otic 11, 41, 49, 116, 117, 119, 125, 127, **128,** 129, 152, 153
petrosal–see Ganglion, inferior, of glossopharyngeal nerve
phrenic 302, 309
pterygopalatine 37–40, 56, 65, 115–117, 119, 125, **127,** 129, 152, 153
nasal branches 37–39, 125, 127
pharyngeal branch 38, 56, 116, 127
renal 322, 323, 326, 387, 388
sacral sympathetic 154, 300
semilunar–see Ganglion, trigeminal
spinal sensory (dorsal root) **155,** 156, 166, 179, 241, 303, 306, 307, 309, 310, 323, 388
spiral–see Ganglion, cochlear (spiral)
stellate–see Ganglion, cervicothoracic (stellate)
submandibular 41, 53, 55, 65, 116, 117, 125, **127,** 152, 153
superior
of glossopharyngeal nerve 119
of vagus nerve 120, 121, 228
of sympathetic trunk
cervical
inferior–see Ganglion, cervicothoracic (stellate)

**Ganglion** *cont.*
middle 65, 124, 152, 154, 214, 215, 228
superior 28, 39, 54, 119, 122, **124, 125–**128, 152, 154, 199, 214, 215, 228
lumbar 156, 216, 300, 322, 323, **380, 381,** 383, 385–388
sacral 154, 300
thoracic 126, 152, 156, 179, 198, 214, 215, **228,** 230, 303, 307, 386, 387
vertebral 124, 152, 214, 215, 228
thoracic sympathetic 126, 152, 156, 179, 198, 214, 215, **228,** 230, 303, 307, 386, 387
trigeminal **40,** 41, 81, 93, 98, 110, 111, 116, 125–129
of vagus nerve–see Ganglion, inferior; superior; of vagus nerve
vertebral sympathetic 124, 152, 214, 215, 228
vestibular 90, 118
Gartner–see Duct, longitudinal, of epoöphoron (Gartner's)
Gasserian ganglion–see Ganglion, trigeminal
**Geniculum** of facial nerve 89, 92, 111, 118
**Genitalia**
female 350, 389
homlogues of 389–390
male 354–356, 361, 389
**Genu**
of corpus callosum 100, 101, 104, 106, 139
of facial nerve
external–see Ganglion, geniculate
internal–see Geniculum of facial nerve
of internal capsule 104
Gerdy–see Tubercle, Gerdy's
Gimbernat–see Ligament, lacunar
**Gingiva** (gum) 51
**Glabella** 1, 2
**Gland**
adrenal–see Gland, suprarenal
anal 365
areolar 167
Bartholin's–see Gland, vestibular, greater
Brunner's–see Gland, duodenal
bulbourethral (Cowper's) 236, 329, 338, 343, 357–359, 390
Cowper's–see Gland, bulbourethral
duodenal 262
gastric 259
intestinal 308
lacrimal 40, 77, 78, 80, 81, 127, 153
lingual 45, 52
of Littré–see Gland, urethral (male)
mammary 167–see also Breast
meibomian–see Gland, tarsal
mucous, of tongue 52
palatine 46, 57, 58
parathyroid 69, 70
parotid **19,** 22, 23, 26, 54, 55, 60, 66, 119, 128, 153, 154

**Gland** *cont.*
accessory 55
pineal–see Body, pineal
pituitary–see Hypophysis (pituitary gland)
preputial 356
prostate–see Prostate
pyloric 259
retromolar 46
salivary 54, 55–see also Gland, parotid; sublingual; submandibular
sebaceous 76, 511
serous (Ebner) 52
Skene's–see Gland, urethral (female)
Stenson's–see Gland, parotid
sublingual 41, 45, 47, 54, 55, 117, 127, 153
submandibular 22, 23, 26, 27, **41,** 47, 54, **55,** 60, 63, 64, 117, 127, 153
suprarenal 153, 154, 185, 255, 257, 261, 270, 279, 281, 311, 313, 324, **325–**327, 360
arteries of 314, 325
cross section of 325, 518, 519, 525
of infant 313
innervation of (schema) 326
nerves of 326
veins of 325
sweat 153, 154, 365, 511
tarsal (meibomian) 76
thymus 200, 218, 219, 514
thyroid 23, 24, 26, 28, 30, 57, 64, **68,** 69, **70,** 184, 186, 195, 524
arteries of 63, 68
veins of 64, 68
Tyson's–see Gland, preputial
urethral
female 353, 390
male 359, 390
vestibular, greater 352, 375, 390
Wharton's–see Gland, submandibular
**Glans** of
clitoris 350, 389
penis 338, 354, 359, 389
Glisson–see Capsule, of liver
Globe–see Eyeball
**Globus** pallidus 102, 104
**Glomerulus** of
kidney 317, 318
olfactory nerves 113
**Glottis**–see Rima glottidis
Goldmann gonioscopic mirror–see Mirror, Goldmann gonioscopic
**Gonad** 360, 390–see also Ovary; Testis
Graffian follicle–see Follicle, vesicular ovarian
**Granulation,** arachnoid 94–96, 103
**Granulosa** of ovarian follicle 349
**Groove**–see also Sulcus
for anterior meningeal vessels 6
atrioventricular–see Sulcus, coronary
of auditory tube–see Sulcus, of pharyngotympanic (auditory) tube
chiasmatic–see Sulcus, prechiasmatic

**Groove** *cont.*
for circumflex scapular vessels 393
costal 171
coronary (for coronary artery) 516
for digastric muscle–see Notch, mastoid
for greater petrosal nerve 6, 92
for inferior petrosal sinus 3, 6
for inferior vena cava, on bare area of liver 270
infraorbital 1
intermuscular anal–see Groove, intersphincteric
for internal carotid artery–see Sulcus, carotid
intersphincteric 364–366
intertubercular, of humerus–see Sulcus, intertubercular, of humerus
interventricular 516
for lesser petrosal nerve 6
mastoid–see Notch, mastoid
for middle meningeal vessels 3, 4, 6
for middle temporal artery 2, 4
mylohyoid 10
for nasopalatine nerve and vessels–see Groove, vomerine
obturator 457
occipital 5
for occipital artery–see Groove, occipital
for occipital sinus 6
for posterior meningeal vessels 6
for radial nerve 393
for sigmoid sinus 3, 6
for subclavian artery 171
for subclavian vein 171
for superior petrosal sinus 3, 6
for superior sagittal sinus 4, 6
for transverse sinus 3, 6
for ulnar nerve 393, 407
urogenital 389
vomerine (for nasopalatine nerve and vessels) 34
**Gubernaculum** 360, 390
**Gum**–see Gingiva (gum)
**Gutter,** paracolic 254, 264, 328, 339, 340
**Gyrus**
angular 99
cingulate 100, 101
dentate 100, 102, 105, 106, 113
frontal 99, 100
of insula 99
lingual 100, 101
marginal 100
occipitotemporal 100, 101
orbital 101
parahippocampal 100–102, 113
paraterminal–see Gyrus, subcallosal
postcentral 99
precentral 99
straight 101
subcallosal 100
supramarginal 99
temporal 99, 101

**H**

**Habenula** 104
**Hair** 511
cuticle 511
follicle 153, 154, 511
matrix 511
shaft 511
Haller–see Artery, to falciform ligament (from superior epigastric)
**Hamate** 422, 423, 425, 426
**Hamulus**
of cochlea–see Hamulus, of spiral lamina (of cochlea)
of hamate–see Hook, of hamate
pterygoid 2, **3,** 5, 8, 9, 33, 41, 44, 46, 49, 58, 59, 62, 93
of spiral lamina (of cochlea) 90
**Hand**
arteries of 435, 438, 442
bones of 426
ligaments of 427
lymph nodes of 452
muscles (intrinsic) of 428–434, 439
nerves of 435–439, 441, 442, 444, 445, 447
veins of 437, 449
**Handle,** of malleus 88
Hartmann–see Infundibulum, of gallbladder
**Haustra** of large intestine 267
**Head**–see also individual regions
of caudate nucleus 104–106, 136, 138
of epididymis 362
of femur 454, 455, 523
of fibula 458–460, 472, 473, 475, 476, 478, **479,** 482–486, 506
of humerus 392, 394
of malleus 89, 118
of mandible 2, 10
of metacarpal bones 426
of metatarsal bones 488
of pancreas 279, 519
of phalanges (hand) 426
of phalanges (foot) 484
of radius 402, 407, 409
of rib 170, 171, 516
of talus 489
**Heart** 120, 153, 154, 200–202, 204, 205, 209–211, **212–**215, 516, 524
arteries of 204–207
chambers of 208, 209, 212
conductive system of 213
cross section of 212, 230, 516, 524, 525
exterior features 201, 202
innervation of (schema) 215
in situ 200
internal features 208–212
nerves of 214
pericardial sac for 200, 203
surfaces of 201, 202
valves of 210, 202
veins of 204

**Helicotrema** of cochlea 87, 90, 91
**Helix** of external ear 88
Helvetius–see Collar, of Helvetius
**Hematoma**
site of epidural–see Interface, dura-skull
site of subdural–see Interface, arachnoid-dura
**Hemisphere,** cerebral 96, 99–101, 104
Henle–see Loop, nephric (Henle's)
Hering–see Ductule, bile
Hering-Breuer–see Reflex, Hering-Breuer
Hesselbach–see Triangle, inguinal
Huebner–see Artery, medial striate
**Hiatus**–see also Opening
adductor 459, 467, 468, 477, 503
anorectal 335
of deep dorsal vein of penis 335
esophageal 181
for greater petrosal nerve 7
for lesser petrosal nerve 7
sacral 145
saphenous–see Opening, saphenous
semilunar, of ethmoid bone 32, 33, 43, 44
for urethra 335
Hilton–see Line, anocutaneous
**Hilum**
of kidney 313, 520
of lung 187, 515
**Hip**
arteries of 470
bone–see Bone, hip
joint 454
ligaments of 454, 455
muscles of 460–462
nerves of 469
**Hippocampus** 102, 104–106
His–see Bundle, atrioventricular (His)
**Homologues**
external genitalia 389
internal genitalia 390
**Hook of Hamate** 412, 418, 422, 424, 426
**Horn**–see also Cornu
anterior, of lateral ventricle–see Horn, frontal, of lateral ventricle
coccygeal–see Cornu, coccygeal
frontal (anterior), of lateral ventricle 102
of gray matter 151
of hyoid bone
greater 9, 62
lesser 9
inferior, of lateral ventricle–see Horn, temporal, of lateral ventricle
lateral, of gray matter 151, 156–see also Nucleus, intermediolateral (IML)
of lateral ventricle–see Horn, frontal; occipital; temporal; of lateral ventricle
occipital, of lateral ventricle 102, 104–106, 136, 139
posterior, of lateral ventricle–see Horn, occipital, of lateral ventricle
temporal, of lateral ventricle 102, 105, 106, 139
sacral–see Cornu, sacral

**Horn** *cont.*
   of thyroid cartilage 62, 71, 223
Houston—see Folds, rectal, transverse
Hunter—see Canal, adductor
**Humerus 392, 393**, 404, 406–408, 420,
   421
**Hydatid** of Morgagni—see Appendix, vesicular
**Hymen** of vagina 345, 350
Hyoid—see Bone, hyoid
**Hypopharynx** 60—see also Laryngopharynx
**Hypophysis** (pituitary gland) 32, 98, 100,
   101, 140
   arteries and veins of 141
**Hypothalamus** 102, 129, 140, 141, 306


**I**


**Ileum** 252, 254, 263–265, 267, 328, 339,
   340, 520–522
**Ilium** 231, 330–332, 335, 453—see also
   individual landmarks
**Impression**
   of liver 270
   of lung 187
   trigeminal 6
   umbilical 521
**Incisure**—see Notch
   angular, of stomach—see Notch, angular (of
      stomach)
   cardiac—see Notch, cardiac (of stomach)
**Incus** 87, 88, 91, 118
Infundibuliform—see Fascia, spermatic,
   internal
**Infundibulum**
   of ethmoid bone—see Infundibulum,
      ethmoidal
   ethmoidal 33
   of gallbladder 276
   of neurohypophysis (pituitary stalk) 108,
      133, 140
**Innervation**
   of abdominal viscera 304–314
   afferent, of mouth and pharynx 56
   autonomic
      of blood vessels 216
      of nasal cavity 39
   of biliary tract 309
   of blood vessels 216
   cutaneous
      of abdomen 240–241
      of back 163, 178, 179
      of back of neck and scalp 163–164
      of head and neck 18
      of lower limb 502–509
      of thorax 166, 174, 179, 240, 241
      of upper limb 441, 443–445, 447–451
   of duodenum 301, 303
   of extrinsic eye muscles 79
   of heart 215
   of intestines 306
   of kidneys 323
   of liver 309

**Innervation** *cont.*
   of pancreas 310
   of reproductive organs
      female 386
      male 387
   segmental, of lower limb movements 507
   segmental, of skin—see Dermatomes
   of stomach 307
   of tracheobronchial tree 199
   of ureters 323, 388
   of urinary bladder 388
**Inscriptions,** tendinous, of rectus abdominis
      muscle 233
**Insertion** of
   arm muscles 392, 393
   forearm muscles 420, 421
   hip muscles 456, 457
   leg muscles 480
   scalene muscles 25, 171
   shoulder muscles 391–393
   thigh muscles 456, 457
**Inspection** of
   larynx 75
   mouth 45
**Inspiration** 75, 183
**Insula** 99, 104, 134
**Interface**
   arachnoid-dura 96
   dura-skull 96
**Intestine**
   innervation of (schema) 306
   intrinsic autonomic plexuses of 308
   large 252, 254, 267—see also Colon
      arteries of **287,** 288
      lymph vessels/nodes of 297
      mesenteric relations of 254
      mucosa of 267
      musculature 267
      nerves of 305
      veins of 292
   small 120, 252, 263, 328, 329—see also
         Duodenum; Ileum; Jejunum
      arteries of 286
      lymph vessels/nodes of 296
      mesenteric relations of 253
      mucosa of 263
      musculature of 263
      nerves of 304
         autonomic (schema) 308
      veins of 291, 292
**Iris** 76, 82, 84–86
**Ischium** 453—see also individual
      landmarks
**Island**
   of Langerhans—see Islet, pancreatic
   of Reil—see Insula
Islet, pancreatic (island of Langerhans) 279
**Isthmus** of
   cingulate gyrus 100, 101
   prostate 358
   thyroid gland 68

**J**

Jacobson—see Nerve, tympanic
**Jaws** 11—see also Mandible
**Jejunum** 252–254, 261–263, 328—see also
      Intestine, small
**Joint**
   acromioclavicular 396
   atlantoaxial 14, 15
   atlantooccipital 14–16
   of back 146, 147
   carpometacarpal 423, 425
   costotransverse 172, 513
   costovertebral 172
   craniovertebral—see Junction,
         craniovertebral—see also Joint,
         atlantoaxial; atlantooccipital
   elbow 407, 408, 442
   facet—see Joint, zygapophyseal
   glenohumeral 394, 397, 403—see Joint,
         shoulder
   hip 454, 458, 459, 462, 470
   intercarpal 423, 425
   intermetacarpal 425
   interphalangeal (finger) 427, 433, 440
   interphalangeal (toe) 492
   intervertebral (symphysis) 13
   knee 472–476
   manubriosternal 171
   metacarpophalangeal 427, 492
   midcarpal 423, 425
   radiocarpal—see Joint, wrist
   radioulnar
      distal 422–425
      proximal 407–409
   sacroiliac 332, 335, 522
   shoulder (glenohumeral) 394, 397, 403
   sternoclavicular 171, 184, 391, 513
   sternocostal **171,** 391
   sternomanubrial—see Joint manubriosternal
   tarsometatarsal 488, 489
   temporomandibular 11, 35, 48, 49
   of thorax 171, 172
   transverse tarsal 488, 489
   vertebral body 13
   wrist (radiocarpal) 422–425
   zygapophyseal (facet) 13–15, 146, 516—see
         also Facet, costal (of vertebra), for rib
**Jugum** of sphenoid bone 6
**Junction**
   anorectal 336—see also Line, anorectal;
         pectinate
   atlantooccipital 16 —see Joint,
         atlantooccipital; see also Junction,
         craniovertebral
   of bile duct with duodenum—see Junction,
         choledochoduodenal
   choledochoduodenal 278
   craniovertebral 16
   duodenojejunal 165—see also Flexure,
         duodenojejunal
   esophagogastric 224, 259, 517, 524

**Junction** *cont.*
  ileocecal 264, 265, 521
  manubriosternal 171, 515
  pharyngoesophageal 223
  rectosigmoid 267, 363, 365, 366
  ureteropelvic 520


# K

Kerckring–see Fold, circular, of
    duodenum; ileum; jejunum
**Kidney** 165, 185, 217, 255–258, 261, 270,
    271, 281, **311–313,** 319, 324, 325, 327,
    360, 371, 518–520
  arteries 318
    internal (intrarenal) 315
    variations 316
  cross sections 313, 323
  innervation (schema) 323
  in situ 311, 312
  lymph vessels anal nodes 321
  microvasculature 318
  nerves 322
  structure
    gross 313
    internal 317, 318
  relations 311, 312, 324
  segments 315
  vasculature 314–see also Kidney,
    microvasculature
Klippel-Feil–see Syndrome, Klippel-Feil
**Knee**
  arteries of 477
  collateral circulation at–see Anastomoses,
    around knee
  cross section of 476
  joint–see Joint, knee
  lymph nodes of 510
  lymph vessels/nodes at–see Lymph nodes,
    popliteal


# L

Labbé–see Vein, anastomotic, inferior
**Labium**–see also Lip
  majus 337, 342, 345, 350, 353, 389
  minus 337, 342, 345, 350, 353, 389
**Labrum**
  of acetabulum 330, 454, 470
  glenoid, of scapula 398
**Labyrinth**
  bony 90–92
  membranous 90–92
  osseous–see Labyrinth, bony
Lacertus fibrosus–see Aponeurosis,
    bicipital
**Lacuna**
  lateral (venous), of superior sagittal sinus
    94, 95
  of Morgagni–see Lacuna urethral
  of urethral gland–see Lacuna urethral

**Lacuna** *cont.*
  urethral 353, 359
Laimer–see Area, of Laimer
**Lake,** lacrimal 76, 77
**Lambda** 4
**Lamina**–see also Layer; Plate
  affixa 105
  cribrosa, of sclera 82
  medullary, of thalamus 105
  osseous spiral, of cochlea 91
  posterior limiting, of cornea (Descemet's
    membrane) 83
  propria, of gingiva 51
  quadrigeminal–see Plate, tectal
  tectal–see Plate, tectal
  terminalis 100, 101, 109, 140
  of thyroid cartilage 61, 71
  of vertebra 13, 143, 144, 146, 147
Langerhans–see Islet, pancreatic (of
    Langerhans)
**Laryngopharynx** 56, 57, 60
**Laryngoscope** 75
**Larynx** 75, 129, 154, 199
  arteries of 70
  cartilages (skeleton) of 71
  inspection of 75
  muscles of 72, 73
    extrinsic (infrahyoid and suprahyoid
      muscles) 24
    intrinsic 72
      action of 73
  nerves of 68, 70, **74**
**Layer**–see also Lamina
  connective tissue, of hair follicle 511
  nuclear, of medulla oblongata 107
  odontoblast 51
  papillary, of dermis 511
  of rectus sheath 235
  reticular, of skin 511
**Leg**
  arteries of 481–485
  bones of 478, 479
  cross sections of 487
  deep fascia of 487, 508–510
  lymph nodes of 510
  muscles of 481–486
  nerves of 481–485, 504–506
  veins of 481–485
**Lens** 76, 82–86
**Leptomeninges** 156
**Ligament**–see also Fold; Raphé
  acetabular, transverse 330, 454
  alar 15
  of ankle 479, 491, 493
  anular
    of fibrous digital sheath–see Part, anular,
      of fibrous digital tendon sheath
    of radius 408
    of trachea 190
  anococcygeal 334, 351, 352, 387, 388
  anterior, of head of fibula 479
  apical, of dens 15, 16, 57, 59

**Ligament** *cont.*
  arcuate
    of diaphragm 181, 246
    popliteal 474, 476
    pubic–see Ligament, pubic, inferior
      (arcuate)
  of atlas 15, 16
  bifurcate (of transverse tarsal joint) 491
  broad 319, 337, 339, 344–346, 390
  calcaneocuboid 491, 500
    dorsal 491
    plantar 492
  calcaneofibular 479, 490, 491
  calcaneometatarsal–see Band, lateral, of
    plantar aponeurosis
  calcaneonavicular, plantar (spring) 491,
    492, 500
  capitotriquetral 424
  cardinal (transverse cervical or
    Mackenrodt's) 341, 344–347
  carpal 416, 417, 424, 427–430, 435, 449
    palmar–see Fiber, transverse, of
      antebrachial fascia
    transverse (flexor retinaculum) 417, 424,
      429–431, 434, 435, 442
  carpometacarpal 424, 425, 427
  cervical
    lateral–see Ligament, cardinal
    transverse–see Ligament, cardinal
  check, of rectus muscles 78
  collateral
    of ankle 491
    of elbow 408
    fibular (of knee) 459, 460, 472–476,
      479, 482, 483, 485, 486
    of finger–see Ligament, collateral, of
      interphalargeal joint, of hand
    of interphalangeal joint
      of hand 427, 433
      of foot 492
    of knee 459, 460, 472–476, 479,
      482–486
    of metacarpophalangeal joint 427
    of metatarsophalangeal joint 492
    radial
      of elbow joint 408
      of wrist joint 424, 425
    tibial (of knee) 459, 472–476, 482–485
    of toe–see Ligament, collateral, of
      interphalangeal joint, of foot
    ulnar
      of elbow 408
      of wrist joint 424, 425
    of wrist 424, 425
  conoid 394, 396
  Cooper's–see Ligament, suspensory, of
    breast; pectineal
  coracoacromial 394, 396, 397, 402
  coracoclavicular 394, 396
  coracohumeral 394
  coronary, of liver 257, 270, 329
  costoclavicular 171, 391, 399

**Ligament** *cont.*
costocoracoid 174, 399
costotransverse 172, 179, 241
costovertebral 172
costoxiphoid 171
craniocervical 14, 15
cricothyroid, median 24, 59, 62, 68, 71,
    190
cruciate
    of atlas 15, 16
    of fibrous digital sheath–see Part,
        cruciate, of fibrous digital tendon
        sheath
    of knee 473–475, 479
cuboideonavicular
    dorsal 491
    plantar 492
cuneocuboid, dorsal 491
cuneonavicular
    dorsal 491
    plantar 492
deep
    posterior sacrococcygeal 331
    transverse metacarpal 427, 434
    transverse metatarsal 492, 500
deltoid–see Ligament, medial (collateral),
    of ankle
denticulate 155
diaphragmatic (of gonad)–see Ligament,
    suspensory, of gonad
of elbow 408
falciform 235, 236, 252, 257, 258, 270,
    288, 293, 327
fibular collateral–see Ligament, collateral,
    fibular
of foot 491, 492
fundiform, of penis 232, 243, 329, 338
gastrolienal–see Ligament, gastrosplenic
gastrophrenic 255, 257, 311
gastrosplenic 255–257, 281, 311, 327
Gimbernat's–see Ligament, lacunar
glenohumeral 394
of hand 427
of head of femur 454
of head of fibula 476, 479
hepatoduodenal 255, 258, 261, 262,
    271, 518
hepatogastric 258, 271
of hip 454, 458, 459, 470
humeral, transverse 394
hyoepiglottic 57, 71
iliofemoral 454, 462, 470
iliolumbar 147, 312, 331
of incus 89
infundibulopelvic–see Ligament,
    suspensory, of ovary
inguinal (Poupart's) 232–234, 242–**245,**
    246, 333,
        339–341, 351, 354, 355, 378, 458,
        464, 466, 467, 508, 510
intercarpal, interosseous 425
intercartilaginous, of trachea 190

**Ligament** *cont.*
interclavicular 171, 391
intercuneiform, dorsal 491
interfoveolar 236
interosseous–see under Ligament,
    intercarpal; sacroiliac; talocalcaneal,
    –see also Membrane, interosseous
interphalangeal
    of hand 427, 433
    of foot 492
interspinous 146, 147
intertransverse 172
ischiofemoral 454, 470
of knee 458–460, 472–760, 479, 482, 483,
    486
lacunar (Gimbernat's) 233, 234, 236, 243,
    244, 246, 510
lateral
    (collateral) of ankle 491
    of temporomandibular joint 11, 35
lienorenal–see Ligament, splenorenal
longitudinal
    anterior 14, 16, 57, 59, 146, 147, 165,
        172, 246, 327–329, 331, 339, 340
    posterior 15, 16, 146, 147
lumbocostal 312
Mackenrodt's–see Ligament, cardinal
of malleus 89
of Marshall–see Fold, of left vena cava
medial (collateral), of ankle 479, 490, 491
meniscofemoral, posterior 474, 475
metacarpal
    dorsal 425
    palmar 424, 427
    transverse
        deep 427, 434
        superficial 428, 449
metacarpophalangeal 427, 433
metatarsal
    dorsal 491, 500
    plantar 492, 496, 500
    transverse
        deep 492, 500
        superficial 496
nuchal–see Ligamentum, nuchae
oblique popliteal 474, 476
of ovary 337, 339, 344–347, 390
palmar
    carpal 416, 417, 424, 428–430, 435,
        449
    carpometacarpal 424, 427
    digital 427, 433, 440
    metacarpal 424, 427
    radiocarpal 424
    radioulnar 424
    ulnocarpal 424
palpebral 76, 78
patellar 458–460, 467, 426–474, 476, 479,
    484–486
pectinate, of iridocorneal angle–see
    Reticulum, trabecular

**Ligament** *cont.*
pectineal (Cooper's) 233, 234, 236, 243,
    244, 246
of pelvis 330, 331
perineal, transverse 333, 335, 338, 342,
    351, 357, 376
phrenicocolic 255, 257
phrenoesophageal 224
pisohamate 424
pisometacarpal 424
plantar
    calcaneocuboid 492
    calcaneonavicular 491, 492, 500
    cuboideonavicular 492
    cuneonavicular 492
    long 491, 492, 500
    metatarsal 492, 500
    short 492 500
    tarsometatarsal 492
popliteal
    arcuate 474, 476
    oblique 474, 476
Poupart's–see Ligament, inguinal
proper ovarian–see Ligament, of ovary
pubic, inferior (arcuate) 231, 337–338,
    341, 342, 351, 357
pubofemoral 454
puboprostatic 342, 343
pubovesical 341–343
pulmonary 187, 197, 218, 219
radial collateral–see Ligament, collateral
    radial, of elbow, wrist joint
radiate
    carpal 424
    of head of rib 172
    sternocostal 391
radiocarpal 425
radioulnar 425
rectosacral–see Ligament, uterosacral
reflected inguinal 233, 234, 243
round
    of femur–see Ligament, of head of femur
    of liver 217, 236, 258, 270, 271, 288,
        293, 328
    of uterus 337, 339, 343–**345,** 347, 351,
        353, 371, 390
sacrococcygeal
    anterior 246, 331, 333, 335, 341
    lateral 147, 330, 331
    posterior 147, 330, 331
sacrogenital–see Ligament, uterosacral;
    Fold, sacrogenital
sacroiliac
    anterior 331
    dorsal–see Ligament, sacroiliac,
        posterior
    interosseous 522
    posterior 147, 330, 331
sacrospinous 147, 330, 331, 334, 336,
    381, 461, 469
sacrotuberous 147, 330, **331,** 334, 336,
    352, 367, 368, 373, 381, 382, 384,
    461, 468, 469, 523

**Ligament** *cont.*
 of scapula 394, 396–398
 scapular, transverse
  inferior 397
  superior 394, 396, 397, 398
 skin (retinacula cutis) 511
 sphenomandibular 11, 35, 49
 spiral, of cochlea 91
 splenorenal 255, 257, 281, 311, 327
 spring–see Ligament, calcaneonavicular,
   plantar (spring)
 sternoclavicular 391
 sternocostal 171, 391
 stylohyoid 9, 53, 58, 59, 62
 stylomandibular 9, 11
 supraspinous 146, 147, 165, 328, 330, 331
 suspensory
  of axilla 399
  of breast 167
  of clitoris 351, 352
  of gonad 360, 390
  of lens–see Zonule, ciliary, see also
    Fiber, zonular
  of ovary 337, 339, 341, 344–346, 371,
    390
  of penis 233, 242, 329, 338
 talocalcaneal 490, 491
 talocrural
  lateral–see Ligament, collateral, of
    ankle
  medial–see Ligament, deltoid
 talofibular 479, 490, 491
 talonavicular 491
 tarsometatarsal
  dorsal 491, 500
  plantar 492
 temporomandibular–see Ligament, lateral,
   of temporomandibular joint
 thyroepiglottic 71
 tibial collateral–see Ligament, collateral,
   tibial, of knee
 tibiocalcaneal–see Part, of medial
   (collateral) ligament, of ankle
 tibiofibular 479, 490, 491
 tibionavicular–see Part, of medial
   (collateral) ligament, of ankle
 tibiotalar–see Part, of medial (collateral)
   ligament, of ankle
 transverse
  acetabular–see Ligament, acetabular,
    transverse
  of atlas 15, 16
  cervical–see Ligament, cardinal
  humeral–see Ligament, humeral,
    transverse
  of knee 475
  metacarpal–see Ligament, metacarpal,
    transverse, deep; superficial
  metatarsal–see Ligament, metatarsal,
    transverse, deep; superficial
  perineal 333 335, 338, 341, 342, 351,
    357, 376

**Ligament** *cont.*
  scapular–see Ligament, scapular,
    transverse
 trapezoid 394, 396
 of Treitz–see Muscle, suspensory, of
   duodenum
 triangular, of liver 257, 270
 ulnar collateral–see Ligament, collateral,
   ulnar, of elbow; wrist
 ulnocarpal 425
 umbilical–see also Fold, umbilical
  medial 217, 234–**236**, 244, 245, 247,
    319, 339–341, 371, 373, 374, 522
  median 236, 244, 245, 329, 341, 342,
    371, 374
 uterine, lateral–see Ligament, broad
 uterosacral 337, 341, 344, 346, 347
 of vertebral column 146, 147
 vocal 71, 72
 of wrist 424, 425
 Y, of Bigelow–see Ligament, iliofemoral
**Ligamentum**
 arteriosum 195, 201, 209, 217, 219
 capitis femoris–see Ligament, of head of
   femur
 flavum 14, 16, 146, 147, 328
 nuchae 14, 16
 teres–see Ligament, round, of liver; of
   uterus
 venosum 217
**Limb**
 of incus 88, 89
 lower 453–510
 of supraventricular crest (parietal and
   septal) 208
 of stapes 87, 88
 upper 391–452
**Limbus**
 of acetabulum–see Margin, acetabular
 of cornea 76
 of fossa ovalis 208
**Limen**
 of insula 99, 134
 nasal 32
**Line**–see also Plane
 anocutaneous–see Groove, intersphincteric
 anorectal 365
 arcuate
  of ilium 231, 330, 331, 333, 335, 453
  of rectus sheath 234, 236, 238, 243, 329
 dentate, of anal canal–see Line, pectinate,
   of anal canal
 gluteal 330, 453
 Hilton's white–see Groove, intersphincteric
 iliopectineal 331, 335, 364
 intermediate, of iliac crest 231, 330,
   331, 453
 intersphincteric anal–see Groove,
   intersphincteric
 intertrochanteric, of femur 454, 455
 McGregor's 16
 mylohyoid 10

**Line** *cont.*
 nuchal
  inferior 5
  superior 5, 160–162
 oblique, of
  mandible 2, 10, 62
  thyroid cartilage 24, 71
  tibia 473, 478
 pectinate, of
  anal canal 365
  femur 459
  pubis 231, 246, 330, 331, 335, 453
 pectineal
  of femur 455
  of pubis–see Pecten pubis
 SchwalbeÕs 83, 84
 semilunar, of abdomen 251
 soleal, of tibia 478
 temporal 2
 transverse sacral–see Ridge, transverse, of
   sacrum
 white, of Hilton–see Line, anocutaneous
 wrinkle, of face 20
 zigzag (Z), of stomach 224, 259
**Linea**
 alba 174, **232**–235, 241–243, 327, 328,
   339, 340, 522
 aspera of femur 455
 semicircularis–see Line, arcuate, of rectus
   sheath
 semilunaris–see Line, semilunar
 terminalis (of pelvis) 145, 331, 339–341,
   345
**Lingula**
 of cerebellum 107, 109, 137
 of left lung 186–189
 of mandible 10
 of pancreas–see Process, uncinate, of
   pancreas
**Lip** 45–see also Labium
 of bicipital groove–see Crest, of humeral
   tubercle
 of iliac crest 231, 330, 331
 Lissauer–see Fasciculus, dorsolateral
 Littré–see Gland, urethral (male)
**Liver** 120, 184, 185, 217, 226, 252, 255,
   258, 261, 269, **270**–272, 274, 276, 324,
   325, 327, 329
 arteries of 282, 284, 288
 bed of 270
 collateral supply of 288
 cross sections of 517–520, 524, 525
 histology of 273–275
 in situ 271
 innervation of (schema) 309
 intrahepatic vascular and duct systems 272,
   273
 lymph vessels and nodes of 298
 segments and lobes 272
 structure (schema) 274
 surfaces 270
 topography 269
 variations in form 271

**Lobe**
cerebellar 107
cerebral 99
ear–see Lobule, of auricle
eparterial–see Bronchus, eparterial
frontal 99
of liver 258, 272
of lung–see Lobe, pulmonary
occipital 99, 114
parietal 99
piriform 113
of pituitary gland 133, 140
of prostate 358, 374
pulmonary 186–189, 194, 230, 517, 525
temporal 99, 134
of thyroid gland 68, 70
**Lobule**
of auricle 88
cerebellar 107, 109, 137
of external ear–see Lobule, of auricle
of mammary gland 167
paracentral, of cerebrum 100
parietal, of cerebrum
inferior 99
superior 99
of testis 362
**Locus** ceruleus 109
**Loop, nephronic** (Henle's) 317, 318
**Lunate** 422–426
of acetabulum–see Surface, lunate
**Lung** 154, 184–**187,** 188, 189, 197, 200,
201, 230, 269, 324
arteries of 194
bronchopulmonary segments 188, 189
cross sections 230, 573–517, 524, 525
external features 184–187
in situ 186
intrapulmonary circulation (schema) 193
lymph vessels and nodes 197
topography 184, 185
veins 194
**Lunula**
of fingernail 440
of semilunar cusp 211
Luschka–see Aperture, lateral, of 4th
ventricle; Muscle, of levator ani,
prerectal rectal fibers of
**Lymphatic duct**–see also Duct, thoracic;
Trunk (lymph); cisterna chyli
right 197, 296
**Lymph follicle**–see Lymphoid nodule
**Lymph node**–see also Lymph vessel
of abdominal cavity 249
aortic
arch 197
lateral 245, 317, 373
apical axillary–see under Lymph node,
axillary
appendicular 297
axillary 66, 169, 399, 525
anterior–see Lymph node, axillary
pectoral
apical 66, 169

**Lymph node** *cont.*
brachial 169
central 169, 399
lateral–see Lymph node, axillary,
brachial
pectoral 169, 399
posterior–see Lymph node, axillary,
subscapular
subscapular 169
of bladder 321
brachial (lateral) axillary–see under Lymph
node axillary
of breast 169
bronchopulmonary 187, 197, 218, 219
buccinator 66
of Calot–see Lymph node, cystic
cardiac (of stomach)–see Lymph node,
gastric, left
carinal–see Lymph node, tracheobronchial
cecal 297
celiac 227, 249, 295, 296, 298, 299
central axillary–see under Lymph node
axillary
cervical 66, 67, 197, 227
Cloquet's–see Lymph node, inguinal, deep,
highest
colic 297
cubital 452
cystic 298, 299
deltopectoral 452
diaphragmatic 227
epicolic 297
epigastric
inferior 249
superficial 249, 378
of esophagus 227
facial 66
gastric, left 227, 295, 299
gastroepiploic–see Lymph node, gastro-
omental
gastro-omental 295
of genitalia 379
hepatic 291, 298, 299
hilar–see Lymph node, bronchopulmonary
hypogastric–see Lymph node, iliac,
internal
ileocolic 297
iliac
common 249, 297, 321, 377, 379
external 249, 297, 321, 377, 379,
510
internal 249, 297, 321, 377, 379
inferior vena cava 298
infracardiac 227
infrapyloric–see Lymph node, subpyloric
inguinal
deep 249, 377–379, 5140
highest 249, 377–379
superficial 249, 297, 377–379, 510
intercalated 66, 67
intercostal 227, 249
internal thoracic–see Lymph node,
parasternal

**Lymph node** *cont.*
interpectoral 169
intestinal–see Lymph node, superior
mesenteric, juxtaintestinal group
intrapulmonary–see Lymph node,
pulmonary
jugular
anterior–see Lymph node, cervical,
anterior superficial
external–see Lymph node, cervical,
lateral superficial
internal–see Lymph node, cervical, deep
lateral
jugulodigastric 66, 67
juguloomohyoid 66, 67
of kidney 321
of large intestine 297
of limb
lower 510
upper 452
of liver–see Lymph node, hepatic
lumbar 249, 321, 377
of lung 197
mandibular 66
mastoid 66
mediastinal 227, 249, 513
mesenteric
inferior 249, 297, 299
superior 249, 295–297, 299
of mouth 66, 67
nasolabial 66
of neck 66, 67
obturator 377
occipital 66
of oral region 66, 67
pancreatic 295, 299
pancreaticoduodenal 299
paracolic 297
parasternal 169
paratracheal 197, 227
paravesical 321
parotid 66
pectoral (anterior) axillary–see under
Lymph node, axillary
of pelvis 377, 379
of perineum 377–379
of pharynx 66, 67
phrenic, inferior 169, 249
popliteal 510
preaortic 249, 297, 379
presacral–see also Lymph node,
sacral, middle
pretracheal 66, 68
promontorial 321, 377, 379
pulmonary 197
pyloric 298 299
rectal 297
retrocardiac 227
retropharyngeal 67
retropyloric 295
of Rosenmüller–see Lymph node, inguinal,
deep, highest

**Lymph node** *cont.*
　Rotter's–see Lymph node, interpectoral
　sacral
　　lateral 249, 377, 379
　　middle 249, 321, 377, 379
　scalene–see Lymph node, cervical, inferior
　　deep
　sigmoid 297
　of small intestine 296
　spinal accessory–see Lymph node, cervical,
　　deep lateral
　splenic 295, 299
　sternocleidomastoid 66
　of stomach 295
　　nodes around cardia 227, 295, 298
　subclavian–see Lymph node, apical axillary
　subinguinal–see Lymph node, inguinal
　submandibular 54, 66, 67
　submental 66, 67
　subparotid 66
　subpyloric 295
　subscapular (posterior) axillary–see under
　　Lymph node, axillary
　supraclavicular 66
　suprahyoid 66
　suprapyloric 295
　thoracic, internal–see Lymph node,
　　parasternal
　thyroid 66
　of tongue 67
　tracheal–see Lymph node, paratracheal
　tracheobronchial 197, 218, 219, 227,
　　249, 514, 515
　transverse cervical 66
　of urinary bladder 321, 379
　of vena cava, inferior 298
　vesical 321, 379
**Lymph nodule**
　of appendix 266
　aggregate of small intestine 263
　of stomach 259
**Lymph trunk**
　bronchomediastinal 197, 249
　intestinal 249, 296
　jugular 66, 197, 249
　lumbar 249, 296, 321
　subclavian 66, 197, 249
**Lymph vessel**–see also Lymph node; Lymph
　　nodule
　anal 297
　of breast 169
　of esophagus 227
　of genitalia
　　female 377
　　male 379
　of hand 452
　of intestine
　　large 297
　　small 296
　of kidneys 321
　of liver 274, 298
　of lower limbs 510

**Lymph vessel** *cont.*
　of lung 197
　of mammary gland 169
　of oral region 66
　of pancreas 299
　perianal 297
　of perineum (female) 378
　of pelvis
　　female 377
　　male 379
　of pharynx
　of posterior abdominal wall 249
　prostatic 379
　of stomach 295
　testicular 379
　of trachea 190
　of upper limb 452
　of urinary bladder 321
Lymphoid nodule
　aggregated
　　of vermiform appendix 266
　　of ileum (Peyer's patches) 263
　solitary
　　of ileum 263
　　of stomach 259

**M**

**Mackenrodt**–see Ligament, cardinal
**Macula** lutea 82, 86, 114
**Magenstrasse**–see Canal, gastric
**Mall**–see Space, periportal (Mall)
**Malleollus** 478, 479, 481–486, 493–495
**Malleus** 87–89, 91, 118
**Malpighian**–see Corpuscle, renal
**Mandible** 1, 2, 9, **10,** 11, 22, 30, 47, 54, 57,
　60, 62
**Manubrium**–see also Handle
　malleus–see Handle, of malleus
　sternum 22, 23, 30, 57, 170, 171, 176,
　　186, 391, 513, 514
**Margin**–see also Border
　acetabular 331, 453
　of heart–see also Border, of heart
　　acute 201
　　obtuse 201
　of pharyngeal constrictor muscles 59
Marshall's ligament–see Vein, oblique, of left
　atrium
**Mater**
　arachnoid 94, 96, 103, 155, 156
　dura 34, 91, 93–97, 103, 148, 149, 155,
　　156, 165
　pia 94, 96, 149, 155, 156
**Matter**
　gray 151, 155
　white 151, 155
**Maxilla** 1–3, 5, 8, 9, 31–34, 42, 44, 46, 50,
　76, 93
McBurney–see Point, McBurney's
McGregor–see Line, McGregor's
**Measurement** of pelvis 332

**Meatus**
　acoustic
　　external 2, 5, 9, 87, 88, 91
　　internal 3, 7, 87, 92, 117, 118
　urethral, external–see Orifice, urethral,
　　external
　nasal
　　inferior 32, 42, 77
　　middle 32, 42, 44
　　superior 32, 44
**Mediastinum** 218–230
　cross section of 230
　lateral views 218–219
　testis 362
**Medulla**
　of kidney 313, 317, 318, 519
　oblongata 39, 100, 109, 118, 128, 129,
　　153, 154, 215, 306, 323
　spinal–see Cord, spinal
　of suprarenal gland 325, 326
Meibomian–see Gland, tarsal
Meissner–see Plexus (nerve), myenteric
**Melanocyte** 511
**Membrane**
　atlantoaxial, posterior 16
　atlantooccipital
　　anterior 14, 16, 57, 59
　　posterior 14, 16
　basilar, of cochlea 91
　costocoracoid 399
　cricothyroid–see Ligament,
　　cricothyroid, median
　Descemet's–see Lamina, posterior limiting,
　　of cornea
　glassy, of hair follicle 511
　intercostal
　　external 166, 174, 175, 177, 179, 241
　　internal 166, 179, 218, 219, 241
　interosseous, of
　　forearm 409, 411, 413, 419, 424,
　　　425
　　leg 476, 477, 479, 483, 485, 487,
　　　490
　obturator 246, 330, 345, 454
　perineal 329, 333, 336, 343, 345,
　　351–353, 355–357, 363, 366, 368,
　　374–376
　pharyngobasilar–see Fascia,
　　pharyngobasilar
　Reissner's–see Membrane, vestibular
　suprapleural 218, 219
　tectorial, of
　　atlantoaxial joint 15, 16
　　cochlea 91
　thyrohyoid 24, 57, 59, 61, 62, 68, 70, 71,
　　223
　tympanic 87–89, 91
　　secondary 91
　vestibular (Reissner's) 91
**Meninges** 94–96, 103, 155, 156
　arteries 95
　veins 94–96
**Meniscus** of knee 473–476

**Mesentery** 165, **252–257,** 261, 263, 291, 308, 328, 329, 339, 340
  relation to intestines 253, 254
**Meshwork,** trabecular, of iridocorneal angle 83
**Mesoappendix** 264, 266, 304
**Mesocolon**
  sigmoid 254, 267, 287, 311, 319, 363
  transverse 252–256, 261, 267, 287, 291, 311, 329
**Mesometrium** (of broad ligament) 346
**Mesosalpinx** (of broad ligament) 344, 346
**Mesovarium** (of broad ligament) 344, 345, 346
Metacarpal–see Bone, metacarpal
Metatarsal–see Bone, metatarsal
**Mirror,** Goldmann gonioscopic 84
**Modiolus,** cochlear 91
Monro–see Foramen, interventricular (Monro)
**Mons** pubis 350
Morgagni–see Column, anal (Morgagni); Appendix, vesicular (hydatid of Morgagni); Lacuna, urethral
Morquio–see Syndrome, Morquio's
**Mouth**
  floor of 47
  glands of 55
  inspection of 45
  lymph nodes of 66, 67
  muscles of 47, 54
  nerves of 56, 65
  roof of 46
  veins of 64
  movement–see Action
**Mucosa**
  of colon 267
  of duodenum 262, 278
  of esophagus 223, 224
  of ileum 263, 308
  of intestine
    large 267, 308
    small 263, 308
  of jejunum 263, 308
  olfactory 38, 113
  pharyngeal 58
  of stomach 224, 259
  of tongue 52
  of trachea 190
Müller–see Muscle, tarsal, superior (Müller)
Müllerian duct–see Duct, paramesonephric (müllerian)
**Muscle**
  abdominal oblique–see Muscle, oblique, external; internal
  of abdominal wall 232–237, 246
  abductor
    digiti minimi (hand) 430, 434, 439, 445
    digiti minimi (foot) 492, 493, 495, 497–500, 505
    hallucis 492, 493, 495, 497–500, 505
    pollicis brevis 430, 434, 435, 444
    pollicis longus 411, 414, 415, 419, 436, 438, 439, 447

**Muscle** *cont.*
  adductor
    brevis 459, 467, 471, 503
    hallucis 492, 499, 501, 505
    longus 458, 459, 466, 467, 471, 503, 523
    magnus **459,** 461, 466–468, 471, 472, 476, 482, 503, 504
      hamstrings (ischiocondylar) part of 503
    minimus 459, 461, 468
    pollicis 429–431, 434, 435, 445
  anal sphincter–see Sphincter, anal
  anconeus 403, 414, 415, 419, 446, 447
  of arm 402, 403
  arrector, of hair 511
  articularis, genus 471, 473, 476, 502
  aryepiglottic 72, 74
  arytenoid
    oblique 61, 72, 74, 223
    transverse 57, 61, 72–74, 223
  auricularis 20, 21
  of back 160–162, 164
  biceps
    brachii 394–397, 399, 401, **402,** 404, 406, 408, 416–418, 442, 443, 513–515
    femoris 460, **461,** 468, 469, 472, 473, 476, 479, 481–486, 504, 506
  brachialis 400, **402,** 404, 406, 416–418, 442, 443, 446
  brachioradialis **402–404,** 406, 414, 415, **416–419,** 442, 446, 447
  buccinator 20, 21, 41, 42, 46, 48, **49,** 54, 55, 59, 62, 63, 117
  bulbocavernosus–see Muscle, bulbo-spongiosus
  bulbospongiosus 329, 338, 343, 345, 351–353, **355,** 357, 367, 368, 375, 376, 388
  ciliary 82, 83, 115, 126
  circular
    of duodenum 262
    esophageal 59, 61–69, 222–224, 229
    intestinal 308
    of rectum 336, 365, 366
    of stomach 224
  coccygeus–see Muscle, (ischio-) coccygeus
  compressor
    –see under Compressor
  constrictor
    pharyngeal
      inferior 22, 59, 61, **62,** 69, 70, 74, 120, 221–223
        cricopharyngeal part–see Muscle, cricopharyngeus
      middle 22, 53, 58, 59, **61,** 62, 69, 120, 223
      superior 35, 46, 49, 53, 54, 58, **59,** 61–63, 69, 120, 223
        glossopharyngeal part 53, 59
    of pupil–see Muscle, sphincter, of pupil
  coracobrachialis 397, 401, 402, 404, 406, 442, 443, 514, 515

**Muscle** *cont.*
  corrugator
    cutis ani 365, 366
    supercilii 20, 21, 31, 117
  cremaster 233, 234, 242, 243, 245, 361, 362
  cricoarytenoid
    lateral 72–74
    posterior 61, 72–74, 223
  cricopharyngeus 59, 61, 62, 69, 70, 74, 221–223
  cricothyroid 24, 62, 68, 72–74, 120
  deltoid 22, 23, 160, 163, 174, 175, 178, 394, **395,** 397, 399, 401, 402–404, 406, 442, 446, 513, 515, 524
  depressor
    anguli oris 20, 21, 48, 117
    labii inferioris 20, 21, 48, 117
    septi nasi 20, 21, 31, 117
  detrusor–see Muscle, of urinary bladder, intrinsic
  digastric
    anterior belly 22–24, 26, 27, 29, 41, **47,** 55, 62
    posterior belly 22–24, 27, 29, 35, 41, **47,** 53–55, 61, 62, 67, 117
  dilator, of pupil 83, 115, 126
  of duodenum–see Muscle, suspensory, of duodenum
  epicranius–see Muscle, occipitofrontalis
  erector spinae 160, **161,** 162, 165, 166, 177–179, 241, 312, 324, 327, 328, 513–522
  of esophagus
    circular 59, 61, 69, 222–224, 229
    longitudinal 59, 61, 69, 222–224, 229
  of expiration 183
  extensor
    carpi radialis brevis 403, **411,** 414–416, 419, 436, 438, 439, 446, 447
    carpi radialis longus 403, 406, **411,** 414–416, 419, 436, 438, 439, 446, 447
    carpi ulnaris 403, **411,** 414, 415, 419, 438, 439, 446, 447
    digiti minimi **411,** 414, 415, 419, 438, 439, 447
    digitorum 403, **411,** 414, 419, 431, 433, 438–440, 446, 447
    digitorum brevis 484–486, 493, **494,** 495, 500, 506
    digitorum longus 460, 473, **484–487,** 493–495, 500, 506
    hallucis brevis 484, 485, 494, 495, 500, 506
    hallucis longus 484–487, 493–495, 500, 506
    indicis 411, 415, 419, 438, 439, 447
    pollicis brevis **411,** 414, 415, 418, 419, 436, 438, 439, 447
    pollicis longus **411,** 414, 415, 419, 431, 436, 438, 439, 447
  of eye 79, 115
    extrinsic
      oblique
        inferior 78, 79, 115

**Muscle** *cont.*
    superior 78, 79, 81, 115
    rectus
        inferior 78, 79, 115
        lateral 78, 79, 81, 82, 115
        medial 78, 79, 81, 82, 115
        superior 78, 79, 81, 115
    intrinsic
        ciliary 88, 83, 115, 126
        dilator, of pupil 83, 115, 126
        sphincter, of pupil 83, 115, 126
    of facial expression 20, 21, 48, 117
    fibularis (peroneus)
        brevis 481–486, 487, 490–495, 499, 500, 506
        longus 460, 472, 473, 481–486, 487, 490–495, 499, 500, 506
        tertius 484, 486, 487, 491, 493–495, 500
    flexor
        carpi radialis 402, 404, **412,** 416–419, 424, 429–431, 442, 444
        carpi ulnaris 403, **412,** 414–419, 424, 429, 430, 434, 442, 445
        digiti minimi brevis (hand) 431, 434, 445
        digiti minimi brevis (foot) 492, 497–500, 505
        digitorum brevis 492, 493, 497–499, 505
        digitorum longus 481–483, 487, 493, 505
        digitorum profundus **413,** 418, 419, 424, 427, 429–433, 440, 442, 444, 445
        digitorum superficialis **413,** 416–419, 424, 427, 429–433, 440, 442, 444
        hallucis brevis 487, 497–500, 505
        hallucis longus 483, 487, 505
        pollicis brevis 418, 430, 434, 435, 444, 445
        pollicis longus **413,** 416–419, 424, 429–431, 442, 444
    of floor of mouth 47
    of foot 494–501
    of forearm 410–418
    frontalis–see Muscle, occipitofrontalis frontal belly
    gastrocnemius 460, 461, 468, 472, 473, 476, **481–**487, 504, 505
    gemellus
        inferior 461, 468, 469, 523
        superior 461, 468, 469
    genioglossus 53, 54, 57, 122
    geniohyoid 24, 30, 47, 53, 57, 59, 122, 123
    glossopharyngeus–see Muscle, constrictor, pharyngeal, superior, glossopharyngeal part
    gluteus
        maximus 160, 163, 237, 312, 336, 352, 355, 346, 367, 368, 381, 382, 384, 460, **461,** 468, 469, 471, 522, 523
        medius 160, 237, 312, 458, 460, **461,** 462, 466–469, 522, 523
        minimus 461, 462, 466–469, 522, 523
    gracilis 458, 459, 461, 466–458, 471–473, 481, 503

**Muscle** *cont.*
    of hand 428–434, 439–see also individual muscles
    of hip 460–462
    hypothenar 428, 429, 431, 434, 445
    hyoglossus 22, 24, 29, 47, 53, 54, 58, 59, 62, 122
    iliacus 236, 246, 311, 341, 364, 458, **462,** 464, 465, 502, 521–523
    iliococcygeus 333–336, 345, 367
    iliocostalis 161, 331
    iliopsoas 236, 243, 458, 459, **462,** 466, 467, 470, 471, 523
    infrahyoid 24–see also individual muscles
    infraspinatus 160, 166, 178, 179, 394–396, 397–399, 403, 446, 513–515
    of inspiration 183
    intercostal 513–520, 524, 525
        external 162, 166, 174, 175, **177,** 179, 183, 186, 218, 219, 233, 238, 241
        innermost 166, 176, 179, 238, 241
        internal 119, 166, 175, 176, 179, 183, 186, 188, 218, 238, 241
    interosseous
        dorsal (of hand) 415, 429, 431, 433, 434, 436, 439, 445
        dorsal (of foot) 492, 494, 495, 500, 501, 505
        palmar 431, 433, 434, 445
        plantar 492, 499–501, 505
    interspinalis
        cervicis 162
        lumborum 162
    intertransversarius, lateral 162
    ischiocavernosus 337, 338, 343, 345, 351, 352, 355–357, 363, 367, 375, 376
    (ischio-)coccygeus 246, 333, 334–336, 369, 373, 381–383, 465
    of larynx 72
    latissimus dorsi **160,** 163, 165, 166, 174, 178, 232, 233, 237, 238, 240, 241, 312, 324, 327, 328, 395, 397, 399, 400, 402, 404, 406, 514–517
    of leg 481–486
    levator
        anguli oris 20, 21, 48, 117
        ani 246, 267, 293, 306, 329, **333–**338, 343, 345, 351–353, 355–357, 363–369, 373, 375, 381, 382, 465, 523
        prerectal fibers of 336
        costorum 162, 177
        labii superioris 20, 21, 48, 60, 117
            alaeque nasi 20, 21, 48, 117
        palpebrae superioris 76, 78, 79, 81, 115
        scapulae 22, 27, 30, 160, 163, 175, 177, **178,** 395, 398, 446
        veli palatini 46, 49, 58, 59, 61, 62, 88, 89, 93, 120
    longissimus 161, 331
        capitis 161, 164
        cervicis 161

**Muscle** *cont.*
    thoracis 161
    longitudinal
        of duodenum 262
        esophageal 59, 69
        intestinal 312
        pharyngeal 59, 223
        of rectum 336, 364–366
        of stomach 224
    longus
        capitis, 22, 25, 54
        colli 25, 30, 220
    lumbrical
        (of foot) 492, 497–500, 505
        (of hand) 429–434, 444, 445
    of Luschka
    masseter 19, 22, 23, 48, 55, 54
    of mastication 48, 49
    mentalis 20, 21, 48, 117
    of mouth 47–49
    Müller's–see Muscle, tarsal, superior (Müller)
    multifidus 162
    mylohyoid 21–23, 26, 27, 29, 41, **47,** 53–55, 59, 62
    nasalis 20, 21, 31, 117
    of neck 23–25
    oblique
        external 160, 161, 163, 165, 167, 174–179, 183, 232–238, 240–243, 245, 246, 312, 324, 327, 328, 339, 340, 354, 355, 395, 460
        inferior 78, 79, 115
        internal 160, 161, 165, 174, 175, 177, 178, 183, 233–238, 240, 242, 243, 246, 312, 324, 328, 339, 340
        superior 78, 79, 81, 115
    obliquus capitis
        inferior 161, 162, 164
        superior 161, 162, 164
    obturator
        externus 459, 467, 503
        internus 236, 246, 333–336, 343, 345, 364, 369, 373, 382, 461, 465, 468, 469, 523
    occipitalis–see Muscle, occipitofrontalis, occipital belly
    occipitofrontalis
        frontal belly 20, 21, 31, 117
        occipital belly 21, 117, 164
    omohyoid
        inferior belly 22–**24,** 26, 27, 122, 123, 174, 175, 395, 398–400
        superior belly 22–**24,** 26, 27, 30, 47, 122, 123, 174, 175, 186
    opponens
        digiti minimi 430, 434, 445
        pollicis 430, 434, 435, 444
    orbicularis
        oculi 20, 21, 76, 117
        oris 20, 21, 31, 48, 54, 117
    palatoglossus 46, 52–54, 58, 120

**Muscle** *cont.*

palatopharyngeus 46, 52–54, 58, 59, 61, 120, 223, 240
palmaris
brevis 428, 445
longus 412, 418–419, 424, 428–430, 444
papillary 516
anterior 208, 209, 211–213, 230
conal–see Muscle, papillary, septal
medial 208, 211, 212
posterior 208, 209, 211–213, 230
septal 208, 211, 212
pectinate 208
pectineus 458, 459, 466, 467, 470, 471, 502, 523
pectoralis
major 22, 23, 26, 167, **174,** 175, 179, 186, 230, 232, 233, 395, 399, 400, 402, 404, 406, 513–516, 524
minor **174,** 175, 186, 397, 399, 400, 402, 404, 513–515, 524
perineal–see also individual muscles of perineum
transverse
deep 329, 333, 337, 342, 345, 352, 357, 363, 375
superficial 333, 334, 351, 352, 355–357, 363, 367, 368, 375, 376
peroneus–see Muscle, fibularis (peroneus)
pharyngeal constrictor–see Muscle, constrictor, pharyngeal
of pharynx 58, 59, 61, 62, 68, 223
piriformis 246, **333**–335, 373, 381–383, 461, 465, 468, 469
plantaris 460, 461, 468, 472, 476, 481, **482,** 483, 487, 504, 505
platysma 20, 21, 23, 26, 30, 117
popliteus 461, 473–**476,** 482, 483, 487, 505
prevertebral 25
procerus 20, 21, 31, 117
pronator
quadratus **410,** 418, 419, 430, 431, 434, 444
teres 402, 404, **410,** 415–419, 442, 444
psoas
major 165, 181, 236, 246–248, 250, 261, 311, 312, 320, 324, 328, 339–341, 371, 458, **462,** 464, 465, 502, 520–523
minor 246, 328, 339, 340, 462
pterygoid
external–see Muscle, pterygoid, lateral
internal–see Muscle, pterygoid, medial
lateral 35, 41, 48, 49
medial 19, 35, 41, 46, 49, 54, 61, 65
pubococcygeus 333–336, 345, 367
puborectalis 329, 333–336, 363, 367, 369, 523
pyramidalis 233, 245
quadratus
femoris 459, 461, 467–469

**Muscle** *cont.*

lumborum 162, 165, **181,** 246–248, 250, 311, 312, 324, 328, 339, 340, 462, 464
plantae 498, 499, 502, 505
quadriceps femoris 458, 502–see also Muscle, rectus femoris; vastus intermedialis; vastus lateralis; vastus medialis
rectococcygeus 246
rectourethralis 246, 336
of rectum 336, 364–366
rectus
abdominis 174, 175, 179, 183, **233**–236, 238, 240, 241, 243, 245, 327–329, 338, 339–341, 351, 517–522
capitis
anterior 25, 67
lateralis 25
posterior (major and minor) 161, 162, 164
of eye
inferior 78, 79, 115
lateral 78, 79, 81, 82, 115
medial 78, 79, 81, 82, 115
superior 78, 79, 81, 115
femoris 458–460, 466, 467, 471, 502, 523
of respiration 183
rhomboid
major 160, 163, 166, 178, 179, 237, **395,** 446, 513–515
minor 160, 163, 178, 399, 450
risorius 20, 21, 117
sacrospinalis–see Muscle, erector spinae
salpingopharyngeus 58, 59, 61, 93, 120
sartorius 234, **458**–461, 466, 467, 471–473, 481, 484, 485, 502, 523
scalene
anterior 22–24, **25,** 27, 28, 30, 63–65, 68, 173, 175–177, 182, 183, 186, 195, 200, 218–220, 398, 400, 524, 525
middle (medius) 22–**25,** 27, 30, 63–65, 173, 175, 177, 183, 220, 525
posterior 22–**25,** 30, 175, 177, 183, 525
semimembranosus 460, **461,** 468, 471, 472, 474, 476, 481–483, 504
semispinalis
capitis 160–162, 164, 395
cervicis 164
thoracis 162
semitendinosus 458, 459, **461,** 468, 469, 471–473, 481, 504
serratus
anterior 160, 166, 167, 174, 175, **177**–179, 232–234, 237, 238, 240, 241, 327, 395, 399, 400, 513–517, 524
posterior inferior 160, 161, 165, 177, 178, 237, 312
posterior superior 160, 161, 177
of shoulder 395–397–see also individual muscles
of soft palate 59

**Muscle** *cont.*

soleus 461, 472, 481–487, 493, 495, 504, 505
sphincter
anal–see Sphincter, anal
of pupil 83, 115, 126
urethrae 236, 333, 336, 338, 342, 343, 351–353, 357–359, 374, 375, 388
spinalis 161, 331
splenius
capitis 22, 160, 161, 164, 177, 178, 395
cervicis 160, 161, 164, 177
stapedius 88, 89
sternalis 174
sternocleidomastoid **22,** 23, 26, 27, 29, 30, 54, 55, 67, 121, 123, 160, 164, 174, 178, 183, 186, 395, 400
sternohyoid 22–**24,** 26, 27, 30, 47, 122, 123, 174–176, 186
sternothyroid 22–**24,** 26, 27, 30, 122, 123, 174–176, 186
of stomach 224, 260
styloglossus 22, 35, 53, 54, 59, 62, 122
stylohyoid 22–24, 27, 29, 35, 41, 47, 53–55, 61, 62, 117
stylopharyngeus 53, 54, 58, 59, 61, 62, 119, 120, 223
subclavius 174, 175, 218, 219, 395, 399, 400, 524
subcostal 241
submucosae ani 365, 366
subscapularis 166, 177, 179, 394, 396, 397, 399, 402, 404, 513–515, 525
supinator 410, 415, 417–419, 442, 447
suprahyoid 24–see also individual muscles
supraspinatus 160, 163, 178, 394–396, 397–399, 403, 446, 525
suspensory, of duodenum 253, 260, 262, 278
tarsal, superior (Müller) 76
temporalis 41, 48
tensor
fasciae latae 237, 458, **460,** 466–469, 471, 523
tympani 41, 88, 89
veli palatini 41, 46, 49, 58, 59, 62, 93
teres
major 160, 163, 166, 177, 178, 237, 395, 397–400, 402–404, 406, 446, 514, 515
minor 160, 163, 178, 394–396, 397–399, 403, 446, 513, 514
thenar 416, 428, 429, 434, 435, 444
of thigh 458–462
of thoracic wall 174–178, 183
thyroarytenoid 72–74
thyroepiglottic 72, 74
thyrohyoid 22–24, 26, 27, 47, 122, 123
tibialis
anterior 460, 472, 473, **484**–487, 491, **492**–495, 500, 506

**Muscle** *cont.*
    posterior 481–**483,** 487, 491, **492,** 493,
        498–500, 505
    of tongue 52–54, 122
    trachealis 190
    transverse perineal–see Muscle, perineal,
        transverse
    transversospinalis 177, 513–see also
        Muscle, longissimus; multifidus;
        semispinalis
    transversus
        abdominis 161, 162, 165, 175–177,
            181, 183, **234**–238, 240, 241, 243,
            245, 246, 250, 311, 312, 327, 328,
            339, 340, 462, 464, 521, 522
        thoracis 166, 175, 176, 179, 180, 230, 238
    trapezius 22–24, 26, 30, 121, 123, **160,**
        163, 164, 166, 174, 175, 178, 179,
        237, 241, 395, 399, 400, 513–517, 525
    triceps brachii 395, 397, 398, 400, **403,**
        404, 406, 408, 414, 416, 446, 513–515
    of urinary bladder, intrinsic 342–344, 353,
        358, 359
    of urogenital diaphragm 352, 358
    uvular 46
    vastus
        intermedius **458,** 459, 467, 471, 473, 502
        lateralis 458–**460,** 466–468, 471–473,
            484, 486, 502
        medialis **458,** 459, 466, 467, 471–473,
            484, 502
    vocalis 72–74
    zygomaticus
        major 20, 21, 48, 117
        minor 20, 21, 48, 117
**Muscle layer**
    of appendix 266
    of colon 265
    of duodenum 260, 262, 278
    of esophagus 61, 69, 260
    of ileum 263, 265
    of jejunum 263
    of large intestine 267
    of stomach 260
**Muscularis** mucosae
    of intestine 308
    of rectum 365, 366
    of stomach 259
**Musculus**
    submucosae ani 365, 366
    uvulae–see Muscle, uvular
**Myometrium** 346


**N**

Naris, posterior–see Choana
**Nasopharynx** 32, 56, 57, 60, 87, 93, 98
**Navicular** 488, 489, 491, 500, 501
Navicular bone–see Navicular
**Neck**
    arteries of 28, 29, 63
    of bladder 338, 343, 353

**Neck** *cont.*
    bones of 9, 12, 13
    cutaneous nerves of 26
    fascial layers of 30
    of femur 454, 455, 523
    of fibula 478
    of gallbladder 276
    of humerus 392, 393, 513
    ligaments of 14, 15
    lymph nodes of 66, 67
    of mandible 10
    muscles of 21–25
    nerves of 18, 26, 27, 65, 123, 124
    of pancreas 279
    of radius 407, 409
    of rib 170, 171, 180, 516
    of scapula 170, 392, 393
    surgical–see Neck, of humerus
    of tooth 51
    veins of
        superficial 26
        deep 64
**Nephron** of kidney 317, 318
**Nerve**
    of abdominal wall 240, 241, 250
    abducent 78, 81, 98, 108, 111, 112, **115**
    accessory 27, 29, 65, 98, 108, 110–112,
        120, **121,** 123, 163, 177, 178
        external branch 121
        internal branch 121
        obturator 250, 463, 464
    alveolar
        inferior 35, 41, 47, 49, 54, 56, 65, 116,
            125, 128, 751
        superior 39, 40, 56, 65, 116
        nasal branch 37
    anal (rectal), inferior 306, 381, 382, 384,
        385, 463, 469
    anococcygeal 382, 384, 463, 465
    antebrachial cutaneous–see Nerve,
        cutaneous, of forearm
    anterior cutaneous branch of femoral–see
        under Nerve, femoral, anterior
        cutaneous branch
    anterior division of
        mandibular 41
        obturator–see Nerve, obturator, anterior
            branch
    of arm 442, 443, 446–448
    of arteries 216
    articular–see Articular branch under Nerve,
        auriculotemporal; fibular (peroneal);
        median; obturator; tibial; ulnar
    auricular
        anterior 116
        branch–see under Nerve, mandibular;
            vagus
        great 18, 26, 27, 123, 163, 164
        posterior 19, 41, 117
            occipital branch 117
        to auricular muscles 117
    auriculotemporal 11, 18, 35, **41,** 49, 55,
        65, 116, 119, 128

**Nerve** *cont.*
    articular branch 116
    parotid branch 116
    autonomic 39, 110–112, 115–117, 119,
        120, **124**–128, 152–154, **198,** 199,
        215, 216, 228, **300**–310, 322, 323,
        326, 380, 381, 383, 385–388
        in abdomen 304
        in head 125
        in neck 124
        in thorax 198
    axillary 396, 397, 400, 401, 403, 443,
        444, **446,** 450
    of back 163
    of bile ducts 153, 313
    of blood vessels 216
    brachial cutaneous–see Nerve, cutaneous,
        of arm
    of bronchus 153, 199
    buccal (of mandibular nerve) 18, 35, 41,
        56, 65, 116
        branch of facial–see Nerve, facial,
            buccal branch
        branch of mandibular nerve–see Nerve,
            buccal (of mandibular nerve)
    calcaneal
        lateral–see Nerve, sural, lateral calcaneal
            branch
        medial–see Nerve, tibial, medial,
            calcaneal branch
    cardiac (sympathetic)
        cervical 63, 124, 125, 152, 198,
            214–216, 228
        thoracic 124, 152, 182, 198, 214–216,
            228
    cardiac (vagal)
        cervical 63, 65, 120, 124, 125, 152,
            198, 214, 215, 228
        thoracic 120, 124, 152, 182, 198, 214,
            215, 228
    caroticotympanic 117, 119
    carotid
        internal 39, 124, 125, 127, 152, 154,
            216
        sinus branch–see Nerve,
            glossopharyngeal, carotid branch
    cavernous 381, 387
    celiac–see Celiac branch under Nerve,
        vagus
    cervical
        branch of facial–see Nerve, facial,
            cervical branch
        transverse 18, 26, 27, 123
    chorda tympani 41, 56, 65, 88, 89,
        116–118, **125,** 127–129, 152
    ciliary
        long 40, 81, 115, 116, 125, 126
        short 40, 81, 115, 116, 125, 126
    of clitoris 250, 384, 385, 463, 469
    cluneal
        inferior 163, 382, 388, 468, 469, 504,
            509
        middle 163, 468, 509

**Nerve** *cont.*
superior 163, 237, 468, 509
coccygeal 148, 149, 465
to coccygeus muscle 250, 463, 465
cochlear 87, 90–92, **118**
communicating–see under Branch,
communicating
cranial 110–122, 125–129–see also
individual nerves
crural, medial cutaneous 506
cutaneous 511–see also individual nerves
antebrachial–see under Nerve,
cutaneous, of forearm
of anterior abdominal wall 240, 241
of arm 447, 448, 450
lateral
inferior 403, 446–448, 450
superior 163, 397, 403, 446–448,
450
medial 240, 400, 401, 404, 406,
442–444, 448, 450
posterior 403, 446, 447, 450
brachial–see under Nerve, cutaneous, of
arm
branch–see under Nerve, femoral;
iliophypogastric; intercostal; spinal;
subcostal
dorsal
intermediate (superficial fibularl) 506,
508
lateral (sural) 494, 495, 504–506, 508,
509
medial (superficial fibular) 506, 508
of face 18
femoral–see under Nerve, cutaneous, of
thigh
of foot 505, 506, 508, 509
of forearm 443, 447, 449, 450
lateral 402, 406, 416–419, 438,
441–443, 448–450
medial 400, 401, 404, 406, 416, 419,
438, 441–444, 448–450
posterior 403, 406, 419, 437, 438,
441, 446–450
of hand 441, 444, 445, 448, 450
of head 18
of leg 502, 506, 508, 509
of lower limb 508, 509
of neck 18, 26
perforating 382, 384, 463, 465, 469, 509
of shoulder 448, 450
sural
lateral 481, 482, 504–506
median 481, 482, 504, 505
of thigh 502–504, 508, 509
lateral 240, 244, 250, 311, 380,
462–464, 466, 467, 471, 502,
503, 508, 509
posterior 148, 384, 463, 465, 468,
469, 471, 504, 509
pudendal branch 384, 469, 504

**Nerve** *cont.*
deep–see under Nerve, fibular (peroneal);
petrosal; temporal–see also Deep
branch under Nerve, plantar, lateral;
radial; ulnar
dental branch–see under Nerve, maxillary
to descending colon 153
of diaphragm 182
digastric–see Digastric branch under
Nerve, facial
digital
dorsal (finger) 436–438, 440, 441, 447,
449, 450
dorsal (toe) 484, 485, 494, 495, 506,
508
palmar
common 428, 429, 431, 435, 441,
442, 444, 445
proper 428, 429, 435, 440–442, 444,
445, 449, 450
dorsal branch to dorsum of middle
and distal phalanges 444, 445
proper (thumb) 429, 435
plantar
common 498, 505
proper 485, 494–499, 505
dorsal branch to dorsum of middle
and distal phalanges 485, 494
to dilator of pupil 115, 153
dorsal
branch of–see under Nerve, radial; ulnar
of clitoris 250, 384, 385, 463, 474
of penis 250, 355, 357, 376, 380–382,
387, 463, 469
scapular–see Nerve, scapular, dorsal
of duodenum 300–303
of esophagus 228, 229
ethmoidal
anterior 18, 37, 38, 40, 81, 115, 116
nasal branch 11, 31, 27, 38, 40, 116
posterior 40, 81, 115, 116
external branch–see under Nerve,
accessory; laryngeal, superior nerve
to eye muscles 78, 81, 112, 115, 126
facial **19,** 26, 29, 35, 39, 41, 54, 55, 65,
87, 89, 92, 98, 108, 110–112,
**117**–119, 125, 127–129, 152, 153
buccal branch 19, 117
cervical branch 19, 117
digastric branch (to posterior belly of
digastric muscle) 19
marginal mandibular branch 19, 26, 117
stylohyoid branch 19
temporal branch 19, 117
zygomalic branch 19, 117
femoral 236, 244, 250, 341, 378, 380,
462–464, 466, 467, 471, **502,** 503,
510, 521–523
anterior cutaneous branch 250, 380,
502, 508, 509

**Nerve** *cont.*
branch–see under Nerve, genitofemoral
lateral, cutaneous–see Nerve, cutaneous,
of thigh, lateral
posterior, cutaneous–see Nerve,
cutaneous, of thigh, posterior
fibular (peroneal)
common 461, 463, 465, 468,
471–473,481–486, 504–**506**
articular branch 504
deep 484, 485, 487, 494, 495, 506
lateral and medial branch 485, 494,
504
dorsal digital branch 494
superficial 484–487, 494, 495, 504,
506, 508
dorsal digital branch 494
of foot 494–499, 504, 505
of forearm 442, 444, 445, 447
frontal 40, 78, 81, 115, 116, 125
of gallbladder 153
ganglionic–see Ganglionic branch under
Nerve, maxillary
gastric branch–see Nerve, vagus, gastric
branch
to geniohyoid muscle 27
genital–see Genital branch under Nerve,
genitofemoral
of genitalia 153, 380, 384, 386, 387
genitofemoral 240, 244, 250, 311, 319,
328, 380, 462–464, 503, 508
femoral branch **240,** 244, 250, 380, 463,
464, 508
genital branch 240, 243–245, **250,** 361,
380, 463, 464, 508
gingival–see Gingival branch under Nerve,
maxillary
glossopharyngeal 29, 56, 58, 63, 65, 98,
108, 110–112, 117, **119,** 120, 124,
125, 127–129, 152–154, 199
branch to stylopharyngeus 119
carotid branch 119, 124, 125
lingual branch 56, 119
pharyngeal branch 119
tonsillar branch 56, 58, 65, 119
gluteal (inferior and superior) 148, 463,
465, 468, 469
of hair follicle 153
of hand 435–438, 440–442, 444, 445,
447, 449
of heart 153, 214, 215
hepatic–see Hepatic branch under Nerve,
vagus
of hip 469
hypogastric 152, 153, 300, 305, 306, 322,
323, **380,** 381, **383,** 385, 386–388
hypoglossal 27, 29, 41, 53, 54, 64, 65, 98,
108, 111, 112, **122,** 123
meningeal branch 122
to iliacus muscle 463, 464

Nerve *cont.*
  iliohypogastric 148, 163, 237, 240, 250,
      311, 312, 328, 380, 385, 462–**464,**
      503, 509
    cutaneous branch 237, 240, 384
  ilioinguinal 148, 240, 245, 250, 311, 312,
      328, 380, 384, 385, 462–**464,** 503, 508
    anterior labial branch of 250, 384
    anterior scrotal branch of 240, 250,
        380, 508
  to inferior gemellus muscle 463, 465, 469
  infraorbital 18, 31, 37, 39, 40, 65, 76, 78,
      115, 116
    nasal branch 37, 39, 40
  infrapatellar–see Infrapatellar branch under
      Nerve, saphenous
  infratrochlear 18, 31, 40, 81, 116
  intercostal 148, 152, 156, 166, 174–177,
      179, 182, 198, 215, 216, 218, 219,
      228, 240, **241,** 303, 323, 327, 401,
      463–see also Nerve, spinal, thoracic
    cutaneous branch 174–177, 179, 240,
        241
  intercostobrachial 175, 177, 240, 400,
      442, 448, 450
  intermediate (nervus intermedius, of facial
      nerve) 56, 98, 108, 117, 118, 129
  intermesenteric–see Plexus (nerve),
      intermesenteric
  internal branch–see under Nerve,
      accessory; laryngeal superior
  internal carotid 39, 124, 125, 127, 152,
      154, 216
  interosseous
    anterior (median) 418, 419, 444
    of leg (tibial) 505
    posterior (radial) 415, 419, 437, 447
  intestinal–see Intestinal branch under
      Nerve, vagus
  of intestine 312
    large 120, 153, 154, 305, 306, 308
    small 120, 153, 154, 304, 306, 308
  ischiatic–see Nerve, sciatic
  of Jacobson–see Nerve, tympanic
  of kidney 153, 326, 327
  labial–see under Nerve, genitofemoral,
      genital branch; ilioinguinal; perineal
  lacrimal 18, 40, 78, 81, 115, 116, 125
    palpebral branch 18
  of lacrimal gland 153
  laryngeal
    inferior, right (anomalous) 74
    recurrent 28, 30, 65, 68–70, 74, 120,
        124, 152, 182, 195, 198, 200, 201,
        214, 219, 220, 223, 228
    superior 56, 59, 61, 65, 68–70, 74, 120,
        124, 125, 129, 152, 199, 223, 228
      external branch 65, 68, 70, 74, 120
      internal branch 59, 65, 68, 70, 74,
          120, 223
  laryngopharyngeal branch of superior
      cervical ganglion–see under Ganglion,
      cervical, superior

Nerve *cont.*
  of larynx 68, 70, 74, 153
  lateral femoral cutaneous–see Nerve,
      cutaneous, femoral, lateral
  to lateral pterygoid muscle 41, 65
  of leg 481–485, 502–506
  to levator ani muscle 250, 463, 465
  to levator scapulae muscle 27, 123
  lingual 11, 35, 41, 45, 47, 49, 53–56,
      65, 116, 117, 125, 127–129, 152
    branch–see under Nerve,
        glossopharyngeal 56, 119
  of liver 153, 309
  long thoracic 174, 175, 177, 240, 400,
      401, 436
  to longus capitis muscle 27, 123
  to longus colli muscle 27, 123, 401
  lumbar splanchnic 152, 153, 300, 305,
      306, 322, 323, 326, 380, 381, 383,
      385–388
  of lung 153, 198, 199
  mandibular 11, 18, 40, **41,** 56, 65, 81, 98,
      112, 115, 116, 119, 125, 127–129
    meningeal branch 41, 81
  marginal mandibular branch–see under
      Nerve, facial
  masseteric 35, 41, 48, 49, 65, 116
  maxillary 18, 38–**40,** 41, 56, 65, 81, 98,
      112, 115, 116, 125, 127–129
    dental branch 40
    ganglionic branch to pterygopalatine
        ganglion 40
    gingival branch 40
    mandibular branch 40, 81, 116
    nasal branch 116
  to medial pterygoid muscle 41, 65, 116
  median 400–402, 404, 406, 416–419, 424,
      428–430, 434, 435, 441–**444,** 449, 450
    articular branch 444
    motor branch to thenar muscle 478, 434,
        425, 442
    palmar branch 416, 417, 428, 429, 435,
        441, 444, 449, 450
  meningeal branch–see under Nerve,
      hypoglossal; mandibular, maxillary;
      spinal; vagus–see also Tentorial
      (meningeal) branch under Nerve,
      ophthalmic
  mental 18, 41, 65, 116
  motor 511
    branch–see under Nerve, median, motor
        branch to thenar muscle
    root of trigeminal–see Nerve, trigeminal,
        motor and sensory roots
  of mouth 56, 65
  musculocutaneous 400–402, 404, 406,
      418, 441–**443,** 444
  to mylohyoid 11, 35, 41, 47, 49, 54, 65, 116
  nasal–see Nasal branch under Nerve,
      alveolar, superior; ethmoidal, anterior;
      palatine, greater; infraorbital;
      maxillary; also under Ganglion,
      pterygopalatine

Nerve *cont.*
  of nasal cavity 37–39
  nasociliary 40, 78, 81, 115, 116, 125, 126
  nasopalatine 37–39, 116
  of neck 23, 26, 27, 65, 123, 124
  obturator 236, 250, 319, 371, 381,
      463–465, 467, 471, 502, **503,** 508,
      509, 521–523
    accessory 250, 463, 464
    articular branch 503
    anterior branch 467, 503
    posterior branch 467, 503
  to obturator internus muscle 463, 465,
      468, 469
  occipital
    branch–see under Nerve, auricular,
        posterior
    greater 18, 123, 163, 164
    lesser 18, 27, 123, 163, 164
    third 18, 163, 164
  oculomotor 78, 79, 81, 98, 108, 110–112,
      **115,** 125, 152, 153
  olfactory 37, 38, 112, 113
  to omohyoid muscle 27–see also Ansa
      cervicalis
  ophthalmic 18, **40,** 41, 81, 98, 112, 115,
      116, 125–129
    meningeal branch–see Nerve,
        ophthalmic, tentorial (meningeal)
        branch
    tentorial (meningeal) branch 40, 81, 116
  optic 42, 78, 79, 81, 82, 86, 98, 101, 112,
      **114,** 126, 136, 137
  of orbit 40, 81
  palatine
    descending 127
    greater 37–40, 46, 56, 65, 116, 125,127
      nasal branch 37, 38, 125, 127
    lesser 37–40, 46, 56, 65, 116, 125, 127
  palmar–see Palmar branch under Nerve,
      median; ulnar
  palpebral–see Palpebral branch under
      Nerve, lacrimal
  of pancreas 153, 313, 314
  parasympathetic–see Fiber (nerve),
      parasympathetic
  parotid–see Parotid branch under Nerve,
      auriculotemporal
  of parotid gland 128
  pectoral
    lateral 174, 399–401
    medial 174, 399–401
  pelvic splanchnic–see Nerve, splanchnic,
      pelvic
  of pelvic viscera 381, 383, 386, 387
  of penis 250, 355, 357, 376,
      380–382, 387, 463, 469
  perforating cutaneous–see Nerve,
      cutaneous, perforating
  pericardial–see Pericardial branch under
      Nerve, phrenic

**Nerve** *cont.*
perineal
branch–see under Nerve, cutaneous, of
thigh, posterior; spinal, sacral
posterior labial branch of 384, 463, 469
posterior scrotal branch of 381, 382,
463, 469
of perineum 382, 384, 386, 387
of peripheral blood vessels 153
peroneal–see Nerve, fibular (peroneal)
petrosal
deep 38, 39, 117, 119, **125,** 127
greater 38, 39, 56, 81, 89, 117–119, 125,
127, 129
lesser 41, 81, 116, 117, 119, 128
pharyngeal–see Pharyngeal branch under
Nerve, glossopharyngeal; vagus; also
under Ganglion, pterygopalatine
of pharynx 56, 65
phrenic
abdominal portion 181, 300, 302, 309, 326
cervical portion 25, 27, 28, 30, 63, 65,
68, 123, 124, 175, 177, 182, 186,
195, 200, 201, 214, 220
thoracic portion 176, 180, 182, 200,
201, 203, 218, 219, 230, 238, 404,
513, 514
pericardial branch 182
to piriformis muscle 463, 465
plantar
lateral 483, 496, 498, 499, 504, 505, 509
cutaneous branch 496
deep branch 498, 499, 505
superficial branch 498, 499, 505
digital branch (common and proper)
497–499
medial 483, 493, 496–499, 504, 505, 509
cutaneous branch 496
digital branch (common and proper)
497–499
posterior
division of
mandibular 41
obturator–see Nerve, obturator,
posterior branch
presacral–see Plexus (nerve), hypo-gastric,
superior
of prostate 153
to psoas muscle 463, 464
to pterygoid muscle 41, 65, 116
of pterygoid canal (vidian) 37–40, 116,
117, 119, 125, 127, 129
pterygopalatine–see Pterygopalatine branch
under Nerve, maxillary
pudendal 148, 250, 306, 322, 381–388,
463, 465, 468, 469, 523
block (anesthesia) of 384
perineal branch–see Nerve, perineal
of pupil
dilator 115, 153
sphincter 115, 153

**Nerve** *cont.*
pyloric–see Pyloric branch under Nerve,
vagus, hepatic branch
to quadratus femoris muscle 463, 465,
469
quadratus plantae 505
radial 397, 400, 401, 403, 406, 414, 415,
417–419, 428, 436–438,
441–444, **446, 447,** 450
deep branch 415, 417–419, 442, 445
dorsal branch 419, 447
superficial branch 414, 417, 419, 428,
436–438, 441, 442, 447, 449, 450
rectal
inferior–see Nerve, anal (rectal), inferior
superior 306
to rectus capitis muscle 27, 123
of rectum 153
recurrent
branch–see under Nerve, fibular
(peroneal), deep; mandibular; spinal
laryngeal–see Nerve, laryngeal, recurrent
sacral splanchnic–see under Nerve,
splanchnic
saphenous 466, 467, 471, 484, 485, 487,
502, 505, 508, 509
infrapatellar branch 466, 467, 502
medial cutaneous branch 502
to scalene muscle 27, 123, 401
scapular, dorsal 400, 401, 446
sciatic 148, 152, 461, 463, 465, 468, 469,
471, **504,** 523
muscular branch 468
scrotal–see Nerve, ilioinguinal, (anterior)
scrotal branch; perineal (posterior)
scrotal branch; genitofemoral, genital
branch
to sebaceous gland 153
sensory 511
root of trigeminal–see Nerve, trigeminal,
motor and sensory roots
of shoulder 446–448
of sigmoid colon 153
of small intestine 153, 304, 306, 308
to sphincter of pupil 115, 153
spinal
cervical 18, 27, 30, 65, 108, 121, 148,
149, 152, 163, 164, 166, 182, 215,
216
cutaneous branch 163, 164, 166, 237,
241
lumbar 147–149, 152, 156, 163, 165,
166, 215, 216, 237, 241, 381, 386, 388
(recurrent) meningeal branch 156, 241,
307
sacral 148, 149, 152, 163, 166, 385
perineal branch of 54, 467, 469
thoracic 126–128, 148, 149, 152, 155,
156, 163, **166,** 178, 179, 215, 216,
237, **241,** 307–see also Nerve,
intercostal

**Nerve** *cont.*
spinosus–see Nerve, mandibular,
meningeal branch
splanchnic
greater 152, 153, 180, 181, **198,** 216,
218, 219, 228, 230, 241, 246, 250,
300–307, 309, 310, 322, 326, 380,
381, 385–387
least 152, 153, 181, 198, 216, 246, 250,
300–307, 322, 323, 326, 327, 380,
381, 385–387
lesser 152, 153, 181, **198,** 216, 241,
246, 250, 300–307, 322, 323, 326,
327, 380, 381, 385–387
lumbar 152, 153, 300, 305, 306, 322,
323, 326, 380, 381, 383, 385–388
pelvic 152–154, 250, 300, 305, 322,
323, 381, 383, 385–388, 463, 465
sacral 152, 153, 305, 306, 322, 381,
383, 388, 465
thoracic–see Nerve, cardiac
(sympathetic), thoracic; splanchnic,
greater; least; lesser
to stapedius muscle 117
to sternohyoid muscle 27–see also Ansa
cervicalis
to sternothyroid muscle 27–see also Ansa
cervicalis
of stomach 153, 300–303
to stylohyoid muscle–see Nerve, facial,
stylohyoid branch
to stylopharyngeus muscle–see Nerve,
glossopharyngeal, stylopharyngeal
branch
to subclavius muscle 405
subcostal 148, 237, 240, 250, 311, 312,
380, 385, 463, 464, 508
cutaneous branch 237, 240, 250
sublingual 41
of sublingual gland 153
of submandibular gland 153
suboccipital 14, 164
subscapular
lower 397, 400, 401, 446
upper 400, 401
superficial branch–see under Nerve,
plantar, lateral; radial, ulnar
to superior gemellus muscle 463, 465,
468, 469
supraclavicular 18, 26, 27, 123, 240, 448,
450
supraorbital 18, 31, 40, 76, 81, 116
of suprarenal gland 153, 326
suprascapular 397, 400, 401, 446
supratrochlear 18, 31, 40, 76, 81, 116
sural 504, 505, 509
calcaneal branch (lateral) 483
communicating branch 500
cutaneous branch:
lateral 468, 481, 482, 487, 504–509
lateral dorsal 494, 495, 504–506,
508, 509

**Nerve** *cont.*
medial 468, 481, 482, 487, 504, 505,
509
of sweat gland 153
sympathetic–see Fiber (nerve), sympathetic
of teeth 40, 41
temporal
branch of facial–see Nerve, facial,
temporal branch
deep 35, 41, 65, 116
to tensor tympani muscle 41, 116
to tensor veli palatini muscle 41, 65, 116
tentorial–see Tentorial (meningeal) branch
under Nerve, ophthalmic
of thigh 466–468, 502–504
thoracic, long 174, 175, 177, 240, 400,
401
of thoracic wall 179
thoracoabdominal 241
thoracodorsal 397, 400, 401
to thyrohyoid muscle 27, 29–see also Ansa
cervicalis
of thyroid gland 68
tibial 461, 463, 465, 468, 471, 481–483,
487, 493, 498, 504, 505
articular branch 504
calcalneal branch (medial) 496–499, 504
of tongue 53, 56
tonsillar–see Tonsillar branch under Nerve,
glossopharyngeal
of trachea 153, 199
of tracheobronchial tree 199
transverse cervical–see Nerve, cervical,
transverse
trigeminal 18, 40, 41, 56, 92, 108,
110–112, **116,** 125, 127–129, 137
motor and sensory roots 41, 125
trochlear 78, 81, 98, 108–112, **115**
tubal, of tympanic plexus 119
tympanic (Jacobson) 89, 117, 119, 128
ulnar 400, 401, 403, 404, 406,
414–419, 424, 429, 430, 434, 435,
437, 441–**445,** 450
articular branch 445
deep branch 417, 418, 424, 428, 429,
434, 435, 442, 445
dorsal branch 414, 416–418, 437, 438,
441, 445, 449
palmar branch 417, 428, 429, 435, 441,
449, 450
superficial branch 417, 428, 429, 439,
442, 445
of ureter 322, 323, 388
of urinary bladder 153, 322, 388
vagus 27–30, 56, 63–65, 68–70, 74, 98,
108, 110–112, 119, **120,** 121, 124,
125, 129, 152–154, 182, 195,
198–201, 214, 215, 218–220, 228,
300–307, 323, 513, 514–see also
Nerve, laryngeal
anterior vagal trunk 120, 220, 300–305
auricular branch 18, 120

**Nerve** *cont.*
cardiac branch
cervical 120, 124, 125, 198, 214, 215, 220
thoracic 120, 198, 214, 215, 220
celiac branch 120, 220, 304, 305
esophageal branch
gastric branch 120, 300–305
hepatic branch 120, 300, 301
pyloric branch 120, 301
intestinal branch 120
meningeal branch 120
pharyngeal branch 119, 120, 124, 152,
228
posterior vagal trunk 220, 300–305
pulmonary branch 199
vestibular 87, 90, 92, 118
vestibulocochlear 87, 90, 92, 98, 108,
110–112, **118,** 125
Vidian–see Nerve, of pterygoid canal
(vidian)
of wrist 441
zygomatic 40, 115, 116
branch of facial nerve–see Nerve, facial,
zygomatic branch
branch of maxillary nerve–see Nerve,
zygomatic
zygomaticofacial branch 18, 40, 65, 116
zygomaticotemporal branch 18, 40, 65, 116
**Nervi erigentes**–see Nerve, splanchnic,
pelvic
**Nervous system**–see System, nervous
**Nervus**
intermedius–see Nerve, intermediate
spinosus–see Nerve, mandibular meningeal
branch
**Neurohypophysis** 133, 140
infundibulum of–see Infundibulum, of
neurohypophysis
**Newborn** (neonate)
circulation of–see Circulation, postnatal
cranium of 8
**Nipple** of breast 167, 184
**Node**
atrioventricular (AV) 213
lymph–see Lymph node
sinuatrial (SA) 204, 213
**Nodule**
Albini's–see Nodule, fibrous, of mitral
valve
Arantii–see Nodule, of semilunar valve
of cerebellum 107, 137
fibrous, of mitral valve (Albini) 211
lymph–see Lymph nodule
of semilunar valve (Arantius) 211
**Nodulus** of cerebellum 109
**Nose**
cartilage of 31
concha of 32–34
external 31
lateral wall of 32, 33
medial wall of 34
septum of 34

**Notch**
acetabular 330, 453
angular, of stomach 258
cardiac, of
of left lung 184, 186, 187
of stomach 224, 258
cerebellar (anterior and posterior) 107
fibular, of tibia 478
inferior–see under Notch, vertebral
interarytenoid 60, 75
intertragic 88
ischiatic–see Notch, sciatic
jugular 23, 170, 184
mandibular 2, 9, 10
mastoid 5
pancreatic 279
preoccipital 99
radial, of ulna 407, 409
scapular–see Notch, suprascapular
sciatic (greater and lesser) 231, 453
of stomach–see Notch, angular; cardiac, of
stomach
superior–see under Notch, thyroid;
vertebral
supraorbital 1, 2, 8
suprascapular 170, 392, 394, 396–398
suprasternal 184–see also Notch,
jugular
of thyroid cartilage 71
trochlear, of ulna 407, 409
of ulna–see Notch, radial; trochlear, of ulna
ulnar, of radius 409
vertebral (inferior and superior) 143, 144
**Nucleus**
abducent 110, 111, 115
accessory oculomotor⇓see Nucleus
oculomotor, accessory
ambiguus 110, 111, 119–121
basal (basal ganglia) 104
caudate 102, 104–106, 134, 138
cerebellar (dentate, emboliform, fastigial,
globose) 107
cochlear (anterior and posterior) 110, 111,
118
of cranial nerve **110, 111,** 115–122
dentate, of cerebellum 107, 109
dorsal
cochlear 110, 111, 118
vagal–see Nucleus, posterior (dorsal), of
vagus nerve
dorsomedial, of hypothalamus 140
Edinger-Westphal–see Nucleus, oculomotor
accessory
emboliform, of cerebellum 107
facial 110, 111
fastigial, of cerebellum 107
geniculate, lateral 114
globose, of cerebellum 107
hypoglossal 110, 111, 122
hypothalamic (dorsomedial; mammillary;
paraventricular; posterior; supraoptic;
tuberal; ventromedial) 140

**Nucleus** *cont.*
  intermediolateral (IML) 126–128–see also
      Horn, lateral, of gray matter
  intralaminar, of thalamus 105
  of lens 83, 85
  lentiform 102, 104, 134
  mammillary, of hypothalamus 140
  mesencephalic, of trigeminal nerve 110,
      111, 116, 129
  motor
      of facial nerve 117
      of trigeminal nerve 110, 111, 116, 129
  oculomotor 115
      accessory 110, 111, 115, 126
  olfactory 113
  paraventricular, of hypothalamus
      140
  pontine, of trigeminal nerve–see Nucleus,
      principal sensory, of trigeminal nerve
  posterior (dorsal)
      of hypothalamus 140
      of vagus nerve 110, 111, 120, 215, 306,
          323
  principal sensory, of trigeminal nerve 110,
      111, 116
  pulposus 144
  red 101, 110, 111
  reticular 105
  ruber–see Nucleus, red
  salivatory
      inferior 110, 111, 119, 128
      superior 39, 110, 111, 117, 127
  sensory, principal, of trigeminal nerve 110,
      111, 116
  septal (pellucidum) 113
  of solitary tract 110, 111, 117, 119, 120,
      129, 215, 327
  spinal
      of accessory nerve 110, 111
      of trigeminal nerve 110, 111, 116, 119,
          120
  supraoptic, of hypothalamus 140
  thalamic 105
  trigeminal–see Nucleus, motor; principle
      sensory; spinal of trigeminal nerve
  trochlear 110, 111, 115
  tuberal, of hypothalamus 140
  vagal, dorsal–see Nucleus, posterior, of
      vagus nerve
  of vagus nerve, posterior (dorsal)–see
      Nucleus, posterior (dorsal), of vagus
      nerve
  ventromedial, of hypothalamus 140
  vestibular 110, 111, 118
      inferior, lateral, medial and superior 118

**O**

Oddi–see Sphincter, of hepatopancreatic
    ampulla

**Olecranon** of ulna 403, 407, 409, 411, 414,
    415, 446
**Omentum**
  greater 252, 255, 256, 258, 271, 328, 329
  lesser 258, 271, 279, 301, 302, 327, 329,
      520
**Opening**–see also Hiatus
  of alveolar duct 192
  of auditory tube–see Opening, pharyngeal,
      of pharyngotympanic (auditory) tube
  of Bartholin's gland 350
  of bladder 342
  of bulbourethral duct 358, 359
  of coronary arteries 211, 212
  of coronary sinus 208
  of ejaculatory duct 358, 359, 390
  of ethmoidal cells 32, 33, 44
  of greater vestibular gland 350
  ileocecal–see Orifice, ileal
  internal acoustic 92
  of maxillary sinus 32, 33, 42–44
  of nasolacrimal duct 32, 33, 43,
      77
  of paraurethral duct 350, 353
  of parotid duct 45
  pharyngeal, of pharyngotympanic
      (auditory) tube 32, 57, 58, 60, 61, 119
  of preputial gland 356
  of prostatic duct 358, 359
  of pylorus–see Orifice, pyloric
  saphenous 232, 233, 239, 242, 244, 351,
      354, 508, 510
  of Skene's ducts 350, 353
  of sphenoidal sinus 32, 33, 43
  of stomach
      cardiac–see Orifice, cardiac, of stomach
      pyloric–see Orifice, pyloric
  of sublingual duct 45, 55
  of submandibular duct 45, 55
  of superior cerebral vein 95
  of Tyson's glands 360
  of ureter–see Orifice, ureteric
  of urethra–see Orifice, urethral
  of urethral gland 357
  of uterine tube 350
  of uterus–see under Os
  of vagina–see Orifice, vaginal
  of vermiform appendix–see Orifice, of
      (vermiform) appendix
  of vestibular canaliculus 90
**Ora** serrata 82, 85, 86
**Orbit** 1, 2, 8, 42, 44, 76–81
  anterior adnexa of 76–77
  arteries of 80
  fascia of 78
  muscles of 79
  nerves of 40, 81
  veins of 80
**Organ**
  reproductive
      female, innervation of 386
      male, innervation of 387
  spiral, of Corti 91

Orifice–see also Opening
  cardiac, of stomach 259
  pyloric 262
  of tricuspid valve 516
  ureteric 343, 353, 358
  urethral external 337, 338, 350, 353, 356,
      359, 363, 389
  vaginal 337, 350
  of (vermiform) appendix 265
**Origin** of
  arm muscles 392, 393
  cremaster muscle 233, 242
  diaphragm 181
  forearm muscles 420, 421
  genioglossus muscle 47
  hip muscles 456, 457
  leg muscles 480
  scalene muscles 25
  serratus anterior muscle 171
  shoulder muscles 171
  subclavius muscle 171
  thigh muscles 456, 457
**Oropharynx** 30, 45, 56–58, 60, 61
**Os**–see also Bone
  of uterus (external internal) 350
**Os** odontoideum 16
**Ossicle,** auditory 88
Ostium–see Opening
**Ovary** 341, 343, 348–350, **353,** 375, 387,
    390, 394
**Ovum** 353

**P**

**Pain,** referred, in
  biliary disease 313
  pancreatic disease 314
**Palate** 34, 42, 44
Palatine bone–see Bone, palatine
**Palpebra** 76
**Pancreas** 102, 165, 255–257, 261, 262, 276,
    278, **279,** 285, 310, 329, 333, 518–520
  arteries of 283–285
  cross sections of 256, 518–520
  duct of 276, 278, 280
  histology of 279
  innervation of (schema)153, 314
  in situ 279
  intrinsic nerve supply 310
  lymph vessels and nodes of 303
  notch of 279
  veins of 294
**Papilla**
  circumvallate–see Papilla, vallate
  dermal 511
  filiform 52
  foliate 52, 129
  fungiform 52, 129
  gingival 51
  of hair follicle 511
  incisive 46

**Papilla** *cont.*
  duodenal
      major 262, 276, 278, 280
      minor 262, 278, 280
  lacrimal 76, 77
  of parotid duct 45
  renal 317
  vallate 52, 129
  of Vater–see Papilla, duodenal, major
**Paradidymis** 390
Parietal bone–see Bone, parietal
**Paroöphoron** 390
**Pars**
  distalis, of adenohypophysis 140
  flaccida, of tympanic membrane 88
  infundibularis, of adenohypophysis 140
  intermedia, of adenohypophysis 140
  nervosa–see Part, optic (visual) of retina
  plana, of ciliary body 85
  tensa, of tympanic membrane 88
  tuberalis, of adenohypophysis 140
**Part**
  anular, of fibrous digital tendon sheath of
      fingers 425, 427, **428,** 431
  atrioventricular, of membranous septum
      209–213
  basilar, of occipital bone 3, 5, 6, 14, 15,
      25, 32–34, 46, 59–61
  cardiac, of stomach 224
  cavernous, of internal carotid nerve
      plexus–see under Plexus (nerve),
      carotid, internal
  central, of lateral ventricle 102
  ciliary, of retina 82, 85
  cricopharyngeal, of inferior pharyngeal
      constrictor–see Muscle,
      cricopharyngeus
  cruciate, of fibrous digital tendon sheaths
      of fingers 425, 427, **428,** 431
  of duodenum 253, 261, 329
  glossopharyngeal, of superior pharyngeal
      constrictor–see under Muscle,
      constrictor, pharyngeal, superior
  hamstrings, of adductor magnus muscle
      503
  of hypothalamus 306
  of inferior frontal gyrus 99
  interarticular, of cervical vertebrae 13
  interchondral, of internal intercostal
      muscle 183
  of interventricular septum 209–213, 230
  ischiocondylar–see Part, hamstrings of
      adductor magnus muscle
  of lacrimal gland 77
  of medial (collateral) ligament of ankle
      tibiocalcaneal 491
      tibionavicular 491
      tibiotalar (anterior and posterior) 491
  membranous, of interventricular septum
      209–213, 230
  muscular, of interventricular system 208,
      209, 211–213

**Part** *cont.*
  optic (visual), of retina 82
  of temporal bone
      petrous 3, 5, 92
      squamous 2, 3
Passavant–see Ridge, Passavant's
**Patella** 458–460, 467, 472, 473, 476, 484,
      486
**Pathway**
  ascending, of spinal cord 151
  autonomic reflex 311
  descending, of spinal cord 126, 151
  lymphatic
      to anterior mediastinal nodes 169
      to inferior phrenic nodes and liver 169
      to opposite breast 169
  of sound reception 87
  taste 129
  visual 114, 126, 126
**Pecten**
  anal 365
  pubis 231, 246, 330, 331, 335, 453
**Pedicle** of
  axis 12
  vertebra 12, 143, 144, 146, 147
**Peduncle**
  cerebral 100, 101, 109, 132, 138
  cerebellar
      inferior 107–109, 118, 137
      middle 107–109, 137
      superior 107–109, 137
**Pelvis**
  arteries of 369, 371–376
      female 371, 373, 375
      male 374
  bony 231, 330–332, 453
  diameters of 332
  diaphragm of 334–336
  false 330, 339, 340
  gender differences of 332
  of kidney–see Pelvis, renal
  ligaments of 330, 331
  lymph vessels and nodes of 325, 377–379
      female 377
      male 379
  measurements of 332
  muscles of–see Diaphragm, pelvic;
      urogenital
  nerves of 381, 387, 386, 387
      female 383, 385
      male  387
  renal 313, 520
  true 330
  veins of 371, 373–376
  viscera of
      female 337, 339, 343–349
      male 338, 340, 343, 358
**Penis** 354–356, 359, 361, 389
**Pericardium** 30, 180, 186, 195, 200, 201,
      203, 218–221
**Pericranium** 96
**Perineum** 337, 338, 350–352, 354, 355, 357,
      376, 378, 382, 384

**Perineum** *cont.*
  (female)
      arteries of 375
      external genitalia (vulva) 350
      deep dissection of 352
      lymph vessels and nodes 377, 378
      nerves of 384
      superficial dissection of 351
      urethra 353
      veins of 375
  (male)
      arteries of 372, 376
      external genitalia 354
      deep dissection of 357
      lymph vessels and nodes 379
      nerves of 380, 382
      scrotum and contents 361
      superficial dissection of 355, 356
      testis, epididymis 362
      urethra 359
      veins of 372, 376
**Periodontium** 51
**Periorbita** 78
**Peritoneum** 165, 224, 234–236, 245, 267,
      304, 311, 324, 325, 337–340, 342, 343,
      345, 351, 363, 364, 368, 371, 383–see
      also Cavity, peritoneal
  parietal 244, 254, 256, 257, 327–329, 340
  of posterior aspect of anterior abdominal
      wall 257
  visceral 256, 263, 266, 308
**Pes**
  anserinus 458, 472, 473
  hippocampi 105, 106
Petit–see Triangle, of Petit
Peyer's–see Lymph nodule, aggregate of small
      intestine
**Phalanges** 420, 421, 426, 427, 433, 440,
      488, 489, 492, 501
**Pharynx**/pharyngeal region 30, 32, 45,
      56–58, 60, 61, 87, 93, 98
  arteries of 63
  lymph vessels and nodes of 66, 67
  mucosa of 60
  muscles of 58, 59, **61, 62,** 68
  nerves of 56, 65
  veins of 64
**Philtrum** 45
**Phonation,** position of glottis during 75
**Pia mater** 94, 96, 102, 155, 156
**Pisiform** 416–418, 422–430, 434, 435
**Pit,** anal 389
**Plane**
  of abdomen 251
  interspinous 251
  intertubercular 251
  lateral rectus 251, 269
  midclavicular 251
  midinguinal–see Plane, lateral rectus
  semilunar–see Plane, lateral rectus
  subcostal 251
  transpyloric 251, 269

PLATE 38

**Plate**–see also Lamina; Surface
cribriform, of ethmoid bone 3, 6, 7, 33, 34, 38, 113
horizontal, of palatine bone 3, 5, 33, 34, 93
lateral pterygoid of sphenoid bone 2, 3, 5, 8, 9, 33, 34, 49, 62, 93
levator 337, 338
limiting, of portal space 274, 275
medial pterygoid of sphenoid bone 3, 5, 33, 34, 44, 46, 49, 58, 59
orbital, of ethmoid bone 1, 2, 8
palmar digital 431, 437, 440
perpendicular, of
ethmoid bone 1, 3, 34
palatine bone 3, 33, 34
plantar digital 492, 500
quadrigeminal–see Plate, tectal
tectal 100, 109
**Pleura**
cervical 184, 185
costal 180, 184–186, 195, 200, 218–220, 236, 269, 316, 327
cupula 184, 185
diaphragmatic 180, 182, 186, 195, 200, 218–220, 236, 269, 327
dome 184, 185
mediastinal 180, 182, 186, 195, 200, 201, 203, 218–220, 230
parietal–see Pleura, cervical; costal; diaphragmatic; mediastinal
pericardial–see Pleura, mediastinal
visceral 193
**Plexus (arterial)**
malleolar 485
patellar 466, 467, 477
pial 157, 158
**Plexus (capillary),** of kidney 318
**Plexus (choroid)** of
lateral ventricle 94, 102, 104–106, 132, 136, 138
3rd ventricle 100, 102, 103, 136
4th ventricle 103, 108, 109
**Plexus (lymph),** subpleural 197
**Plexus (nerve)**
alveolar, superior–see Plexus, dental, superior
aortic 152, 198, 250, 300, 303, 322, 384, 381, 383, 385–388–see also Plexus (nerve), intermesenteric
of appendicular artery 304. 305
Auerbach's–see Plexus (nerve), myenteric
autonomic, intrinsic, of intestines (schema) 308
brachial 22, 25–27, 65, 148, 168, 173, 175, 177, 182, 186, 195, 200, 216, 218–220, 399–**401,** 404
cardiac 120, 152, 153, 198, 214, 215, 228
of carotid artery
common 124, 125
external 124, 125, 127
cavernous part 115
internal 81, 115, 117, 119, 125, 126, 152

**Plexus (nerve)** *cont.*
cavernous–see under Plexus (nerve)
carotid, internal
of cecal arteries 309
celiac 120, 152, 228, **300–303,** 304, 305, 322, 323, 326, 381, 386
cervical 18, **27,** 122, 123, 148–see also Ansa cervicalis
coccygeal 463, 465
of colic arteries
left 304, 305, 306
middle 304, 305
right 304, 305
dental
inferior 116
superior 40
of ductus deferens 380, 381, 387
enteric 307, 308
esophageal 120, 152, 195, 198, 218–220, 228, 230, 303
of facial artery 125
of gastric arteries
left 300–305, 381
right 301–304
of gastroduodenal artery 302, 304, 309
of gastro-omental artery 301, 302
of hepatic artery 120, 300–302, 304, 309, 327
hypogastric
inferior 152, 153, 300 305, 306, 322, 323, 380, 381, 383, 385–388
superior 152, 153, 300, 305, 306, 322, 323, 339, 340, 380, 381, 383, 385–388
of iliac arteries
common 300, 383
external 300, 383
internal 300, 305 383
of ileocolic artery 304, 305
intermesenteric 152, 153, 250, 300, 304–306, 322, 323, 328, 380, 381, 383, 385–388
intrinsic, of intestines (schema) 308
jejunal 301
lumbar 148, 216, 250, 328, **462, 463,** 464, 502, 503, 521
lumbosacral 463
of marginal artery 305
of maxillary artery 125
Meissner's–see Plexus (nerve), submucous
mesenteric
inferior 152, 300, 305, 306, 381
superior 152, 300–302, **304,** 306, 310, 381
of middle meningeal artery 125
myenteric (Auerbach's) 229, 308
ovarian 300, 322, 383, 386
of pancreaticoduodenal arteries
anterior inferior 301, 302
anterior superior 301, 302
inferior 301, 304, 305
posterior inferior 302

**Plexus (nerve)** *cont.*
posterior superior 302
parotid, of facial nerve 19
patellar 508
pelvic 152, 300, 305, 306, 320, 323, 380, 381, 383, 385–388
periglandular 308
perivascular 307–see also name of specific artery under Plexus (nerve)
pharyngeal 56, 65, 119, 120, 124, 125
phrenic, inferior 300–302, 304, 305, 326, 381
prostatic 152, 322, 381, 387, 388
pulmonary 120, 152, 153, 198, 199, 228
pyloric 301
rectal 152, 305, 306, 322, 381, 383
of rectal arteries
middle 305
superior 300, 305, 381
of rectosigmoid artery 305
renal 300, 305, 322, 323, 326, 381, 388
sacral 148, 216, 250, 300, 305, 322, 323, 381, 386–388, **463, 465**
of sigmoid arteries 305
of splenic artery 300–302
submucous (Meissner's) 229, 308
subserous 308
suprarenal 300, 305
testicular 300, 322, 380, 387
tympanic 89, 117, 119, 126, 128
ureteric 300, 322, 381
uterovaginal 383, 385, 386
uterine 383, 385, 386
vaginal 383, 385, 386
of vertebral artery 124
vesical 152, 305, 322, 381, 383, 385, 387, 388
**Plexus (venous)**
anal 364
areolar 239
basilar 97, 98
epidural–see Plexus (venous), vertebral, internal
esophageal 226
pampiniform 239, 361, 372, 374
paravesical 343
pial 159
prevesical 342, 374
prostatic 374
pterygoid 64, 80
pudendal 248
rectal
external 296, 365, 366, 370
internal 365, 366, 370
perimuscular 248, 296, 370
retropubic 342, 374
submucous 226
urethral 353
vertebral
external 159
internal (epidural) 156, 159
vesical 338
vesicourethral 248

**Plica**–see also Fold
  semilunaris, of conjunctiva 76, 77
**Point**
  anthropometry 1, 2, 4
  central, of perineum–see Tendon, central,
    of perineum
  McBurney's 266
Poirier–see Space, of Poirier
**Pole** of cerebrum 99, 101
  of kidney 313, 518, 519
**Pons** 100, 108, 109, 128, 129
**Pore**
  interalveolar (Kohn) 192
  of sweat gland 511
**Porta** hepatis 270, 273
**Position** of
  appendix 266
  stomach 258
  uterus 348
**Postnatal circulation** 217
**Pouch**
  of Douglas–see Pouch, rectouterine
  Rathke's 44
  rectouterine 337, 339, 341, 344, 346, 363
  superficial perineal–see Space, perineal,
    superficial
  vesicouterine 341, 345, 346, 367
Poupart–see Ligament, Poupart's
**Precuneus** 100
**Prenatal circulation** 217
**Prepuce** of
  clitoris 351, 389
  penis 338, 389
Pre–rolandic–see Artery, pre–rolandic
**Process**
  accessory, of lumbar vertebra 144
  alveolar, of maxilla 1–3, 9, 33, 42
  articular, of
    sacrum, superior 145
    vertebra
      inferior 12, 13, 143, 144, 146, 147
      superior 143, 144, 146, 147
  caudate, of liver 270, 272
  ciliary 82, 83, 85
  clinoid
    anterior 3, 6
    posterior 6
  condylar, of mandible 2, 9, 10
  coracoid, of scapula 170, 174, 175,
    392–394, 396–400, 402, 404
  coronoid, of
    mandible 2, 9, 10
    ulna 407, 409, 413
  ethmoidal, of inferior nasal concha
    33
  frontal, of
    maxilla 1, 2, 31, 33, 76
    zygomatic bone 1
  infundibular, of neurohypophysis
    140
  jugular, of occipital bone 25
  lenticular, of incus 89

**Process** cont.
  of malleus anterior 89
  mammillary, of lumbar vertebra 144
  mastoid, of temporal bone 2, 5, 9, 19,
    22–25, 29, 47, 53, 93, 162
  muscular, of arytenoid cartilage 71,
    72
  odontoid–see Dens of axis
  orbital, of palatine bone 1, 33
  palatine, of maxilla 3, 5, 32–34, 46, 93
  papillary, of liver 270
  pterygoid, of sphenoid bone 2, 3, 5, 8, 9,
    33, 34
  pyramidal, of palatine bone 5, 8, 9
  sphenoid, of palatine bone 33
  spinous, of
    axis 162
    sphenoid bone–see Spine, of sphenoid
      bone
    vertebra 12–14, 16, 143, 144, 146, 147,
      160, 162, 163, 165, 177, 185
  styloid, of
    radius 413, 426
    temporal bone 2, 5, 8, 9, 11, 22, 24, 25,
      29, 47, 53, 61, 62
    ulna 409, 422
  of talus, posterior 491, 492
  temporal, of zygomatic bone 1, 2
  transverse, of
    atlas 12, 25, 162
    axis 12, 25
    cervical vertebra 12, 13, 25, 130
    coccyx 145
    lumbar vertebrae 144, 146, 147, 165,
      181, 231
    thoracic vertebrae 143, 172
  uncinate, of
    cervical vertebrae 13
    ethmoid bone 32, 33, 43, 44
    pancreas 279, 520
  vocal, of arytenoid cartilage 71, 72
  xiphoid 170, 171, 174, 176, 184, 186,
    231, 232, 517
  zygomatic, of
    maxilla 1, 5
    temporal bone 2, 5, 8
**Prominence**
  of facial canal 89
  laryngeal 71
  of lateral semicircular canal 87, 89
**Promontory**
  sacral 145, 231, 330–333, 337, 339, 340,
    344, 383, 522
  of tympanic cavity 87–89
**Prostate** 154, 236, 329, 336, 382, 343, 357,
    **358,** 359, 363, 390, 523
**Protuberance**
  mental 1, 10
  occipital
    external 2, 3, 5, 178
    internal 6
**Pterion** 2
Pubis–see Bone, pubic

Pulley–see Part, anular; cruciate, of fibrous
  digital tendon sheaths of fingers
**Pulp,** dental 51
**Pulvinar** 101, 104, 105, 108, 109, 132,
  136–138
**Puncta,** lacrimal 76, 77
**Pupil** 76, 84
Purkinje–see Fiber, Purkinje
**Putamen** 102, 104
**Pylorus** 258–262, 298, 299, 301, 518
**Pyramid** of
  cerebellum 107, 109, 137
  kidney 313, 317, 318
  medulla 108

## Q

**Quadrants** of abdomen 251

## R

**Radiograph** of
  appendix 266
  ileum 263
  jejunum 263
**Radius** 407–**409,** 410–413, 415, 418–425,
  430, 434, 439
**Ramus**
  communicans
    gray 27, 124, 126–128, 152–156, 166,
      179, 198, 215, **216,** 218, 219, 228,
      241, 250, 300, 303, **306,** 307, 322,
      323 381, 383, 385–388, 463–465
    white 126–128, 152–**154,** 155, 156,
      166, 179, 198, 215, **216,** 218, 219,
      228, 241, 250, 300, 303, **306,** 307,
      323, 381, 383, 385–388, 463, 464
  ischiopubic 336, 338, 351, 352, 354–358
  of ischium 453
  of lateral sulcus 99
  of mandible 1, 2, 9, 10, 19, 22, 54
  pubic
    inferior 231, 330, 331, 334, 337, 343,
      345, 453
    superior 231, 243, 330, 331, 335, 337,
      338, 356, 357, 453, 454, 459, 462,
      465
  of spinal nerve
    dorsal 18, 155, 156, 164, 166, 179, 241
    ventral 155, 156, 166, 179, 241,
      323–see also Nerve, intercostal;
      Plexus (nerve), brachial; cervical;
      lumbar; sacral
**Raphé**–see also Ligament
  iliococcygeal 333, 334
  median, of
    levator ani muscle 333, 334
    mylohyoid muscle 47
  of palate 46
  penoscrotal 389

**Raphé** *cont.*
 perineal 350, 389
 pharyngeal 61, 69, 222
 pterygomandibular 9, 35, 46, 49, 54, 58,
   59, 62
 urethral 389
Rathke–see Pouch, Rathke's
**Ray,** medullary, of kidney 317
**Recess**–see also Space; Fossa; Pouch
 anterior, of ischioanal fossa–see under
   Fossa, ischioanal
 cochlear, of vestibule 90
 costodiaphragmatic 180, 184, 185, 195,
   218, 219, 312, 324, 327, 517, 524, 525
 costomediastinal 180
 duodenal 253
 elliptical, of vestibule 90
 epitympanic 87–89
 ileocecal 264
 ileocolic–see Recess, ileocecal
 infundibular, of 3rd ventricle 102
 intersigmoid 254, 319
 lateral, of 4th ventricle 102, 109
 of lesser sac–see Recess, of omental bursa
 of maxillary sinus 42
 mesentericoparietal 253
 of omental bursa (superior) 255, 257, 270,
   329
 optic, of 3rd ventricle–see Recess,
   supraoptic, of 3rd ventricle
 paraduodenal 253
 pharyngeal 32, 58, 60
 pineal, of 3rd ventricle 102
 piriform–see Fossa, piriform
 rectovesical–see Pouch, rectovesical
 retrocecal 250, 260
 sphenoethmoidal 32, 33
 spherical, of vestibule 90
 subpopliteal 473, 474
 supraoptic, of 3rd ventricle 100, 102
 suprapineal, of 3rd ventricle 102
 of 3rd ventricle 100, 102
 of 4th ventricle, lateral 102, 109
 vesicouterine–see Pouch, vesicouterine
 of vestibule 90
**Rectum**/anal canal 153, 246, 254, 257, 267,
   311, 329, 333, 334, 336–342, 351, 358,
   **363–368,** 369–371, 383
 arteries 369
 external sphincter (female and male) 367
 in situ (female and male) 363
 veins of 370
**Reflex**
 autonomic 307
 cough 199
 Hering-Breuer 199
 sneeze 199
**Region**
 of abdomen 251
 epigastric 251
 femoral 242, 244
 flank 251
 groin 251

**Region** *cont.*
 hypochondriac 251
 hypogastric–see Region, pubic
 iliac–see Region, groin
 iliocecal 264, 265
 inguinal 242–245–see also Region, groin
 lateral, of abdomen–see Region, flank
 lumbar, of back 251
 oral/pharyngeal
   arteries of 63
   lymph vessels and nodes of 66–67
   nerves of 65
   muscles of 61–62
   veins of 64
 pubic 251
 umbilical 251
Reil–see Insula
Reissner–see Membrane, Reissner's
**Relations** of spinal nerve roots to vertebrae
   149
**Respiration** 183
Rete–see Plexus
**Rete** testis 362
**Retina** 82, 83, 86, 114
**Retinaculum**
 extensor
   inferior 484, 486, 493, 494, 506
   superior 484, 486, 493, 494
   of wrist 414, 415, 436–439
 fibular
   inferior 483, 486, 490, 491, 493
   superior 481–483, 486, 491, 493
 flexor, of
   ankle 481–483, 493, 498, 499, 505
   wrist–see Ligament, transverse carpal
 patellar
   lateral 458–460, 472–474, 484–486
   medial 458, 459, 467, 472–474, 484,
     485
 peroneal–see Retinaculum fibular
**Retrocession** of uterus 348
**Retroversion** of uterus 348
Retzius–see Space, of Retzius; Vein,
   retroperitoneal
**Rib** 170, 171, 173, 180, 184, 185, 231,
   513–520, 524, 525
 cervical 173
**Ridge**–see also Fold; Crest
 Passavant's 59
 transverse, of sacrum 145
**Rima glottidis** 75
**Ring**
 common tendinous 78, 79, 81, 115
 femoral 236, 243, 244, 339–341, 510
 fibrous, of heart 210
 inguinal
   deep 234, 236, 242, 243, 339–341,
     344, 360
   superficial 232, 242, 243, 245, 351,
     355, 360, 361
Riolan–see Arc of Riolan
**Rod** of retina 114
Rolandic artery–see Artery, central sulcal

**Roof** of mouth 46
**Root**
 of accessory nerve
   cranial 120, 121
   spinal 121
 of ansa cervicalis
   cervical–see Root of ansa cervicalis,
     inferior
   hypoglossal–see Root of ansa cervicalis,
     superior
   inferior 27, 29, 65, 68, 122, 123
   superior 27, 29, 65, 68, 122, 123
 of brachial plexus 401
 of ciliary ganglion
   nasociliary–see Root, of ciliary ganglion,
     sensory
   oculomotor–see Root, of ciliary
     ganglion, parasympathetic
   parasympathetic 81, 115
   sensory 81, 115, 116, 125, 126
   sympathetic 81, 115, 125, 126
 of lung 182, 201
 of mesentery 253, 257, 261, 279, 291, 319
 of pterygopalatine ganglion–see Nerve,
     maxillary, ganglionic branch
 of spinal nerve
   arteries of 157–158
   dorsal 108, 127, 128, 149, 155, 156,
     166, 241, 307, 388
   relation of, to meninges 155–156
   relation of, to vertebrae 149, 156
   veins of 159
   ventral 108, 127, 128, 149, 155, 156,
     166, 179, 241, 303, 307, 388
 of tongue 52, 57, 60, 75, 223
 of tooth 51
 of trigeminal nerve
   motor 41, 125
   sensory 41, 125
Rosenmüller–see Lymph node,
   Cloquet's
Rosenthal–see Vein, of basal
**Rostrum** of corpus callosum 100, 134, 138
Rotter–see Lymph node, interpectoral
**Ruga**–see also Fold
 gastric 224, 259, 517
 palatine 46
 vaginal 345


## S

**Sac**
 alveolar 192
 endolymphatic 91
 lacrimal 76, 77
 lesser peritoneal–see Bursa, omental
 scrotal 364
**Saccule** of internal ear 87, 90, 91, 118
**Sacrum** 142, **145,** 147, 149, 231, 330, 334,
   335
Santorini–see Duct, pancreatic,
   accessory

**Scala**
   tympani of cochlea 87, 90, 91
   vestibuli of cochlea 87, 90, 91
**Scapha** of external ear 88
**Scaphoid** 422–426, 436
**Scapula** 24, 28, 166, 170, 177, 179, **392, 393,** 399, 513–516, 525
Scarpa–see Fascia, Scarpa's
Schlemm–see Sinus, venous, scleral
Schwalbe–see Line, Schwalbe's
**Sclera** 76, 78, 82, 83, 85, 86
**Scrotum** 338, 360–362, 367, 376, 389
**Segment**
   bronchopulmonary 188, 189
   of kidney–see Segment, renal
   of liver 272
   of lung–see Segment, bronchopulmonary
   renal 319
Segmentation, dermal–see Dermatomes
**Sella** turcica 3, 6, 32, 34, 57
**Septum**
   atrioventricular 210, 213, 230
   Denonvilliers'–see Fascia, rectovesical
   interalveolar 10
   interatrial 208, 516
   intercavernous, of Buck's fascia 355
   interlobular, of pancreas 279
   intermuscular
      anterior, of leg 487
      lateral
         of arm 402, 403, 406, 415, 418, 446
         of thigh 471
      medial
         of arm 402–404, 406, 415–418
         of thigh 471
      posterior, of leg 487
      transverse, of leg 487
   interventricular 208–213, 516
   of lung 193
   nasal 32, **34,** 37, 38, 42, 44, 57, 60
   orbital 76
   pellucidum 100, 102, 104–106, 134, 136, 138, 140
   of penis 359
   rectovesical–see Fascia, rectovesical
   of scrotum 338, 361, 362, 367, 376
   transverse fibrous, of ischioanal fossa 364–367
**Serosa** 308–see also Peritoneum, viscera
   of appendix 266
   of small intestine 263
Sesamoid–see Bone, sesamoid
**Shaft**
   of clitoris–see Body, of clitoris
   of femur 455, 462
   of humerus 513–515
   of penis–see Body, of penis
**Sheath**
   bulbar–see Sheath, fascial, of eyeball
   carotid 23, 30, 54
   of eye muscles–see Fascia, muscular of eye muscles

**Sheath** *cont.*
   fascial, of eyeball 78, 82
   femoral 233, 234, 236, 244, 466, 510
   flexor–see also Sheath, tendon, fibrous; synovial
      common (ulnar bursa) 429–432
   of hair follicle (external, internal) 511
   of optic nerve 78, 82
   rectus 175, 232–235, 243, 327–329
      anterior layer of 174, 240, 242, 338, 351, 395
      posterior layer of 238, 240
   tendon/tendinous
      of ankle 493
      fibrous digital
         of foot 497, 498
         of hand 427, 429, 431, 432, 435, 440
            anular and cruciform parts of 429, 431, 432
      synovial
         (extensor) of wrist/dorsum of hand 439
         (flexor) of fingers 427, 429, 431, 432, 435, 440
         of flexor carpi radialis 430
         of flexor pollicis longus (radial bursa) 429–431
         of foot 487, 498,
      of thyroid gland–see Capsule, fibrous of thyroid gland
**Shoulder**
   arteries of 28, 398
   bones of 391–393
   cross sections of 394, 513–515
   fasciae of 399
   joints of 391, 394
   lymph vessels and nodes of 452
   muscles of 395–397
   nerves of 446
Sibson–see Fascia, Sibson's
**Sinus**–see also Recess
   anal 365
   aortic 211, 212
   carotid 119, 124, 125, 130, 199
   cavernous 80, 98, 130, 133
   confluence of 97, 98, 137, 138
   coronary 202–204, 209, 211, 230, 516, 524, 525
   dural 97, 98, 137, 138
   of epididymis 362
   ethmoidal–see Cell, ethmoidal
   frontal 3, 32–34, 42–44, 57
   intercavernous (anterior and posterior) 97
   maxillary 39, 40, 42–44
   occipital 97, 137
   paranasal 42–44–see also individual paranasal sinuses; Cell (air)
      changes with age 44
   pericardial
      oblique 203, 230, 516
      transverse 201, 203, 208, 209
   petrosal
      inferior 97, 98

**Sinus** *cont.*
   superior 92, 97, 98
   prostatic 358, 359
   pyloric 258
   rectal–see Sinus, anal
   renal 313
   sagittal
      inferior 94, 97, 98, 137–139
      superior 94–98, 100, 103, 137, 138
   sigmoid 92, 97, 98
   sphenoidal 3, 32–34, 42–44, 57, 58, 78, 98
   sphenoparietal 97, 98
   straight 97, 98, 100, 137–139
   tarsal 488, 489
   transverse, of dura 97, 98, 137, 138
   urethral–see Sinus, prostatic
   urogenital 390
   of Valsalva–see Sinus, aortic
   venosus sclera–see Sinus, venous, scleral
   venous 97, 98–see also individual venous sinuses
      dural 97, 98
      scleral 83
**Sinusoid** of liver 273–275, 298
Skeleton–see Bone
Skene–see Duct, Skene's; Gland, Skene's
**Skin** 235, 511
   cross section of 511
   of penis 355, 356, 361
   of scrotum 361
**Skull**–see Cranium
**Slit,** nasal 7
**Sneeze** 199
**Snuffbox,** anatomical 414, 436, 438, 439
**Space**–see also Recess; Pouch; Fossa
   of Burns–see Space, suprasternal
   of Disse–see Space, perisinusoidal
   endopelvic 341
   epidural 94, 96, 156
      cranial–see Interface, dura-skull
      vertebral 156
   episcleral 78, 82
   of Fontana–see Space, of iridocorneal angle
   interglobular 51
   interproximal, between teeth 51
   intervaginal, of optic nerve 82
   of iridocorneal angle (Fontana) 83
   lumbar
      inferior–see Triangle, lumbar
      superior–see Triangle, auscultatory
   of Mall–see Space, periportal (Mall)
   midpalmar 429, 431, 432
   paravesical 343
   perianal 364, 365, 368
   perichoroidal 82, 83
   perineal (superficial) 338, 345, 351, 352, 355–357, 368, 375, 376, 382
   perineopelvic 368
   periportal (Mall) 274, 298
   perisinusoidal (Disse) 274, 298
   of Poirier 424

**Space** *cont.*
    postanal 368
    prerectal 368
    presacral (potential) 341, 368
    prevesical 234, 329, 336, 338, 341, 342,
       368
    quadrangular 397, 398
    rectovaginal (potential) 341
    rectovesical 338, 368
    retropharyngeal 30, 54, 57, 59
    retroprostatic 368
    retropubic 329, 336, 338, 341, 342, 368
    of Retzius–see Space, retropubic
    subarachnoid 94, 96, 103, 155, 156
    subdural 94, 96
    submucous 364, 368
    suprachoroidal 82, 83
    suprasternal (Burns) 23, 30, 57
    thenar 429, 431, 432
    triangular 397, 398
    vesicocervical (potential) 341, 344
    vesicovaginal (potential) 341, 344
**Sphenoid**–see Bone, sphenoid
**Sphincter**
    anal
       external 267, 306, 329, 333, 337, 338,
         342, 351, 352, 355–357, 363–365,
         366–369, 375, 389
       internal 364–366
    of Boyden–see Sphincter, of (common) bile
       duct
    of (common) bile duct 278
    esophageal
       inferior 221
       superior
    external anal–see sphincter, anal external
    of hepatopancreatic ampulla 278, 309
    ileocecal 265
    of Oddi–see Sphincter, of hepatopancreatic
       ampulla
    palatopharyngeal 59
    of pancreatic duct 278
    of pupillae–see Muscle, sphincter, of pupil
    pyloric–see Pylorus
    urethrae–see Muscle, sphincter urethrae
    urethral
       external–see Muscle, sphincter urethrae
       internal 353
    urethrovaginalis 333, 342, 345, 351, 352
**Spine**–see also Column, vertebral
    iliac
       anterior
         inferior 231, 246, 330, 331, 335, 453,
          454, 458, 459
         superior **231**–234, 242, 243, 245,
          246, **330**, 331, 352, 354, **453,**
          454, 458–460, 462, 466
       posterior
         inferior 147, 330, 453
         superior 147, 330, 331, 453

**Spine** *cont.*
    ischial 147, 231, 246, 330–335, 369, 382,
       384, **453,** 454, 469
    mental 10, 47
    nasal
       anterior, of maxilla 1, 2, 3, 31, 33, 34
       of frontal bone 33, 34
       posterior, of palatine bone 5, 33, 34
    of scapula 160, 163, 170, 178, 185, 393,
       395–399
    of sphenoid bone 5, 9, 93
**Spleen** 184, 185, 255, 256, 258, 271, 279,
    **281**, 325, 327, 517–519, 525
    arteries of 282–284
    cross sections 281, 517–519, 525
    in situ 281
    surfaces 281
    veins of 290, 293
**Splenium** of corpus callosum 100, 101, 104,
    106, 109, 136–139
**Spur,** scleral 82, 84
**Stage** of development
    of ovum 349
    of paranasal sinuses 44
**Stalk,** pituitary–see Infundibulum, of
    neurohypophysis
**Stapes** 87–89, 91
**Stem,** infundibular, of neurohypophysis
    140
**Stensen**–see Duct, parotid
**Sternum** 24, 57, 166, 170, 174, 176, 179,
    180, 221, 230, 329, 395, 517, 518, 524, 525
**Stomach** 184, 220, 221, 224, 225, 252, 255,
    256, **258**–260, 270, 271, 276, 279, 281, 327
    arteries of 282–283
    bed of 257, 261
    cross sections of 256,259, 517, 518, 524,
       525
    innervation of (schema) 303
    in situ 258
    mucosa of 259
    musculature of 260
    nerves of 301, 302
    variations in form of 258
    veins of 294
**Stratum**
    basale 511
    corneum 511
    granulosum 511
    lucidum 511
    spinosum 511
**Stria**
    medullaris of thalamus 100, 105, 109
    olfactory 113
    terminalis 102, 105, 106
**Striatum** 104
**Submucosa**
    of esophagus 223, 224, 229
    of ileum 263
    intestinal 308
    of jejunum 263
    of stomach 259

**Substance**
    gelatinous 151
    interpeduncular–see Substance, perforated,
       posterior
    perforated
       anterior 101, 113
       posterior 108
**Substantia**
    adamantina 51
    eburnea 51
    gelatinosa–see Substance, gelatinous
    nigra 101
    ossea 51
**Sulcus**–see also Groove
    calcarine (cerebral) 99–101, 105, 114
    carotid 6
    central (cerebral) 99, 100
    cerebral 99, 101, 134
    cingulate (cerebral) 100
    collateral (cerebral) 100, 101
    coronal, of glans, penis 389
    coronary 201, 202
    of corpus callosum 100
    frontal (cerebral) 99
    hippocampal 106
    hypothalamic 100, 109, 140
    for inferior vena cava on liver–see Groove,
       for inferior vena cava on bare area of
       liver
    of insula 99
    interparietal, (cerebral) 99
    intertubercular, of humerus 392
    interventricular, of heart
       anterior 201
       posterior 202, 203
    lateral (cerebral) 99, 101, 134
    limitans of 4th ventricle 109
    lunate, of cerebrum 99
    median, of
       tongue–see Groove, midline, of tongue
       4th ventricle 109
    occipital, transverse (cerebral) 99
    occipitotemporal (cerebral) 100, 101
    olfactory (cerebral) 101
    orbital (cerebral) 101
    paracentral (cerebral) 100
    paracolic–see Gutter, paracolic
    parieto-occipital (cerebral) 99, 100
    of pharyngotympanic (auditory) tube 5
    postcentral (cerebral) 99
    precentral (cerebral) 99, 100
    prechiasmatic 6
    rhinal (cerebral) 100, 101
    of Rolando–see Sulcus, central
    of spinal cord
       dorsal
         intermediate 151
         lateral 151
         median 109, 151, 155
       ventral lateral 151
    sylvian–see Sulcus, lateral
    temporal 99, 101

**Sulcus** *cont.*
   terminalis 52, 202
   transverse occipital 99
   of 4th ventricle 109
**Surface**–see also Plate
   of heart 201, 202
   of liver 270
      diaphragmatic 270, 272
      parietal–see Surface, of liver,
         diaphragmatic
      visceral 270, 272
   lumbosacral articular 145
   lunate, of acetabulum 454
   of lung 187
      costal 184–186
      diaphragmatic 187
      mediastinal 187
   nasal, of maxilla 3
   orbital, of frontal bone 6
   patellar, of femur 455
   of sacrum
      auricular 145, 147
      dorsal 145
      pelvic 145
   of tibia, articular 474, 478, 479
**Sustentaculum** tali 489–492
**Suture**
   coronal 1–4, 8
   frontoparietal–see Suture, coronal
   intermaxillary 31
   interparietal–see Suture, sagittal
   lambdoid 2–4, 8
   median palatine 5
   parietooccipital–see Suture, lambdoid
   sagittal 4, 8
   sphenooccipital–see Synchondrosis,
      sphenooccipital
   squamous 8
   transverse palatine 5
**Swelling,** labioscrotal 389
Sylvian sulcus–see Sulcus, lateral
**Symphysis,** pubic **231,** 243, 245, 246,
      330–336, 338, 341, 342, 351, 354, 357,
      373, 523
Synapsis–see also Terminal, nerve
   adrenergic 154
   cholinergic 154
**Synchondrosis**
   of first rib 391
   manubriosternal 171, 391
   sphenooccipital 57
   xiphisternal 171
**Syndrome**
   Down's 16
   Klippel-Feil 16
   Morquio's 16
**System**
   anterolateral (ALS) 151
   biliary, intrahepatic (schema) 275
   conducting, of heart 213
   dorsal column 151

**System** *cont.*
   nervous, autonomic (ANS) 39, 115–117,
      119, 120, **124**–128, 152–154, **198,**
      199, 215, 216, 228, **300**–310, 322,
      323, 326, 380, 381, 383, 385–388
   schema 153
   synapses of 154
   topography of 152
   nervous, parasympathetic 39, 115–117,
      119, 120, 126–128, 152–154, 199,
      215, 303, 306, 307, 309, 310, 323,
      385–388
   nervous, sympathetic 39, 115–117,
      126–128, 152–154, 199, 215, 216,
      303, 306, 307, 309, 310, 323, 326,
      385–388
   reproductive–see Organ, reproductive
**Systole** 210


**T**

**Tag,** epithelial, of glans 389
**Tail of**
   caudate nucleus 102, 104, 106
   pancreas 279, 281, 311
**Talus** 488–490
Tarsal bone–see Bone of foot
Tarsus–see Bone, of foot
   of eyelid 76, 78, 79
**Taste** 52, 56, 117, 119, 129
Tectum–see Lamina, quadrigeminal; tectal
**Teeth** 44, 50, 51, 221
**Tegmen** tympani 87
**Tegmentum,** midbrain 109
**Tela** choroidea of 3rd ventricle 102, 105, 138
**Tendon**–see also individual muscles
   Achilles 481–483, 486, 491, 493
   of ankle 491, 493–495
   anular, common–see Ring, common
      tendinous
   calcaneal 481–483, 486, 491, 493
   central, of
      diaphragm 180, 181, 246
      perineum–see Body, perineal
   common
      anular–see Ring, common tendinous
      extensor 411, 414, 415
      flexor 412, 413, 416
   conjoined–see Falx, inguinal
   digastric–see Tendon, intermediate, of
      digastric muscle
   extensor, common 411 413, 415
   flexor, common 412, 413, 416
   intermediate, of digastric muscle 23, 24,
      47, 53, 54
   patellar–see Ligament, patellar
   plantaris 461, 481, 482, 487
   popliteal 473–475
   quadriceps femoris 467, 471–473, 476,
      484–486
**Tenia**
   of colon
      free 254, 264, 265, 267, 363, 366

**Tenia** *cont.*
      libera–see Tenia, of colon, free
      mesocolic 264, 265, 267
      omental 264, 267
   of 4th ventricle 109
Tenon–see Sheath, fascial, of eyeball
**Tentorium** cerebelli 81, 97, 98, 100, 137, 138
**Terminal, nerve**–see also Synapsis
   adrenergic 199
   cholinergic 199
**Testis** 329, 338, 360–362, 376, 387, 390
**Thalamus** 100, 102, 104, **105,** 106, 108,
      109, 137, 138, 140, 306
Thebesian–see Valve, of coronary sinus; Vein,
      smallest, of heart (venae cordis minimae)
**Theca** of ovarian follicle 349
**Thigh**
   arteries of 466–468, 477
   bones of 455–457
   cross section of 471
   lymph nodes of 510
   muscles of 458–462
   nerves of 466–468, 502–504
**Thorax**
   arteries of 176, 179, 225–see also
      arteries of individual organs
   bones of 170, 171
   cross sections of 230, 513–516, 524, 525
   joints of 171, 172
   lymph vessels and nodes of 169, 197, 227
   muscles of 174–178, 183
   nerves of 174, 178, 179, 198–see also
      nerves of individual organs
   veins of 176, 226–see also veins of
      individual organs
   viscera of–see individual organs
**Tibia** 474, 476, **478, 479,** 484, 459, 487,
      490, 491, 493–495
**Tissue**
   adipose 30, 232–see also Tissue,
      subcutaneous
   alar fibrofatty 31, 33
   fatty, of anterior mediastinum 187
   subcutaneous 511
      fatty (Camper's) layer, of abdomen 232,
         235, 329, 338, 351, 354
      membranous layer
         of abdomen (Scarpa's) 232, 235, 351
         of perineum (Colles')–see Fascia,
            perineal, superficial (Colles')
**Tongue** 32, 34, 42, **52–55,** 57, 58, 60, 67,
      119, 122, 129
   arteries of 53
   cross sections of 54, 57
   dorsum of 52
   histology of 52
   lymph vessels and nodes of 67
   muscles of 53
   veins of 53
**Tonsil**
   of cerebellum 107, 109, 137
   lingual 52, 57, 58, 75
   palatine 45, 46, 52, 54, 57, **58,** 60

**Tonsil** *cont.*
pharyngeal 32, 57, 58, 60, 61
**Topography** of
abdominal viscera 251
autonomic nervous system 152
esophagus 221
gallbladder 269
kidney 312
liver 269
lung 184, 185
perineum 354
spinal nerve 148, 166
thyroid gland 68
**Torus** tubarius 32, 58, 60
**Trabecula**
carneae 208
fibrous, of adenohypophysis 140
of iridocorneal–see Meshwork, trabecular,
of iridocorneal angle
septomarginal 208, 211, 212
**Trachea** 9, 23, 24, 30, 57, 59, 62, 68–71, 75,
120, 154, 184, 186, **190,** 191, 194–196,
200, 218, 220–222, 225, 513, 514, 524,
525
**Tract**
biliary 276–278
innervation (schema) 309
comma 151
corticospinal 151
dorsolateral 151
fiber, principle, of spinal cord 151
gastrointestinal 154
hypothalamohypophyseal 140
iliopubic 243, 341
iliotibial 458, **460,** 461, 468, 471–474,
479, 481, 484–486
of Lissauer–see Fasciculus, dorsolateral
mammillothalamic 140
olfactory 38, 100, 101, 108, 113
optic 101, 102, 106, 108, 114, 132, 137
pontoreticulospinal 151
pyramidal 151
reticulospinal 151
rubrospinal 151
of spinal cord 151
spinal, of trigeminal nerve 110, 111, 116,
119, 120
spinocerebellar 151
spinohypothalamic 151
spinomesencephalic 151
spinoolivary 151
spinoreticular 151
spinotectal 151
spinothalamic 151
supraopticohypophyseal 140
tectospinal 126, 151
tuberohypophyseal 140
vestibulospinal 151
**Tragus** of external ear 88
**Trapezium** 422, 423, 426, 427, 430, 436
**Trapezoid** 422, 423, 425, 426
**Treves**–see Fold, bloodless, of Treves
**Triad,** portal 273, 298, 518

**Triangle**
anal 354
auscultatory 237, 395 516
of Calot 284–see Triangle, cystohepatic
cervical 21, 30, 160, 164, 174, 178
cystohepatic 284, 290
deltopectoral 395
Hesselbach's–see Triangle, inguinal
inguinal 236, 243
lumbar 160, 178, 237
lumbocostal–see Triangle, lumbocostal
perineal–see Triangle, urogenital
of Petit–see Triangle, lumbar
sternocostal 181
suboccipital 164
urogenital 354
**Trigone**–see also Triangle
collateral 105
fibrous, of heart 210
habenular 105, 109
hypoglossal 109
lumbocostal 181
olfactory 113
of urinary bladder 338, 342, 343, 353,
358, 359
vagal 109
vertebrocostal 181
**Triquetrum** 422–426
**Trochanter of femur**
greater 231, 454, 455, 458, 459, 461, 462,
468, 469, 523
lesser 231, 246, 458, 455, 462
**Trochlea**
fibular 488–490
of humerus 392, 393, 407
peroneal–see Trochlea, fibular
of superior oblique muscle 79
of talus 488, 489
**Trolard**–see Vein, of Trolard
**Tropism**–see Facet, tropism
**Trunk (arterial)**
brachiocephalic 28, 68–70, 130, 131, 176,
**182,** 195, 200–202, 220, 225
celiac 152, 181, 217, 220, 225, 247, 253,
257, 261, 279, **282–**286, 288–290,
292, 303, 306, 310, 311, 314, 329,
381, 518, 519
celiacomesenteric 288
costocervical 27, 28, 63, 130, 131
gastrophrenic 288
hepatogastric 288
hepatolienomesenteric 288
hepatomesenteric 288
lienogastric 288
lienomesenteric 288
meningohypophyseal 95
pulmonary 194, 195, 201, 203, 208, 212,
213, 217, 515, 525
thyrocervical 27–29, 63, 65, 68–70, 130,
131, 220, 225, 398
of corpus callosum 100, 134
**Trunk (lymphatic)**–see also Duct, thoracic
bronchomediastinal 197, 249

**Trunk (lymphatic)** *cont.*
intestinal 249, 296
jugular 66, 197, 249
lumbar 249, 300, 325
subclavian 66, 197, 249
**Trunk (nerve)**
of brachial plexus 401
lumbosacral 250, 381, 462–465, 502, 503,
521, 522
sympathetic
cervical 30, 39, 63, 65, 119, **124–**128,
152, 216, 228
lumbar 152, 181, 216, 246, **250,** 300,
305, 306, 322, 326–328, 339, 340,
380, 381, 383, 385–387, 463–465
sacral 152, 326, 463, 465
thoracic 39, 126–128, 152, 179, 180,
**198,** 216, 218, 219, 228, 230, 241,
300, 303, 306, 307, 309, 310,
385–387
vagal
anterior 120, 152, 198, 220, **228,** 229,
246, 300–305, 309, 310, 322, 326,
381
posterior 120, 152, **228,** 229, 246,
300–305, 309, 310, 322, 326, 381
**Tube**
auditory–see Tube, pharyngotympanic
Eustachian–see Tube, pharyngotympanic
fallopian–see Tube, uterine
pharyngotympanic (auditory) 5, 32, 46, 49,
57–61, 87–89, 91, **93,** 199, 120
uterine 337, 339, 344–347, 371, 383, 386,
390
**Tuber**
of cerebellum 107, 109, 137
cinereum 100, 101, 108, 140
parietal 8
**Tubercle**
adductor 455, 459, 467, 468, 472,
475
anal 389
anterior
of atlas 12, 15, 16, 32
of C6–see Tubercle, carotid
thalamic 105
of transverse process of cervical
vertebra 13
articular, of temporal bone 2, 5, 11, 49
of atlas, for transverse ligament 12
auricular 88
carotid 14
conoid, of clavicle 391
corniculate 60, 61, 72, 75
cuneate 108, 109
cuneiform 60, 61, 72, 75
dorsal, of radius 422
of external ear–see Tubercle, auricular
genital 389
Gerdy's 460, 473, 475, 478
gracile 108, 109

**Tubercle** cont.
of humerus
greater 392–394, 397, 402, 403
lesser 392–394 402
of iliac crest–see Tuberculum, of iliac crest
infraglenoid of scapula 392, 393
intercondylar, of tibia 478, 479
mental, of mandible 1, 10
olfactory 113
pharyngeal, of basilar part of temporal
bone 5, 14, 34, 57–59, 61
posterior
of atlas 16, 161, 162
of transverse process of cervical
vertebra 13
pubic **231,** 233, 234, 242, 245, 246, 330,
331, 335, 336, 351, 356, 453, 458, 459
of radius–see Tubercle, dorsal, of radius
of rib 170, 171
of scaphoid 422, 424, 426
supraglenoid, of scapula 392
of talus 488
of trapezium bone 422, 424, 426
trigeminal 109
of Vater–see Papilla, duodenal, major
**Tuberculum** sellae 6
of iliac crest 231, 453
**Tuberosity**
calcaneal 481, 482, 489, 490, 492,
496–499
of cuboid bone 489, 492, 500
deltoid 392, 393
gluteal, of femur 455
iliac 231, 453
ischial 147, 231, **330–332,** 334, 336, 351,
352, 354–357, 364, 367, 369, 384,
**453,** 454, 461, 468, 469
maxillary 2, 9
of metatarsal bone
1st 489, 492–494
5th 488, 489, 499–501
navicular 488, 489, 492, 495, 500
parietal–see Tuber, parietal
radial 402, 407, 409
sacral 145
tibial 458, 459, 472–476, 478, 479, 484, 486
of ulna 402, 407, 409
**Tubule**
collecting, of kidney 317, 318
dentinal 51
mesonephric 390
seminiferous 362
Tunic dartos–see Fascia, dartos
**Tunica**
albuginea
of corpora cavernosa penis 355, 359
of corpus spongiosum penis 355, 359
of ovary 349
of penis–see Tunica, albuginea, of
corpora cavernosa penis;
spongiosum
testis 362

**Tunica** cont.
vaginalis, of testis 329, 361, 362
**Tunnel,** carpal 424
Turbinate–see Concha, nasal
Tyson–see Gland, Tyson's

## U

**Ulna** 407–**409,** 410–415, 419–425, 430, 434,
439
**Umbilicus** 236, 288
**Umbo** of tympanic membrane 88
**Uncus**
of brain 100, 101, 106, 113
of cervical vertebrae 13
**Urachus** 235, **236,** 244, 245, 257, 329,
338–342, 344, 351, 371, 374
Urinary bladder–see Bladder urinary
**Ureter** 236, 244, 248, 254, 257, 300, 311,
313, **319,** 321, 328, 337–342, 344–346,
358, 363, 364, 371–375, 381, 383, 388,
520–522
**Urethra** 154, 246, 333, 334, 336, 342, 343,
351–**353,** 355, 357–**359,** 390, 523
female 342, 343, 351, 352, **353**
male
bulbous portion–see under Urethra,
spongy
cavernous part–see Urethra, spongy
intermediate part 359
membranous part–see Urethra,
intermediate part
pendulous (penile) portion–see under
Urethra, spongy
prostatic 343, 359, 523
spongy 358, 359
bulbous portion 343, 358, 359
pendulous (penile) portion 358, 359
**Uterus** 337, 339, 342, 344–**346,** 347, 348,
351, 363, 371, 383, 385, 386, 390
**Utricle**
prostatic 358, 359, 390
of vestibular labyrinth 87, 90, 91, 118
**Uvula** 45, 58, 60, 61
of bladder 343, 358, 359
of cerebellum 107, 109, 137

## V

**Vagina** 333, 334, 337, 342, 343, **345**–347,
351–353, 363, 367, 371, 386, 389, 390
**Vallecula,** epiglottic 52, 58, 75
Valsalva–see Sinus, of Valsalva
**Valve**
anal 365
aortic 209–213, 524
atrioventricular 211
of coronary sinus 208
eustachian–see Valve, of inferior vena cava
of foramen ovale 209
of heart 210, 211

**Valve** cont.
Houston's–see Fold, transverse, of rectum
of inferior vena cava 208
mitral 209–213, 230, 516, 524
pulmonary 208, 210, 213
rectal–see Fold, transverse, of rectum
thebesian–see Valve, of coronary sinus
tricuspid 208, 210–212, 230, 516, 524
**Variation** in
arteries
bronchial 196
cardiac–see Variations in, arteries,
coronary
celiac–see Variations in, trunk, celiac
colic 289
coronary 205
esophageal 225
hepatic 288
renal 316
blood supply of heart 205
colon, sigmoid 268
ducts
bile 278
hepatic 277
cystic 277
pancreatic 278, 280
liver, form of 271
nerves, of esophagus 229
sigmoid colon, position of 268
stomach, form of 258
trunk, celiac 288
uterus, position of 348
veins
cardiac 205
portal 294
renal 316
**Vas** deferens–see Ductus, deferens
**Vasa** rectae
of kidney 318
of small intestine–see Artery, straight
(arteriae rectae)
Vasculature, visceral 282–303
Vater–see Papilla, duodenal, major
**Vein**–see also Sinus, venous
of abdominal wall 235, 244
accessory
cephalic 448, 493
hemiazygos 196, 219, 226
saphenous 508, 509
acromial–see Acromial branch under Vein,
thoracoacromial
alveolar
inferior 54, 64
posterior superior 64
of anal canal 370
anastomotic
inferior (Labbé) 96, 138
superior (Trolard) 96
angular 17, 64, 80
antebrachial, median 419, 448, 449
appendicular 296, 297
arcuate, of kidney 318
ascending lumbar 248, 314

**Vein** *cont.*

atrial 139
auricular, posterior 17, 64
axillary 175, 186, 239, 399, 452, 524, 525
azygos 180, 181, 194–196, 198, 218, 220, **226,** 230, 246, 327, 514–517
basal (Rosenthal) 137–139
basilic 400, 406, 419, 437, 448, 449, 452
basivertebral 159
brachial 400, 406
  lateral 137
brachiocephalic 64, 68, 69, 176, 195, 197, 200, 201, 218–220, 226, 513, 524
of brain 137–139, 141
bronchial 196
capsular, of kidney 318
cardiac 204, 205
caudate 138, 139
cecal 292, 293
central
  of liver 273, 274
  retinal 82, 86
  of spinal cord 159
cephalic 174, 175, 239, 395, 399, 400, 406, 419, 437, **448,** 449, 452, 524
cerebellar 137
cerebral
  anterior 137–139
  deep 94, 96, 98, 137–139
  direct lateral 138, 139
  great, (Galen) 97, 98, 100, 109, 137–139
  internal 94, 102, 105, 137–139
  superficial 94–**96,** 98, 138
cervical, transverse 64, 163
choroidal, superior 94, 138, 139
ciliary, anterior 83, 86
of ciliary body 86
circumflex humeral 448
of clitoris, deep dorsal–see Vein, dorsal, deep, of clitoris
colic
  left 292–294
  middle 279, 290–294
  right 291–294, 328
of colon 292
communicating, between
  anterior and internal jugular veins 26, 64
  lumbar and hemiazygos veins 314
of conjunctiva 86
coronary 226–see also Vein, gastric, left
of cranial fossa, posterior 137
cremasteric 245, 372
cubital, median 448, 452
cystic 294
deep, of thigh 471
deferential 292
digital
  dorsal (foot) 508
  dorsal (hand) 437, 449
  palmar 449
diploic **94,** 96

**Vein** *cont.*

dorsal
  deep
    of clitoris 248, 333, 334, 337, 341, 342
    of penis 338, 355, 357, 372, 374, 376
  superficial, of penis 355
of duodenum 290
emissary 94, 96
  mastoid 17, 94
  occipital 94
  parietal 17, 94
  of Vesalius 64
epigastric
  inferior 234, 236, **239,** 243–245, 248, 257, 328, 339, 340, 371, 372, 374
  superficial 232, 239, 242, 248, 466, 508
  superior 175, 176, 234, 239, 327
episcleral 86
esophageal 226, 290, 293, 294
of eye 86
of eyelids 80
facial 17, 26, 27, 53–55, 64, 80
  deep 17, 64
  transverse 17, 64
femoral 233, 234, 239, 242, 244, 245, 248, 354, 372, 378, 459, **466,** 467, 471, 508, 510, 523
  deep–see Vein, deep, of thigh
fibular (peroneal) 481, 487
of Galen–see Vein, cerebral, great, (Galen)
gastric
  left 226, **290–294,** 327
  right 226, 290–294
  short 226, 257, 281, 290, 292–294, 327
gastroepiploic–see Vein, gastro-omental
gastro-omental 226, 281, 290, 292–294
gluteal 248, 292
of hand 437, 449
of head, superficial 17
of heart, 204, 205
hemiazygos 180, 181, 226, 230, 515
  accessory 196, 219, 226
hemorrhoidal–see Vein, of anal canal; rectal
hepatic 217, 220, 226, 248, 257, 270, 273, 290
  portal–see Vein, portal (hepatic)
hippocampal 139
hypophyseal 133, 141
hypothalamic 141
ileal 291, 292, 294
ileocolic 291–294
iliac
  common 248, 254, 370, 372, 374, 383, 522
  deep circumflex 236, 244, 248, 341, 374
  external 236, 243–245, 248, 254, 264, 292, 337–**341,** 344, 364, 370, 372, 374, 467
  internal 248, 292, 341, 345, 370, 372, 374

**Vein** *cont.*

superficial circumflex 232, 239, 242, 248, 466, 508
iliolumbar 248
infraorbital 17, 64
innervation of 216
innominate–see Vein, brachiocephalic
intercalated, of liver–see Vein, of liver, sublobular
intercapitular 437, 449
intercostal
  anterior 176, 239
  highest–see Vein, intercostal, superior
  posterior 218, 219, 226, 239, 327
  superior 218, 219, 226
interlobar, of kidney 318
interlobular, of kidney 318
intervertebral 159
intestinal 291, 292, 294
  large 292
  small 291
intraculminate 137
intrapulmonary 193
jejunal 291, 292, 294
jugular
  anterior 26, 64, 68, 239
  external 17, 26, 55, 64, 68, 186, 195, 200, 226, 239, 524
  internal 17, 23–30, 53–55, **64,** 67–70, 122, 175, 176, 186, 195, 197, 200, 201, 220, 226, 239, 524
of kidney 313, 314, 318–see also Vein, renal
of Labbé–see Vein, anastomotic, inferior
labial 64
laryngeal, superior 64, 223
of left ventricle, posterior 204
of leg 481–485
lingual 17, 53–55, 64–see also Vena comitans, of hypoglossal nerve
  deep 45, 53, 64
  dorsal
of liver
  central 273, 274
  intercalated–see Vein, of liver, sublobular
  sublobular 273, 274
of lower limb, superficial 508, 509
lumbar 248, 314
  ascending 248, 314
of lung 194, 195
macular–see Venule, macular
Marshall–see Vein, oblique, of left atrium
maxillary 64
medullary, anterior 137
meningeal, middle 94, 96
mental 64
mesencephalic 137, 139
mesenteric
  inferior 226, 253, 279, 290, **292–**294, 299, 328, 370

**Vein** *cont.*

superior 165, 226, 257, 261, 262, 279, 286, 290, **291–294**, 299, 324, 328, 519, 520
metacarpal, dorsal 437, 449
metatarsal, dorsal 508
of mouth 64
musculophrenic 175, 176, 239
nasal
   dorsal 17
   external 64
   of retina–see Venule, retinal, nasal
nasofrontal 17, 64, 80
of neck 26, 64
oblique, of left atrium 202–204, 209
obturator 236, 248, 226, 370, 374
occipital 17, 64
   internal 139
ophthalmic
   inferior 80
   superior 64, 78, 80, 98
of orbit 80
ovarian 248, 292, 311, 314, 319, 328, 339, 341, 344, 346, 349, 371, **375**
   tubal branch of 374
palatine, external 64
pancreatic 290, 292, 294
pancreaticoduodenal 290, 292–294
paraumbilical 236, 239, 293
of pelvic viscera 371, 373–376
of penis
   dorsal
      deep 232, 239, 248, 336, 338, 355, 357, 372, 374, 376
      superficial 232, 239, 355, 374
   lateral superficial 355
pericallosal 137, 139
pericardiacophrenic 176, 180, 195, 200, 201, 203, 218, 219, 230
perineal 376
peroneal–see Vein, fibular
petrosal 98, 137
of pharynx 64
phrenic, inferior 226, 248, 257, 314
pontine, transverse 137
pontomesencephalic, anterior 137
popliteal 461, 468, 471, 481, 482, 510
portal (hepatic) 217, 226, 256, 261, 262, 270–273, 276, 279, 282, 284, 290–**293, 294,** 299, 327, 329, 518, 519
   anastomoses (portacaval) 293
   branch of 274, 275
   variations and anomalies of 294
of posterior cranial fossa 137
precentral 137
preculminate 137
prepyloric 290, 292
profunda femoris–see Vein, deep, of thigh
prostatic–see Plexus (venous), prostatic
pubic 244, 248
pudendal
   external 239, 248

**Vein** *cont.*

deep 372, 466
   superficial 232, 372, 378, 476, 508
internal 248, 292, 364, 370, 376, 523
pulmonary 187, 193–195, 201–203, 208, 209, 212, 213, 217–219, 230, 294, 516, 525
radicular 159
rectal 370
   inferior 292, 293, 370
   middle 248, 292, 293, 370
   superior 257, 292, 293, 370
rectosigmoid 292, 293, 370
renal 226, 248, 281, 311, 313, **314,** 316, 320, 324, 325, 329, 371, 372, 520
of retina–see Venule, retinal
retromandibular 17, 26, 53–55, 64, 80
retrotonsillar 137
of Rosenthal–see Vein, basal (Rosenthal)
sacral
   lateral 248
   median 248, 292, 344, 370, 371, 374
saphenous
   accessory 508, 509
   great 232, 233, 239, 242, 248, 354, 378, 471, 487, 508–510
   small 468, 481, 487, 508–510
of scalp 17
scrotal, anterior 239
septal 138, 139
sigmoid 257, 292, 293, 328, 370
of skull 94
spermatic
   external–see Vein, cremasteric
   internal–see Vein, testicular
spinal 137, 159
splenic 226, 256, 257, 281, 286, **290**–294, 299, 325, 327, 329, 518, 519
stellate, of kidney 313, 318
of stomach 290
straight 291
subclavian 25, 27, 28, 64, 68, 69, 175–177, 186, 195, 197, 200, 201, 218–220, **226,** 239, 400
subcostal 248
subcutaneous 511
subependymal 139
sublingual 53, 55
sublobular, of liver 273, 274
submental 64
sulcal (anterior and posterior) 159
superficial
   of arm 448
   cerebral 96
   of head 17
   of lower limb 508, 509
   of neck 26
   of shoulder 458
   of trunk 239
supraorbital 17, 64, 80
suprarenal 226, 248, 314, 325
suprascapular 64
supratrochlear 17, 64, 80

**Vein** *cont.*

temporal
   deep 94
      middle 17, 94
   of retina–see Venule, retinal, temporal
   superficial 17, 55, 64, 94, 96
terminal–see Vein, thalamostriate, superior
testicular 243–245, 248, 257, 292, 311, 314, 319, 328, 340, **372**
thalamic, superior 139
thalamostriate 94, 139
   caudate 139
   inferior 137, 139
   superior 102, 105, 138, 139
of thigh 508, 509
   deep 471
thoracic
   internal 69, 175, 176, 180, 186, 201, 230, 239, 514–516
   lateral 239
thoracoacromial 448
thoracoepigastric 232, 239
thyroid
   inferior 64, 68, 69, 186, 200, 226
   middle 64, 68
   superior 26, 64, 68
tibial
   anterior 487
   posterior 481, 482, 487
of Trolard 96
of trunk, superficial 239
tubal branch of ovarian–see Vein, ovarian, tubal branch
umbilical 217
uncal 138
uterine 248, 292, 344–346, 370, 375
vaginal 296, 374
vermian 137, 139
of vertebrae 159
vertebral 226
vesalian–see Vein, emissary, (Vesalius)
vesical 248, 292, 370
vorticose 80, 86
zygomaticofacial 17
zygomaticotemporal 17
**Velum**
medullary, of cerebellum
   inferior 100, 107
   superior 100, 107–109
of palate 45, 60
**Vena cava**
inferior 165, 180, 194, 195, 198, 202, 203, 208, 209, 211, 213, 217, 218, 220, 226, 230, **248,** 255–257, 261, 270, 272, 279, 290, 294, 311, 312, 314, 316, 324, 325, 327, 328, 339, 340, 369–374, 383, 517–521, 524
superior 68, 69, 182, 194, 195, 200–203, 208, 212, 213, 217, 218, 226, 514–516, 524
**Vena** comitans

**Vena** *cont.*
of hypoglossal nerve 53, 54, 64
of radial artery 429
of ulnar artery 429
of vagus nerve 226
**Vena** recta–see Vein, straight
Vena terminalis–see Vein, thalamostriate,
superior
**Ventricle**
of brain 102
lateral 94, **102,** 104, 106, 132, 136, 139
3rd **102,** 105, 109, 139
4th 100, 102, 107, **109,** 136, 137, 139
of heart
left 194, 201–203, **209,** 212, 230, 516, 525
right 194, 201–203, **208,** 212,
230, 516, 525
of larynx 75
**Venule**
macular 86
rectae, of renal parenchyma 322
retinal 82
nasal 86
remporal 86
**Vermis** of cerebellum 107, 109
**Vertebra**
cervical 9, 12–14, 25, 30, 142, 148, 149,
185, 221
coccygeal–see Coccyx
lumbar 142, 144, 146–149, 156, 221
prominens 14
sacral–see Sacrum
thoracic 9, 142, 143, 148, 149, 156, 221
**Verumontanum**–see Colliculus, seminal
Vesalius, vein of–see Vein, emissary,
(Vesalius)
**Vesicle,** seminal 338, 340, 358, 390
**Vessel**
blood–see Artery; Vein
lymph–see Lymph vessel
**Vestibule**
of bony labyrinth 87, 90, 91
laryngeal 75
nasal 32, 34
of vagina 345, 350, 390
Vidian–see Nerve, of pterygoid canal
**Vinculum** 433
**Viscera** 258–268–see also individual organs
**Vision** 114
**Vomer** 1, 3, 5, 34

**W**

**Wall**
abdominal 231–250
anterior 232–236, 238–240
arteries of 238
dissection of 232–234
deep 234
intermediate 233

**Wall** *cont.*
superficial 232
internal view 236
nerves of 240
peritoneum of 236
veins of 239
posterior 246–250
arteries of 247
internal view 246
lymph vessels and nodes of 249
nerves of 250
peritoneum of 257
veins of 248
posterolateral 237
nasal
lateral 32, 33
medial 34–see also Septum, nasal
thoracic 174–179
anterior 174–176
cross sections of 179, 513–517
cutaneous nerves of 174
muscles of 174–179
posterior 178
Wharton–see Duct, submandibular;
Gland, submandibular
**Window**
cochlear–see Window, round
oval 8, 87–91
round 8, 87–91
vestibular–see Window, oval
**Wing** of
central (cerebellar) lobule 107
ilium 231, 330, 335, 453
sacrum 145
sphenoid bone
greater 1–3, 5, 6, 8
lesser 1, 3, 6
Winslow–see Foramen, omental (epiploic)
Wirsung–see Duct, pancreatic, principal
Wolffian duct–see Duct, wolffian
**Wrist**
arteries of, 430, 442
bones of 422, 426
dissection of
superficial 428, 436–438
deep 429
ligaments of 424, 425
movements of 423
nerves of 430, 441
tendons of 430, 439

**X**

X-ray–see Arteriogram; Radiograph
Xiphoid–see Process, xiphoid

**Y**

**Y ligament–see Ligament, Y, of Bigelow**

**Z**

Zinn–see Ring, common, tendinous;
Zonule, ciliary (Zinn)
**Zona**
orbicularis, of hip joint 454
pellucida of ovarian follicle 349
**Zone**–see also Area; Region
of cutaneous innervation of face 18
of stomach 259
subcapsular, of kidney 317, 318
**Zonule,** ciliary (of Zinn) 82, 83, 85, 86